SCOPE 20

Methods for Assessing the Effects of Chemicals on Reproductive Functions

SCOPE 20

Methods for Assessing the Effects of Chemicals on Reproductive Functions

Edited by
Velimir B. Vouk
*National Institute of Environmental Health Sciences,
Research Triangle Park, North Carolina, USA*

and

Patrick J. Sheehan
*Institute of Environmental Medicine,
New York University Medical Centre,
New York, USA*

Prepared by
Scientific Group on Methodologies for the
Safety Evaluation of Chemicals
(SGOMSEC)

*Published on behalf of the
Scientific Committee on Problems of the
Environment (SCOPE) of the International Council of
Scientific Unions (ICSU), and the
International Program on Chemical Safety (IPCS) of the
World Health Organization (WHO),
the United Nations Environment Programme (UNEP)
and the International Labour Organization (ILO)
by*

JOHN WILEY & SONS
Chichester · New York · Brisbane · Toronto · Singapore

Library of Congress Cataloging in Publication Data:
Main entry under title:

Methods for assessing the effects of chemicals on
   reproductive functions.

   'Published on behalf of the Scientific Committee on
Problems of the Environment (SCOPE) of the International
Council of Scientific Unions (ICSU) and the International
Program on Chemical Safety (IPCS) of the WHO/UNEP/ILO.'
   Includes the Joint report of the Workshop on Methods
for Assessing the Effects of Chemicals on Reproductive
Function, Ispra, Italy, May 3–8, 1981, sponsored by the
Scientific Group on Methodologies for the Safety Evalua-
tion of Chemicals.

   Includes bibliographies and index.
   'SCOPE 20.'
   1. Reproduction—Congresses. 2. Toxicology—Congresses
I. Vouk, Velimir. II. Sheehan, Patrick J.
III. Scientific Committee on Problems of the Environ-
ment. IV. International Program on Chemical Safety.
V. Workshop on Methods for Assessing the Effects of
Chemicals on Reproductive Function (1981; Ispra, Italy)
VI. Scientific Group on Methodologies for the Safety
Evaluation of Chemicals.
QP251.M44   1983   574.2'16   82-13529

ISBN 0 471 10538 4

British Library Cataloguing in Publication Data:

Methods for assessing the effects of chemicals on
   reproductive functions.—(SCOPE; 20)
   1. Reproduction   2. Environmentally induced
   diseases   3. Pollution—Physiological effect
   I. Vouk, Velimir B.   II. Sheehan, Patrick J.
   III. Series
   616.85'83   QH471

ISBN 0 471 10538 4

Photosetting by Thomson Press (India) Limited, New Delhi and
Printed by Page Bros., (Norwich) Ltd

Acknowledgements

The editors would like to acknowledge the assistance they received from:

G. C. Butler

K. G. Davey

Robert L. Dixon

W. LeRoy Heinrichs

Arne Jensen

A. G. Johnels

V. Landa

Thaddeus Mann

Norton Nelson

D. A. T. New

D. B. Peakall

J. H. Slater

SCOPE 1: Global Environmental Monitoring 1971, 68pp (out of print)

SCOPE 2: Man-Made Lakes as Modified Ecosystems, 1972, 76pp

SCOPE 3: Global Environmental Monitoring System (GEMS): Action Plan for Phase 1, 1973, 132pp

SCOPE 4: Environmental Sciences in Developing Countries, 1974, 72pp

Environment and Development, proceedings of SCOPE/UNEP Symposium on Environmental Sciences in Developing Countries, Nairobi, February 11-23, 1974, 418pp

SCOPE 5: Environmental Impact Assessment: Principles and Procedures, 1975, 160pp

SCOPE 6: Environmental Pollutants: Selected Analytical Methods, 1975, 277pp (available from Butterworth & Co. (Publishers) Ltd., Sevenoaks, Kent, England)

SCOPE 7: Nitrogen, Phosphorus, and Sulphur: Global Cycles, 1975, 192pp (available from Dr Thomas Rosswall, Swedish Natural Science Research Council, Stockholm, Sweden)

SCOPE 8: Risk Assessment of Environmental Hazard, 1978, 132pp

SCOPE 9: Simulation Modelling of Environmental Problems, 1978, 128pp

SCOPE 10: Environmental Issues, 1977, 242pp

SCOPE 11: Shelter Provision in Developing Countries, 1978, 112pp

SCOPE 12: Principles of Ecotoxicology, 1979, 372pp

SCOPE 13: The Global Carbon Cycle, 1979, 491pp

SCOPE 14: Saharan Dust: Mobilization, Transport, Deposition, 1979, 320pp

SCOPE 15: Environmental Risk Assessment, 1980, 176pp

SCOPE 16: Carbon Cycle Modelling, 1981, 404pp

SCOPE 17: Some Perspectives of the Major Biogeochemical Cycles, 1981, 175pp

SCOPE 18: The Role of Fire in Northern Circumpolar Ecosystems, 1983, 344pp

SCOPE 19: The Global Biogeochemical Sulphur Cycle, 1983, 496pp

SCOPE 20: Methods for Assessing the Effects of Chemicals on Reproductive Functions, 1983,

Funds to meet SCOPE expenses are provided by contributions from SCOPE National Committees, an annual subvention from ICSU (and through ICSU, from UNESCO), an annual subvention from the French Ministère de l'Environnement et du Cadre de Vie, contracts with UN Bodies, particularly UNEP, and grants from Foundations and industrial enterprises.

International Council of Scientific Unions (ICSU)
Scientific Committee on Problems of the Environment (SCOPE)

SCOPE is one of a number of committees established by a non-governmental group of scientific organizations, the International Council of Scientific Unions (ICSU). The membership of ICSU includes representatives from 68 National Academies of Science, 18 International Unions, and 12 other bodies called Scientific Associates. To cover multidisciplinary activities which include the interests of several unions, ICSU has established 10 scientific committees, of which SCOPE, founded in 1969, is one. Currently, representatives of 34 member countries and 15 Unions and Scientific Committees participate in the work of SCOPE, which directs particular attention to the needs of developing countries.

The mandate of SCOPE is to assemble, review, and assess the information available on man-made environmental changes and the effects of these changes on man; to assess and evaluate the methodologies of measurement of environmental parameters; to provide an intelligence service on current research; and by the recruitment of the best available scientific information and constructive thinking to establish itself as a corpus of informed advice for the benefit of centres of fundamental research and of organizations and agencies operationally engaged in studies of the environment.

SCOPE is governed by a General Assembly, which meets every three years. Between such meetings its activities are directed by the Executive Committee.

R. E. Munn
Editor-in-Chief
SCOPE Publications

Executive Secretary: Ms V. Plocq

Secretariat: 51 Bld de Montmorency
75016 PARIS

Contents

Contents
xiii

PART B CONTRIBUTED PAPERS

Contents

Foreword

One of the very troublesome and growing problems in environmental management is how best to assess the consequences of releasing chemicals into natural and modified ecosystems. The number and production of chemical compounds increase. The technological capacity to identify and measure their presence enlarges. As knowledge of organism and ecosystem processes is deepened, the complexity of tracing out their effects multiplies.

In these circumstances the wise choice of methods for examining the effects of chemicals in the environment has become a matter of urgency. Upon the method selected and its proper application may rest a series of decisions as to industrial production, government regulation, and consumer choice. Recognizing the need for careful appraisal of the grounds for making those decisions about tests, SCOPE began exploring in 1978 the ways in which the experience and judgment of the scientific community could be marshalled to the task.

Under the creative leadership of Norton Nelson, and building on the thinking embodied in the *Principles of Ecotoxicology* (SCOPE 12) edited by Gordon C. Butler, a plan was developed for a Scientific Group on Methodologies for the Safety Evaluation of Chemicals. This was established jointly with the World Health Organization. Subsequently the United Nations Environment Programme and the International Labour Organization associated themselves with the effort, within the framework of the International Programme on Chemical Safety (IPCS), sponsored by those three United Nations Organizations.

In the typical mode of SCOPE activities, the work was interdisciplinary and international, and it sought to provide objective scientific advice for the benefit of governments and international organizations. It drew heavily upon the research and judgment of scientists in more than a dozen countries. Financial support came from their home institutions as well as from a variety of organizations.

This volume is the first in a projected series, and exemplifies the approach to be taken in examining various facets of evaluating chemicals in the environment. It is a cooperative exploration of an enlarging problem and is helpful in outlining what we don't know as well as what we do know. It thereby strengthens the base for sound environmental management.

GILBERT F. WHITE

xv

Foreword

The International Programme on Chemical Safety (IPCS), a joint project of the United Nations Environment Programme (UNEP), the International Labour Organisation (ILO), and the World Health Organization (WHO), aims at protecting human health and the environment from the adverse effects of the ever-increasing number of chemicals on the market and in the environment, to which the population at large may be exposed and which also reach other biota.

The IPCS is therefore anxious to evaluate the degree of risk presented by such chemicals but, as the usefulness of any evaluation greatly depends on the quality and reliability of the experimental techniques used for determining toxic effects, the IPCS is encouraging their development and validation with a view to recommending those that produce internationally comparable results. Consequently, the IPCS actively supported the review of methods for assessing the effects of chemicals on reproductive function, carried out by the Scientific Group on Methodologies for the Safety Evaluation of Chemicals (SGOMSEC).

It is hoped that the report of this scientific group and the individual papers included in the present publication will prove to be useful additions to the methodology available in the complex field of toxicology. The publication, of course, represents the personal views of the scientists involved, but all participating in the IPCS will doubtless consult their work with great interest.

MICHEL. J. MERCIER
Manager, International
Programme on Chemical Safety

Preface

This publication reports the first endeavour of the Scientific Group on Methodologies for the Safety Evaluation of Chemicals (SGOMSEC). SGOMSEC grew out of an organizational meeting sponsored by the Rockefeller Foundation in Bellagio, Italy, 15–17 June 1978. The proposals developed at that meeting have been endorsed by the World Health Organization (WHO), the Scientific Committee on Problems of the Environment (SCOPE) and the United Nation Environment Programme (UNEP). The Scientific Group operates under their general sponsorship, guided by an Executive Committee.

The objective of SGOMSEC is to examine methods for the predictive evaluation of the adverse effects of chemicals on humans and other forms of life. It is the intention of SGOMSEC to review the methods which are in an initial stage, have not yet become routine procedures, but are urgently needed in the assessment of the effects of industrial and environmental chemicals. Such reviews will be concerned mainly with laboratory procedures and also with epidemiological approaches and field studies, and with up-to-date diagnostic methods where these are required.

Because of widespread concern throughout the world regarding chemical assaults on human health and the natural environment in the widest sense, there is a growing need for reliable methods to evaluate possible adverse effects. National and international agencies and individual scientists need precise methods to establish priorities, develop controls, and plan regulations.

SGOMSEC undertakes these studies to support scientists in their endeavours to select methods for assessing potential chemical injury. In many cases, of course, adequate methods are not available, and this report undertakes to identify the gaps and suggest research that may be needed to fill them.

Whilst injury to the reproductive function in the individual is of major concern in humans and farm animals, in other animals and in plants the concern is with the survival of the entire species or population rather than of individuals. Both areas are obviously very broad and some omissions had to be made. In the case of mammalian reproductive function, the study group has decided to give very little attention to the two areas, germ cell injury and teratology. This does not imply the unimportance of these fields, but some restriction is imperative, the more so as these areas have been extensively reviewed elsewhere.

The breadth of the non-mammalian areas is so vast that even with the

xvii

deliberate omission of some important areas, the present review can only be regarded as a beginning. As such, we hope it will provide a solid base for future more detailed examinations of the methods available.

The development of this publication has extended over a year and has involved scientists from many parts of the world, individually in the review of their fields, and collectively in the preparation of the joint conclusions and recommendations. This report thus consists of two main parts: 24 contributed papers, each representing the efforts of individual scientists, and a Joint Report which represents the collective conclusions and recommendations of the scientists working together at a Workshop in Ispra, Italy, 4–8 May 1981. The authors alone are responsible for opinion expressed in the signed contributions.

The Joint Report was drafted by the work groups listed in each section of the report, and reviewed at the closing plenary session of the Workshop. The comments and suggestions of the plenary session were incorporated into the drafts of work group reports. Scientific editing was carried out in consultation with an Editorial Committee whose members were Gordon C. Butler (Co-Chairman), W. LeRoy Heinrichs, V. Landa, Thaddeus Mann, Norton Nelson (Co-Chairman), J. Pařizek and J. Piotrowski; and assisted by K. G. Davey, Robert L. Dixon, Rune Eliasson, Arne Jensen, A. G. Johnels, J. B. Kerr, Donald Mattison, D. A. T. New and Linda R. Wudl.

Those responsible for organizing this activity are well aware of the effort put into the preparation of the individual papers and the Joint Report and wish to express their appreciation of the time, effort and skills that have contributed to this publication. They are also grateful to the sponsoring agencies, WHO, SCOPE and UNEP, to those organizations that sent working representatives to the Workshop, the Organization for Economic Cooperation and Development (OECD) and the Commission of the European Communities (CEC), and to the Joint Research Centre for their generosity in providing facilities for the Workshop in Ispra. Thanks also are due to agencies who provided the funding for this activity, WHO, SCOPE, the Rockefeller Foundation, A. W. Mellon Foundation, the National Institute of Environmental Health Sciences, and the Research Division and the Occupational Health Programme of the Commission of the European Communities.

The assistance of Ms. Judith H. Edmonds, Ms. Joyce McManus, Ms. B. Rosenfeld, Ms. Vickie Englebright and Ms. Susan Schrag in the preparation of typescripts is gratefully acknowledged.

NORTON NELSON
*Chairman, Scientific Group on
Methodologies for the Safety
Evaluation of Chemicals*

Scientific Group on Methodologies for the Safety Evaluation of Chemicals

N. P. Bočkov, Director, Institute of Medical Genetics and Secretary, Academy of Medical Sciences of the USSR, Kaširskoe šossé 6a, Moscow 115478, USSR

*****Gordon C. Butler**, Division of Biological Sciences, National Research Council of Canada, Ottawa, Ontario K1A OR6, Canada (*Vice Chairman*)

*****Miki Goto**, Professor, Department of Chemistry and Director, Institute of Ecotoxicology, Gakushuin University, 1-5-1 Mejiro, Toshima-ku, Tokyo 171, Japan

C. R. Krishna Murti, Director, Industrial Toxicology Research Centre, Mahatma Gandhi Marg, Post Box No. 80, Lucknow 226001 U.P., India

V. Landa, Director, Institute of Entomology, Czechoslovak Academy of Sciences, Viničná 7, 128 00 Praha 2, Czechoslovakia

Aly Massoud, Professor and Chairman, Department of Community, Industrial and Environmental Health, Ain Shams University, P.O. Box 38, Abbassia, Cairo, Egypt

*****Norton Nelson**, Professor, New York University Medical Center, Institute of Environmental Medicine, 550 First Avenue, New York, New York 10016, USA (*Chairman*)

*****A. G. Johnels**, President, Royal Swedish Academy of Sciences, The Swedish Museum of Natural History, S-10405 Stockholm 50, Sweden

*****Blanca Raquel Ordoñez**, Coordinator of the Environmental Health Research Programme, Universidad Autonoma Metropolitana, Boulevard Manuel Avila Comacho 90 Naucalpan, Z. P. 10, Apartado Postal 325, Mexico 1, D. F. Mexico

J. Pařizek, Scientist, International Programme on Chemical Safety, Division of Environmental Health, World Health Organization, 1211 Geneva 27, Switzerland (*Secretary*)

Dennis V. Parke, Professor of Biochemistry, University of Surrey, Guildford, Surrey GU2 FXH, England, United Kingdom

J. Piotrowski, Chief, Department of Toxicological Chemistry, Institute of Environmental Research and Bioanalysis, Medical Academy of Łodz, Narutowicza 120a, 90–145 Łodz, Poland

*Member of the Executive Committee

Patrick J. Sheehan, New York University Medical Center, Institute of Environmental Medicine, 550 First Avenue, New York, New York 10016, USA (*SCOPE Liaison Officer*)

E. Somers, Director General, Environmental Health Directorate, Department of National Health and Welfare, Ottawa, Ontario K1A OL2, Canada

Velimir B. Vouk, Visiting Scientist, National Institute of Environmental Health Sciences, P.O. Box 12233, Research Triangle Park, North Carolina 27709, USA

Participants of the Workshop on Methods for Assessing the Effects of Chemicals on Reproductive Function, Ispra, Italy, 3–8 May, 1981

Yusuf Ahmad, Pakistan Council of Scientific and Industrial Research, Proass Centre Building, P.O. Box 672, Shahrah-e-Kamal Ataturk, Karachi 39, Pakistan (*WHO Temporary Adviser*)

Bertil Åkesson, Professor, Department of Zoology, University of Göteborg, Box 250 59, S-400 31, Göteborg, Sweden

B. L. Bayne, Institute for Marine Environmental Research, Prospect Place, The Hoe, Plymouth, PLl-3DH, Devonshire, United Kingdom

* **B. Bennetová**, Institute of Entomology, Czechoslavak Academy of Sciences, Viničná 7, 128 00 Praha 2, Czechoslovakia

Gordon C. Butler, Division of Biological Sciences, National Research Council of Canada, Ottawa, KlA OR6, Canada (*Co-chairman*)

David J. Clegg, Head, Pesticide Section, Toxicology Evaluation Division, Food Directorate, Department of National Health and Welfare, Ottawa, Ontario KlA OL2 Canada (*Representing Health and Welfare Canada*)

H. Crose, United Nations Environment Programme, P.O. Box 30552, Nairobi, Kenya (*Representing UNEP*)

K. G. Davey, Professor and Chairman, Department of Biology, York University, 4700 Keele Street, Downsview, Ontario M3J IP3, Canada

D. R. Dixon, N.E.R.C. Institute for Marine Environmental Research, Prospect Place, The Hoe, Plymouth PL1-3DA, Devonshire, United Kingdom

Robert L. Dixon, Chief, Laboratory of Reproductive and Developmental Toxicology, National Institute of Environmental Health Sciences, National Institutes of Health, P.O. Box 12233, Research Triangle Park, NC 27709, USA

Richard Doherty, Departments of Pediatrics, Genetics, Obstetrics, and Radiation Biology and Biophysics, University of Rochester School of Medicine, Box 777, Rochester, New York 14642, USA

E. M. Donaldson, Vancouver West Laboratory, Resource Services Branch,

*Did not attend the Workshop

Department of Fisheries and Oceans, West Vancouver, B. C. V6V 1N6, Canada

Rune Eliasson, Reproductive Physiology Unit, Department of Physiology, Karolinska Institutet, Box 60 400, S-104 01 Stockholm, Sweden

* **Merrit Gadallah,** Visiting Scholar, Stanford University School of Medicine, Stanford, California 94350, USA

* **I. Gelbič,** Institute of Entomology, Czechoslovak Academy of Sciences, Viničná 7, 128 00 Praha 2, Czechoslovakia

Miki Goto, Professor, Department of Chemistry and Director, Institute of Ecotoxicology, Gakushuin University, 1-5-1 Mejiro, Toshima-ku, Tokyo 171, Japan

W. LeRoy Heinrichs, Professor and Chairman, Department of Gynecology and Obstetrics, Stanford University, Stanford, California 94304, USA

K. Jayasena, Professor and Head, Department of Pharmacology, Medical School, Peradeniya, Sri Lanka (*WHO Temporary Adviser*)

Richard Jelínek, Institute of Experimental Medicine, Czechoslovak Academy of Sciences, CE 128 00 Praha 2, Czechoslovakia

Arne Jensen, Institute of Marine Biochemistry, University of Trondheim, N-7034 Troudheim, NTH, Norway

***Arne Jernelöv,** Swedish Water and Air Pollution Research Laboratory (IVL), Box 21060, 10031 Stockholm, Sweden

Jan E. Jirásek, Institute for Mother and Child Care, nábr. K. Marxe 157, 147 10 Praha 4-Podoli, Czechoslovakia

Alf G. Johnels, President, Royal Swedish Academy of Sciences, The Swedish Museum of Natural History, S-10405 Stockholm 50, Sweden

Jeffrey B. Kerr, Department of Anatomy, Monash University, Clayton, Victoria, Australia 3168

* **J. E. Kihlström,** Professor of Ecotoxicology, Institute of Zoophysiology University of Uppsala, Box 560, S-751 22 Uppsala, Sweden

* **Jennie Kline,** Psychiatric Institute, New York State and Gertrude H. Sergievsky Center, School of Public Health, Columbia University, New York, New York, USA

* **David M. de Kretser,** Professor, Department of Anatomy, Monash University, Clayton, Victoria, Australia 3168

V. Landa, Institute of Entomology, Czechoslovak Academy of Sciences, Viničná 7, 128 00 Praha 2, Czechoslovakia

Vincenzo G. Leone, Istituto di Zoologia, Università di Milano, Via Celoria 10, 20133 Milano, Italy (*Representing University of Milan*)

B. V. Leonov, Head, Laboratory for Experimental Embryology, All-Union Research Institute of Obstetrics and Gynecology, c/o Ministry of Health of the

USSR, Rahmanovskij pereulok 3, Moscow, USSR (*WHO Temporary Adviser*)

* **H. F. Linskens**, Professor, Botanisch Laboratorium, Fakulteit der Wiskunde, Katholieke Universiteit, Toernooiveld, Nijmegen, The Netherlands

Cecilia Lutwak-Mann, Endocrinology and Reproduction Research Branch, National Institute of Child Health and Human Development, National Institute of Health, Bethesda, Maryland 20205, USA

Thaddeus Mann, Endocrinology and Reproduction Branch, National Institute of Child Health and Human Development, National Institutes of Health, Bethesda, Maryland 20205, USA

Otakar Marhan, Research Institute for Pharmacy and Biochemistry, Konárovice, Czechoslovakia

AnnLouise Martin, Swedish Water and Air Pollution Research Laboratory (IVL), Aneboda, S-360 30 Lammhult, Sweden

* **S. Matolín**, Institute of Entomology, Czechoslovak Academy of Sciences, Viničná 7, 128 00 Praha 2, Czechoslovakia

Donald R. Mattison, Senior Investigator, Pregnancy Research Branch, National Institute of Child Health and Human Development, National Institutes of Health, Building 10, Room 5B04, Bethesda, Maryland 20205, USA

Michel Mercier, Manager, International Programme on Chemical Safety, Division of Environmental Health, World Health Organization, 1211 Geneva 27, Switzerland (*Representing WHO*)

Margaret Merlini, Joint Research Centre (JRC), Commission of the European Communities, 21020 Ispra, Varese, Italy (*Representing JRC, Ispra*)

Victor Morganroth, Food and Drug Administration, 200 C Street, S. W. Washington, DC 20204, USA (*Representing OECD*)

Norton Nelson, Professor, New York University Medical Center, Institute of Environmental Medicine, 550 First Avenue, New York, New York 10016, USA (*Co-Chairman*)

D. A. T. New, Physiological Laboratory, University of Cambridge CB2 3EG, England, United Kingdom

Blanca Raquel Ordoñez, Universidad Autonoma Metropolitana, Boulevard Manuel Avila Comacho 90 Naucalpan, Z. P. 10, Apartado Postal 325, Mexico 1, D. F., Mexico

J. Pařizek, Scientist, International Programme on Chemical Safety, Division of Environmental Health, World Health Organization, 1211 Geneva 27, Switzerland

David B. Peakall, Chief, Wildlife Toxicology Division, National Wildlife Research Centre, Ottawa, Ontario K1A OE7, Canada

*Did not attend the Workshop

Paul L. Pfahler, Agronomy Department, 304 Newell Hall, University of Florida, Gainesville, Florida, USA

Jerzy K. Piotrowski, Chief, Department of Toxicological Chemistry, Institute of Environmental Research and Bioanalysis, Medical Academy of Lodz, Narutowicza 120a, 90-145 Lodz, Poland (*Representing UNEP*)

D. Michael Pugh, Faculty of Veterinary Medicine, Bullsbridge, Dublin 4, Ireland (*Representing CEC Health and Safety Directorate*)

Oscar Ravera, Joint Research Centre, Commission of the European Communities, 21020 Ispra (Varese), Italy (*Representing CEC Joint Research Centre, Ispra*)

* **Griff T. Ross**, Deputy Director, The Clinical Center, National Institutes of Health, Building 10, Room 5B04, Bethesda, Maryland 20205, USA

* **A. S. M. Saleuddin**, Department of Biology, York University, 4700 Keele Street, Downsview, Ontario M3J IP3, Canada

* **I. V. Sanockij**, Institute of Work Hygiene and Occupational Diseases, Academy of Medical Sciences, 31 Majerovskij projezd, Moscow, E-275, USSR

E. Scherer, Freshwater Institute, Department of Fisheries and Oceans, Winnepeg, Manitoba R3T 2N6, Canada

Patrick Sheehan, New York University Medical Center, Institute of Environmental Medicine, 500 First Avenue, New York, New York 10016, USA (*SCOPE Liaison Officer*)

* **Michael I. Sherman**, Department of Cell Biology, Roche Institute of Molecular Biology, Nutley, New Jersey 07110, USA

J. Howard Slater, Department of Environmental Sciences, University of Warwick, Coventry CV4 7AL, England, United Kingdom

* **T. Soldán**, Institute of Entomology, Czechoslovak Academy of Sciences, Viničná 7, 128 00 Praha 2, Czechoslovakia

* **C. G. H. Steel**, Department of Biology, York University, 4700 Keele Street, Downsview, Ontario M3J IP3, Canada

* **Zena Stein**, Psychiatric Institute, New York State and Gertrude H. Sergievsky Center, School of Public Health, Columbia University, New York, New York, USA

Robert G. Tardiff, Executive Director, Board of Toxicology and Environmental Health Hazards, National Academy of Sciences, 2101 Constitution Avenue, Washington, DC 20418 (*Representing National Academy of Sciences/National Research Council*)

M. Th. Van der Venne, Health and Safety Directorate, Commission of the European Communities, Jean Monet Building, Luxembourg (G.D.) (*Representing CEC Health and Safety Directorate*)

Velimir B. Vouk, Visiting Scientist, National Institute of Environmental Health

---

*Did not attend the Workshop

Sciences, National Institutes of Health, P.O. Box 12233, Research Triangle Park, NC 27709, USA (*WHO Temporary Adviser*)

Dorothy Warburton, Associate Professor in Pediatrics (Human Genetics and Development), Columbia University College of Physicians and Surgeons, 622 West 168th Street, New York, New York 10032, USA

* **R. A. Webb**, Department of Biology, York University, 4700 Keele Street, Downsview, Ontario M3J IP3, Canada

Linda R. Wudl, Research Biologist (Genetic Toxicology), Corporate Medical Affairs Division, Allied Chemical Corporation, Morristown, New Jersey 07960, USA

*Did not attend the Workshop

PART A

JOINT REPORT

Methods for Assessing the Effects of Chemicals on Reproductive Functions
Edited by V. B. Vouk and P. J. Sheehan
© 1983 SCOPE

1 Introduction, General Conclusions and Recommendations*

1.1 INTRODUCTION

The interest in and importance of both human and non-human reproduction are obvious. In both of these subjects there are complexities and conflicting elements.

The reproduction of many non-human species is of economic importance to human beings and necessary for their nutrition. Obvious examples are domestic animals, fish and cereals. In some cases the food is actually a part of the reproductive process, e.g. eggs and seeds.

Other examples of human dependence on non-human populations are intestinal bacteria and pollinating insects of which it is important to have an appropriate kind and quantity.

On the other hand, human beings may wish to reduce the reproduction of populations that interfere with their health or well-being, for example: vermin that eat human food or carry disease; biting insects; insects that carry disease; plants that overgrow waters or soil; and pathogenic bacteria.

In addition to these homocentric considerations there are important ecological implications of non-human reproduction. The condition of an ecosystem depends on the rate of reproduction of a multitude of species in relation to the death rate of each species and to the interactions between species. The relations between species and ecosystems are complex and largely unknown. The extermination of a species represents an irretrievable loss and, since its long-term consequences cannot be predicted, man's activities should not be permitted to have this result.

In the present report the discussions of methods for evaluating the effects of chemicals on reproductive functions are divided into two parts, one dealing with mammalian, the other with non-mammalian targets. This seemed justified because of the appreciable differences in basic concepts and experimental approaches. Although there was some criticism of the approximately equal space and attention being devoted to the two groups of biota, considering the enormous variety and number of phyla (divisions), classes, families, genera and

---

* This section was prepared by a Workgroup co-chaired by Norton Nelson and Gordon C. Butler. The members were Thaddeus Mann, LeRoy Heinrichs, David B. Peakall, V. Landa, J. H. Slater, J. Parizek, J. Piotrowski, Patrick Sheehan and Velimir Vouk.

species, and the innumerable individuals in the non-mammalian group of animals, plants and microorganisms in comparison with one class of mammals, it was manifestly impossible to allocate attention on this basis.

Another justification for the choice of the subject for this SGOMSEC study arises from the notable lack of methods for assessing the effects of chemicals on reproductive function; additionally, such methods are rarely included in a standard battery of toxicological tests, and if so, only to a limited extent. It appeared during the discussions in this Workshop that for many reproductive functions, especially human, the tests consisted of qualitative assessment of morphology rather than of quantitative methods for measuring specific biological functions.

The Workshop concentrated on test procedures that would assist scientists in giving advice to governmental control and regulatory agencies, industries and research-supporting organizations. It was assumed that these scientists know most of the science basic to the methodology. For this reason the reader will find only a minimum coverage of this material in the Joint Report which concentrates as far as possible on the tests of the effects of chemicals on reproduction where they exist, their suitability, their shortcomings and, possibly, their lacks. In the assessment of the known tests, a number of attributes were considered including the following.

Relevance to practical problems As far as possible methods should be suitable for assessing and illuminating problems involving chemicals, species and effects that have created difficulties and may do so again. An example that comes to mind is the effect of accumulated chlorinated hydrocarbons on the reproduction of birds of prey.

Economy Wherever possible the procedures should not require too much expenditure of effort and money, especially if they are to be routinely and widely used. Frequently, some compromise with this principle will be required. For example, *in vivo* laboratory tests may be the cheapest, but expensive population investigations under field conditions may be considered the most relevant. A serious limitation in studies of large mammals is that the number of individuals studied is frequently limited to samples too small to give statistical confidence.

Predictive ability It is difficult to decide *a priori* which tests may lead to confident predictions. However, a few generalizations are possible. As mentioned above, population studies of effects under field conditions are often the most relevant. If tests can be found that are valid for a whole class of chemicals, they are likely to be more efficient and economical. To assist prediction, tests should permit quantitative assessment of the response to graded dosing. There are many difficulties in these quantifications. In epidemiological studies the doses are rarely if ever known, even approximately, and, as mentioned above, many histological effects are described without quantification.

Another problem of quantitative testing is the difficulty of knowing how long to continue the exposure, how to express it (concentration × time, concentration in target tissue, amount absorbed systemically, etc.) and how long to continue observing the response (hours, days, a lifetime, more than one generation). Nevertheless it is the dose and the relative sensitivity of the receptor to a chemical that determine the relative hazard.

Acceptability This concept applies to a method that may find general acceptance because it is relevant to practical problems, is economical, has predictive ability, is easy to perform, and gives comparable results. The advantage of widely accepted methods performed uniformly and with widely accepted results is obvious. Many such tests exist already, with or without validation. Where possible these are listed, described and assessed.

Reservations were generally expressed about the applicability of tests on a single part of the reproductive process, performed on a single species with a single pure chemical. In real life several toxins or stresses may be operating simultaneously and there may be considerable interspecies reactions such as competition and predation.

Methods for testing the reproductive effects on mammals are discussed in two sections of the Joint Report, one dealing with females, the other with males. The section on females includes integrated reproduction studies which reflect the overall reproductive capability of the mammalian species, and a discussion of epidemiological investigations applicable, in principle, to both the female and male function. This is followed by a section on methods for testing the effects of chemicals on vertebrates other than mammals, separate subsections being devoted to birds, fishes, reptiles, and amphibians. The report on invertebrates is divided differently: one subsection is devoted to field studies and analyses of field-collected material, the other to laboratory studies covering Platyhelminthes, Cnidaria, Aschelminthes, Annelida, Arthropoda, Mollusca, and Echinodermata. In the last section, methods applicable to higher plants, algae and microorganisms are reviewed. Lists of references cited in the Joint Report are attached to each section and so are the specific conclusions and recommendations for further development of methods and for the methodological research required.

1.2 GENERAL CONCLUSIONS AND RECOMMENDATIONS

(1) Toxicology of reproductive function is a rapidly developing field and requires continuous updating. Methods for laboratory testing and field studies discussed in this report need to be reviewed and, if necessary, revised within the next 3–5 years.

(2) National and international scientific organizations should be informed of the conclusions and recommendations of this meeting so that the whole scientific community becomes aware of the areas of greatest priority for research.

(3) Working groups concerned with effects of chemicals on reproductive function of microorganisms, plants and animals other than mammals require an extensive specialized expertise to be able to consider adequately the many species, genera, families, orders, classes and phyla involved. This should be taken into account when convening future workshops.

(4) Within the International Programme on Chemical Safety a system should be developed for international cooperation in the field of chemical effects on reproduction in non-human targets, including domestic and agricultural animals and plants.

(5) An international organized interlaboratory comparison programme should be established to validate the available tests under a variety of conditions. For many species, generally used sets of methods and procedures are available; however, their applicability under different conditions should be verified.

(6) Interlaboratory comparison and validation projects require reference chemicals known to affect reproductive function in different species. An international bank of such chemicals should be established so that samples become readily available, on request, to research laboratories and field stations in every part of the world.

(7) Field studies are necessary for most species of plants and animals in order to ascertain the relationship between effects observed in the laboratory or in individual case studies and effects that arise under real field conditions. They are also required to identify the most sensitive indicator species and species suitable for laboratory studies (test species).

(8) The main problem in field studies, including epidemiological investigations, is the proper assessment of exposure. Without effective methods for estimating exposure such studies are difficult to interpret. This is a problem common to all toxicological field studies.

(9) More effort must be directed towards developing test procedures for assessing reliably, quantitatively, and with precision the fate and effects of chemicals within defined ecosystems.

(10) When developing tests for effects on reproductive function one should not overlook the possibility of biological conversion of chemicals into more toxic forms.

Methods for Assessing the Effects of Chemicals on Reproductive Functions
Edited by V. B. Vouk and P. J. Sheehan
© 1983 SCOPE

2 Mammals: Reproductive Function of Females*

The great complexity of the female reproductive system of mammals not only provides multiple targets for chemical injury, but also offers many endpoints for evaluating its function. A single permanent set of oocytes formed during embryogenesis must serve the entire reproductive lifetime. Biological changes in the female reproductive system of most mammals can be documented in early fetal life, at birth and during puberty. The system seems to be relatively quiescent during the late fetal and prepubertal periods. After the development of an integrated reproductive function during puberty, in most mammals cyclic and dynamic changes characterize the pituitary and ovarian activity, and the responses of target tissues. Assessments of reproductive capacity at any time after puberty and before menopause are therefore always related to the stage of development of the follicle or corpus luteum. Practically, however, the definitive and ultimate test of reproductive capacity is conception and successful pregnàncy which depend upon an additional and even more complex set of integrated functions.

Reproductive performance by female mammals also depends on the development of sexual receptivity, coitus, and gamete and zygote transport within the reproductive tract to a proper site where the implantation of the embryo can produce a placenta for adequate nutritional exchange. Maternal physiological functions must adjust to promote the remarkable growth of the fetus to maturity. After sudden explosive uterine contractions terminate the pregnancy, once again a new set of integrated functions is activated in the postpartum female to provide for nurturing of the progeny.

Testing for reproductive toxicity must necessarily include some of the methods used in teratology and genetic toxicology. Reproduction failures such as abortion and reduced fetal growth may reflect primary injury of either the fetus or the mother or both, which may be produced by similar or different mechanisms. Occasionally, as with anencephaly in primates, a primary fetal

---

* This section was prepared by a Workgroup chaired by W. LeRoy Heinrichs. The rapporteur was D. S. T. New, and other members were Yusuf Ahmad, David J. Clegg, Richard Doherty, K. Jayasena, Richard Jelinek, Jan E. Jirásek, B. V. Leonov, Donald R. Mattison, Margaret Merlini, Victor Morganroth, Blanca Ordoñez, J. Piotrowski, D. M. Pugh, Dorothy Warburton and Linda Wudl.

injury may result in secondary impairments, such as disturbances in maternal physiology (delayed parturition in this case). Our inability to discriminate between the effects on mother and the fetus *in vivo* requires in some cases an *in vitro* confirmation, usually carried out by teratogenicity or mutagenicity tests. The assessment of female reproductive function *in vivo* usually depends on inferential and indirect observations, since the gonad and the developing progeny are practically inaccessible for direct evaluation. Evaluation of toxicity to reproductive function is further complicated by a unique endocrine physiology of some mammalian classes or species, and by different forms of metabolism and placentation that occur in various mammals. Extrapolation of data from one species to another may therefore be difficult and subject to error. None the less, batteries of screening tests can be devised that provide qualitative and quantitative assessments of specific reproductive processes and deviations from the normal function. Specific tests are directed toward probing and defining distinct physiological impairments, and sometimes mechanisms by which an injury has been produced. Testing of these obligatory and correlated functional activities separately is arbitrary and tends to obscure their functional integration.

2.1 INTEGRATED REPRODUCTION STUDIES IN ANIMALS

Integrated studies are designed to provide a broad spectrum of data related to the effects of a test substance on reproductive function of mammals. The data generated vary according to the type of test, ranging from information on the total reproductive function, including postpartum effects, to data concerned with very specific time periods of the reproductive process. The tests may have wide variations in protocols depending upon the anticipated use of the results. Thus, data required for regulatory purposes vary according to the country, or even the agency to which the data will be submitted. Several attempts have been made to harmonize the required methods (OECD, 1981; IRLG, 1981); with moderate success to date. Therefore, this report does not provide detailed specific protocols, but an attempt has been made to discuss common elements associated with integrated testing of reproductive capacity. In addition, some major areas of contention between different protocols are considered.

All methods listed below are currently in use and are included in bioassays of chemicals, when necessary. Thus, there is a large body of data indicating that the tests described are practicable and reproducible.

2.1.1 Multigeneration Studies

Studies of this category are intended to provide data on gonadal function, oestrous cycle, mating behaviour, conception, implantation, abortion, parturition, postnatal survival, lactation, maternal behaviour, postpartum growth to

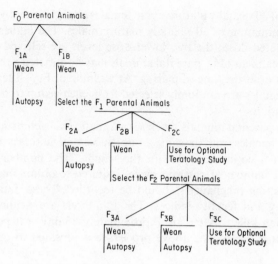

Figure 2.1 Protocol for a three-generation reproduction and teratogenicity study. (Adapted from Collins, 1978)

weaning, and, in part, abnormal fetal or embryonic development, over a period of more than one generation, with one or more litters per generation.

The classical three-generation reproduction study (see for example Collins, 1978) requires continuous exposure of the parental generation (F_0) from weaning until termination of lactation following generation of the second (F_{1B}) litter. Offspring in each generation are continuously exposed to the test substance. The experimental scheme can be diagrammatically represented as follows (Figure 2.1). The inclusion of 'C' subgroups for teratological studies is optional.

There are several variations on this classic scheme (e.g. NAS, 1977), and recent data indicate that no more than two generations are required (Clegg, 1979) or scientifically justified. In a single generation test, the offspring (F_1) are usually discarded after weaning and are not themselves bred. The parental generation is treated from weaning through pregnancy and lactation of the F_1. No test animals are exposed during their own gestation and suckling periods. Thus, the chemical exposure does not include fertilization, embryogenesis, weaning and sexual maturation, and these processes may be particularly vulnerable to chemical toxicity. Certain chemicals, particularly those thought likely to interfere with the development and functional maturation of the reproductive and endocrine systems, should be subjected to a two-generation study. The postnatal effects of diethylstilboestrol provide an important example of the functional results of subtle gestational effects (McLachlan and Dixon, 1976; Stenchever et al., 1981).

In multigeneration experiments there are usually three treatment groups and a control group. As recommended in one guideline published by NAS (1977), each group consists of 20 sexually mature virgin females (most frequently rats or mice) mated with a minimum of 10 sexually mature males. The highest dose is the maximum tolerated dose; the two lower dose levels are selected in geometric progression. Treatment of F_0 parental animals may be initiated either on the day of implantation or at the time of pairing. At weaning of F_{1A} litters, at least 10 males and 20 females are randomly selected from each group to become the F_1 parental generation.

When the F_1 parental animals reach sexual maturity, each male is randomly mated with two females from the same group. Successful mating is determined by the presence of a copulation plug in the vagina. The number of observed copulations, the number of oestrous cycles required to obtain mating, and the number of resulting pregnancies should be recorded. These data are used to calculate mating and fertility indices. The F_{2A} litters are weaned at 21 days postpartum, then killed. After an approximately 15-day rest period, the F_1 females are mated again. The above procedure is repeated to obtain the F_{2B} litters.

All offspring (F_{1A}, F_{2A}, F_{2B}) are examined for physical abnormalities at birth. On the day 4 of lactation, litters with more than 10 offspring may be reduced to that number by killing randomly selected individual animals.

After the second litter (F_{2B}) has been weaned (following approximately 33 weeks of testing for the rat), 10 male and 10 female F_1 parental animals from each group are killed and gross pathological observations are made. If histological changes are noted, the target organs of the next lower dose group of animals are also examined. Throughout gross and microscopic examination particular attention is paid to the reproductive organs.

A gross internal examination is made of any offspring appearing abnormal. In addition, 10 male and 10 female offspring, randomly selected from the F_{2B} litters of each test group and the control group, are killed at weaning and subjected to a complete gross examination. Tissues are obtained and preserved as for F_1 parental animals. Histopathological examinations are conducted on the weanlings of the control and highest-dose group. If abnormalities are noted, the target organs of the next lower dose group of animals are also examined.

The advantages of multigeneration studies include a wide experience available in performing such tests, generation of data on a wide range of reproductive processes, the quantitative nature of the data obtained, and the possibility of observing behavioural effects of prolonged exposure. In view of the extensive information gained, such studies are probably cost effective.

Although these tests have been used for the last 20 years, there is still a considerable debate within the scientific community on a number of points pertaining to both the design of the studies and the interpretation of data. A few of these points are discussed below.

(1) A major area of contention is the number of generations which should be included in the study. Guidelines exist for 1, 2, 3 or more generations. It appears

that one-generation studies are adequate for screening of chemicals, for testing for fertility, and for substances where human exposure is limited and of short duration. This last situation is often encountered in the case of pharmaceuticals. The need for multiple generation studies exceeding two generations arises only when the generated data indicate an increasing toxicity of the test substance during the first two generations.

(2) A traditional multigeneration study requires two litters per generation because the first litters produced by adolescent mothers often show a great deal of variation. Because of this variation, data based on the first litters are less useful than data from the second litters which are more uniform in size and health. A number of the proposed guidelines recommend only one litter, but the animals should not be bred until they have fully matured. In addition, guidelines exist which continue to recommend multiple litters in one or more generations. At least one guideline recommends that the option of producing a second litter should depend on the variability of control data obtained in the first breeding. There are several studies indicating that in at least one generation a second litter facilitates the evaluation of the complete study (Clegg, 1979).

(3) Some guidelines recommend commencement of dosing of the F_0 generation immediately after weaning. However, others propose a later date for initiation of dosing with different times of commencement for males and females. All guidelines propose that the interval between initiation of dosing and pairing should be adequate to ensure dosing throughout the period of at least one spermatogenesis cycle for the male, and at least four oestrous cycles for the female.

(4) The ratio of male to female pairing varies in different guidelines. In general, the ratio of one male to two females is used. However, there is a contention among scientists with regard to the cost effectiveness of obtaining additional data from 1:1 matings. All authors are in agreement that sibling matings must be avoided.

(5) Whenever possible, the route of administration should reflect human exposure. However, even after the decision regarding route has been made, there are still potential problem areas such as dose levels and how the dose should be administered (by gavage, water or diet). This decision should be made in the light of pharmacokinetic considerations.

(6) The guidelines available recommend that pairing should start earlier than 15 weeks postpartum for the first litter. The possibility of investigating differences in sensitivity that may be related to the age of the animals of the parental generation is thus eliminated. A question that still remains to be answered is whether or not such potential effects should be investigated.

(7) There is also a question concerning the standardization of litter sizes, and whether culling should be done at all. The reduction in litter size could obscure the observation of adverse effects which may be due to either increased litter size or decreased lactation capacity of the dam. Further, reduction in litter sizes may result in reduced statistical variation, and thus add a bias due to culling methods.

It is recommended that culling should not be routinely done although a number of current guidelines suggest the procedure.

(8) Animals may be assigned to dose groups by stratified random sampling based on consideration of body weight and other variables. This procedure is used because it reduces the variability in animal weight and in other relevant variables at the beginning of the experiment and may be used later to assure that litter mates are not cross-mated.

(9) It is questionable whether offspring should be weighed individually or collectively, and assigned individual identification numbers. It is recognized that collection of data on individuals is time consuming and expensive.

(10) Questions have been raised as to whether nesting material should be used and if so, what kind. Although use of nesting materials may reduce maternal stress by allowing the dam to act out nesting instincts, the animal may ingest or inhale contaminants contained in the material.

(11) There are a number of questions regarding dose levels, e.g. whether the highest dose selected should cause deaths among the dams, whether it should be significantly toxic to fetal development, or whether it should have adverse effects on the mother and the fetus; another question is whether the low dose should produce no effects or minimal effects, or whether it should simulate likely human exposure.

(12) The recommendations on autopsy after the completion of the experiment vary in different guidelines ranging from full histopathological examination to discarding the animals without any examination. Current practice favours gross examination of animals in the experiment with special attention to the reproductive system and preservation for possible future microscopic examination of at least the complete reproductive system in both sexes.

(13) The number of parental animals per test group determines the statistical power of the study. Most guidelines recommend that at least 20 litters be produced per generation. It is advisable that more than 20 mating pairs be used to produce the recommended number of litters. Several guidelines suggest that half the dams of the final litter be killed prior to delivery. This procedure is of questionable value. It may provide some information regarding possible embryotoxicity of the test material but at the expense of the statistical power of the test.

2.1.2 Fertility Tests

The purpose of such tests is to determine the level of fertility. They are also used as screening tests for effects on reproduction which may result from premating exposure.

There are at least two guidelines for the fertility test, one which terminates exposure to the test substance shortly after implantation and the other which continues the exposure throughout gestation and lactation. The former procedure provides a more precise prediction of fertility and preimplantation

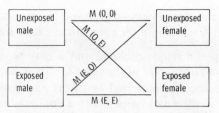

Figure 2.2　Reciprocal- or cross-mating studies. E, exposed; O, not exposed; M, mating

toxicity, since the data generated by the latter procedure may be confounded by embryotoxicity arising from a prolonged dosing period.

There is another difference between these two procedures. In the long-term exposure studies one-half of the mated females (presumably one mated to each male) are killed at midpregnancy to permit the count of corpora lutea and the examination of uterine contents.

Neither option appears to provide an adequate basis for determining fertility. It is suggested that a more informative test should consist of exposure of one-half of the animals up to the mating and the other half up to the time of implantation followed by the sacrifice of mated females at about day 12.

2.1.3 Reciprocal- or Cross-mating Studies

The purpose of these studies is to determine whether adverse effects on reproduction are associated with male or with female dysfunction.

Pairing is carried out according to the diagram shown in Figure 2.2.

Recommendations for the duration of dosing vary. The length of dosing will depend on the end-points (e.g. fertility, embryotoxicity, etc.) under investigation.

Selection of appropriate dose levels is again the major problem. In this type of study, the maximum dose levels may be different for males and females, because of different sensitivities, or for pregnant and non-pregnant females.

Other difficulties associated with this type of study include points (1), (2), (3), (4), (5), (7), (8), and (13) discussed in the section (2.1.1.) multigeneration studies on, as well as the time of sacrifice of the females.

2.1.4 Tests for Selective Embryotoxicity

These tests aim at detecting congenital malformations, abortions, resorptions, delayed development, sex ratios, and early and late embryonic death.

Mated females are exposed from the time of implantation to the termination of organogenesis, and sacrificed before parturition. Detailed guidelines on these methods are available in the testing guidelines of both OECD (1981) and IRLG (1981). These guidelines differ only in language, not in scientific detail.

The advantages of selective embryotoxicity tests include the capacity to detect and quantitate adverse effects of a test substance on the mother–fetus interaction after implantation, the ease of performance and the potential to simulate routes of human exposure. A number of the contentious issues are summarized below.

(1) Extrapolation is a major problem and it may be extremely difficult to extrapolate even from one strain of the same species to another. Variations are due largely to differences in maternal and fetal pharmacokinetics and metabolism. Variability in placental types is also a confounding factor.

(2) Toxicity to the mother limits the dose which reaches the fetus. Furthermore, adverse effects on the mother can cause fetal changes which are a reflection of the maternal effects rather than of direct effects of the test substance on the fetus or the placenta.

(3) Identification of malformations can occasionally be extremely difficult and controversial. For instance, difficulties in detecting minor changes in the ear ossicles are considerable. However, these malformations can result in a major defect, deafness. Similarly, the significance of such phenomena as sternal ossification defects, delayed digital ossification and 14th rib development is difficult to determine. Many investigators ignore these effects (even when dose-related incidences are observed), while others argue that they may be of considerable significance. There is general agreement that at worst such phenomena are a reflection of increased maternal stress.

(4) Route and type of administration as well as the frequency of, and time interval between, doses are other areas of concern. Basically, this has been addressed in the section on multiple-generation studies.

(5) The use of positive controls is a feature of many teratogenicity guidelines. In general, this is an unnecessary requirement. Positive results obtained with such control animals would indicate only that the test animals are susceptible to induction of terata by a substance already known to be teratogenic. They are of no value in predicting the susceptibility of the test animals to the substance under investigation.

(6) In evaluating data from teratogenicity studies, a major confusion arises from differences in terms used to describe the same defect. It is essential that as soon as possible a list of agreed terms be prepared to describe malformations. At least a detailed listing of alternative terms for the various terata is urgently required.

(7) Interlaboratory variability in test results using the same test substance in identical strains of test species appears to indicate the influence of external factors such as animal husbandry and/or the environmental conditions in the animal house which may exert a considerable impact on the final outcome of the test. This appears to require more consideration than it currently receives.

2.1.5 Perinatal and Postnatal Studies

The purpose of such studies is to investigate perinatal and postnatal effects in the absence of the confounding effects of early toxicity to reproductive function. The test substance is administered after the termination of organogenesis (i.e after the closure of palatal shelves) until weaning.

There are problems in interpreting such data because it is difficult to differentiate between the adverse effects on lactation of mothers and the effects on offspring due to transfer of the chemical via the milk.

2.2 EPIDEMIOLOGICAL INVESTIGATIONS

When exposure to a potentially toxic chemical has occurred in a human population, for example through an accident, occupational exposure, or therapeutic or illegal drug use, or when a widely available compound has come under suspicion (e.g. caffeine), an epidemiological approach may be used to look for effects on reproduction.

The epidemiological investigation of reproductive failure is subject to many problems, including low statistical power because of small population size, difficulties in defining exposure, bias in reporting and multiple end-points to be considered. The epidemiological approach also does not provide information about the mechanisms of action of the toxic agent.

An ideal study would include laboratory methods for refining the information on the outcome (e.g. semen analysis, chromosomal analysis of aborted fetuses) and on the exposure (e.g. biochemical tests, bioassays in man).

Statistical aspects to be considered in epidemiological studies include power, sample size, significance level and the magnitude of the effect. For a detailed discussion of these issues see Armitage (1971), Hill (1977) and Warburton *et al.* (1983, this volume).

Ethical considerations concerning privacy of medical and other information and informed consent for participation in studies must be a part of any epidemiological investigation.

In spite of these difficulties, there is no substitute for epidemiological studies since only they can provide information required to validate laboratory tests on experimental animals as predictors of human reproductive performance.

2.2.1 Definition of Exposure

Definition and quantitative assessment of exposure are very difficult and are often the limiting factors in many epidemiological studies of the effects of chemicals on health. The presence of exposure may be inferred by interviews or by identifying and specifying the place of work or residence, or determined by objective measures of exposures such as chemical analysis of body tissues and biological indicators such as chromosome aberrations or sperm abnormalities. Recall bias must be suspected whenever the major source of information on exposures is interview data. Validation of exposures by other methods (medical records or biochemical tests) for at least a part of the sample may indicate the extent of the problem. Another approach is to use several control groups, including one which has experienced another adverse outcome not likely to be the result of the same exposure as the one under investigation (e.g. Down's syndrome as a control for neural tube defects).

The relationship between chemical exposures and effects on reproduction is complex. To cause an effect, exposure may have to occur before fertilization (perhaps many years) or during gestation. It may act through the male parent or through the female parent, or both.

Once a chemical is released into the environment it is extremely difficult to relate any long-term effects of exposure to specific chemicals, because exposure to a multiplicity of other compounds occurs at the same time. An initial approach is to examine high-exposure groups (normally those in the manufacturing area), ensuring long-term clinical follow-up of exposed individuals. There will still be confounding effects due to the multiple exposure to various chemicals, but the probability of detecting the substance causing the adverse effect will be substantially increased, compared with general population studies. Once a tentative identification of a compound causing adverse effects has been made at this level, epidemiological studies of other exposed populations can be initiated.

2.2.2 Type of Studies

There are three possible levels of epidemiological investigations. At level I, the investigator looks only at readily accessible sources of data. Level II studies include full-scale epidemiological field investigations (case control or cohort). This may involve acquiring laboratory or interview data, or undertaking more extensive record searching than at level I. At level III, long-term follow-up studies of a population are undertaken.

2.2.2.1   *Studies Using Readily Accessible Data*

A level I analysis will consist of a comparison of the observed frequencies of reproduction events with available baseline data in order to decide whether a significant increase in an adverse outcome has occurred.

Only certain reproduction end-points routinely recorded in vital records or screening programmes will be available for this type of study. In most parts of the world these will consist of late fetal loss, birthrate, incidence of low birth weight and some congenital malformations. Newborn or prenatal screening programmes may also be used when available, the latter being especially valuable in providing an early warning of increases in some kinds of reproductive failures (for further discussion of reproduction end-points see Warburton *et al.*, 1983, this volume).

If a level I investigation leads to a clear-cut negative result, proceeding with further investigations may be unwarranted. When level I studies provide evidence for a positive effect, it may be advisable to undertake a more complete investigation and look at other end-points which might result.

2.2.2.2 *Epidemiological Field Studies*

Two basic experimental designs are used to demonstrate an association between a hazardous exposure of a population and reproductive failures. In a case control study the frequency and intensity of an exposure are compared between those who have experienced the outcome considered (cases) and those who have not (controls). In a cohort study the frequency of a reproductive outcome is compared between those who were exposed to a chemical or another environmental factor and those who were not exposed. A cohort study is usually prospective, but it may be retrospective as well.

2.2.2.3 *Long-term Follow-up Studies*

The effects of chemical exposures on reproductive function and the predictive value of laboratory and clinical observations can best be assessed by following up groups of individuals over their whole reproductive period. Any follow-up study is bound to include a considerable number of individuals who will be lost during the follow-up period, and it is important to consider biases which may be introduced if such a loss is not independent of the outcome.

2.3 IMPAIRMENT OF SPECIFIC FEMALE REPRODUCTIVE PROCESSES

2.3.1 Oogenesis and Ovulation

2.3.1.1 *Toxicity to the Developing Ovary*

Adverse effects of chemicals on the developing ovary will impinge upon the formation of the follicle complex. These adverse effects may occur during: the development of the ovary; primordial germ cell proliferation or migration; oogonial differentiation or proliferation; or formation of the primordial follicle. The rapid development of knowledge of ovarian embryology will greatly enhance investigations of the mechanisms of toxicity of chemicals to the developing ovary.

The mechanisms of mammalian oogenesis and folliculogenesis are presently understood in outline form (Haffen, 1977; Zuckerman and Baker, 1977, Gondos, 1978; Hardesty, 1978; Merchant-Larios, 1978). Methods, applicable to experimental animals, that are presently available to assess the effects of test compounds on oogenesis and/or folliculogenesis include histological determination of oocyte/follicle number which is a direct measure of toxicity (Dobson and

Cooper, 1974; Baker, 1976; Dobson *et al.*, 1978; Felton *et al.*, 1978). Fertility after prenatal treatment can also be assessed (Reimers and Sluss, 1978; Reimers *et al.*, 1980; Mackenzie and Angevine, 1981). Exposure during specific stages of gestation (or postnatally, depending on species) allows identification of the actual stage of disruption of oogensis or folliculogenesis (Mandl, 1964; Chen *et al.*, 1981; Mattison *et al.*, 1981). Although there are species differences in susceptibility and in the temporal sequence of disruption of oogenesis and folliculogenesis, a demonstration of toxicity in rodents generally indicates toxicity in primates (Mandl, 1964; Sieber and Adamson, 1975; Baker and Neal, 1977; Dobson *et al.*, 1978; Ash, 1980). The method is applicable to test animals, but not to women, and can be easily added to the standard multigeneration screening tests.

Indirect measures of toxicity to oogenesis and folliculogenesis in experimental animals include assessment of ovarian function, age of vaginal opening, age of reproductive senesence and age of total reproductive capacity (Heinrichs *et al.*, 1971; Gellert *et al.*, 1972; Gellert *et al.*, 1974; Kimbrough 1974; Kupfer, 1975; Gellert and Heinrichs, 1975; Gellert *et al.*, 1975; Gellert, 1978). The indirect measures are much less sensitive than direct oocyte/follicle counting; however, they are useful in human clinical assessment.

The extension of morphological techniques allowing qualitative and quantitative assessment of primordial germ cell number, migration, oogonial proliferation, and urogenital ridge development that are currently used in research may be useful for detailed evaluation of specific susceptible stages. The development of embryo culture methodology will allow *in vitro* assessment of disruption of oogenesis/folliculogenesis. This technique will permit separation of maternal metabolism from the metabolism of conceptus in studies designed to explore mechanisms of ootoxicity of chemicals. Additional areas for future research include *in vitro* techniques to evaluate primordial germ cell proliferation, migration and differentiation as well as folliculogenesis. Interaction of the developing ovary with other organ systems such as the thymus is also an area which deserves further consideration (Nishizuka and Sakakura, 1971; Lintern-Moore and Pantelouris, 1975a,b, 1976a,b,c; Michael, 1979; Ways *et al.*, 1980; Thompson, 1981).

Methods available to assess toxicity to human oogenesis/folliculogenesis are predominantly based on indirect measures of follicular function. These assays are well validated and used clinically. Clinical assessment of pubertal milestones (Tanner, 1962; Yen and Jaffe, 1978; Frantz, 1981; Ross and Vande Wiele, 1981) is useful only if the toxicity results in oocyte depletion before the onset or completion of puberty. Additional data, including quantitative determination of serum gonadotropins and ovarian steroids, will help identify other causes of disordered pubertal progression such as hypothalamic–pituitary dysfunction. Documentation of the presence of oocytes/follicles may become available by using a laparascopic ovarian biopsy technique, but because it requires a surgical procedure it is not extensively used (Taylor, 1979). Ovarian biopsy will differentiate the resistant ovary syndrome from oocyte depletion. Prenatal galactosaemia may represent a useful model for toxicity to the developing ovary (Hoefnagel *et al.*, 1979; Kaufman et al., 1979, 1981; Chen *et al.*, 1981; Coulam, 1981).

The age of menopause, with clinical signs of ovarian failure, is easily determined, and in suitable epidemiological investigations it may be useful for identifying disorder of oogenesis/folliculogenesis due to chemical toxicity.

The development of ultrasound equipment and techniques with increased resolution may allow non-invasive evaluation of ovarian fine structure (Robertson *et al.*, 1979; O'Herlihy *et al.*, 1980a,b; Renaud *et al.*, 1980; Smith *et al.*, 1980). At the present time ultrasound techniques can be used to evaluate ovarian size which is roughly proportional to the number of growing follicles. Serum assays for peptides (i.e. inhibin-like substances) produced by resting follicles would obviate the necessity for ovarian biopsy; however, this promising method remains to be developed.

2.3.1.2 *Toxicity to the Developed Ovary*

Adverse effects of chemicals on the developed ovary include direct effects on oocyte or follicle, disordered follicular growth, abnormal steroid hormone synthesis, interruptions of the hypothalamic–pituitary–ovarian control mechanisms, and inhibition of the release of the oocyte and of the formation of the corpus leteum. As these processes are crucial for fertility, a host of assay methods with varying degrees of specificity is available. Test substances altering any of these reproductive events in experimental animals would be identified in the multigeneration screens presently used in reproductive toxicity testing. However, species differences in endocrine control mechanisms along the hypothalamic–pituitary–ovarian axis may make extrapolation to primates difficult (Gorski, 1971; Knobil, 1974, 1980; Hutchinson and Sharp, 1977; Richards, 1978; Yen, 1978; DiZerega and Hodgen, 1981a,b).

Follicle growth Direct methods to assay follicular growth in experimental animals such as rodents include uptake of ^{3}H-thymidine, response of ovarian weight to pregnant mares' serum gonadotropin, and measurement of follicle kinetics (Zuckerman and Mandl, 1952; Pedersen and Peters, 1968; Pedersen, 1970; Goldenberg *et al.*, 1972; Harman *et al.*, 1975; Louvet *et al.*, 1975; Faddy *et al.*, 1976; Hillier *et al.*, 1980). These assays have been widely used; they signal direct adverse effects on follicular growth as well as indirect effects altering clearance of gonadotropins.

As follicular growth is associated with the production of oestrogens, indirect assays which determine serum levels of oestrogen or oestrogenic effects on target tissues have also been used as measures of follicular growth. These indirect assays include time of vaginal opening in immature rats, uterine weight, endometrial morphology and serum levels of follicle-stimulating hormone and luteinizing hormone (FSH/LH). The interpretation of these assays is complicated by the fact that they are indirect measures of follicular growth: compounds altering the metabolism or clearance of oestrogens can alter the response (Welch *et al.*, 1969, 1971). Additionally, compounds which alter follicular growth and also have oestrogen agonist or antagonist properties will complicate the use and interpretation of these indirect methods.

Methods which should be developed include measurement of xenobiotics in follicular fluid; this will have to be developed in animals larger than rodents (McNatty, 1978). Granulosa cell culture techniques presently being developed may allow direct screening of test substances for their ability to inhibit granulosa cell proliferation and/or oestrogen production (Hillier *et al.*, 1977; Zeleznik *et al.*, 1979). Factors involved in the recruitment of follicles from the resting pool, the first step in follicular growth, have not been completely elucidated and additional research is essential. The role of other organ systems in modulating the clearance of oestrogens and decreasing or increasing serum levels also needs further evaluation. Test substances altering peripheral levels of oestrogen indirectly by induction or suppression of hepatic monooxygenases or changes in gut flora (see Slater, 1983, this volume) will have adverse effects on the endocrine feedback mechanisms along the hypothalamic–pituitary–ovarian axis.

Methods to monitor follicular growth in women are widely available and have been used extensively in clinical assessment of ovarian function. Clinical assessment of cyclic menstrual function in women reflects assessment of the integrated functioning of the reproductive system (Ross, 1974; Ross and Lipsett, 1978; Wentz, 1979; DiZerega and Hodgen 1981a). Measurement of serum oestrogen and progesterone levels throughout the menstrual cycle indirectly monitors follicular growth and steroid synthesis (Yen, 1978). Clinically useful indirect measures of oestrogen production include changes in quantity and quality of cervical mucus (Billings *et al.*, 1972, 1977; Billings and Billings, 1973) and timely cyclic menstrual flow. As indirect measures, they cannot distinguish mechanisms altering follicular growth from those altering clearance, end organ response to or effectiveness of oestrogens. Measurement of serum gonadotropins throughout the menstrual cycle also demonstrates appropriate hypothalamic–pituitary function and intact feedback mechanisms.

As previously mentioned, enhancement of the resolution of ultrasound technology may allow indirect assessment of follicular development (see section 2.3.1.1). The use of laparoscopy to assess follicular growth by biopsy or direct visualization may also have applicability in selected situations. Human granulosa cell culture techniques may provide accurate and directly applicable screening techniques to determine the effects of xenobiotic chemicals on granulosa cell proliferation and/or steroid production.

Ovulation Ovulation reflects the successful functioning of the hypothalamic–pituitary–ovarian axis including follicle growth, steroid hormone production, LH surge, follicle rupture and oocyte release.

Direct methods to assess ovulation in experimental animals include collection of oocytes from uteri or fallopian tubes in spontaneous or stimulated ovarian cycles (Orberg and Kihlström, 1973; Linder *et al.*, 1974; Weir and Rowlands, 1977; Espey, 1978). The presence of oocytes in the uterus or tubes in stimulated overian cycles in rodents, or reflex ovulation is a direct measure of follicle growth, rupture and oocyte release. This assay has been used extensively in reproduction biology to assay compounds like the prostaglandin synthetase inhibitors, which inhibit follicle rupture (Mori *et al.*, 1980), or other compounds like phenobarbitone or the cannabinoids which block the LH surge (Barraclough and Sawyer, 1957; Cordova *et al.*, 1980; Kostellow *et al.*, 1980).

Indirect measures of ovulation are also useful in experimental assay systems, including embryo flushing and implantation site quantitation (Hammer and Mitchell, 1979; Shani *et al.*, 1979; Yoshinaga *et al.*, 1979). Embryo flushing quantitates both ovulation and fertilization, and implantation site quantitation additionally assays implantation of the embryo and endometrial development under the control of both oestrogens and progesterone. Implantation site assays have the advantage of direct visual scoring. Additional methods include release of uterine fluid and thermogenic responses resulting from progesterone production, signalling the development of a functional corpus luteum following ovulation.

Methods requiring killing of the test animals, although expedient in rodents, may not be applicable to larger animals including non-human primates. In these cases, serum progesterone assay or thermogenic responses will be useful. Ultrasound examination to demonstrate follicle rupture or direct laparoscopic visualization may also be useful in non-human primates (see section 2.3.1.1). These assay systems have been useful in reproduction biology and can be adapted to toxicology.

Methods assaying ovulation in women are indirect, and monitor progesterone production by the corpus luteum, which forms following ovulation, or the effects of progesterone on responsive end organs. The least invasive technique involves monitoring changes in the fluidity, air drying pattern and elasticity of cervical mucus. This technique has been widely developed, can be easily taught, and is used to monitor ovulation and signal fertile and non-fertile portions of the menstrual cycle (Billings *et al.*, 1972, 1977; Billings and Billings, 1973; Wentz, 1979). Endometerial biopsy for morphological evaluation of ovulation has also been extensively used in women (Noyes *et al.*,1950). The changes in endometrial morphology are characteristic; however, the necessity for a biopsy decreases the potential for broad application. Endometrial aspiration tehcniques, however, may prove useful in field studies (Smith, 1960).

As with larger animals, hysteroscopic or laparoscopic harvesting of oocytes or ultrasound examination may prove useful. Broad screening is also possible with assays for urinary oestrogens and progestogens (Evans *et al.*, 1980).

Corpus luteum function Corpus luteum formation and function in experimental animals can be assessed by measurement of serum progesterone following spontaneous or induced ovulation. As the follicle is the precursor of the corpus luteum, subtle disorder of follicular growth may be manifest in abnormal luteal function. Ovarian weight and morphological and morphometric analysis following ovulation have been used to monitor corpus luteum formation (Stouffer and Hodgen, 1980).

Some indirect measures of progesterone production have been discussed in the ovulation section. An additional indirect measure is decidualization of the pseudo-pregnant rodent uterus. This assay has been successfully used in toxicological studies by several investigators (e.g. Card and Mitchell, 1978). As with other end organ responses, interference at the progesterone receptor, or alterations in hepatic or renal clearance of progesterone may interfere with the interpretation of the assay.

Development of in vitro assay systems, granulosa cell differentiation or luteal cell function may provide rapid reliable screening systems.

Methods to assess human corpus luteum function were discussed in the ovulation section and include thermogenic response, serial progesterone measurement, cervical mucus changes and endometrial biopsy. Urinary steroid assays will aid the development of epidemiological studies which are essential in reproductive toxicology.

Atresia Currently used methods to monitor oocyte and/or follicle destruction in experimental animals include serial oocyte counts (Jones and Krohn, 1961; Pedersen and Peters, 1968; Pedersen, 1970; Faddy *et al.*, 1976). These methods are quantifiable and reliable and have been used to explore the effects of oocyte and follicle toxins (Jick *et al.*, 1977; Mattison and Thorgeirsson 1978a,b, 1979; Mattison, 1980; Mattison and Nightingale, 1980; Mattison *et al.*, 1981). Lifetime breeding studies, which have also been useful, are generally insensitive and appear to require extensive oocyte destruction before they can be easily scored as positive. Age at reproductive failure in larger animals is a useful screening end-point and may be applicable to field studies.

Methods of human surveillance for oocyte destruction include monitoring populations for changes in the age of menopause. This has been used with success in patients treated with ovotoxic drugs, as well as in environmental exposure studies (Tokuhata, 1968; Pettersson *et al.*, 1973; Sieber and Adamson, 1975; Jick *et al.*, 1977; Vessey *et al.*, 1978; Mattison *et al.*, 1980). This method should be used more extensively in population monitoring. Clinical assessment of oocyte destruction has generally focused on the ovarian failure end-point, with little information available concerning assay techniques to monitor increased rates of destruction before ovarian failure. Assessment of ovarian failure in women includes clinically established techniques that measure follicular and corpus luteum function as previously discussed.

2.3.2 Gamete Transport, Fertilization, Zygote Transport and Implantation

Disruption of any one component of that phase of the reproductive process which begins with gamete transport and ends in implantation would impair the reproductive function, and would be revealed in an integrated whole animal reproductive study. Identification of the cause of impairment or the exact stage at which failure occurs could be regarded as a goal that is relevant to basic research rather than to screening for regulatory purposes. Nevertheless, some *in vivo* and *in vitro* methods currently used to investigate mechanisms of early reproductive failure hold promise as pre-screening procedures to replace costly long-term whole animal testing.

The successful function of the reproductive tract depends on the participation of a number of appropriately phased activities. These include motility (muscular or ciliary), secretion (luminal fluids in response to internal and external signals), and adaptive cell growth and turnover (cyclic structural changes of oestrus and of pregnancy). Xenobiotics may interfere directly or indirectly with one or more of these activities of the female genital tract. It is possible to inspect, assess or measure each of these activities in the various components of the female genital tract. While the tract is important in that it provides the environment in which the fertilized egg develops from a single cell to the implanting blastocyst and beyond, xenobiotics can, in addition, act directly on the developing zygote, and these effects can also be studied by simple inspection, assessment or measurement.

Within the phase of the reproductive process which begins with gamete transport and ends with the attachment and implantation of the embryo, relatively simple procedures exist for studying sperm transport, fertilization, the rate of tubal transport of the zygote, the rate of development of the embryo, the morphological normality of the developing embryo, implantation and the spacing of fetuses along the uterine horns. These techniques have been developed for establishing the pattern of normal reproductive activity, but could be applied to dosed females and F_1 female progeny, e.g. as pre-screening tests prior to a multigeneration study.

2.3.2.1 *Existing Tests*

At the regulatory level there are no recognized alternatives to the fertility test or one-, two- or three-generation reproduction studies (see, e.g. NAS, 1977; OECD,

1981; sections 2.1.1 and 2.1.2) for testing the effects of chemicals on those reproduction events which culminate in implantation. The Workgroup was not aware of the established use of alternative test procedures in other situations, with the possible exception of the mouse dominant lethal test which was designed to detect heritable chromosomal damage but which, with minor modifications, would also suffice as a one-generation reproduction study in the male. It does not offer an advantage to reproduction studies in the female.

2.3.2.2 *Established Research Methods With Testing Potential*

The stages of female reproductive function and early embryogenesis have been studied extensively by researchers. The techniques used, although not presently considered routine test procedures, are appropriate for use in evaluating the effects of chemicals on reproductive processes. Oocyte maturation, ovulation, transport of ovulated oocytes to the oviducts, sperm transport and fertilization can all be measured with a high degree of sensitivity and reproducibility using inbred strains of mice, and possibly rabbits and rats. Induced ovulation followed by artificial insemination (West *et al.*, 1977), subsequent timed removal from the oviducts, and analysis of numbers of fertilized, ovulated eggs would yield information regarding these processes. An additional advantage of artificial insemination is that by using the mixed semen from treated and untreated males (of two phenotypically distinguishable mouse strains), it is possible to determine their relative fertilizing ability by comparing F_1 phenotype ratios with control values. This technique eliminates uncertainties caused by interanimal variability and also enables one to distinguish between sperm dysfunction and the presence of inhibitors in the seminal fluid (see also section 3.3.2).

Two- or four-cell embryos can be removed from oviducts and cultured up to and including peri-implantation stages (Whitten, 1971). Such a procedure would yield information concerning the ability of fertilized eggs derived from treated parents to cleave, develop through preimplantation stages, hatch, attach and outgrow on artificial substrata or on uterine monolayers (Sherman and Wudl, 1976). These later stages of observation (i.e. hatching through implantation) are, of course, only model systems for events occurring in the female reproductive tract. However, they have been shown to be valid methods for determining embryonic viability and development. Biochemical markers can also be used as determinative end-points for these developmental stages. The effects of xenobiotic chemicals on preimplantation embryo development *in vitro* can also be determined. Such treated embryos, transferred into a suitable foster mother (McLaren and Michie, 1956), can be observed for later developmental defects.

There are also established *in vivo* methods by which the development of the zygote can be studied. These procedures rely on killing the pregnant female and inspecting the genital tract and its contents at precisely timed intervals after mating. For test purposes these methods would require a colony in which there is normally a high frequency of successful mating. It is possible to establish a time scale in which the location of the zygote in the genital tract correlates well with its stage of development. Deviation from the norm would identify an effect on the rate of transport of the embryo and/or an effect on cleavage rate. Similarly, once the interval between mating and implantation has been determined for the strain being used, the absence of decidual swellings 48 hours or more beyond the expected time of implantation would suggest anti-implantation action (provided it had been previously established that the chemical under study does not affect development to the expanded blastocyst stage). This technique would also reveal an effect on the spacing of embryos along the uterine horns or their existence in ectopic sites. Comparisons between these *in vivo* analyses and *in vitro* studies outlined above allow the distinction between indirect (i.e. maternal) and direct (embryotoxic) actions of chemicals.

More sophisticated techniques have been used to study aspects of female reproductive function in laboratory animals (including non-human primates) and domestic species. While these could be useful in determining the precise cause of infertility, it is unlikely that such relatively complex and expensive method will be developed for screening purposes.

Direct evaluation of early embryonic stages through implantation in the woman is not yet feasible. However, difficulties in this phase would appear as failure to conceive. Tests capable of discriminating among all the causes of failure to conceive or early failure of pregnancy are not yet available (Warburton, personal communication).

2.3.3 Embryonic Differentiation and Fetal Development

2.3.3.1 *Whole Animal Tests*

Current methods with whole animals are used for screening chemicals for embryotoxicity by determining the extent of fetal loss and fetal abnormality. Although these methods are relatively easy to use, they lead to many difficulties of interpretation (see section 2.1.4). There are considerable errors of prediction resulting from interspecies variations, particularly from differences in maternal metabolism of xenobiotics. It is therefore difficult to use experimental animals in tests for specifically human metabolites. Other problems arise from differences in placental transfer of compounds in different species, and failure of some test animals to reveal embryotoxicity because of atypically severe effects of particular chemicals on the mother. Practical limitations are the high cost and relatively large quantities of test substances required.

For these reasons, consideration of alternatives is recommended. It is suggested that particular attention be given to methods using chick embryos, and rat and mouse embryos *in vitro*.

2.3.3.2 *Embryo Culture Methods*

Xenobiotics can be tested in chick embryos of all stages of development (Jelínek, 1979). Rat and mouse embryos can be maintained in culture at all stages of organogenesis (New, 1978; 1983, this volume). During the period from head-fold to early limb-bud stage (9 1/2–11 1/2 days of gestation in the rat) they grow exceptionally well and at the same rate as *in vivo*. Because this is the most critical period of development, in which minimum damage leads to maximum defects, embryos provide a particularly sensitive test for the toxicity of xenobiotic chemicals.

The use of embryos avoids all the problems of whole animal tests arising from variations in maternal metabolism. They can be used for testing of metabolites of xenobiotics produced specifically in man, or in any selected animal.

These methods are cheap, reliable and can be used routinely. They require a somewhat higher level of skill than whole animal tests but are sufficiently simple that large numbers of embryos can be processed in a short time. A number of studies with known teratogenic and other agents have shown that the embryo culture methods provide an efficient and sensitive test for embryotoxicity.

Serum can be added to chick embryos in the egg or after explantation. Rat and mouse embryos are grown in serum. Chemicals may be tested in any of the following ways:

(1) by direct addition of the agent to the serum;
(2) by direct addition of the agent to the serum together with components of the activating systems (Fantel *et al.*, 1979);
(3) by using serum from animals exposed to the agent (Klein *et al.*, 1980; Kitchin *et al.*, 1981a, b); or
(4) by using serum from human subjects exposed to the agent (see Chatot *et al.*, 1980).

In the case of chick embryos, chemicals can also be administered without serum (Jelínek, 1977, 1979).

Routine examination of the embryos for toxic effects can include observations of heart rate, glucose consumption and lactate production, size and gross morphology, histology, total protein and DNA, protein of parts of the embryo (e.g. head/body ratios for microcephaly, Cockroft and New, 1978), and cellular damage, e.g. sister chromatid exchange (see Wudl and Sherman, 1983, this volume).

More critical comparisons of effects of known embryotoxic agents in the whole animal and in alternative systems would provide further information on the predictive value of tests with chick embryos or cultured rat/mouse embryos compared with whole animal tests, and on relative costs. Examination of the many end-points that may be used in assessing toxicity requires further study in order to select the best end-points for routine use.

2.3.3.3 *Human Studies*

The effects of chemical exposure on human embryonic differentiation and fetal development can be most directly ascertained by clinical and epidemiological studies. Possible end-points and the available and potential methods to determine these end-points include the following:

Embryonic and fetal loss Loss after implantation but before clinically recognized pregnancy (10 days to approximately 28 days after conception) could be determined by pregnancy tests. Pregnancy can be detected as early as 10 days after conception by radioimmunoassay (RIA) or radioreceptor assay (RRA) of the B subunit of human chorionic gonadotropin (hCG) in maternal serum or urine. Continuation or loss of pregnancy is determined by a pregnancy test after the time of the next expected menses. Such a study would have to be done prospectively on a group of women attempting to become pregnant. This procedure would be expensive and difficult to apply on a large population sample. Also, little is known about the causes of these early losses and how they relate to other reproductive end-points. However, the test would be powerful even with a small population sample, as it has been suggested that there is a high rate of very early losses (about 20%) in the unexposed population.

Loss of clinically recognized pregnancy (later than about 28 days after conception) is considered to be a spontaneous abortion. Such losses could be studied by examining hospital records or other medical records or by retrospective interviews. In the first two cases, the verification of the pregnancy by pathological examination would be possible, and information could be obtained on

(1) the gestation period (sometimes available from the local medical practitioner);
(2) morphology of the abortion product of conception (empty sac, disorganized embryo, malformed embryo or fetus, grossly normal embryo or fetus, etc.);
(3) placental abnormalities; and
(4) karyotype through culture of fetal tissues.

In a prospective study, additional information on the time of death of the conceptus might be obtained from ultrasound studies of heart beats.

Hospital and medical records may seriously underestimate the incidence of early spontaneous abortion, since many will not come to medical attention. The proportion will depend upon the availability and use of services, and the quality of record keeping. In some cases, information on spontaneous abortion may be available from vital statistics records, but it is rare for such data to be collected on early pregnancy losses. More accurate data can be obtained by retrospective interviews of the mother (though not from other informants such as the husband). However, these data are subject to the bias of recall and inaccuracies of self-diagnosis.

Prenatal studies Prenatal monitoring of the fetus is possible by ultrasonography. Using real time ultrasound imaging, embryonal heart beat can be visualized, beginning at gestational week 7. Information on the general appearance of the conceptus and the site of implantation can be obtained approximately a week earlier. At midgestation (gestational weeks 18–20), ultrasound screening makes it possible to detect multiple pregnancies and some gross malformations of the fetus, such as anencephalies. Ultrasonic anthropological measurements made at this period can be used as a starting point for prospective growth evaluations. Abnormalities in placental localization and structure can be recognized at the same time, and this may prevent prenatal losses. The evaluation of fetal growth should be based on at least two additional ultrasonic measurements performed around gestational weeks 29 and 35.

The method is currently regarded as safe. Screening of the whole population is possible and the results can be statistically evaluated. Ultrasonic screening could eventually be used to detect differences in pregnancy outcome in exposed and non-exposed populations in cases of industrial accidents. The cost of ultrasound testing is considerable.

Transabdominal monitoring of fetal behaviour (fetal heart rate, fetal movements) is possible during the third trimester of pregnancy. In some cases, the registered changes may reflect immediately the exposure to xenobiotics.

These methods are used in evaluating fetal well-being and are regarded as completely safe. The cost is comparably low and the results are immediately available.

X-ray radiography in human prenatal screening should be limited to strictly indicated cases. The method poses risks of serious long-term consequences, and even gross defects are difficult to detect. The expenses are considerable. X-ray radiography should not be applied if the fetus is expected to survive, and its use should be confined to experimental animal studies.

Cultivation of amniotic cells and their karyotyping is a routine method for detecting structural and numerical chromosomal abnormalities. The method is reliable and useful but expensive.

Chemical tests elucidating hormonal levels are used for sex prediction and for diagnosis of some endocrine disorders. Tests based on the concentration of alpha-fetoprotein (AFP) in the amniotic fluid and within maternal circulation have been used in large population studies for screening of open neural tube defects. The risk of complications related to amniocentesis may be less than 0.5%. The optimal period for amniocentesis is between 16 and 18 gestational weeks. Usually 5–20 ml of fluid are withdrawn from a total of 120–300 ml. Biological testing of amniotic fluid requires skill and is time consuming. Screening of AFP may be done at reasonable cost.

Perinatal deaths Frequencies of late fetal deaths, stillbirths and deaths of newborns are available from vital statistics data in most countries. This is an accurately recorded and easily accessible end-point. However, it is subject to variation due to levels of perinatal care, and this must be controlled in the study.

Weights of newborns and placenta Birth weight is accurately and regularly recorded on birth certificates in many countries. It is also available in hospital and physician's records, or, retrospectively, from maternal history. Placental weight is available from medical records. Birth weight is a sensitive indicator of maternal and fetal exposures. Low birth weight is highly correlated with perinatal death, congenital malformations, chromosomal abnormalities and developmental delay, and, in the absence of other data on these end-points, birth weights can be used instead. This information is also accurately recorded and not subject to bias of recall. Placental weight is less accurately measured and recorded, but generally correlates highly with birth weight. However, change in placental weight/birth weight ratio may be informative.

Congenital malformations In term births, congenital malformations are usually incompletely and inaccurately recorded on birth and death certificates. To determine malformations, infants should be examined by a paediatrician preferably trained in dysmorphology. Age at examination must be controlled because rates and types of malformation will vary with age. Congenital malformations should be classified as far as possible into aetiological categories. Laboratory tests may be required to make specific diagnosis. The variety of malformations makes it usually necessary to group them for analysis. Methods of doing so are imprecise, and classification may produce misleading results. Interview data on malformations and exposure status may introduce bias.

Delayed effects Follow-up studies of offspring of exposed mothers can reveal effects which cannot be detected at birth. These include developmental delays, behavioural abnormalities and transplacentally induced cancers. Tests of developmental status, intelligence and behaviour would have to be used to assess these end-points. Cancers can be ascertained by follow-up studies or through searches of cancer registries and death registries. These follow-up studies are expensive and many subjects will be lost during the follow-up study. Although difficult to investigate, these are significant end-points.

2.3.3.4 *Parturition*

Two major effects of chemical agents on parturition have to be considered:

Premature labour and delivery A preliminary screening of chemicals for this effect can be performed by testing for uterotonic activity *in vitro*. There are three optional methods:

(1) the *in vitro* rat uterine strip test for uterotonic activity. The isolated uterine horn of an oestrogen-primed virgin rat (Sprague-Dawley or Wistar strain) is suspended in de Jalons' solution or Munsick's solution. The advantage of this test is that it is simple, sensitive and inexpensive. The potency of the test substance can be expressed in relation to oxytocin by means of a 4 × 4 point bioassay. Although the validity of this test in relation to human uterus has not been established, all the known oxytocic agents have a demonstrable effect on the rat uterus.

(2) an alternative would be to use premenopausal human myometrium strips *in vitro*. While this test would be more relevant when testing for possible uterotonic effects in women, premenopausal human uteri are difficult to obtain in some countries.

(3) the *in vitro* rabbit uterine test is also useful for detecting uterotonic activity. This entails the recording of changes in intrauterine pressures caused by contractions induced in the uterus. A rubber balloon or a nylon sponge coupled to a pressure transducer is used for recording the changes on a polygraph. Although this preparation is sensitive to all known oxytocic agents, inherent disadvantages of the system are that a considerable amount of time is necessary to set up the assay and, even more so, it is susceptible to spontaneous contractions which are sometimes difficult to distinguish from those induced by the test substance. This makes the preparation unsuitable for quantitative assays when it is necessary to express the potency of the test substance in relation to a standard oxytocic substance such as oxytocin.

Delayed parturition This effect of chemicals would result in exposure of the fetus (and mother) to the well-known hazards of postmaturity. Although it is not an established method, *in vitro* inhibition of oxytocin or prostaglandin activity in the isolated uterus from an oestrogen primed rat could probably be used to identify chemicals capable of delaying parturition. The procedure would consist of determining whether the contractions normally induced by oxytocin and/or prostaglandin are inhibited when the test substance is present in the bath in which the uterus is suspended. Since several factors are involved in the induction of labour, the validity of this test is open to question.

Delay in parturition could be best tested in a whole animal experiment using pregnant rats. The average duration of pregnancy in this species is well established and, by administering the suspected chemical or drug to pregnant rats, it would be easy to determine whether parturition is delayed.

The problem is that there are no accepted guidelines on dosing and/or duration of treatment with the test substance. The route of administration also needs consideration. Oral administration is easy but becomes problematic when the test substance is insoluble in water. In such cases, the substance could be suspended in gum acacia or 'complexed' with polyvinylpyrrolidine (PVP). For 'complexation' with PVP, the test substance is first dissolved in a non-aqueous solvent such as ethanol, mixed with 4 parts of PVP and the solvent removed by lyophilization. The residue will now dissolve or form a suspension with water. Subcutaneous injections should be administered in different areas of the abdominal wall each day to prevent ulceration and induration which would result if the injections were given to the same area daily. Intraperitoneal injections are not recommended as they may cause adhesions. The test could also be designed to determine whether an anti-implantation effect is produced and whether the chemical causes fetal resorption. For this purpose, the chemical would have to be administered for 10 days from the date of conception as determined by the presence of sperm in a vaginal smear or a copulation plug, and the autopsy performed on day 16 of pregnancy. An analysis of the number of corpora lutea, the number of implantation sites and the number of normal fetuses would then be determined.

When a chemical agent is strongly suspected of affecting parturition, it may be necessary to resort to experiments with primates. This is, however, very expensive and can be performed only at a few specialized centres.

The procedures described above can be regarded only as a general guideline, as there are very few chemical agents which are abortifacient (e.g. ergot alkaloids, quinine) or which delay parturition (e.g. alcohol, isoxsuprine).

Other complications of parturition Animal models are not currently available for testing for retention of placenta, abnormal bleeding of third trimester and parturition, or dysfunctional labour. Epidemiological methods described in section 2.2 could be used to evaluate these complications.

2.3.3.5 *Effects of Chemical Agents on Lactation*

Inhibition of lactation (physiological/behavioural) can be evaluated by a whole animal study, using litter survival and growth to weaning as end-points; the species used is mouse or rat.

Postnatal effects of chemical agents may be mediated directly via chemical content of milk, or indirectly through the effects on the mother (neglect of offspring). A cross-foster design (Figure 2.3) can separate fetal effects (parental exposure) from postnatal effects due to transmission of the contaminant in milk, or due to the effects on maternal lactation or behaviour (Keller and Doherty, 1980). Analytical and other methodological requirements include a radiolabelled chemical, or a specific, reliable analytical method sufficiently sensitive to measure the chemicals quantitatively in a small volume of mouse blood (0.100–1.00 ml), plasma (0.050–0.500 ml) and milk (0.150–0.250 ml) (samples can be pooled from

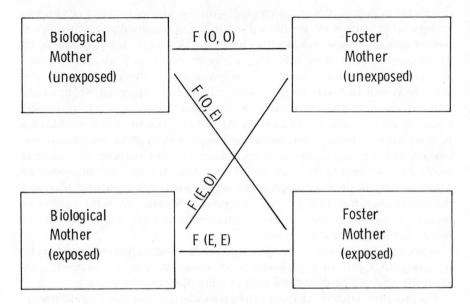

Figure 2.3　Litters cross-fostering study. F designates cross-fostered litters. The letters in parentheses represent exposure of biological mother (first letter) and foster mother (second letter). E, exposed; O, not exposed

groups of mice); a bleeding technique (insertion of capillary tube into orbital sinus); and a milking technique (milk collection is aided by subcutaneous injection of 0.3 U of synthetic oxytocin 15 minutes before hand expression of milk into constant bore capillary tubes). The dosing route has to be as similar as possible to the human route of exposure. The dose level should be in the non-toxic range. An option of intravenous route (mouse tail vein injection) is possible for pharmacokinetic studies.

   A similar (non-radioactive) method can be used for measuring accidental or occupational exposures, or for monitoring chronic exposures of widespread chemical contaminants of the human environment, such as PCBs and lead.

2.3.3.6 *Effects of Chemical Agents on Maternal Behaviour*

Chemical agents may affect maternal behaviour to the offspring, such as lactation and nesting. The best way of studying this effect would be by means of a cross-fostering design experiment (see section 2.3.3.5). The end-points would include litter survival, litter weight, evidence of cannibalism, nesting and general behaviour of the mothers. Since there are few recorded observations of the effects of chemicals on mothering, detailed experimental protocols need to be developed.

Test procedures discussed in section 2 are summarized in Table 2.1.

2.4 CONCLUSIONS AND RECOMMENDATIONS

(1) Most of the currently available methods for determining female reproductive end-points have not been validated for adverse effects caused by xenobiotic agents.

(2) For new products or products already present in the human environment, which must be evaluated in terms of human health hazard, test procedures are required which are applicable to routine screening of large numbers of compounds in experimental laboratory animals. Sensitive procedures are also necessary for the retrospective evaluation of the effects of chemicals on human populations or domestic animals. In addition, there is a need for continued monitoring of compounds which have already been tested and released for use.

(3) The Workgroup felt that the development of population screening procedures to monitor reproduction end-points based on non-invasive techniques is an area which requires further attention.

(4) The difficulties of applying the results of *in vitro* or *in vivo* laboratory studies of female reproductive functions to human health risk estimation are the same as in other branches of predictive toxicology.

(5) The Workgroup strongly encouraged continuous surveillance and critical re-evalution of standard tests of toxicity to female reproductive function. Biologically appropriate targets, toxicological validity and cost effectiveness of tests are aspects that require re-evaluation, so that non-efficacious procedures can be appropriately modified or eliminated from standard testing protocols as new information becomes available.

(6) The Workgroup noted that reliable methods are now available for using rat and mouse embryos *in vitro* and chick embryos in testing for embryotoxicity of chemicals. These methods appear to have several advantages over the standard whole animal tests and should be further examined to assess their predictive value and cost effectiveness in comparison with other procedures.

(7) When evaluating the effects of environmental chemicals, the potential of farm animals as indicator species should not be overlooked. Domesticated animals can be especially valuable as their reproductive activities are in most cases accurately recorded. This constitutes a valuable source of information for retrospective epidemiological surveys.

(8) There are certain aspects of female reproductive function in which effects of xenobiotics are not known. For example, there are no laboratory or animal models to study such effects as abnormal placentation (placenta praevia) and postpartum hemorrhage. Research is required to develop valid test methods for such adverse changes.

Table 2.1 Methods for assing the effects of chemicals on female reproductive function of mammals

Stage of reproductive process	Method	Established	Screen	Quantitative risk evaluation
A. Epidemiological and clinical studies				
(1) All stages	Epidemiology			
	Level I	Yes	+	−
	Level II	Yes	−	+
	Level III	Yes	−	+
(2) Oogenesis/Ovulation				
(a) Follicle growth	Levels of serum oestrogen, progesterone, gonadotropins and other cyclic changes	Yes	+	−
	Ultrasound, laparoscopy	No	−	−
(b) Ovulation	Cyclic changes in cervical mucus and endometrial morphology	Yes	+	−
	Levels of urinary or serum oestrogens and progesterone	Yes	+	−
	Thermogenic response	Yes	+	−
	Ultrasound, laparoscopy, hysteroscopy	No	−	−
(c) Corpus luteum function	Same as (b)			
(d) Atresia	Population monitoring for age of menopause	Yes	−	+

(3) Gamete transport → fertilization → implantation	None	—	—
(4) Postimplantation to birth* (none for early pregnancy)			
Ultrasonography	No	—	—
Transabdominal monitoring	Yes	—	—
X-rays	Yes	—	—
Amniocentesis	Yes	(+)	+
Milk contamination	No	—	+
(5) Parturition/lactation			

*Note: Effects on postimplantation processes until birth, including birth weights and abnormalities, may be studied epidemiologically.

Table 2.1. (*contd.*)

Test Procedures

Stage	Method	Estab-lished	Pre-screen	Approval testing	New compounds	Environ-mental pollutants	Comments
B. Laboratory animal models							
(1) All stages	♂, ♀ Reproduction (2 generations)	Yes	–	+	+	+	
(2) Oogenesis/ Ovulation							
(a) Follicle Growth	(i) Uptake of ³H-thymidine & ovarian weight in response to gonadotropin (alternatives: serum oestrogen, time of vaginal opening, uterine weight, endometrial morphology, serum FSH/LH)	Yes	+	–	+	+	
	(ii) Granulosa cell culture (to measure inhibition of proliferation or oestrogen production)	No	+	–	+	+	
(b) Ovulation	Collection and counting of oocytes (normal or induced ovulation)	Yes	+	–	+	+	
(c) Corpus luteum	(i) Serum progesterone	Yes	+	–	+	+	
	(ii) Morphological analysis	Yes (some species)	+	–	+	+	
	(iii) Decidualization of pseudo-pregnant rodent	Yes	–	–	+	+	
(d) Atresia	(i) Direct counts of ovarian serial sections	Yes	+	–	+	+	
	(ii) Life time breeding	Yes					

...port→fertili-zation→implantation (mouse)

Method						Comments
(a) Ovulation→Fertilization (gamete transport)						
Induced ovulation/artificial insemination with timed counts of fertilized eggs	No	+	−	+	+	
(b) Preimplantation						
In vivo: uterus flushing	No	+	−	+	+	
In vitro: culture from 2 to 4 cell stage	No	+	−	+	+	Embryo or parent can be treated prior to culture
(c) Implantation						
In vivo: number, spacing	No	+	−	+	+	
In vitro: number, cell number per embryo, differentiation	No	+	−	+	+	Embryo or parent can be treated prior to culture
(4) Postimplantation to birth						
In vitro culture of rat or mouse midgestation embryos	No	(+)†	(−)†	+	+	
Chick embryos	No	(+)†	(−)†	+	+	
(5) Parturition/lactation						
In vitro rat/rabbit uterine strip test	Yes	+	−	+	+	
Cross-fostering	Yes	−	+	−	+	
Determination of chemical contaminants in milk	Yes	−	+	−	+	

† Parentheses indicate that the utility of the method as a pre-screen or approval testing procedure is not clearly established.

(9) The development of a more accurate and extensive data base on human reproductive end-points should be encouraged. The present routinely available vital and health statistics services should be upgraded, particularly with respect to rapid data analysis and feedback to those responsible for data recording. Also to be encouraged are centralized data banks (local or national level) on occupational, health and reproduction statistics organized in such a way that data linkage is possible.

2.5 REFERENCES

Armitage, P. (1971). *Statistical Methods in Medical Research*, 504 pages. Blackwell Scientific Publications, Oxford and Edinburgh.

Ash, P. (1980). The influence of radiation on fertility in man. *Br. J. Radiol.* 53, 271–278.

Baker, T. C. (1976). The effects of ionizing radiation on the mammalian ovary with particular reference to oogenesis. In Greep, R. O. and Astwork, E. G. (Eds.) *Handbook of Physiology. Endocrinology II*, Part I, pp. 349–361. American Physiological Society, Washington, DC.

Baker, T. C. and Neal, P. (1977). Action of ionizing radiations on the mammalian ovary. In Zuckerman, S. J. and Weir, B. J. (Eds.) *The Ovary*, 2nd edn. Vol. III, pp. 1–58. Academic Press, New York.

Barraclough, C. A. and Sawyer, C. H. (1957). Blockade of the release of pituitary ovulating hormone in the rat by chlorpromazine and reserpine: possible mechanisms of action. *Endocrinology (Philadelphia)* 61, 341–351.

Billings, E. L. and Billings, J. J. (1973). The idea of the ovulation method. *Aust. Fam. Physician* 2, 81–85.

Billings, E. L., Billings, J. J., Brown, J. B. and Burger, H. G. (1972). Symptoms and hormonal changes accompanying ovulation. *Lancet* ii, 282–284.

Billings, E. L., Billings, J. J. and Catarinich, M. (1977). *Atlas of the Ovulation Method*, 3rd edn. Advocate Press, Melbourne.

Card, J. P. and Mitchell, J. A. (1978). The effects of nicotine administration on deciduomer induction in the rat. *Biol. Reprod.* 19, 326–331.

Chatot, C. L., Klein, N. W., Piatek, J. and Pierro, L. J. (1980). Successful culture of rat embryos on human serum: use in the detection of teratogens. *Science (Washington, DC)* 207, 1471–1473.

Chen, Y. T., Mattison, D., Feigenbaum, L., Fukui, H. and Schulman, J. D. (1981). Reduction in oocyte number following prenatal exposure to a high galactose diet. *Pediatr. Res.* 15, 642.

Clegg, D. J. (1979). Animal reproduction and carcinogenicity studies in relation to human safety evaluation. In Deichman, W. B. (Ed.) *Toxicology and Occupational Medicine*, pp. 45–59. Elsevier/North Holland, New York, Amsterdam, Oxford.

Cockroft, D. L. and New, D. A. T. (1978). Abnormalities induced in cultured rat embryos by hyperthermia. *Teratology* 17, 277–284.

Collins, T. F. X. (1978). Multigeneration studies of reproduction. In Wilson, J. G. and Fraser, F. C. (Eds.) *Handbook of Teratology: Research Procedures and Data Analysis*, Vol. 4, pp. 191–219, Plenum Press, New York and London.

Cordova, T., Ayalon, D., Lander, N., Mechoulam, R., Nir, I., Puder, M. and Lindner, H. R. (1980). The ovulation blocking effect of cannabinoids: structure activity relationships. *Psychoneuroendocrinology (Oxford)* 5, 53–62.

Coulam, C. B. (1981). Hormonal status of galactosaemia homozygotes. *Lancet* i, 165.

DiZerega, G. S. and Hodgen, G. D. (1981a). Folliculogenesis in the primate ovarian cycle. *Endocrine Rev.* **2**, 27–49.

DiZerega, G. S. and Hodgen, G. D. (1981b). Luteal phase dysfunction infertility: a sequel to aberrant folliculogenesis. *Fertil. Steril.* **35**, 489–499.

Dobson, P. L. and Cooper, M. F. (1974). Tritium toxicity: effects of low-level ^{3}HOH exposure on developing female germ cells in the mouse. *Radiat. Res.* **38**, 91–100.

Dobson, P. L., Koehler, C. G., Felton, J. S., Kwan, T. C., Wuebbles, B. J. and Jones, D. L. C. (1978). Vulnerability of female germ cells in developing mice and monkeys to tritium, gamma rays, and polycyclic aromatic hydrocarbons. In Mahlum, D. D., Sikor, M. R., Hackett, P. L. and Andrew, F. D. (Eds.) *Development Toxicology of Energy-Related Pollutants.* DOE Symposium Series 47: Conference 771017, Washington, DC.

Espey, L. L. (1978) Ovulation. In Jones, R. E. (Ed.) *The Vertebrate Ovary: Comparative Biology and Evolution*, pp. 503–532. Plenum Press, New York and London.

Evans, J. J., Stewart, C. R. and Merrich, A. Y. (1980). Oestradiol in saliva during the menstrual cycle. *Br. J. Obstet. Gynaecol.* **87**, 624–626.

Faddy, M. J., Jones, E. L. and Edwards, R. G. (1976). An analytical model for ovarian follicle dynamics. *J. exp. Zool.* **197**, 173–185.

Fantel, A. G., Greenaway, J. C., Juchau, M. R. and Shepard, T. H. (1979). Teratogenic bioactivation of cyclophosphamide *in vitro. Life Sci.* **25**, 67–72.

Felton, J. S., Kwan, T. C., Wuebbles, B. J. and Dobson, R. L. (1978). Genetic differences in polycyclic aromatic hydrocarbon metabolism and their effects on oocyte killing in developing mice. In Mahlum, D. D., Sikov, M. R., Hackett, P. L. and Andrew, F. D. (Eds.) *Developmental Toxicology of Energy-Related Pollutants.* DOE Symposium Series 47: Conference 771017, Washington, DC.

Frantz, A. G. (1981). The breast. In Williams, R. H. (Ed.) *Textbook of Endocrinology*, 6th edn, pp. 400–411. W. B. Saunders Company, Philadelphia.

Gellert, R. J. (1978). Uterotrophic activity of polychlorinated biphenyls (PCB) and induction of precocious reproductive aging in neonatally treated female rats. *Environ. Res.* **16**, 123–130.

Gellert, R. J. and Heinrichs, W. L. (1975). Effects of DDT homologs administered to female rats during the perinatal period. *Biol. Neonate* **26**, 283–290.

Gellert, R. J., Heinrichs, W. L. and Swerdloff, R. S. (1972). DDT homologs: estrogen-like effects on the vagina, uterus and pituitary of the rat. *Endocrinology (Philadelphia)* **91**, 1095–1100.

Gellert, R. J., Heinrichs, W. L. and Swerdloff, R. (1974). Effects of neonatally administered DDT homologs on reproductive function in male and female rats. *Neuroendocrinology* **16**, 84–94.

Gellert, R. J., Wallace, C. A., Weismeier, E. M. and Shuman, R. M. (1975). Topical exposure of neonates to hexachlorphene: longstanding effects on mating behavior and prostatic development in rats. *Toxic. appl. Pharmac.* **43**, 339–349.

Goldenberg, R. L., Vaitukaitis, J. L. and Ross, G. T. (1972). Estrogen and follicle stimulating hormone interactions on follicle growth in rats. *Endocrinology (Philadelphia)* **90**, 1492–1498.

Gondos, B. (1978). Oogonia and oocytes in mammals. In Jones, R. E. (Ed.) *The Vertebrate Ovary: Comparative Biology and Evolution*, pp. 83–120. Plenum Press, New York and London.

Gorski, R. A. (1971). Gonadal hormones and the perinatal development of neuroendocrine function. In Martini, C. and Ganong, W. F. (Eds.) *Frontiers in Neuroendocrinology*, pp. 237–290. Oxford University Press, Oxford, London, Glasgow, New York.

Haffen, K. (1977). Sexual differentiation of the ovary. In Zuckerman, S. J. and Weir, B. J.

(Eds.) *The Ovary*, 2nd edn, Vol. I, pp. 69–112. Academic Press, New York, San Francisco, London.

Hammer, R. E. and Mitchell, J. A. (1979). Nicotine reduces embryo growth, delays implantation and retards parturition in rats. *Proc. Soc. exp. Biol. Med.* **162**, 333–336.

Hardesty, W. M. (1978). Primordial germ cells and the vertebrate germ line. In Jones, E. R. (Ed.) *The Vertebrate Ovary: Comparative Biology and Evolution*, pp. 1–45. Plenum Press, New York and London.

Harman, S. M., Louvet, J. P. and Ross, G. T. (1975). Inhibition of the ovarian augmentation reaction by a chemical antiestrogen. *Endocrinology (Philadelphia)* **96**, 1119–1122.

Heinrichs, W. L., Gellert, R. J., Bakke, J. L. and Lawrence, N. L. (1971). DDT administered to neonatal rats induces persistent estrus syndrome. *Science (Washington, DC)* **173**, 642–643.

Hill, Sir Austin Bradford (1977). *A Short Textbook of Medical Statistics*, 325 pp. Hodder and Stoughton, London, Sydney, Auckland, Toronto.

Hillier, S. G., Knazek, R. A. and Ross, G. T. (1977). Androgenic stimulation of progesterone production by granulosa cells from preantral ovarian follicles: further *in vitro* studies using replicate cell cultures. *Endocrinology (Philadelphia)* **100**, 1539–1549.

Hillier, S. G., Zeleznik, A. J., Knazek, R. A. and Ross, G. T. (1980) Hormonal regulation of preovulatory follicle maturation in the rat. *J. Reprod. Fertil.* **60**, 219–229.

Hoefnagel, D., Wurster-Hill, D. and Cheld, E. L. (1979). Ovarian failure in galactosaemia. *Lancet* **ii**, 1197.

Hutchinson, J. S. M. and Sharp, P. J. (1977). Hypothalamus-pituitary control of the ovary. In Zuckerman, S. J. and Weir, B. J. (Eds.) *The Ovary*, 2nd edn, Vol. III, pp. 227–304. Academic Press, New York, San Francisco, London.

IRLG (1981). *Recommended Guidelines for Teratogenicity Studies in the Rat, Mouse, Hamster and Rabbit.* Interagency Regulatory Liaison Group, Washington, DC.

Jelínek, R. (1977). The chick embryotoxicity screening test (CHEST). In Neubert, D., Merker, H.-J. and Kwasigroch, T. E. (Eds.) *Methods in Prenatal Toxicology*, pp. 381–386. G. Thieme, Stuttgart.

Jelínek, R. (1979). Embryotoxicity assay on morphogenetic systems. In Benešová, O., Rychter, Z. and Jelinek, R. (Eds.) *Evaluation of Embryotoxicity, Mutagenicity and Carcinogenicity Risks in New Drugs*, pp. 195–205. Univerzita Karlova, Praha.

Jick, H., Porter, J. and Morrison, A. S. (1977). Relation between smoking and age of natural menopause. *Lancet* **i**, 1354–1355.

Jones, E. C. and Krohn, P. L. (1961). The relationship between age, numbers of oocytes and fertility in virgin and multiparous mice. *J. Endocrinol.* **21**, 469–495.

Kaufman, F. R., Kogut, M. D., Donnell, G. N., Gobelsmann, U., March, C. and Koch, R. (1981). Hypergonadotropic hypogonadism in female patients with galactosemia. *New Engl. J. Med.* **304**, 994–998.

Kaufman, F., Kogut, M. D., Donnell, G. N., Koch, R. and Geobelsmann, U. (1979). Ovarian failure in galactosaemia. *Lancet* **ii**, 737–738.

Keller, C. A. and Doherty, R. A. (1980). Lead and calcium distributions in blood, plasma and milk of the lactating mouse. *J. Lab. clin. Med.* **95**, 81–89.

Kimbrough, R. D. (1974). The toxicity of polychlorinated polycyclic compounds and related chemicals. *CRC Crit. Rev. Toxicol.* **2**, 445–498.

Kitchin, K. T., Sanyal, M. K. and Schmid, B. P. (1981a). A coupled microsomal-activating/embryo culture system: toxicity of reduced β-nicotinamide adenine dinucleotide phosphate (NADPH). *Biochem. Pharmacol.* **30**, 985–992.

Kitchin, K. T., Schmid, B. P. and Sanyal, M. K. (1981b). Teratogenicity of cyclophosphamide in a coupled microsomal activating/embryo culture system. *Biochem. Pharmacol.* **30**, 59–64.

Klein, N. W., Vogler, M. A., Chatot, C. L. and Pierro, L. J. (1980). The use of cultured rat embryos to evaluate the teratogenic activity of serum: cadmium and cyclophosphamide. *Teratology* **21**, 199–208.

Knobil, E. (1974). On the control of gonadotropin secretion in the rhesus monkey. *Recent Progr. Horm. Res.* **30**, 1–46.

Knobil, E. (1980). The neuroendocrine control of the menstrual cycle. *Recent Progr. Horm. Res.* **36**, 53–88.

Kostellow, A. B., Ziegler, D., Kunar, J., Fujimoto, G. I. and Morrill, G. A. (1980). Effect of cannabinoids on estrous cycle, ovulation and reproductive capacity of female A/J mice. *Pharmacology* **21**, 68–75.

Kupfer, D. (1975). Effects of pesticides and related compounds on steroid metabolism and function. *CRC Crit. Rev. Toxicol.* **4**, 83–124.

Linder, R. E., Gaines, T. B. and Kimbrough, R. D. (1974). The effect of polychlorinated biphenyls on rat reproduction. *Food Cosmet. Toxicol.* **12**, 63–77.

Lintern-Moore, S. and Pantelouris, E. M. (1975a). Ovarian development in athymic nude mice. I. The size and composition of the follicle population. *Mech. Ageing Dev.* **4**, 385–390.

Lintern-Moore, S. and Pantelouris, E. M. (1975b). Ovarian development in athymic nude mice. II. The growth of the oocyte and follicle. *Mech. Ageing Dev.* **4**, 391–398.

Lintern-Moore, S. and Pantelouris, E. M. (1976a). Ovarian development in athymic nude mice. III. The effect of PMSG and oestradiol upon the size and composition of the ovarian follicle population. *Mech. Ageing Dev.* **5**, 33–38.

Lintern-Moore, S. and Pantelouris, E. M. (1976b). Ovarian development in athymic nude mice. IV. The effect of PMSG and oestradiol in the growth of the oocyte and follicle. *Mech. Ageing Dev.* **5**, 155–162.

Lintern-Moore, S. and Pantelouris, E. M. (1976c). Ovarian development in athymic nude mice. V. The effects of PMSG upon the numbers and growth of follicles in the early juvenile ovary. *Mech. Ageing Dev.* **5**, 259–265.

Louvet, J. P., Harman, S. M. and Ross, G. T. (1975). Effects of human chorionic gonadotropin, human interstitial cell stimulating hormone and human follicle-stimulating hormone on ovarian weights in estrogen-primed hypophysectomized immature female rats. *Endocrinology* (*Philadelphia*) **96**, 1179–1186.

Mackenzie, K. M. and Angevine, D. N. (1981). Infertility in mice exposed in vitro to benzo(a)pyrene. *Biol. Reprod.* **24**, 183–191.

Mandl, A. M. (1964). The radiosensitivity of germ cells. *Biol. Rev. Cambridge Phil. Soc.* **39**, 288–371.

Mattison, D. R. (1980). Oocyte destruction by zenobiotic compounds. *Contemp. Obstet. Gynecol.* **15**, 157–169.

Mattison, D. R., Chang, L., Thorgeirsson, S. S. and Shiromizu, K. (1981). The effects of cyclophosphamide, azathioprine, and 6-mercaptopurine on oocyte and follicle number in C57BL/6N mice. *Res. Commun. Chem. Pathol. Pharmacol.* **31**, 155–161.

Mattison, D. R. and Nightingale, M. S. (1980). The biochemical and genetic characteristics of murine ovarian aryl hydrocarbon (benzo(a)pyrene) hydrozylase activity and its relationship to primordial oocyte destruction by polycyclic aromatic hydrocarbons. *Toxic. appl. Pharmac.* **56**, 399–408.

Mattison, D. R. and Thorgeirsson, S. S. (1978a). Gonadal aryl hydrocarbon hydroxylase in rats and mice. *Cancer Res.* **38**, 1368–1373.

Mattison, D. R. and Thorgeirsson, S. S. (1978b). Smoking and industrial pollution, and their effects on menopause and ovarian cancer. *Lancet* **i**, 187–188.

Mattison, D. R. and Thorgeirsson, S. S. (1979). Ovarian aryl hydrocarbon hydroxylase activity and primordial oocyte toxicity of polycyclic aromatic hydrocarbons in mice. *Cancer Res.* **39**, 3471–3475.

Mattison, D. R., White, N. B. and Nightingale, M. S. (1980). The effect of benzo(a)pyrene on fertility, priomordial oocyte number, and ovarian response to pregnant mare's serum gonadotropin. *Pediatr. Pharmacol.* **1**, 143–151.

McLachlan, J. A. and Dixon, R. L. (1976). Transplacental toxicity of diethylstilbestrol: a special problem in safety evaluation. In Mehlman, M. A., Shapiro, R. E. and Blumenthal, H. (Eds.) *Advances in Modern Toxicology: New Concepts in Safety Evaluation*, pp. 423–448. Hemisphere Publishing Corp., Washington, DC.

McLaren, A. and Michie, D. (1956). Studies on the transfer of fertilized mouse eggs to uterine foster mothers. I. Factors affecting the implantation and survival of native and transferred eggs. *J. exp. Biol.* **33**, 394–416.

McNatty, K. P. (1978). Follicular fluid. In Jones, R. E. (Ed.) *The Vertebrate Ovary: Comparative Biology and Evolution*, pp. 215–260. Plenum Press, New York and London.

Merchant-Larios, H. (1978). Ovarian Differentiation. In Jones, R. E. (Ed.) *The Vertebrate Ovary: Comparative Biology and Evolution*, pp. 47–81. Plenum Press, New York and London.

Michael, S. D. (1979). The role of the endocrine thymus in female reproduction. *Arthritis Rheum.* **22**, 1241–1245.

Mori, T., Kohda, H., Kinoshita, Y., Ezahi, Y., Morimoto, N. and Nishimura, T. (1980). Inhibition by indomethacin of ovulation induced by human chorionic gonadotropin in immature rats primed with pregnant mare serum gonadotropin. *J. Endocrinol.* **84**, 333–341.

NAS (1977). *Principles and Procedures for Evaluating the Toxicity of Household Substances. A Report Prepared by the Committee for the Revision of NAS Publication 1138*, pp. 99–110. National Academy of Sciences, Washington, DC.

New, D. A. T. (1978). Whole-embryo culture and the study of mammalian embryos during organogenesis. *Biol. Rev. Cambridge Phil. Soc.* **53**, 81–122.

Nishizuka, Y. and Sakakura, T. (1971). Ovarian dysgenesis induced by neonatal thymectomy in the mouse. *Endocrinology* (*Philadelphia*) **89**, 886–893.

Noyes, R. W., Hertig, A. T. and Roch, J. (1950). Dating the endometrial biopsy. *Fertil. Steril.* **1**, 3–25.

OECD (1981). *OECD Guidelines for Testing of Chemicals*, 700 pp. Organization for Economic Cooperation and Development, Paris.

O'Herlihy, C., DeCrespigny, L. J. Ch., Lopata, A., Johnston, I., Hoult, I. and Robinson, H. (1980a). Preovulatory follicular size: a comparison of ultrasound and laparoscopic measurements. *Fertil. Steril.* **34**, 24–26.

O'Herlihy, C., DeCrespigny, L. J. Ch. and Robinson, H. P. (1980b). Monitoring ovarian follicular development with real-time ultrasound. *Br. J. Obstet. Gynaecol.* **87**, 613–618.

Orberg, J. and Kihlström, J. E. (1973). Effects of long-term feeding of polychlorinated biphenyls (PCB, Clophen A 60) on the length of the oestrous cycle and on the frequency of implanted ova in the mouse. *Environ. Res.* **6**, 176–179.

Pedersen, T. (1970). Follicle kinetics in the ovary of the cyclic mouse. *Acta Endocrinol.* (*Copenhagen*) **64**, 304–323.

Pedersen, T. and Peters, H. (1968). Proposal for a classification of oocytes and follicles in the mouse ovary. *J. Reprod. Fertil.* **17**, 555–557.

Pettersson, F., Fries, H. and Nillius, S. J. (1973). Epidemiology of secondary amenorrhea. I. Incidence and prevalence rates. *Am. J. Obstet. Gynecol.* **117**, 80–86.

Reimers, T. J. and Sluss, P. M. (1978). 6-Mercaptopurine treatment of pregnant mice. Effects on second and third generations. *Science* (*Washington, DC*) **201**, 65–67.

Reimers, T. J., Sluss, P. M., Goodwin, J. and Seidel, G. E. (1980). Bigenerational effects of 6-mercaptopurine on reproduction in mice. *Biol. Reprod.* **22**, 367–375.

Renaud, R. L., Macier, J., Dervain, I., Ehret, M-C., Aron, C., Plas-Roser, S., Spira, A. and Pollack, H. (1980). Echographic study of follicular maturation and ovulation during the normal menstrual cycle. *Fertil. Steril.* **33**, 272–276.

Richards, J. S. (1978). Hormonal control of follicular growth and maturation in mammals. In Jones, R. E. (Ed.) *The Vertebrate Ovary: Comparative Biology and Evolution*, pp. 331–360. Plenum Press, New York.

Robertson, R. D., Picker, R. H., Wilson, P. C. and Saunders, D. M. (1979). Assessment of ovulation by ultrasound and plasma estradiol determinations. *Obstet. Gynecol. (New York)* **54**, 686–691.

Ross, G. T. (1974). Gonadotropins and prenatal follicular maturation in women. *Fertil. Steril.* **25**, 522–543.

Ross, G. T. and Lipsett, M. B. (1978). Hormonal correlates of normal and abnormal follicle growth after puberty in humans and other primates. *Clin. Endocrinol. Metab.* **7**, 561–575.

Ross, G. T. and Vande Wiele, R. L. (1981). The ovaries. In Williams, R. H. (Ed.) *Textbook of Endocrinology*, 6th edn, pp. 355–399. W. B. Saunders, Philadelphia.

Shani, J., Amit, M. and Givant, Y. (1979). Effect of the timing of perphenazine administration on pregnancy in the rat. *J. Endocrinol.* **80**, 409–411.

Sherman, M. I. and Wudl, L. R. (1976). The implanting mouse blastocyst. In Poste, G. and Nicolson, G. L. (Eds.) *The Cell Surface in Animal Embryogenesis and Development*, pp. 81–125. Elsevier/North-Holland, Amsterdam, New York, Oxford.

Sieber, S. M. and Adamson, R. H. (1975). Toxicity of antineoplastic agents in man: chromosomal aberrations, antifertility effects, congenital malformations, and carcinogenic potential. *Adv. Cancer Res.* **22**, 57–155.

Smith, D. H., Picker, R. H., Smosich, M. and Saunders, D. M. (1980). Assessment of ovulation by ultrasound and estradiol levels during spontaneous and induced cycles. *Fertil. Steril.* **33**, 387–390.

Smith, S. E. Jr. (1960). Plastic tube aspiration of the endometrium. *Obstet. Gynecol.* **16**, 375–376.

Stenchever, M. A., Williamson, R. A., Leonard, J., Karp, L. E., Ley, B., Shy, K. and Smith, D. (1981). Possible relationship between *in utero* diethylstilbestrol exposure and male fertility. *Am. J. Obstet. Gynecol.* **140**, 186–193.

Stouffer, R. L. and Hodgen, G. D. (1980). Induction of luteal phase defects in rhesus monkeys by follicular fluid administration at the onset of the menstrual cycle. *J. clin. Endocrinol. Metab.* **51**, 669–671.

Tanner, J. M. (1962). *Growth at Adolescence*. Charles C. Thomas, Springfield, Illinois.

Taylor, P. J. (1979). Gynecologic laparoscopy. *Obstet. Gynecol. Ann.* **8**, 333–368.

Thompson, E. A. Jr. (1981). The effects of estradiol upon the thymus of the sexually immature female mouse. *J. Steroid Biochem.* **14**, 167–174.

Tokuhata, G. M. (1968). Smoking in relation to infertility and fetal loss. *Archs Environ. Health* **17**, 353–359.

Vessey, M. P., Wright, N. H., McPherson, K. and Wiggins, P. (1978). Fertility after stopping different methods of contraception. *Br. med. J.* **1**, 265–267.

Ways, S. C., Blair, P. B., Bern, H. A. and Stronskawicz, M. O. (1980). Immune responsiveness of adult mice exposed neonatally to diethylstibestrol, steroid hormones, or Vitamin A. *J. Environ. Pathol. Toxicol.* **3**, 207–220.

Weir, B. J. and Rowlands, I. W. (1977). Ovulation and atresia. In Zuckerman, S. J. and Weir, B. J. (Eds.) *The Ovary*, 2nd edn, Vol. 1, pp. 265–302. Academic Press, New York, San Francisco, London.

Welch, R. M., Levin, W. and Conney, A. H. (1969). Estrogenic action of DDT and its analogs. *Toxic. appl. Pharmac.* **14**, 358–367.

Welch, R. M., Levin, W., Kuntzman, Jacobson, M. and Conney, A. H. (1971). Effect of halogenated hydrocarbon insecticides on the metabolism and uterotropic action of estrogens in rats and mice. *Toxic. appl. Pharmac.* **19**, 234–246.

Wentz, A. C. (1979). Physiologic and clinical considerations in luteal phase defects. *Clin. Obstet. Gynecol.* **22**, 169–185.

West, J. D., Frels, W. L., Papaioannou, V. I., Karr, J. P. and Chapman, V. M., (1977). Development of interspecific hybrids of Mus. *J. Embryol. exp. Morphol.* **41**, 233–243.

Whitten, W. K. (1971). Nutritional requirements for the culture of preimplantation embryos *in vitro. Adv. Biosci.* **6**, 129–142.

Yen, S. S. C. (1978). The human menstrual cycle (integrative function of the hypothalamic-pituitary-ovarian-endometrial axis). In Yen, S. S. C. and Jaffe, R. B. (Eds.) *Reproductive Endocrinology: Physiology, Pathophysiology and Clinical Management*, pp. 126–151. W. B. Saunders, Philadelphia.

Yen, S. S. C. and Jaffe, R. B. (1978). *Reproductive Endocrinology: Physiology, Pathophysiology and Clinical Management.* W. B. Saunders, Philadelphia.

Yoshinaga, K., Rice, C., Krenn, J. and Pilot, R. L. (1979). Effects of nicotine on early pregnancy in the rat. *Biol. Reprod.* **20**, 294–303.

Zeleznik, A. J., Hillier, S. G., Knazek, R. A., Ross, G. T. and Coon, H. G. (1979). Production of long-term steroid producing granulosa cell cultures by cell hybridization. *Endocrinology (Baltimore)* **105**, 156–162.

Zuckerman, S. and Baker, T. G. (1977). The development of the ovary and the process of oogenesis. In Zuckerman, S. J. and Weir, B. J. (Eds.) *The Ovary*, 2nd edn, Vol. I, pp. 42–68. Academic Press, New York, San Francisco, London.

Zuckerman, S. and Mandl, A. M. (1952). The growth of the oocyte and follicle in the adult rat. *J. Endocrinol.* **8**, 126–132.

Methods for Assessing the Effects of Chemicals on Reproductive Functions
Edited by V. B. Vouk and P. J. Sheehan
© 1983 SCOPE

3 Mammals: Reproductive Function of Males*

There is an increasing concern that exposure to chemicals may adversely affect male reproductive function. This concern has triggered an intensified scientific interest, and several reports have recently become available dealing with the physiology, biochemistry and toxicology of mammalian reproduction, and the evaluation of underlying biological processes and their susceptibility to exogenous chemicals (Dixon, 1980a, b; Amann, 1981; Bedford, 1981; Burger and de Kretser, 1981; Hansson et al., 1981; Mann and Lutwak-Mann, 1981).

The structures and processes which are involved in male reproductive function and which may be influenced by exogenous chemicals, directly or indirectly, include the hypothalamic–pituitary–gonadal axis, the testes, efferent ducts, epididymis and male accessory organs, the formation and composition of semen, sexual behaviour, and the processes of erection and ejaculation.

An attempt has been made both to assess critically existing testing and evaluation procedures and to suggest applications of more recent research methods. For this reason, perhaps more than usual degree of speculation has been permitted.

3.1 STRUCTURE AND PHYSIOLOGY BACKGROUND

3.1.1 Hypothalamic–Pituitary–Gonadal Axis

Follicle stimulating hormone (FSH) and luteinizing hormone (LH) are glycoproteins synthesized and released from a subpopulation of the basophilic cells of the pituitary gland termed gonadotropic cells (gonadotrophs, gonadotropes). Central regulation of the pituitary gland is mediated by the hypothalamus, communicating by way of a specialized vascular system called the hypophyseal portal system. Hypothalamic neuroendocrine neurons secrete specific releasing or release-inhibiting factors, called hypophysiotropic hormones, into the hypophyseal portal system. These hormones are carried in the blood of the portal

*This section was prepared by a Workgroup chaired by Thaddeus Mann, with Robert L. Dixon as rapporteur. Other members of the Workgroup were R. Eliasson, J. B. Kerr, C. Lutwak-Mann, A. Massoud, J. Pařizek, and R. G. Tardiff.

system to the adenohypophysis where they act upon their target cells to stimulate or inhibit the release of anterior pituitary hormones. Luteinizing-hormone-releasing hormone (LHRH) acts upon gonadotropic cells, thereby stimulating the release of FSH and LH. Purified preparations of native LHRH possess intrinsic FSH-stimulating properties, thus suggesting that LHRH and follicle-stimulating-hormone-releasing hormone (FSHRH) were one and the same substance. Synthetic forms of LHRH stimulate the release of both gonadotropic hormones, thereby leading to the proposal that this compound be termed gonadotropin-releasing hormone (GnRH).

The neuroendocrine neurons have nerve terminals containing monoamines (norepinephrine, dopamine, serotonin) impinging upon them. The effects of reserpine or chloropromazine and other agents which alter or modify the content or actions on reproductive function of brain monoamines are well documented. Dopamine is known to cause the release of LHRH.

The release of hormones by the adenohypophysis involves a chain of events which greatly multiplies the original signal. Hormones released from the target gland, such as the testis, may produce dramatic behavioural and other changes in the organism which are the end result of the hypothalamic release of transmitters. The peripherally released hormones act by way of a feedback mechanism on the brain to modify the concentrations of transmitters in the hypothalamus.

This sensitive and complex system presents several targets for environmental and industrial chemicals, and there are many drugs thought to exert significant effects on or to alter the normal functional state. It is clearly established that the effects of toxic agents on endocrine processes in the brain or pituitary gland may indirectly inhibit spermatogenesis, alter steroidogenesis, cause abnormal sexual behaviour and/or result in sterility. Alterations not so severe as to result in infertility may be detected by measurements of FSH, LH and testosterone concentrations in the blood. In contrast to semen or testicular tissue, blood is relatively easy to obtain, and measurements of these serum hormone concentrations provide specific indicators of toxicity to the reproductive function. FSH probably acts primarily on the Sertoli cells, but it also appears to stimulate the mitotic activity of spermatogonia. LH stimulates steroidogenesis. A defect in the function of the testis (in the production of spermatozoa or testosterone) will tend to be reflected by increased levels of FSH and LH in serum because of lack of the 'negative feedback' effect of testicular hormones. Conversely, if a defect occurs in hypothalamic or pituitary function, blood levels of FSH and LH will tend to decrease. A LHRH test has been demonstrated to be capable of detecting mild degrees of primary testicular dysfunction insufficient to elevate basal hormone levels above the normal range.

Testosterone and other steroids such as danazol and various progestational compounds have an antispermatogenic action mediated via the pituitary gland. The antispermatogenic action of methallibure, certain siloxanes, and chlormadinone as well as that of certain new synthetic agonists of the hypothalamic gonadotropin-releasing hormones are mediated by the pituitary gland (Mann and Lutwak-Mann, 1981).

3.1.2 Testis

The testis can be divided into two major compartments, the interstitium (interstitial space) and the seminiferous tubules. These compartments have different embryological origins, unique cell populations and distinct functions. The major function of the interstitium is the production of steroids by Leydig cells. The two major contributions of the seminiferous tubules are the spermatozoa which develop from the spermatogonial stem cells, and the products of Sertoli cells. The function of both the interstitial tissue and seminiferous tubules is closely inter-related with that of the pituitary gland and hypothalamus.

There are a number of variables to be considered in the assessment of effects of a chemical on testicular functions: pharmacokinetics, routes of administration, multiple exposures, time of exposure, genetic versus epigenetic damage, species differences, age and stage of development (fetal, neonatal, prepubertal, pubertal, adult, senescent) (Dixon and Lee, 1980; Dixon, 1981). Direct adverse effects generally occur in the cells of the seminiferous epithelium; the hypothalamic–pituitary–gonadal axis, sperm maturation or sperm transit may be affected indirectly.

3.1.2.1 *Interstitium*

The Leydig cells are the main site of testosterone synthesis and are closely associated with the blood vessels and the lymphatic space of the testis which facilitate the transport of testosterone from the Leydig cells into the tubules. LH stimulates steroidogenesis in part by increasing the hydrolysis of cholesterol esters to free cholesterol. Cholesterol is probably the source of all testicular steroid hormones. Androgens, the dominant steroids secreted by the testis, are essential for spermatogenesis, the growth and secretory activity of accessory sex organs, somatic masculinization, male behaviour and various metabolic processes. Leydig cell function is further discussed in section 3.2.1.

3.1.2.2 *Seminiferous Tubules*

The primary cellular components of the seminiferous tubules are the germ cells (spermatogonia, primary spermatocytes, secondary spermatocytes, and spermatids) and the Sertoli cells. Spermatogenesis takes place in the seminiferous epithelium where cellular replication of stem cells and stem cell differentiation lead to the formation of spermatozoa. The function of the Sertoli cells is multifaceted and less clear. They do not divide in adult animals, apparently play an important role in meeting the nutritional requirements of the developing sperm, and are involved in fluid secretion. Among the secretory products of the Sertoli cells are the androgen-binding protein (ABP) and inhibin. The Sertoli cells are also critical elements of the blood–testis barrier.

Seminiferous epithelium The primary role of the seminiferous epithelium is the production of sperm. Spermatogenesis is initiated during postnatal development and allows for transmission of genetic material between generations. Specifically, it results in the formation of spermatozoa which contain a haploid number of chromosomes and which are capable—after completing subsequent maturation—of locomotion and penetration of the egg. Spermatogenesis is characterized by the conversion of a specific undifferentiated stem cell into a highly differentiated cell type while retaining a spermatogonial reserve. It involves a complicated set of mitotic divisions and meiosis. Because of these varied characteristics, the process is highly susceptible to cytotoxic chemicals. As the number of spermatozoa ejaculated greatly exceeds the number needed to ensure fertility, comprehensive semen analysis is a more sensitive end-point for identifying adverse effects of chemicals than are mating procedures.

In a laboratory animal such as the rat, numerous spermatogonia in particular regions of the seminiferous tubules divide synchronously, and the cohorts of cells which result differentiate in unison. Intercellular bridges persist between the cytoplasms of the germinal cells after the nuclei divide. Thus, adjacent cross-sections through the seminiferous tubules appear different. Detailed analyses have defined as many as fourteen different cellular association stages in the rat and six stages in man. Each cellular association contains four or five types or layers of germ cells associated in a specific pattern. The complete series of cellular associations is termed the seminiferous epithelial cycle. This cycle ranges from 8 to 16 days depending on species. It is 13 days for the rat and 16 days for man. The relative duration of each stage of the cycle can be estimated histologically or with tritiated thymidine pulse labelling. However, for each species the seminiferous epithelial cycle is a biological constant and unaffected by sexual activity (Amann, 1981).

In contrast to laboratory animals, only a few adjacent cohorts of germ cells develop synchronously in man, and the cellular patterns are much less distinct. Degeneration of potential germ cells likely contributes to this phenomenon.

Shortly after completing DNA synthesis, the developing germ cells leave the basal compartment of the seminiferous tubule and enter the adluminal compartment. There the developing germ cells experience a unique chemical environment which is apparently essential for the completion of meiosis. Theoretically, four spermatids are produced from each preleptotene spermatocyte. Spermatids, in contrast to their round cell precursors, have a highly condensed nucleus, scant cytoplasm, and a flagellum. Based on changes in the spermatid acrosome, spermatogenesis can be considred as a continuum consisting of four different phases of maturation in the testis. The final products of spermatogenesis, the spermatozoa, are released into the lumen of the seminiferous tubule. Prior to release, the germ cells are called spermatids, and after spermiation, they are called spermatozoa or sperm.

The duration of spermatogenesis is the interval between the time when a stem spermatogonium becomes committed to produce a cohort of spermatids and the time of release of the resulting sperm from the seminiferous epithelium. The duration of spermatogenesis is equal to about 4.5 cycles of the seminiferous epithelium. Stem spermatogonia periodically produce differentiating spermatogonia. This periodicity defines the duration of the seminiferous epithelial cycle. Thus, each cycle of mature spermatids released from the seminiferous epithelium originates from spermatogonia committed to differentiation approximately 4.5 cycles earlier. Because cohorts of developing germ cells in different regions within the tubules complete spermatogenesis at different times, spermatozoa are continuously released from the seminiferous epithelium.

Various drugs and environmental chemicals can produce specific lesions that result in degeneration of all germ cells at the point of attack and eventually eliminate those more advanced forms which would have differentiated from the affected cells.

Sertoli cells The Sertoli cells control the immediate environment around the spermatocytes and spermatids and are essential to normal spermatogenesis. Many chemicals affecting spermatogenesis probably act via an effect on the Sertoli cells rather than directly on the germ cells. The Sertoli cells deserve more attention as a target for testicular toxicity.

The Sertoli cells appear to be the host cells for the developing germ cells. Sertoli cells and spermatogonia line the basal lamina of the seminiferous tubule with other germinal cells either situated between adjacent pairs of Sertoli cells or embedded in the luminal margin of the Sertoli cell cytoplasm. Specialized junctions form where adjacent Sertoli cells meet. These junctions supposedly constitute an essential component of the blood–testis barrier, dividing the extracellular space inside the tubule into a basal compartment and an adluminal compartment. The basal compartment is situated between the Sertoli cells and spermatogonia; the adluminal compartment is located between the Sertoli cells and the spermatocytes and spermatids.

Spermatogonial cell mitosis takes place in the basal compartment, and the spermatogonia, preleptotene and leptotene spermatocytes are observed there. At the end of the leptotene phase of meiosis, the primary spermatocytes pass between the Sertoli cells and enter the adluminal compartment. Here the zygotene primary spermatocytes continue to develop through the pachytene and diplotene phases of meiosis and then divide to form secondary spermatocytes followed by a second division yielding round spermatids, thus completing meiosis.

The Sertoli cells secrete a fluid and synthesize proteins, inhibin, and other products. Recent studies also suggest that the Sertoli cells may play a role in the genetic induction of testicular differentiation. Although the occurrence and role of androgen-binding protein (ABP) has been rather extensively studied in laboratory animals, the role of ABP in humans is unclear.

3.1.3 Efferent Ducts and Testicular Plasma

The fluid produced in seminiferous tubules moves into a system of spaces called rete testis which are confluent with the efferent ducts, the latter opening into the caput epididymidis; at the point of entry into the epididymis, the testicular fluid is designated as testicular plasma. Rete testis fluid is characterized by unique proteins and a total protein concentration much lower than that of the plasma. Glutamic acid, alanine, glycine, lysine, aspartic acid and serine occur in higher concentrations in rete testis fluid than in the blood plasma of rats, bulls and rams. Androgen-binding protein (ABP) appears to play a role in the transport of androgens to the epididymis, and inhibin apparently contributes to the regulation of spermatogenesis by suppressing FSH production following absorption from the epididymis. Testosterone, dehydroepiandrosterone, dihydrotestosterone and oestrogens are also found in the rete testis fluid of most laboratory species. Protein synthesis within the seminiferous tubules, active transport mechanisms, and the presence of the blood–testis barrier play obvious roles in maintaining these gradients.

Although the rete testis fluid normally contains inhibin, ABP, transferrin, γ-glutamyl transferase, myoinositol, steroids, amino acids and various enzymes, only ABP and inhibin appear to be specific products and useful functional indicators for the seminiferous epithelium or Sertoli cells. However, the relative concentrations of other constituents may indicate alterations in membrane barriers or active transport processes. The concentration of chemicals in the rete testis fluid relative to unbound plasma concentration may be used to estimate the permeability of the blood–testis barrier for selected chemicals (Okumura *et al.*, 1975).

3.1.4 Epididymis

From the rete testis, testicular semen enters efferent ducts and then the epididymis. Here the sperm are subjected to a changing chemical environment as they move through segments of the organ. Conventionally divided macro-scopically into head (caput), body (corpus), and tail (cauda), these three gross regions in part reflect the histological variations of the organ.

The first two sections (proximal part) are generally regarded together as making up that part of the epididymis involved with sperm maturation, while the terminal (distal) segment is regarded as the site of sperm storage. There are, however, differences in the position and extent of the segments in various species of mammals. The epididymides of rats have a distinctive microscopic structure while those of rams, bulls, dogs and hamsters bear a close resemblance to each other.

In most species between 1.8 and 5.4 days are required for sperm to move through the caput and corpus epididymidis where maturation takes place. In contrast, the transit time for sperm through the cauda epididymidis in sexually rested males differs greatly among species and ranges from 3.6 to 13.6 days with an average transit time of about 6 days for a 21–30-year-old man. The number of sperm in the caput and corpus epididymides is similar in sexually rested males and in males ejaculating daily, while the number of sperm in the cauda epididymidis is lower and transit time increases in males ejaculating regularly. As a result, animals with a large reserve of sperm in the cauda epididymidis can successfully impregnate more females in a short interval.

Important functions of the epididymis are resorption and metabolism of rete testis fluid components, epithelial secretion, sperm maturation and storage of sperm. Thus, it is likely that the composition of the epididymal plasma plays an important role in both sperm maturation and sperm storage and that environmental chemicals may produce adverse effects. Yet, few examples of chemical effects on epididymal function are known.

Active transport processes are suggested by the fact that the amount of fluid flowing through the epididymis is only a small fraction of the volume produced from a cannula inserted into the rete testis. Much of the fluid produced by the testis is apparently absorbed in the initial segment of the epididymis. Fluid absorption increases the relative concentration of sperm. The effects on fertility of altering this active process have not been well studied.

The epididymides produce glycerylphosphorylcholine (GPC), the synthesis of which is androgen dependent. GPC concentration increases progressively in epididymal plasma as it passes from the proximal to distal portion of the epididymis, and the vas deferens of the ram and bull. In contrast, the concentrations of sodium and chloride decrease. GPC might perhaps be partly responsible for the long survival periods of sperm in the epididymis and for the process of sperm maturation.

The epididymides of most laboratory and domestic species also contain large concentrations of carnitine. In the rat epididymis, an androgen-dependent active transport process appears to concentrate carnitine from the blood. Carnitine concentrations contribute to the total osmotic pressure of the fluid and redress the loss of ions in the proximal region of the duct. Epididymal sperm also contain high levels of carnitine along with the enzyme carnitine acetyltransferase. The role of carnitine as a cofactor in fatty acid oxidation is well established.

Another androgen-dependent constituent of the epididymides is sialic acid, an amino sugar, which occurs in particularly high concentrations in the plasma of cauda epididymidis of the rat. It is possible that sialic acid forms part of the glycoprotein in epididymal fluid which acts as a lubricant for the densely packed sperm in the cauda.

Motility is acquired by the sperm gradually during epididymal passage. From the epididymides, sperm move into the vas deferens where glandular secretions are added to the seminal fluid.

Extraneous chemicals such as chlorhydrin may affect the properties of the two major components of epididymal semen, sperm and epididymal plasma.

3.1.5 Accessory Organs

The seminal plasma functions as a vehicle for conveying the ejaculated sperm from the male to the female reproductive tract. The seminal plasma is produced by the secretory organs of the male reproductive system which, apart from epididymides, include the prostate, seminal vesicles and bulbourethral (Cowper's) glands, and urethral (Littré's) glands. An abnormal function of these organs can be reflected in altered seminal characteristics. Seminal plasma is normally an isotonic, neutral medium which in many species contains sources of energy such as fructose and sorbitol that are directly available to sperm. The function of the other constituents such as citric acid and inositol is not known. In general, the secretions emanating from the prostate and seminal vesicles apparently contribute little to fertility even though the pregnancy rate for vesiculectomized males of certain species (e.g. boar) is greatly reduced.

Because all the accessory organs are androgen dependent, they serve as indicators of the Leydig cell function. The weights of the accessory sex glands are an indirect measure of circulating testosterone levels. The ventral prostate of rats has been used as a model to study the actions of testosterone and to investigate the molecular basis of androgen-regulated gene function. The prostate is a common focus of human diseases. Benign prostatic hypertrophy is rather common among older men and the occurrence of prostatic malignancies is not rare. However, although progress is being made, the chemical composition of the semen offers little to differentiate between the benign condition and the onset of malignancy.

It appears that human semen emission initially involves the urethral and Cowper's glands, with the prostatic secretion and sperm following next and the seminal vesicle secretion delivered last. There is a considerable overlap between the pre-sperm, sperm-rich and post-sperm fractions. Thus, even if the ejaculate is collected in as many as six fractions, the split ejaculate method (section 3.2.4.2) seldom makes it possible to obtain a sperm-free fraction consisting exclusively of prostatic or vesicular secretion. Using acid phosphatase and citric acid as markers for prostatic secretion and fructose for the vesicular secretion, it is estimated that 15–30% of the entire human ejaculate is contributed by the prostate and 50–80% by the seminal vesicles. Semen varies both in volume and composition between species. Human, bovine and canine species have a relatively small semen volume (1–10 ml); semen of stallions and boars is ejaculated in much larger quantities.

Glycerylphosphorylcholine (GPC) occurs in the seminal plasma of all animals thus far investigated. Although sperm do not utilize GPC, an enzyme in the secretions of the female genital tract breaks GPC down into phosphoglycerol which is metabolized via the glycolytic pathway. Thus, GPC may be an energy source for sperm in the female tract.

The vas deferens (ductus deferens) transports sperm from the distal portion of the epididymis to the urethra. In some species, including man, the final segment of the vas deferens becomes thicker because of the presence of glands in the wall that form the ampulla. Both the vas deferens and the seminal vesicles apparently secrete prostaglandins in mice, rats and rams.

The semen of some animals, including rodents and man, tends to coagulate on ejaculation. The clotting mechanism involves enzymes and substrates from different accessory organs. In rodents, semen coagulation and copulatory plug formation are brought about by an enzyme–substrate interaction between secretions produced in the coagulating glands and the seminal vesicles. Thus, clotting presumably accomplishes a sealing mechanism in these animals.

3.1.5.1 *Prostate*

Although all male mammals have a prostate, the organ differs anatomically, physiologically and chemically between species, and differences between lobes in the same species may be pronounced. The dorsolateral prostate in the rat differs from the ventral lobes because it produces fructose in addition to citric acid. Also, zinc is concentrated preferentially in the lateral lobes of the dorsolateral prostate and appears to be under hormone control. The rat prostate is notable for its complex structure and its prompt response to castration and androgen stimulation. The human prostate is a tubuloalveolar gland made up of two prominent lateral lobes which contribute about 30% of the ejaculate fluid. Dogs ejaculate semen which is largely composed of prostatic secretion because they have no seminal vesicles.

Prostate secretion in man and many laboratory species contain acid phosphatase, zinc and citric acid. The prostatic secretion is the main source of acid phosphatase in human semen; its concentration provides a convenient method for the assessment of the functional state of the prostate. The human prostate also produces spermine. Certain proteins and enzymes (acid phosphatase, γ-glutamyl transpeptidase, and glutamic-oxaloacetic transaminase), cholesterol, inositol, zinc and magnesium have also been proposed as indicators of human prostatic secretory function.

Using electrophoretic patterns, normal human prostatic fluid obtained by rectal massage has been found to contain about 2% protein. There are at least, four major protein components. In the ventral prostate of the rat, nearly 50% of the total cytosolic protein has non-specific androgen-binding properties and has been used as an indicator of androgen activity.

Testosterone and dihydrotestosterone elicit two types of cellular responses in the accessory tissues, namely cellular proliferation and secretory activity. The accumulation of zinc within the prostatic epithelial cells and the synthesis of zinc-binding protein are regulated by dihydrotestosterone which, in turn, is controlled apparently by zinc levels.

3.1.5.2 *Seminal Vesicle*

As with the prostate, the structure of the seminal vesicle is diverse across animal species. The seminal vesicle is more fittingly described as a seminal or vesicular gland, since it consists of compact glandular tissue arranged in the form of multiple lobes which surround secretory ducts. The seminal vesicles are absent in the dog and cat. The seminal vesicle has been used to study epithelial and stromal interactions.

The seminal vesicle is a useful indicator of Leydig cell function. The vesicular glands can be weighed as an indirect measure of circulating testosterone levels. However, in addition to the major role played by testosterone in the control of seminal vesicle secretion, other factors such as age, blood supply, ejaculation frequency and storage capacity must also be considered.

In man, the seminal vesicle contributes about 60% of the seminal fluid. The seminal vesicles also produce more than half the seminal plasma in laboratory and domestic animals such as the rat, guinea pig and bull. The seminal vesicle secretion is usually more alkaline, has a higher dry weight, and contains more potassium, bicarbonate, acid-soluble phosphate and protein than does prostatic fluid. Another feature of the seminal vesicle secretion is that it has a high content of reducing substances, including sugars and ascorbic acid.

In man, bull, ram and boar (but not rat), the bulk of seminal fructose is secreted by the seminal vesicles and consequently, in these species, the chemical assay of fructose in semen is a useful indicator of the relative contribution of the seminal vesicles to whole semen. Seminal vesicle secretion is also characterized by the presence of proteins and enzymes, phosphorylcholine and prostaglandins. Because vasectomy does not interfere with secretion from the ampullae, seminal vesicles or the ejaculatory ducts, fructose is found in the seminal plasma of vasectomized men. However, their ejaculate, in addition to being sperm-free, also contains less than normal amounts of carnitine and glycerylphosophoryl-choline which comes mainly from the epididymis.

3.1.6 Sexual Behaviour and Libido

One of the first questions to answer in any reproduction study is whether the animals actually mate. In rats, this can be determined by inspecting females each day for vaginal plugs. The number of mountings, thrusts and ejaculations can each be quantified as indicators of reproductive behaviour. It is also important to determine whether the male animal mounts females or other males. If the male copulates and is still sterile, then one should look at the indicators of male fertility. If he does not copulate, then the emphasis of further investigations must be on neuromuscular and/or behavioural deficits.

In humans, loss of libido may occur as a result of either psychological or somatic factors. The loss may be complete in individuals with serious organic diseases or in advanced age. On the other hand, diminished libido may occur sometimes in relation to a particular person, which suggests the involvement of psychological factors. In instances such as these, it is not unusual for a patient to experience nocturnal penile erection and emission of semen.

Excessive libido may occur in conjunction with serious neurological diseases such as encephalitis or brain tumour, as well as with psychological and emotional disturbances. Because appropriate clinical tests generally do not exist and reliable animal models are not available, few studies have attempted to determine the potential role of environmental and occupational factors on sexual behaviour.

3.1.7 Erection and Ejaculation

Since few laboratory and clinical studies have been available, relatively little is known concerning the effects of chemicals on erection or ejaculation (Woods, 1979). Impotence, the failure to obtain or sustain an erection, is rarely of endocrine origin. Attaining an erection depends upon rather complex neurological and circulatory pathways. The occurrence of nocturnal or early-morning erections implies that the neurological and circulatory pathways involved in attaining an erection are intact and indicates that more emphasis should be placed on finding a psychological cause. Impairment of the parasympathetic nerve activity prevents the development of tumescence of the penile corpora cavernosa. The ejaculatory process involves the sympathetic nervous system. Many drugs affect the autonomic nervous system.

In mammals, ejaculation is usually initiated by strong contractions, probably emanating in the efferent ducts of the testis, and quickly spreading along the entire length of the tract. First the prostate, next the ampullae and finally the seminal vesicles contract in an orderly fashion, thus determining the chemical sequence of the various seminal fractions represented in a split-ejaculate. Chemical analysis of the different seminal fractions enables one to decide whether the ejaculatory pattern is normal, slightly altered or seriously disturbed. In an extreme case of ejaculatory sterility, semen is ejaculated into the bladder, and this state of retrograde ejaculation is diagnosed by analysis of urine.

3.1.8 Paternally Related Birth Defects

Reproductive problems and increased incidences of birth defects in their children have been reported by Vietnam veterans exposed to the defoliant 'Agent

Orange'. As a result, increasing attention is being focused upon paternal chemical exposure and perinatal outcome. This rather controversial area has been reviewed recently by Soyka and Joffe (1980) and Strobino and co-workers (1978). Although there have been few systematic studies of the effects of paternal drug exposure on offspring in humans, an association with birth defects has been reported for lead, narcotics, caffeine, ethanol, anticonvulsants, anaesthetic gases and smoking. In mice, progeny number and their survival rates were lower in litters sired by ethanol-treated males than by control males. The role of male factors with regard to birth defects must be carefully studied using standard techniques for evaluation of morphological as well as postnatal functional changes. Retrospective analyses of data on men occupationally exposed must be done carefully to identify and control such confounding variables as the potential toxicity to mother's reproductive function and offspring of a chemical brought home on the husband's garments.

3.2 GENERAL EVALUATION OF FUNCTION AND MORPHOLOGY

3.2.1 Endocrinological Evaluation

The endocrine function of the testis is reflected in serum levels of gonadotropins and androgens. The methods used to determine serum hormone levels are sufficiently sensitive to detect changes of 20% in mean concentrations of FSH and LH. The values for testosterone are more variable, even in the normal male. Hormone levels may be measured in single blood samples, but because of diurnal rhythms, the time of day should be standardized. FSH, LH, and testosterone can be analysed with radioimmunoassay (RIA) techniques and compared with normal ranges from the same laboratory. Any significant difference between hormone levels of control and exposed animals can be accepted as strong evidence for an adverse effect on reproduction. If such an effect is detected in animal studies, a similar effect may be expected in man.

With chemicals acting directly on the testis, LH and, particularly, FSH levels in serum would increase. With a mild toxic action on the testis, blood FSH levels after LHRH administration might exceed normal responses, even when basal FSH levels are normal. If the toxic action is directed primarily at the pituitary gland or central nervous system, LH and FSH levels would tend to decrease. FSH measurements are useful adjuncts to sperm counts and may indicate a direct action of toxic agents on pituitary function. However, despite its wide variability in man, sperm concentration appears to be a more sensitive measure of testicular damage than are elevated FSH levels.

Levels of FSH in blood serum provide a simple index of spermatogenic activity, because destruction of the seminiferous epithelium or dysfunction of Sertoli cells is commonly associated with elevated FSH levels. An elevated FSH level is almost invariably associated with severe oligozoospermia or azoospermia.

LH and testosterone levels provide an index of Leydig cell function, and testicular damage associated with Leydig cell dysfunction is reflected in low serum testosterone and elevated serum LH levels. The combination of normal testosterone and elevated LH levels may indicate a Leydig cell dysfunction compensated for by an increased production of LH. A more accurate and sensitive assessment of the secretory capacity of Leydig cells can be obtained by measuring serum testosterone following hCG administration *in vivo* (see Kerr and de Kretser, 1983, this volume). As the structure of hCG closely resembles that of LH, hCG has been used in many studies instead of LH because it is more readily available. The ability of Leydig cells to secrete testosterone is judged by the incremental increase in testosterone production in hCG-stimulated animals as compared with control animals. Since testicular damage *in vivo* may be associated with altered blood flow to the testis, *in vitro* hCG stimulation of testicular suspensions is also necessary for the assessment of the steroidogenic properties of Leydig cells (see Kerr and de Kretser, 1983, this volume).

Because androgen production is controlled by the action of LH on the Leydig cells, a decreased number of LH receptors associated with Leydig cells is another important measure of testicular damage. This can be assessed by measuring the binding of ^{125}I-hCG to testicular tissue *in vitro* (Kerr and de Kretser, 1983, this volume).

3.2.2 Histological Examination

Histological analyses are performed either on whole testes (animal models) or on biopsy specimens (e.g. man). Light and electron microscopy of damaged testes have demonstrated that structural alterations in Sertoli cells occur often in association with disturbances in the spermatogenic process. Quantitative assessment of the numbers of germ cells provides an objective measure of the effects of chemical agents upon spermatogenesis. Testicular tissue must be fixed immediately in Bouin's fluid (10% formalin is not satisfactory). Slides should be stained with haematoxylin and eosin for simple analyses and with PAS-haematoxylin if more precise staging of spermatids is required. Histological evaluation and enumeration of the number of leptotene spermatocytes per Sertoli cell assist diagnosis.

In laboratory studies, the number of spermatids can be easily quantified with simple equipment and without extensive training of technicians. Homogenization-resistant spermatid nuclei are counted in testicular homogenates and provide a simple, accurate and sensitive method for measuring sperm production. The nuclei of elongated spermatids are resistant to mechanical and chemical disruption and are easily identified after physical disruption of testicular tissue. Resistant nuclei are counted in a cytometer. The interval from the time when spermatids acquire this resistance until spermiation is constant for different species or strains. Thus, the number of resistant spermatids is a direct measure of the production of spermatozoa by the testis and spermatid differentiation. A representative sample taken at necropsy, the entire testes (for rats and rabbits), or biopsy material (20 mg or more) can be homogenized or disrupted ultrasonically. Counts are then made and expressed on both a per testis basis and a per milligram tissue basis. Values from treated animals should be compared with concurrent control counts.

When examining the seminiferous tubules, the following characteristics can be noted: occurrence of lymphoid cell or macrophage infiltration; presence of germ cells of each stage in seminiferous tubules (spermatogonia, spermatocytes, spermatids, sperm); and presence of large numbers of degenerating, multinucleate, or otherwise abnormal germ cells. When evaluating testicular histology, sections representing at least two loci should be examined. The diameter of tubules are measured, and the percentage of seminiferous tubule cross-sections having mature spermatids lining the tubule lumen and the percentage of tubules devoid of germ cells other than spermatogonia are quantified and compared with normal testes. Measurements of diameters should be taken on essentially round tubule cross-sections cut perpendicularly to their long axis.

The end products of spermatogenesis are the 'mature' spermatids about to become detached from the Sertoli cells. Tubules with spermatids aligned at the lumen can be easily recognized and are species specific. The number of preleptotene and early leptotene spermatocytes (stage VIII) per Sertoli cell can be quantified because of a characteristic nuclear morphology. An abnormal number of spermatocytes per Sertoli cell is a sensitive measure of testicular damage.

Depending on the biological and biochemical processes which support them, the various spermatogenic cells are differentially susceptible to chemicals which exert specific effects. Certain spermatogenic cell types uniquely synthesize DNA, some cells divide while others do not, both mitotic and meiotic processes are involved, and certain cells differentiate without further cell division.

Thus, chemicals with selective mechanisms of action can produce degeneration of the seminiferous epithelium and azoospermia without affecting stem spermatogonia. If stem cells remain, eventual recovery of the seminiferous epithelium may occur. Recovery of the seminiferous epithelium and fertility generally requires from 6 to 12 cycles (155 days for rats and 128 days for rabbits).

A number of recent advances with respect to tissue preservation and tissue preparation have contributed significantly to the histopathological evaluation of the testis (Kerr and de Kretser, 1981). In the past, formalin fixation and paraffin embedding were the most widely used methods. However, because no fixative will adequately penetrate more than a few millimetres of solid tissue in a 24-hour period, optimal preservation can be achieved only by delivering the fixative directly into the vascular system. The perfusion method, originally proposed by Christensen (1965) and further modified by Vitale *et al.* (1973), is the most promising new technique. A cannula may be introduced into the lower thoracic aorta and the testis perfused through the testicular artery, or a very fine needle can be inserted directly into the testicular artery. Glutaraldehyde is an excellent fixative for these procedures (Russell and Burguet, 1977).

An improvement in tissue preparation will allow higher resolution with light microscopy. This has been achieved by embedding perfusion-preserved tissue samples in plastic. Generally, the plastic-embedded samples become hardened upon polymerization and allow the cutting of very thin sections similar to those used for electron microscopy. 'Semi-thin' sections of $0.5-1 \mu m$ can be stained with toluidine blue and then evaluated using light microscopy with high resolution even at $1000 \times$ magnification.

3.2.3 Sertoli Cell Function

Analysis of Sertoli cell function previously relied upon morphological analyses using light and electron microscopic techniques. Recent advances in the understanding of Sertoli cell function have allowed the development of simple tests to measure Sertoli cell secretory properties. Calculations of the total amount of androgen-binding protein (ABP) per testis have demonstrated diminished secretory capacity of Sertoli cells in all conditions of spermatogenic damage (Kerr and de Kretser, 1983, this volume). Decreases in ABP produced by damaged testes have been found to be proportional to the severity of spermatogenic disruption (Rich and de Kretser, 1977).

An estimate of fluid production by Sertoli cells can be obtained by ligating the efferent ducts and then comparing the weight of the ligated testis with that of the non-ligated testis. As with the association between ABP secretion and spermatogenic disruption, the total volume of fluid secreted by damaged testis is diminished in proportion to the severity of spermatogenic damage (Kerr and de Kretser, 1983, this volume).

A disturbance of Sertoli cell function can also be expected to alter the production of inhibin. This alteration, in turn, will be reflected in elevations of FSH secretion from the pituitary which can be measured easily using radioimmunoassay of serum FSH (section 3.2.1). A quantitative bioassay of inhibin using cultures of anterior pituitary cells can provide a more direct and precise measurement of inhibin production.

3.2.4 Testicular Semen Analysis

Examination of testicular semen in animals provides an additional means of assessing changes in testicular function. Testicular semen represents a dilute suspension of testicular sperm in testicular plasma. In laboratory animals it is obtained by collecting sperm following incision of the testicular parenchyma. In the bull and ram, testicular semen can be obtained from the rete testis or efferent ducts by cannulation, thus allowing direct sampling for acute studies, or continuing samples during chronic tests. Quantitative analysis of testicular semen performed over a period of time permits one to assess sperm production and relate it to the sperm output in ejaculated semen. This method is obviously not applicable to man. To assess testicular function either in the laboratory or clinic, a longitudinal study is preferred. With the cycle length of the seminiferous epithelium as the divisor, daily sperm production per testis can be estimated.

3.2.5 Epididymal Function

Epididymal function has been most commonly studied using rodents and rabbits. Weight and gross appearance are easily monitored. The distal portion (half corpus plus cauda of the epididymis provides a ready source of mature sperm for evaluation. Sperm can be expressed from the severed end of the epididymis. In some animals, the epididymis can be cannulated which makes it possible to obtain epididymal semen samples not only from the whole organ but from its different segments as well.

Both the number of epididymal sperm and their motility and morphology are useful indicators of a possible toxic influence. The percentage of progressively motile sperm in standardized concentrations can be determined using a phase-contrast microscope, and the incidence of abnormal sperm recorded. Some investigators prepare differentially stained epididymal sperm for detailed morphological evaluation. Sperm in the distal half of the epididymis can be quantified by counting sperm heads following tissue homogenization. The rate at which sperm acquire motility and fertilizing ability in the epididymis can be monitored, as well as the levels of chemical constituents such as glycerylphos-phorylcholine and carnitine in epididymal plasma.

For human subjects an assessment of epididymal function may be obtained from measurements of carnitine in the ejaculate and the incidence of cytoplasmic droplet retention on spermatozoa, the latter indicating a disturbance of sperm maturation during epididymal transit.

3.2.6 Function of Accessory Organs

The rabbit is a particularly useful animal for assessing the effects of chemicals on the function of accessory organs since ejaculates can be collected at frequent time intervals using an artificial vagina. In other laboratory animals, such as mouse, rat, hamster and guinea pig, the direct dissection and examination of male accessory glands and analysis of their secretions provide the best way of assessing effects of chemicals. Because male accessory organs are strictly androgen-dependent, a reduction in either androgen concentration or tissue responsiveness to androgenic stimuli can be detected by analysing the tissues and their secretory products.

In man, the seminal vesicle secretion is characterized by fructose, pro-staglandins and certain enzymes; prostatic fluid is characterized by the presence of citric acid, acid phosphatase, zinc, magnesium and some other enzymes and proteins. The determination of these chemical constituents in the seminal plasma makes it possible to detect and follow up adverse effects produced by extraneous chemicals on the secretory output of the seminal vesicle and the prostate, respectively. There is no evidence that blood analysis could provide useful information.

In farm animals, the methods of assessing adverse effects on secretory function of male acessory organs are similar to those used in man. An additional advantage with some of them such as the boar and stallion, is that split ejaculates can be obtained more easily, and semen is available in larger quantities than with common laboratory species.

3.2.7 Semen Analysis

When evaluating reproductive function in man, semen analysis should be the initial test. Semen is a complex mixture of products of the testes, epididymides, vasa deferentia and ampullae, prostate gland, vesicular glands, bulbourethral glands and urethral glands.

The function of the testis can be examined by analysing semen with respect to sperm number, motility and morphology. As pointed out in section 3.2.1, blood is analysed with respect to FSH, LH and testosterone. Alterations imply disturbed function. In the clinic, such findings usually indicate that the patient should undergo further clinical examinations, and that the potential usefulness of a testicular biopsy should be considered (Belsey *et al.*, 1980; Eliasson, 1981).

In man, farm animals, and certain others mammals including some laboratory animals (rabbit in particular), examination of sperm and seminal plasma in the ejaculate provides the simplest, safest and most reliable method of detecting and quantifying adverse effects of an extraneous chemical agent on the final product of testicular and accessory organ function. A special advantage of semen analysis is that it can be obtained repeatedly in the same individual. Frequency of ejaculation must be considered, and the semen handled carefully prior to examination. In some instances, a split ejaculate, which aids in identifying the route of entry of extraneous chemicals and in assessing affected organs, can be collected and analysed. To define the entry route and target organ more precisely, separate examination of the testis and individual accessory organs is usually necessary.

The technical aspects of semen analysis are detailed later in this section. However, it is necessary to emphasize the importance of standardizing the period of abstinence, the method of collection and the types of analyses. Of further importance is the availability of a well-trained technician capable of providing an accurate analysis of sperm motility and morphology. The human donors should be informed that the semen analyses are requested to study the possible effects of environmental factors on the reproductive organs and that the main emphasis will be on organ function and not on fertility or reproductive potency. In most instances, such an objective approach facilitates participation.

The predictive value of a single semen analysis with respect to male reproductive function is very low. Repeated semen analyses over a period of months are generally required. If possible, it is best to obtain semen samples before exposure to the chemical agent and then continue to obtain them for a period of time after the exposure ceases. Such a design allows the relationship between chemical exposure and testicular function to be more accurately predicted. Ideally, at least two semen samples should be analysed within a 2-week period before exposure and at least three semen samples should be analysed at monthly intervals following the exposure.

The standard analyses include semen volume, viscosity and liquefaction, and number, motility and morphology of the sperm. Human semen is usually collected by masturbation or in a condom following sexual intercourse. With few exceptions, the biochemical composition of semen does not reflect testicular function but rather the functionality and relative contributions of the epididymides and accessory sex glands. The composition of seminal plasma is also influenced by the interval since previous ejaculation and by the extent of sexual excitement prior to ejaculation.

Animal species from which semen can be collected artifically are most useful for toxicity studies. An artificial vagina can be used with the rabbit, cat, bull, ram, boar and stallion. Electroejaculation is used with the monkey, cat, dog, rat, mouse and guinea pig. It is also sometimes used for bulls and rams.

Studies with rabbits and bulls reveal a large coefficient of variation for total sperm number per ejaculate and point out the inadequacy of small experimental groups. The coefficient of variation for total sperm number per ejaculate for bulls is about 35%. Thus, to detect a 10% difference in total sperm per ejaculate, 50 ejaculates from each of 50 bulls per treatment would be necessary. Since the coefficient of variation for total sperm per ejaculate for man is even greater than for the rabbit or bull, even more ejaculates and individuals would be required.

Semen collections in rabbits may be examined as follows:

(1) determination of spermatozoa number by haematocytometer counts and volume measurements;
(2) observation of sperm morphology after staining with aniline blue–crystal violet;
(3) estimation of sperm motility using freshly collected semen diluted with physiological saline; and
(4) testing the fertility of the collected semen by deposition into the vagina of females simultaneously injected with an ovulating dose of luteinizing hormone.

3.2.7.1 *Sperm Concentration, Morphology and Motility*

The term sperm concentration is preferable to those of sperm count or sperm density. Sperm concentration should be determined accurately so that the total number of sperm per ejaculate can be calculated. Sperm concentration should be determined using a calibrated spectrophotometer or electronic cell counter (if contaminating cells or debris are not a problem) because of their accuracy and precision. If extraneous material is present in the semen, time-consuming visual counts using a cytometer with a phase-contrast microscope are necessary. More than six replicate counts are needed to exceed 90% precision for a single sample.

Although sperm morphology has long been regarded as an important indicator of fertility, there is no commonly accepted method of assessment. A minimum requirement should be that the sperm are assessed with attention to the head (plasmalemma, acrosome and nucleus), midpiece (mitochondria), protoplasmic droplets, and tail. Eliasson (1981) suggests that coiled tails are an important indicator of altered function; exposure to organic solvents (glues, paints, and cleaning fluids) correlates with a high incidence of coiled tails. Esposure to lead can cause a significant increase in the percentage of sperm with morphological defects including binucleated, amorphous and tapered forms. Lead-exposed men also have a higher frequency of semen samples with low sperm concentration and poor sperm motility. A variety of other chemicals and stressors have been associated with morphological changes.

Evaluation of sperm morphology is subjective with large variations between laboratories and technicians. The problem is especially difficult with human sperm because of the great variability and high percentage of abnormal sperm usually found in the ejaculate.

Because the morphological characteristics of germ cells are an essential part of a complete semen assessment, slides must be prepared from fresh semen specimens to be useful. Several staining methods are available. Any nuclear stain such as fast green, Wright's, Giemsa or eosin Y-nigrosin is adequate for the evaluation of gross sperm abnormalities (Belsey *et al.*, 1980). Semen from infertile men is characterized by an unusually great diversity of abnormal sperm sizes and shapes. If objective, morphometric data describing sperm size and shape (e.g. head length, width, area, circumference; tail; midpiece width) were obtained from individuals at risk, they could be compared statistically with data from a matched control group and, thus, perhaps aid in human health risk analysis.

Sperm morphometry can be performed using living sperm cells or stained seminal smears. Methods are becoming increasingly automated. Flow cytometry has been used (Gledhill *et al.*, 1979), and a video monitor integrated to a minicomputer allows shape tracings to be automatically converted to morphometric indices of sperm and then stored in the computer memory. Flow cytometry of heated sperm nuclei reveals a significant decrease in resistance to *in situ* denaturation of sperm DNA in samples from animals and men with low fertility and may provide a new and independent determinant of male fertility (Evenson *et al.*, 1980).

Sperm motility should be evaluated with respect to at least three characteristics: progressive motility, percentage of motile sperm, and time after ejaculation. Both quantitative and qualitative aspects must be taken into consideration. Percentage of motile sperm is a widely used measure of sperm quality. Proportion of motile sperm is estimated to the nearest 10%, and velocity is estimated using an arbitrary scale. Sperm motility is usually determined visually, although quantitative methods are also available. The percentage of sperm that are progressively motile, circularly motile, or backwardly motile is conventionally estimated as a subjective observation of sperm in a diluted sample of semen viewed with a phase-contrast microscope. Motility can also be evaluated objectively by measurements made on time exposure negatives (Janick and MacLeod, 1970) or on a videotape recording (Katz and Overstreet, 1981). Sperm motility and morphology measurements are much more constant within species and individuals than is sperm concentration. A decline in motility can be caused by bacterial toxins or by deficiencies in the seminal fluid.

Along with sperm concentration, motility and morphology, particulate debris, agglutination and sperm viability are also important. LDH-X is a sperm-specific isoenzyme of lactic dehydrogenase and can be monitored using RIA techniques or electrophoretically after release from sperm as an indicator of genotypic changes or enzyme inhibition (Belsey *et al.*, 1980).

3.2.7.2 *Split Ejaculate*

When semen is collected by the split-ejaculate method, it is frequently possible to identify fractions of the ejaculate originating in distinct parts of the male reproductive tract such as the epididymis, seminal vesicle, prostate, Cowper's gland and urethral gland. In man, the activity of acid phosphatase, the concentration of citric acid and zinc levels provide sensitive markers of the prostatic secretory activity. Fructose and prostaglandins, among other substances, serve as markers for seminal vesicle secretions. Carnitine is sometimes used to determine the contribution of the epididymal secretion to semen (Mann and Lutwak-Mann, 1981).

3.2.7.3 *Sperm Viability*

Sperm viability, the number of live spermatozoa, can be determined by using one of several supravital staining procedures; one of these is 0.5% eosin in distilled water. Sperm are assessed using phase-contrast microscopy. Another method involves staining the sperm first with 1% eosin in distilled water and then counterstaining with 10% nigrosin in distilled water. These sperm can be observed using a brightfield light microscopy (Belsey *et al.*, 1980).

3.2.7.4 *Acrosome Reaction*

In the presence of calcium ions, the plasma and outer acrosome memberanes of capacitated sperm fuse in the process known as the acrosome reaction. The acrosome reaction is a prerequisite for fertilization in mammalian species and must occur just prior to the penetration of the zona pellucida by the sperm. Although the acrosome is easily seen by phase-contrast microscopy in many laboratory species, it is too small to be visualized by this method of microscopy in human sperm. A method for rapidly quantifying the acrosome reaction in human sperm has been published recently (Talbot and Chacon, 1981). Both capacitation and the acrosome reaction are required for fertilization. In the acrosome reaction, the membrane fusion produces vesicles, and the acrosome contents are released while the limiting membrane about the sperm head remains intact. The acrosome contains a mucolytic enzyme, hyaluronidase, and proteolytic and other enzymes. Some of the enzymes released from the acrosome help individual sperm to pass through the matrix of the cumulus oophorus and penetrate the zona pellucida (Belsey *et al.*, 1980).

3.2.7.5 *In Vitro Tests*

Increased attention is being directed to the development of *in vitro* test procedures. Chemicals can be screened economically by incubating sperm *in vitro* under standard conditions in a protein-containing buffer at 37 °C for 4–8 hours. Sperm can be exposed to the agent briefly (10–30 minutes) or throughout the incubation period. A dose–response curve can be established using subjective methods of evaluation. The decline in percentage of motile sperm over time is an often used criterion, but integrity of the acrosome and plasma membrane, oxygen consumption, ATP content, or degree of agglutination might also be used. Compounds that are spermicidal *in vitro* at concentrations that could be anticipated or shown to be present in blood or seminal fluid should be carefully studied *in vivo*.

3.2.7.6 *Sperm Dilution Experiments*

Laboratory animals and men can have a considerable reduction in sperm concentrations and still be fertile. To determine 'fertility thresholds', semen should be serially diluted and an artificial insemination performed. The sperm dilution at which fertility is altered can be determined and compared either with pretreatment values or with controls.

3.2.7.7 *Foreign Chemicals in Semen*

Foreign chemicals may be excreted in semen. After ingestion, alcohol, salicylates, sulphonamides, ampicillin, erythromycin and other antibiotics are found in human and animal semen (Mann and Lutwak-Mann, 1981). Thalidomide and its metabolites readily find their way into semen and become firmly attached to the sperm. In studies of drugs in semen, sufficient care must be exercised to exclude contamination of semen by traces of urine.

3.2.7.8 *Sperm–Cervical Mucus Interaction*

The cervical epithelium comprises different types of secretory cells which vary in their nature and abundance of secretory granules. Secretions from these cells contribute to the cervical mucus. The rate of mucus secretion is a function of the secretory activity and responsiveness of the secretory cells to circulating hormones. Cyclic alteration in the constituents of cervical mucus influences sperm penetration and survival. The survival of sperm in the secretions of the female reproductive tract is critical to their maintenance and function. Although there is no practical method available at present for evaluating the effects of human uterine and tubal fluids on sperm, cervical mucus is readily accessible for sampling and study. Thus, evaluation of sperm–cervical mucus interaction should be included in any complete investigation of infertility (Belsey *et al.*, 1980; Alexander, 1981).

3.2.7.9 *Data Interpretation*

The following findings with respect to semen analysis indicate altered testicular function and, thus, suggest decreased fertility in humans (Eliasson, 1981):

(1) sperm concentration below 10 million per millilitre of ejaculate;
(2) less than 30% motile spermatozoa particularly if the progressive motility has been assessed as 'poor' or 'none';
(3) more than 30% defective midpieces including the occurrence of protoplasmic droplets;
(4) more than 30% defective tails including coiled tails or other tail defects such as too short, or too thick; and
(5) the occurrence of many immature spermatogenic cells, e.g. spermatids and primary spermatocytes.

In interpreting semen analysis data, it should be taken into account that the seminiferous epithelium is sensitive to various non-chemical influences, e.g., heat, fever, allergic reactions, virus infection and severe psychological stress. Thus, careful control and follow-up of the men included in the study and properly selected control groups from the same society groups are important.

Infections in the accessory genital glands can sometimes cause significant changes in the quality of semen. Since such infections may produce only minor symptoms, a careful clinical examination is necessary. A cytological examination of expressed prostatic fluid should be carried out if there is a suspicion of an infection or an inflammation in the accessory genital organs. When two or more of the following changes in the semen are present, one should suspect an infection and/or inflammation in the accessory genital glands:

(1) more than occasional leucocytes;
(2) prolonged liquefaction time;
(3) low sperm motility;

(4) more than 25% coiled tails;
(5) low concentrations of the organ specific markers; and/or
(6) large variations in the volume and properties of semen samples collected after similar periods of abstinence, e.g., 3–5 days.

3.3 SOME LABORATORY TESTS OF REPRODUCTIVE CAPACITY

Although several species might be used in fertility assessment, rodents and rabbits offer several advantages in comparison with dogs and subhuman primates. The rabbit is particularly useful. Male rabbits have a high, predictable libido that may be useful in assessing hazards to sexual behaviour. More importantly, all sequential phases of the conception process such as endocrine function, spermatogenesis, sperm maturation, ejaculation, sperm capacitation in the female and fertilization are easily evaluated, quantified and manipulated in the rabbit. The ability to characterize the whole ejaculate quantitatively and qualitatively and the ability to collect the ejaculate using an artificial vagina make the rabbit a key test model for sensitive assessment of possible harmful effects of environmental agents on male reproduction. The rat is the second animal of choice.

Only two procedures for fertility assessment are discussed here: serial mating and competitive fertility tests. For multigeneration studies see section 2.1.1.

3.3.1 Serial Mating Fertility Profile

The serial mating technique using mice and rats is a useful test of dominant lethal mutations as well as of male reproductive function (Jackson *et al.*, 1961; Lee and Dixon, 1972). After treatment with the selected chemical, each male is housed singly with a virgin female for a defined period, usually 7 days. This duration ensures that the female experiences one oestrous cycle during the breeding period. During each mating period, female animals are examined daily for vaginal plugs to ensure that the treatment does not interfere with ejaculation and mating capability. After the mating period, the female animal is replaced. These breeding studies are usually continued for 70 days.

Nine days after the end of the mating period, when a female could be approximately 12.5 days pregnant, the females are killed, uteri and fetuses examined, and the number of dead and viable fetuses recorded. Fertility profiles can be drawn from these data and presented in the form of a graph in which the ordinate expresses the percentage of males determined to be fertile as indicated by pregnant females, and the days after treatment are marked on the abscissa. Serial mating assesses the biological functioning of sperm cells and produces fertility patterns which are related inversely in time to the phase of spermatogenesis damaged by the treatment.

In order to identify the relationship between a chemical agent's effect on fertility and the type of spermatogenic stage affected as well as the possible biochemical effects, it is important to understand the underlying biology of the discrete stages of spermatogenesis.

Precise classification of the various spermatogenic cell types in the seminiferous tubules requires light and low-power electron microscopy. Progressive alterations are noted in the nucleus, in the acrosome of developing spermatids and in changing cellular associations. The kinetics of the spermatogenic cycle can be determined by following the progression of ^{3}H-thymidine in pulse-labelled spermatogonia as they differentiate.

Functional changes resulting from adverse effects of chemicals on specific spermatogenic stages are delayed depending on the cell type affected. In the rat, damage to epididymal sperm appears in 1–2 weeks; to spermiogenic cells in 3–5 weeks; to spermatocytes in 6–7 weeks; and to spermatogonia in 8–10 weeks. In man, effects of damage to epididymal sperm would appear in 1–4 weeks; to spermiogenic cells in 5–10 weeks; and to the premeiotic stage in 11–15 weeks.

It is important to bear in mind that fertility is a crude assessment of testicular function, as even a small amount of active spermatogenic tissue can maintain a normal level of fertility. These tests involve all-or-none events and do not detect subtle changes. Since sperm production, especially in test species, is greatly in excess of that required for fertility, even significant reductions in sperm production may not be detectable by breeding studies.

3.3.2 Competitive Fertility

Another potentially useful test approach involves competitive fertility (Beatty *et al.*, 1969). Sperm obtained from untreated males are mixed with sperm from treated animals. The ratio of fertilization by the control and the treated sperm after artificial insemination is determined using chemical or phenotypical markers. The same approach can be used with *in vitro* fertilization. However, these tests are limited to determining the capacity for sperm–egg interactions and not other variables such as sperm transport. Thus, the test provides more limited information than *in vivo* insemination. Oviductal or uterine insemination is another test approach which should be further developed to determine its reliability. Sperm from an untreated male are inseminated into one oviduct and the sperm of a treated male are inseminated into the other. Fertilization rates of superovulated females are then compared (see also section 2.3.2.2).

3.4 CLINICAL EXAMINATION AND EVALUATION

3.4.1 Clinical Examination

The minimal requirements of a clinical examination include a careful medical history and examination of the external genital organs, the prostate and the seminal vesicles.

The size of the testis is a good measure of the spermatogenic cell population, and correlates well with the number of sperm produced. Lack of usual firmness may indicate a loss of seminiferous epithelium.

The size of the testis can be determined with an orchidometer. Length and width of the testes can be measured in species such as rabbit, dog, bull and horse. In animals with a pendulous scrotum, scrotal circumference can also be easily determined (Mann and Lutwak-Mann, 1981). Measurement of testis size should be made biweekly or weekly with animal models, and can be made part of an annual physical examination given to men working in a hazardous environment.

In men, the size of the dorsal part of the prostate can be estimated by rectal examination, but healthy seminal vesicles cannot be felt by palpation. Vesiculography, ultrasonic scanning and computer tomography provide additional means for determining the position, shape and condition of these organs.

3.4.2 Clinical Assessment of Male Fertility

Clinical assessment of male fertility using epidemiological approaches is problematic. The expense and organization involved in collecting data on large samples of geographically widespread males is nearly overwhelming. Prospective studies are cumbersome, and the ethics of clinical trials with specific substances may be questioned. As a result, so-called clinical tests must rely on retrospectively collected epidemiological data such as the incidence of specific birth outcomes and the role of potentially confounding variables.

To aid in data collection, the Chemical Industry Institute of Toxicology (CIIT) in the United States has designed a questionnaire on reproduction to be used uniformly by major industries (Levine *et al.*, 1980). The format will allow collection of reproduction data on workers (approximately 20% female) and their spouses. Adequate background information and control of confounding variables are necessary to make this a useful tool in the epidemiological investigation of male fertility.

3.4.3 *In Vitro* Fertilization

Currently, the most promising approach to the clinical assessment of reproductive effects of chemicals involves *in vitro* fertilization. Improved *in vitro* fertilization techniques with mice, rats, hamsters and rabbits have resulted in an increased understanding of the basic biological mechanisms of fertilization and the role of exogenous chemicals in altering the fertilization process. Conditions have been developed which allow sperm capacitation and a successful extracorporeal union of male and female gametes.

These *in vitro* methods, whether using laboratory animals or the heterologous system (hyman sperm/Golden hamster ova) should help to determine how chemicals interfere with the events surrounding fertilization and to identify those chemicals with a potential to affect humans. There is increasing evidence from animal studies that certain chemicals may inhibit the fertilizing ability of sperm, with no marked effects on any of the common semen characteristics.

Because semen analysis as a predictor of male reproductive capacity is generally unreliable and human *in vitro* fertilization cannot itself be used as a test, a number of investigators have sought to develop a heterologous (interspecies) *in vitro* fertilization test system which uses substitutes for the human ovum. These substitutes include the zona pellucida of stored human follicular ova and the zona-free hamster ovum (Yanagimachi *et al.*, 1976, 1979).

Studies of the penetration by human sperm of zona pellucida-free ovum have identified certain individuals as subfertile who have a routinely determined normal sperm concentration, motility and morphology (Barros *et al.*, 1978; Hall, 1981). These data suggest that the usual semen analysis variables are unsure predictors of male subfertility; only the most extreme semen abnormalities reliably indicate subfertility. Thus, the *in vitro* penetration of laboratory animal ova by human sperm appears to be a useful technique to aid in assessing human fertilization potential.

The following steps are involved in the heterologous test. A human semen sample is obtained and a standard analysis is performed. The spermatozoa are washed in Tyrode's medium, centrifuged, and resuspended at a concentration of 4–8 million sperm per millilitre. Motility is assessed and an aliquot of this stock solution, usually containing a million motile sperm per millilitre, is incubated under oil for 15–18 hours to capacitate the sperm.

While the sperm are being prepared, ova are collected from the oviducts of superovulated test animal females. This superovulation is induced by interaperitoneal injection of pregnant mere's serum gonadotropin followed by human chorionic gonadotropin 2 days later. Ova are recovered from the oviducts and placed in Tyrode's medium. The ova are treated with hyaluronidase to remove the cumulus cells and then washed. Trypsin treatment removes the zona pellucida. Zona pellucida-free hamster ova are added to the dish containing control or experimental sperm, and fertilizing capacity is assessed by measuring sperm binding to the ova, decondensed sperm heads, and/or the pronucleus with the corresponding sperm tail in the ovum's cytoplasm. A consistent failure to penetrate 10% of zona-free hamster ova by human sperm is generally used to categorize semen donors as infertile (Hall, 1981).

Although termed 'fertilization', the process studied is the penetration of the sperm into the ovum with subsequent decondensation of the sperm. Further events of normal fertilization, such as genetic union of the cells, do not occur under these controlled artificial conditions. Cleavage of the hamster ovum penetrated by human sperm has never been observed. It is thought that heterologous tests may form a basis for exploring the effect of drugs that interfere with the process of sperm penetration of the egg and fertilization.

In situations where *in vitro* testing of human sperm fertility is indicated, the use of a double-fluorescent-label competitive sperm penetration assay with the zona-free hamster ovum might increase the sensitivity of the test. The sensitivity of the hamster ovum penetration assay is also increased by counting the total number of sperm per penetrated hamster vitellus as well as the percentage of penetrated eggs.

In vitro fertilization can also be coupled with preimplantation embryo culture, transfer of blastocysts to pseudo-pregnant recipients and evaluation of 'pregnancy outcome' to identify critical early development targets of environmental and other chemicals. Male and female gametes can be exposed to chemicals either *in vitro* or *in vivo* and then be used for *in vitro* fertilization.

3.4.4 Testicular Biopsy

In both large domestic animals and man it is possible to obtain testicular biopsies, but the procedure is not without risk, and it is used on relatively rare occasions.

A biopsy of the human testis will rarely give predictive information if the ejaculate contains more than 20 million sperm per millilitre. The method of securing and examining biopsy specimens has been described in detail (de Kretser and Holstein, 1976). A small incision in the tunica albuginea allows the testicular tissue to protrude and to be excised by a sharp scalpel blade held parallel to the surface of the testis. The tissue must be handled gently and placed in Bouin's or Cleland's fixative prior to processing.

One advantage of performing a testicular biopsy and of examining the specimens histologically is that spermatogenic failures can be related directly to lesions in the seminiferous epithelium. Some of the disadvantage of testicular biopsy are that the method is invasive, can be uncomfortable, and is not free of risks such as haematomas and infections (Eliasson, 1981).

3.5 CONCLUSIONS AND RECOMMENDATIONS

It is readily apparent that the male reproductive function is a set of carefully balanced and sensitive processes. However, little is presently known as to how exogenous chemicals affect these processes and alter functions, although in recent years important advances have been made. The task that faces reproduction biologists, toxicologists, clinicians and epidemiologists is to develop and validate rapid, inexpensive and predictive laboratory and clinical toxicity tests. A second challenge is to apply experimental data in defining the hazard and estimate reproductive function risk to men associated with exposure to chemicals at occupational and ambient environmental concentrations. Some more specific conclusions and recommendations for further work are summarized below.

(1) Radioimmunoassays are available for determining the gonadotropin-releasing hormone and gonadotropins, and for measuring changes in their levels

as a response to administered drugs and chemicals. These approaches should be carefully considered for their application to toxicological studies.

(2) Evaluation of sperm morphology could be made less subjective by developing a classification system based on morphometric standards.

(3) Major improvements in the predictiveness of semen analysis could be made by:

(a) more accurate determination of sperm concentration;
(b) routine determination of the total number of sperm per ejaculate;
(c) more precise determination of the percentage of progressively motile sperm; and
(d) more critical evaluation of sperm morphology by using phase-contrast or differential interference contrast microscopy for careful examination of wet preparation as well as stained smears.

(4) More attention should be directed to studying exogenous chemicals in semen and their effects on sperm. Where applicable, the split-ejaculate technique may be useful for this purpose. The levels of chemicals in semen might be a reliable and easily obtainable measure of exposure.

(5) Functional properties of spermatozoa determine their fertilizing ability, and better methods are required to assess these properties. At the present, sperm motility is the only functional property evaluated in routine analyses. Increased attention should be paid to other functional properties such as the release of enzymes from the spermatozoa, the zinc content, resistance to sodium dodecyl sulphate (SDS), sperm motility in normal cervical mucus, and the interaction between seminal plasma and spermatozoa.

(6) Methods for assessing Sertoli cell functions should be further developed and validated.

(7) Rodent species might be made more predictive for humans by artificially inseminating a limited number of sperm or by decreasing normal sperm production by prenatal (or early postnatal) esposure to ionizing radiation or selected chemicals.

(8) Better laboratory animal models and tests are required for evaluating the effects of chemicals on erection and ejaculation processes.

3.6 REFERENCES

Alexander, N. J. (1981). Evaluation of male infertility with an *in vitro* cervical mucus penetration test. *Fertil. Steril.* **36**, 201–208.

Amann, R. P. (1981). A critical review of methods for evaluation of spermatogenesis from seminal characteristics. *J. Androl.* **2**, 37–58.

Barros, C., Gonzales, J., Herrera, E. and Bustos-Obregon, E. (1978). Fertilizing capacity of human spermatozoa evaluated by actual penetration of foreign eggs. *Contraception* **17**, 87–92.

Beatty, R. A., Bennett, G. H., Hall, J. G., Hancock, J. L. and Steward, D. L. (1969). An experiment with heterospermic insemination in cattle. *J. Reprod. Fertil.* **19(3)**, 491–502.

Bedford, J. M. (Ed.) (1981). *Assessment of Risks to Human Reproduction and Development of the Human Conceptus from Exposure to Environmental Substances*. Draft Report. Oak Ridge National Laboratory, Oak Ridge, Tennessee.

Belsey, M. A., Eliasson, R., Gallegos, A. J., Moghissi, K. S., Paulsen, C. A. and Prasad, M. R. N. (1980). *Laboratory Manual for the Examination of Human Semen and Semen–Cervical Mucus Interaction*, 43 pages. Based on consultations held within the WHO Special Programme of Research, Development and Research Training in Human Reproduction. Press Concern, Singapore.

Burger, H. and de Kretser, D. M. (Eds.) (1981). *Comprehensive Endocrinology: The Testis*, 442 pages. Raven Press, New York.

Christensen, A. K. (1965). The fine structure of testicular interstitial cells in guinea pigs. *J. Cell Biol.* **26**, 911–935.

de Kretser, D. M. and Holstein, A. F. (1976). Testicular biopsy and abnormal germ cells. In Hafez, E. S. E. (Ed.) *Human Semen and Fertility Regulation in Man*, 615 pages. Mosby, St. Louis.

Dixon, R. L. (1980a). Toxic responses of the reproductive system. In Doull, J. Klaassen, D. C. and Amdur, M. O. (Eds.) *Casarett and Doull's Toxicology: The Basic Science of Poisons*, 2nd edn, pp. 332–354. Macmillan Publishing Co., Inc., New York.

Dixon, R. L. (1980b). *Reproductive Toxicology Workshop Recommendations*. Sponsored by National Toxicology Program/National Institute of Environmental Health Sciences, Research Triangle Park, NC (unpublished document).

Dixon, R. L. (1981). The role of pharmacokinetic, adaptive and homeostatic factors in testicular toxicity and risk assessment. In Richmond, C. R., Walsh, P. J. and Copenhaver, E. D. (Eds.). *Proceedings of the Third Life Sciences Symposium on Risk Analysis*, pp. 196–212, Franklin Institute Press, Philadelphia, Pennsylvania.

Dixon, R. L. and Lee, I. P. (1980). Pharmacokinetic and adaptation factors in testicular toxicity. *Fedn Proc., Fedn Am. Soc. exp. Biol.* **39**, 66–72.

Eliasson, R. (1981). Analysis of semen. In Burger, H. and de Kretser, D. (Eds.) *The Testis*, pp. 381–399, Raven Press, New York.

Evenson, D. P., Darzynkiewicz, Z. and Melamed, M. R. (1980). Relation of mammalian sperm chromatin heterogenicity to fertility. *Science (Washington, DC)* **210**, 1131–1133.

Gledhill, B. L., Lake, S. and Dean, P. N. (1979). Flow cytometry and sorting of sperm and other male germ cells. In Melamed, M. R., Mullaney, P. F. and Mendelsohn, M. L. (Eds.) *Flow Cytometry and Sorting*, pp. 471–484, John Wiley and Sons, Inc., Chichester, New York, Brisbane, Toronto.

Hall, J. L. (1981). Relationship between semen quality and human sperm penetration of zona-free hamster ova. *Fertil. Steril.* **35**, 457–463.

Hansson, V., Aakvaag, A. and Purvis, K. (Eds.) (1981). *Molecular and Cellular Endocrinology of the Testis* (1st European Workshop) *Int. J. Androl. Suppl. 3*, 143 pages. Scriptor, Copenhagen.

Jackson, H., Fox, B. W. and Craig, A. W. (1961). Antifertility substances and their assessment in the male rodents. *J. Reprod. Fertil.* **2**, 447–465.

Janick, J. and MacLeod, J. (1970). The measurement of human sperm motility. *Fertil. Steril.* **21**, 140–146.

Katz, D. F. and Overstreet, J. W. (1981). Sperm motility assessment by videomicrography. *Fertil. Steril.* **35**, 188–193.

Kerr, J. B. and de Kretser, D. M. (1981). The cytology of the human testis. In Burger, H. G. and de Kretser, D. M. (Eds.) *The Testis*, pp. 141–169. Raven Press, New York.

Lee, I. P. and Dixon, R. L. (1972). Antineoplastic drug effects on spermatogenesis studied by velocity sedimentation cell separation. *Toxic. appl. Pharmacol.* **23**, 20–41.

Levine, R. J., Symons, M. J., Balogh, S. A., Arndt, D. M., Kaswandik, N. T. and Gentile,

J. W. (1980). A method for monitoring the fertility of workers. *J. occup. Med.* **22**, 781–791.

Mann, T. and Lutwak-Mann, C. (1981). *Male Reproductive Function and Semen: Themes and Trends in Physiology, Biochemistry and Investigative Andrology,* 495 pages. Springer-Verlag, New York.

Okumura, K., Lee, I. P. and Dixon, R. L. (1975). Permeability of selected drugs and chemicals across the blood–testis barrier of the rat. *J. Pharmac. exp. Ther.* **194**, 89–95.

Rich, R. A. and de Kretser, D. M. (1977). Effect of differing degrees of destruction of the rat seminiferous epithelium on levels of serum FSH and androgen binding protein. *Endocrinology (Philadelphia)* **101**, 959–968.

Russell, L. and Burguet, S. (1977). Ultrastructure of Leydig cells as revealed by secondary tissue treatment with a ferrocyanide–osmium mixture. *Tissue and Cell* **9**, 751–766.

Soyka, L. F. and Joffe, J. M. (1980). Male mediated drug effects on offspring. In Schwarz, R. H. and Yaffe, S. J. (Eds.) *Drug and Chemical Risks to the Fetus and Newborn,* pp. 49–66, Alan R. Liss, Inc., New York.

Strobino, B. R., Kline, J. and Stein, Z. (1978). Chemical and physical exposure of parents: effects on human reproduction and offspring. *Early Hum. Dev.* **1**, 371–399.

Talbot, P. and Chacon, R. S. (1981). Triple stain technique for evaluating normal acrosome reactions of human sperm. *J. exp. Zool.* **215(2)**, 201–208.

Vitale, R., Fawcett, D. W. and Dym, M. (1973). The normal development of the blood–testis barrier and the effects of clomiphene and estrogen treatment. *Anat. Rec.* **176**, 333–344.

Woods, J. S. (1979). Drug effects on human sexual behavior. In Woods, N. F. (Ed.) *Human Sexuality in Health and Illness,* 2nd edn, pp. 364–382. C. V. Mosby Company, St. Louis, Missouri.

Yanagimachi, R., Lopata, A., Odom, C. B., Bronson, R. A., Mahi, C. A. and Nicolson, G. L. (1979). Retention of biologic characteristics of zona pellucida in highly concentrated salt solution: the use of salt-stored eggs for assessing the fertilizing capacity of spermatozoa. *Fertil. Steril.* **31**, 562.

Yanagimachi, R., Yanagimachi, H. and Rogers, B. J. (1976). The use of zona-free ova as a test-system for the assessment of the fertilizing capacity of human spermatozoa. *Biol. Reprod.* **15**, 471.

Methods for Assessing the Effects of Chemicals on Reproductive Functions
Edited by V. B. Vouk and P. J. Sheehan
© 1983 SCOPE

4 Vertebrates Other Than Mammals*

There is a wide difference in the information available on the classes of animals under consideration in this section. Birds and fishes have been extensively studied, whereas no tests for the effects of chemicals on the reproduction of reptiles and amphibians are available, and the discussion of these two classes is little more than a list of proposed species and a brief outline of possible test procedures.

Birds have been widely studied because these conspicuous and widely liked creatures have been shown to act as 'early-warning' systems for environmental problems on a number of occasions. Pesticide-induced eggshell thinning caused the extinction of the peregrine falcon in eastern North America and a marked reduction of this and other predatory species in many parts of the world. Fish have a great economic value and sport fishing has a wide following. Beyond these immediate concerns, fish represent the upper trophic, bioaccumulatory level of ecosystems whose primary element, water, acts globally as a most effective transport medium and sink for environmental toxicants. Acid precipitation in eastern North America and northern Europe has prevented the reproduction of fish and as a consequence caused the destruction of freshwater fish populations over wide geographic areas. Reptiles and amphibians have been little studied, apparently due to the fact that they are inconspicuous, have no large-scale group of interested persons and have only slight economic importance. Nevertheless, there is good evidence that some members of these classes are threatened by pollution, perhaps most critically amphibians by increasing acidification of the small bodies of water in which they breed. The development of tests for these two classes is an urgent matter.

A laboratory test species should meet as many as possible of the following criteria:

(1) it should be readily available, and breed easily and reproducibly in captivity;
(2) the production of eggs and young should be capable of quantification;
(3) it should not be insensitive to the chemical or group of chemicals being tested; and
(4) it should be representative of species of ecological or commercial importance.

* This section was prepared by a Workgroup chaired by D. B. Peakall. The rapporteur was A. G. Johnels, and members were E. M. Donaldson, M. Goto, A. L. Martin and E. Scherer.

In field tests the last three criteria also apply, with the additional criterion that (5) the collection of data does not affect the test itself.

Field studies have the advantage that one can test the target species under natural conditions, which aids in the assessment of the impact of chemicals on natural populations. However, there are a number of difficulties to be overcome. It is often not easy to expose the target organism to a chemical, especially if chronic dosing is required. If studies are done by putting organisms into polluted areas and then measuring their reproductive function, the problem is that it is rare for only one pollutant or even one class of pollutants to be present. There is a lack of control of the experiment, and factors such as weather, predation, availability of food and vandalism may have to be taken into account. Another problem is the influence that the observer and the experimental procedures may have on the reproduction of the animals being studied. Nevertheless, despite the difficulties and the cost, the combination of laboratory and field studies is necessary to elucidate major pollutant problems.

4.1 BIRDS

4.1.1 Currently Used Methods

4.1.1.1 *Reproductive Cycle Tests*

The purpose of these tests is to determine the effects of chemicals on the overall reproductive success. Adult birds are paired off and test chemicals introduced into the diet before egg follicle formation. Number of eggs per female, fertility, hatchability and survival of young up to 14–21 days are measured. Eggs are artificially incubated, and eggshell thickness and residue levels measured.

This method is being actively considered as a standard method for the mallard (*Anas platyrhynchos*) and two species of quail (*Colinus virginianus* and *Coturnix coturnix*) by the Organization for Economic Cooperation and Development (OECD) and the American Society for Testing and Materials (ASTM). These species are readily obtainable, breed easily and reproducibly and can be used routinely at the present state of knowledge. They are comparatively inexpensive, and no special training of assistants is required.

This method is a good screening test, as eggs are incubated artificially and young are precocial. However, it gives little information on the effects of pollutants on reproductive behaviour.

Other tests have been considered in order to extend the information obtained by the 'standard' test to other species more closely related to the target species. The procedures are similar to the 'standard' test except that the young are usually reared by parents. Several species have been proposed for such tests.

The black duck (*Anas rubripes*) breeds readily and reproducibly (Longcore and Stendell, 1977) but seems to offer little advantage over the readily available mallard to which it is very closely related.

The American kestrel (*Falco sparverius*), a small falcon, has been bred in captivity for toxicological studies (Porter and Wiemeyer, 1969). Both the barn owl (*Tyto alba*), a medium-sized flesh-eating owl, and the small screech owl (*Otus asio*) have also been bred successfully (McLane and Hall, 1972). All these species require large-size cages and skilled assistants to maintain a reproducible colony breeding. Since the main dietary requirement is meat, these species are too expensive for routine testing. Initial collection of wild birds is necessary and this requires permits. This test is predictive of the effects of chemicals on predatory birds which are particularly vulnerable to pollutants, due to their position in the food chain.

The ring dove (*Streptopelia risoria*) breeds readily in captivity in small cages. Small clutch size (two eggs) requires more birds in order to obtain adequate sample size than for the 'standard' test species, which have large clutch sizes, and young must be reared by parents. The ring dove is comparatively inexpensive, and no special training of assistants is needed. Breeding behaviour has been very well studied (Lehrman, 1964) and has been used to demonstrate behavioural alterations caused by chemicals (Peakall and Peakall, 1973). Doves frequent farmland, but have a low position in food chains.

The starling (*Sturnus vulgaris*) can be bred in captivity although the supply of insect food for small young causes difficulties. The clutch is large and readily available. Hole-nesting makes behavioural observations difficult, but reproductive success is high and reasonably consistent (Powell and Gray, 1980).

4.1.1.2 *Multigeneration Studies*

Most avian toxicology studies are carried out over less than a full life cycle, and effects caused in offspring and carried on to the next generation will not be observed.

Multigeneration studies have been carried out using ring doves, quail and mallards. Tests do not differ from reproductive cycle tests for the same species except in length and, therefore, cost. Several experiments (Peakall *et al.*, 1972; Carnio and McQueen, 1973; Heinz, 1979) showed that the effects are greater in the second and third generations; in some cases they are much greater than the effects observed in the first generation. These findings point out the inadequacies of the 'standard' reproduction cycle test which is not a true full cycle test.

4.1.1.3 *Egg Injection Experiments*

The egg injection test is a simple screening method to test for the effects of chemicals on the developing avian embryo. Dissolved chemicals are injected into the yolk of fertile chicken eggs (McLaughlin *et al.*, 1963; Dunachie and Fletcher,

1969). Artificially incubated eggs are candled at intervals to check on development.

This is by far the most rapid and inexpensive of the avian tests, although it only checks a single part of the reproductive cycle. If the chemical is placed on the air sac membrane, the question is whether or not the chemical is absorbed into the yolk; direct injection into the yolk causes appreciable mortality which can be offset by increasing the sample size.

The technique can be used in the field on target species or near congeners (Gilman *et al.*, 1978), although the pigmentation of many species makes the candling of eggs, to determine whether development is in progress, virtually impossible.

4.1.2 Potential Test Methods

4.1.2.1 *Cytogenetics*

The purpose of cytogenetic tests is to look for genetic damage in birds that may be caused by chemicals. In preparations made from rapidly proliferating tissue of the avian embryo, chromosomes can be examined after cell division has been arrested with Colcemid, and breaks and other abnormalities determined (Bloom *et al.*, 1972). Also the rates of sister-chromatid exchange can be determined in cells from the allantoic sac of avian embryos (Bloom, 1978). Neither of these techniques has been used extensively, although chromosomal abnormalities have been associated with reproductive failure in ring doves caused by poly-chlorinated biphenyls (PCBs) (Peakall *et al.*, 1972). These techniques could be added to the protocols for the reproductive cycle and the egg injection tests.

Cytogenetic methods are fairly rapid and reproducible but call for skilled technical assistants. The possibility of correlating the degree of cytogenetic damage with the degree of reproductive failure would be valuable. Cytogenetic techniques are capable of being used under field conditions, and rates of sister-chromatid exchange in gull embryonic material have been shown to be fairly consistent from colony to colony (Ellenton, personal communication). In field studies, cytogenetic changes cannot be linked to a specific chemical with certainty even if chemical analysis for residue levels is undertaken.

4.1.2.2 *Liver Enzyme Induction*

The purpose of this test is to determine the degree of hepatic enzyme induction in embryos and relate it to the degree of exposure to toxic chemicals. Livers from late embryos or young chicks are removed and microsomal fractions isolated. The rate of metabolism of specific substrates (usually labelled) is measured and related to the protein content of the microsomal fraction (Conney and Klutch, 1963).

This technique is fairly rapid and reasonably reproducible but calls for skilled technical support. It could be added to the reproductive cycle or the egg injection technique. Hepatic enzyme induction is a response to foreign chemicals and although there are differences in the induction processes by different classes of chemicals, more work is needed to relate enzyme induction caused by specific chemicals to the metabolism of a specific substrate. This specificity could be used to indicate what chemical(s) the bird had been exposed to, and thus it could be employed in field studies. The induction of hepatic enzymes can affect circulating steroid levels; it does not seem to be correlated with breeding success.

4.1.2.3 *Hormonal Cycle*

The purpose of this test is to determine the changes in hormonal cycle caused by chemicals as an indication of effects of chemicals on reproduction. Circulating hormone levels can be measured in samples of blood collected at fixed time intervals. Analysis is carried out by radioimmunoassay techniques.

This method is fairly rapid and reproducible but calls for skilled technical support. Changes in steroid hormone levels should be predictive of the changes in the reproductive cycle but may not add much to the information obtained from the reproductive cycle test. For example, delayed onset of breeding has been found to be caused by organochlorine compounds, and this correlates with a slower rise of oestrogen levels (McArthur, 1980), but changes of hormone level are not more sensitive than direct observation.

4.1.2.4 *Adrenocortical Function*

The effects of chemicals on the adrenocortical function of birds may be evaluated by determining the weight and histological changes of adrenals (Holmes and Gorsline, 1981). Measurement of levels of corticosteroids in blood may be performed by radioimmunoassay.

Histological work is time consuming and requires the sacrifice of individual animals. Determination of levels of circulating corticosterone is relatively rapid but also requires skilled assistance. The relationship of the levels of circulating hormones to exposure to chemicals is obscure, as Cavanaugh and Holmes (1982) found a decrease in mallard exposed to oil, whereas Peakall *et al.* (1981) found an increase in gulls and guillemots also exposed to oil.

4.1.2.5 *Egg Exchange Experiments*

The objective of this type of test is to separate direct embryotoxic effects from effects caused by behavioural abnormalities. Eggs laid by females exposed to a chemical are moved and put under control females, while eggs from control females are put under females exposed to the chemicals.

Under field conditions this is a difficult and complex experiment which has been carried out on ospreys (*Pandion haliaetus*) (Wiemeyer *et al.*, 1975) and herring gulls (*Larus argentatus*) (Peakall *et al.*, 1980). Under laboratory conditions it can be done quite readily (Peakall and Peakall, 1973) and could be easily used when reproductive cycle tests indicate that hatchability of eggs under the natural parent is decreased by a chemical, in order to determine the importance of the behavioural component.

4.1.3 Field Experiments on Reproductive Cycle

The objective of field experiments is to test the effects of chemicals on avian reproduction under natural conditions. Adults are treated with chemicals and allowed to continue their breeding cycle. Long-term dosing is a problem which has been tackled by putting out contaminated prey (Enderson and Berger, 1970).

A technique that has promise of wide application is implantation of the material under the skin. Osborn and Harris (1979) successfully implanted PCBs contained in open plastic tubes in seabirds and were able to simulate known levels of this pollutant.

While this approach tests chemicals under realistic conditions and allows the target species or near congeners to be tested, it is a difficult and expensive technique. It may well be the only feasible approach when species cannot be bred successfully in captivity (i.e., pelagic seabirds). There are legal complications since permits are usually required. Field experiments suffer from a lack of control over the experiment (weather, predation, vandalism, etc.) and from considerable variability of results; it is often not feasible to increase the sample size enough to compensate for this. And, lastly, there is the problem of the effect of the biologist on the system being studied.

Another comparatively simple, currently used field procedure is to obtain an index of the reproductive success of bird colonies breeding under natural conditions. Colonies are visited three times during the breeding season (mid-incubation, two visits to mark young) and the numbers of nests, eggs and young counted on each visit and the total production (young/pair) is calculated. The number of visits should be reduced to a minimum both to reduce the cost and to minimize the disturbance of the colony which can cause appreciable mortality. Additional visits give more information but three visits are considered adequate for the calculation of an index of breeding success (Weseloh *et al.*, 1979). This method does not test the effect of any given chemical but gives an indication of environmental quality of a certain area. It is necessary to have information on the feeding and migratory habits of the birds being studied. Breeding success can be affected by factors other than toxic chemicals such as weather and availability of food. This method has been used successfully as part of the Great Lakes Water Quality Surveillance Program.

4.2 FISH

4.2.1 Currently Used Methods

Up to the early and mid-seventies, only acute lethal tests were standard tests for fish (e.g. 96-hour LC_{50} for rainbow trout, *Salmo gairdneri*). However, the need to determine impairment of physiological functions, including reproduction, in order to assess the environmental risk of chemicals is now well recognized (Donaldson and Scherer, 1983, this volume). As with toxicological testing with other phyla and classes of organisms, a number of years is required to allow tests based on observed effects to develop into 'proposed' or 'tentative' and finally 'accepted' or 'standard' methods.

4.2.1.1 *Standard Life-Cycle Tests*

Two partial- and two complete-life-cycle tests are described in *Standard Methods for the Examination of Water and Waste Water* which is an official handbook used by regulatory agencies in North America (APHA *et al.*, 1981). A partial-life-cycle bioassay usually includes one to two life stages of the fish, such as egg and alevin, fry, juvenile, or adult, while a complete-life-cycle test covers more than a generation, for example, exposed adult, egg, fry, juvenile, and adult to eggs. Tests for two freshwater species, the brook trout (*Salvelinus fontinalis*) and the fathead minnow (*Pimephales promelas*), and two estuarine/marine species, the sheeps-head minnow (*Cyprinodon variegatus*) and the Atlantic silverside (*Menidia menidia*), are described. The tests are presented as tentative (i.e. still under investigation) and consist of partial-life-cycle bioassays with the brook trout and silverside and complete-life-cycle bioassays with the sheepshead and fathead minnow. The rationale for choosing these species was to arrive at the best possible compromise between availability of species, ease of handling, holding and culturing, availability of background data on reproduction and development, and sensitivity of eggs, embryos, larvae and adults to chemicals. Criteria for reproductive impairment to be measured are: number of spawnings and eggs; time till hatching; percentage of eggs hatching; number and percentage of larvae surviving; frequency of deformities; and growth and mortality of larvae.

4.2.1.2 *Standard Early-Life-History Tests*

The US Environmental Protection Agency (EPA), in cooperation with the American Society for Testing and Materials (ASTM), has prepared draft guidelines for conducting toxicity tests with the early life stages of fishes alone (ASTM, 1981). These guidelines are expected to become standard methods for routine testing.

A review by McKim (1977), analysing the results of 56 complete-life-cycle tests with 34 different organic and inorganic chemicals, had concluded that 'embryolarval and early juvenile life stages were the most, or among the most, sensitive in whole life cycle tests' (see also Macek and Sleight, 1977). If supported and verified by future experience, there will be a strong tendency to forego costly and time-consuming complete-life-cycle methods in favour of testing these early life stages only. For the same amount of cost and effort, a far greater number of species may be tested. Indeed, some 15 possible test species from freshwater and marine habitats are suggested by ASTM (1981). End-points used to measure the effects of chemicals are: percentage survival of embryos to hatching; heart beat and movement, if visible through the chorion; time of hatching; time to swim-up (salmonids only); behaviour of larvae (ventilation rate, rate and coordination of movement); deformities; growth; and mortalities.

Standard tests for routine use will always have to strike a balance between reliability, predictive value and ecological significance on the one hand, and practicality and cost efficiency on the other. Many of the economically and ecologically important fish species, especially those from the marine environment, are difficult to culture. As a consequence, a number of easy-to-handle species with short life cycles have been suggested for routine use in partial- and complete-life-cycle and multigeneration tests, e.g. the flagfish, *Jordanella floridae* (Smith, 1973; ASTM, 1981), the guppy, *Poecilia reticulata* (Pierson, 1981) and the zebrafish, *Brachydanio rerio* (Kihlström *et al.*, 1971; Laale, 1977; Lillie *et al.*, 1979).

4.2.2 Potential Test Methods

4.2.2.1 *Gamete Test*

In most teleosts, gametes are released into the aquatic environment where they are exposed to pollutants in water prior to and during fertilization. In this test, eggs and spermatozoa are exposed separately for up to 1 hour in media in which their ability to be fertilized and fertilizing capacity, respectively, are maintained. After exposure, treated eggs are fertilized with normal spermatozoa and treated sperm, and tested for their ability to fertilize normal ova. Percentage fertilization is determined by examining intact or cleared eggs hours or days after the fertilization, depending on species and incubation temperature (Billard, 1978a, b; Billard *et al.*, 1978)

This type of test is particularly appropriate where the fish are likely to be exposed to a particular pollutant on the spawning ground. The test has the advantage of being rapid and relatively simple to conduct. A disadvantage of the method is that insufficient research has been conducted to relate this artificially extended exposure of gametes to pollutants to the relatively brief exposure period which normally occurs between gamete release and fertilization. The methods available to date have been developed using rainbow trout (*Salmo gairdneri*) gametes; however, the technique could be applied to other species such as herring

(*Clupea sp.*) which also migrate to specific spawning locations, and whose spawning is also characterized by marked seasonality.

4.2.2.2 Medaka Embryo Test

The medaka (*Oryzias latipes*) species has the advantages of producing eggs each day and of producing eggs which are transparent, permitting observation of embryonic development.

In the medaka embryo test, eggs (10) are placed in test solution (20 ml) in screw top vials (23 ml) soon after fertilization. Mortalities and developmental abnormalities are noted until and including hatching (Stoss and Haines, 1979).

This technique is rapid and the use of closed exposure vials is inexpensive. The transparency of eggs permits observation of embryonic abnormalities prior to hatching, and the method may provide a rapid and simple tool for estimating maximum acceptable toxicant concentration (MATC).

4.2.2.3 Cytogenetics

There is a pressing need for a field technique to assess the effect of pollutants on the reproductive successes of marine species having pelagic eggs. Examination of planktonic eggs for cytogenetic abnormalities has been proposed as an appropriate approach to this problem.

Fish eggs are collected during the breeding season using plankton tows at specific depths. Eggs are preserved in a suitable fixative for karyological studies. Water samples and, if possible, egg samples are collected at the same time for chemical analysis. The presence of cytogenetic and cytological abnormalities in the embryo and yolk sac membrane are correlated with the presence of pollutants (Longwell and Hughes, 1980).

This technique shows promise as a field method; however, laboratory studies are needed to confirm whether the changes observed in the field are in fact caused by specific pollutants and, if so, which pollutants are responsible. The work reported to date has been conducted on the Atlantic mackerel (*Scomber scombrus*).

4.2.2.4 Histopathological Tests

The histopathological examination of male and female gonads in exposed fish provides a means of assessing chemical effects on reproductive development in maturing fish during gonadal development. Fish are either exposed in the laboratory or collected from field locations where exposure to xenobiotics is suspected. At autopsy the gonadosomatic index is determined. The testes and ovaries are examined for gross changes in colour and appearance, and portions of ovarian and testicular tissue are prepared for histological assessment. Criteria for chemical damage include reduced gonadal size, abnormal appearance, inhibition of vitellogenesis, increase in the proportion of atretic oocytes, inhibition of spermatogenesis and abnormal appearance of spermatozoa (this observation requires the use of an electron microscope).

The method has the benefit of providing direct evidence of impact on gonadal development but has the disadvantage of requiring extensive histological work to quantify the histopathological response. The test has been applied in different forms to several species including the flagfish (*Jordanella floridae*) (Ruby *et al.*, 1977, 1978), the cod (*Gadus morhua*) (Freeman *et al.*, 1980) and the brook trout (*Salvelinus fontinalis*) (Sangalang and O'Halloran, 1973).

4.2.2.5 *Inhibition of Spawning*

Inhibition of spawning has been shown to be a critical end-point for certain types of chemicals tested in life-cycle tests (McKim, 1977). Thus it is possible that inhibition of spawning can be used as a test in its own right. This type of test involves exposure of fish during sexual maturation to a chemical pollutant in an environment which would be normally conducive to natural spawning. Suitable test end-points include delay in maturation, inhibition of spawning and reduction in eggs produced per female (Curtis and Beyers, 1978).

This test has the advantage of being as sensitive as, or more sensitive than, the early-life-history test for certain chemicals while being less costly and time consuming than the full- or partial-life-cycle tests. The medaka (*Oryzias latipes*), the bluegill (*Lepomis macrochirus*), the flagfish (*Jordanella floridae*) and the fathead minnow (*Pimephales promelas*) are some of the species in which spawning inhibition has been investigated.

4.2.2.6 *Mutagenicity Tests*

Examination for mutagenicity is a particularly important aspect of toxicity testing. Conduct of the test with a viviparous fish permits evaluation of embryo production and embryo mortality. Male guppies (*Poecilia reticulata*) are exposed in water or by injection. The males are then mated with normal females 24 hours after initiation of treatment, and after 10 days the females are autopsied and the number of live and dead embryos determined (Mathews *et al.*, 1978). The injected fish are more sensitive than immersed fish, but the latter treatment more closely reflects environmental exposure. This test using the guppy is the only test for chemical mutagenicity in fish that could be located in the literature. It has the advantages of simplicity and rapidity.

4.2.2.7 *Tests Based on Hormonal Control Mechanisms*

While some chemicals have direct effects on gonadal tissue, others may have indirect deleterious effects on gonadal development which are mediated by effects on the hormonal control of reproductive development. Measurement of the concentration, turnover or production rate of reproductive hormones thus provides a means of testing for effects of chemicals on reproduction before morphological or histological changes are observed or before failure to reproduce is noted. The measurement of corticosteroid hormones has already been used to quantify the stress response of fish to pollutants (for a review see Donaldson, 1981). Test fish are exposed to the chemical for a period during gonadal development, and blood samples are collected for evaluating the plasma concentration of appropriate hormones by radioimmunoassay techniques. Hormones which have been shown to be, or are potential indicators of reproductive impairment include gonadotropin-releasing hormone, gonadotropins, oestrogens, androgens and progestogens. It is evident from the literature on fish that pollutants not only can change the concentration of hormones in the plasma and in the endocrine glands, but also can modify the timing of the cyclic changes in hormone concentration which are associated with normal reproductive development. Thus two key end-points for this type of test are changes in hormone concentration and changes in timing of hormone production and/or release.

The advantage of this type of test is that it may be expected to have predictive value with respect to longer term effects such as failure to spawn. A disadvantage is the requirement for relatively sophisticated analytical equipment. However, recent advances in analytical biochemistry have simplified the procedures and reduced the volume of plasma required for hormone analysis. Tests of this type have been conducted on the brook trout (*Salvelinus fontinalis*) (Sangalang and Freeman, 1974), the rainbow trout (*Salmo gairdneri*) and common carp (*Cyprinus carpio*) (Sivarajah *et al.*, 1978) and the Indian catfish (*Heteropneustes fossilis*) (Singh and Singh, 1980).

4.2.2.8 *Spawning Behaviour Tests*

None of the standard or potential tests delineated above, with the exception of those life cycle tests which include natural spawning, provides any measure of the effect of chemicals on migration to spawning locations, aggregation of mature conspecifics, spawning habitat selection, courting behaviour and spawning performance. Specific methods are not available to examine the effects of chemicals on some of these behavioural aspects of fish reproduction.

A maze technique has been developed to assess the effect of chemicals on the response of zebrafish (*Brachydanio rerio*) to a sexual aggregating pheromone produced by conspecifics (Bloom *et al.*, 1978). Methods are also available for testing attraction to or avoidance of polluted waters by fish (Höglund, 1953; Sprague, 1964; Hansen, 1969; Scherer and Nowak, 1973), and chemosensory impairment by chemicals (Hara, 1979). While quantitative behavioural tests on fish require a significant commitment of resources, these tests provide a measure of impacts on reproduction that would not be detected using other test methods.

4.3 REPTILES

Geographical distribution is one criterion for the selection of test species. Lizards and snakes (order Squamata) are chiefly tropical, although some species are found in temperate regions. The order Squamata, with some 4800 species, is the most numerous and widely distributed of all the reptiles (Kaplan, 1974). The turtles (order Chelonia) are most abundant in the north and south temperate zones, while the crocodiles are largely tropical. The latest control list of the Convention on International Trade in Endangered Species, as agreed in Delhi in 1981, contains 74 species of reptiles which are considered to be rare or endangered.

No standard methods for assessing effects of chemicals on reproductive functions of reptiles have been developed.

Kaplan (1974) gives some information on reproduction processes of reptiles, but much of the information is based on field data. Campbell and Busack (1979) recently described laboratory maintenance of turtles, but they consider largely non-breeding individuals, and Ewert (1979) dealt with maintaining eggs in the laboratory.

The choice of species to represent the class of Reptilia would be:

(1) a freshwater turtle, *Trionyl sinensis*, which is bred for human consumption in Japan; alternatives are *Mauremys japonicus* and/or *Thinemys reevesi*, which are both bred in Japan for pet trade; or
(2) a lizard, where the alternatives are *Anolis carolinensis, Lacerta* sp., or *Cnemidophorus exsanguis; Anolis carolinensis* is routinely bred for experimental use in the USA and its breeding biology has been well studied (see Licht, 1971).

Species belonging to the genus *Lacerta* might be another choice, being present in nature over large parts of the world, and being easy to handle in laboratories. Breeding colonies of *Cnemidophorus exsanguis* have been established, and have shown consistent reproductive success and very little genetic variation (Cole and Townsend, 1977).

4.3.1 Test Methods

No standard methods exist, and only potential methods can be suggested. Some similarity—egg laying—between reptiles and birds suggests the possibility for similar test methods. Many reptiles are fairly slow to reach sexual maturity, which will initially restrict test programmes to partial-life-cycle tests.

A partial-life-cycle test could be carried out by exposing adults to chemicals through food and water or by injection. Reproduction end-points that could be used include egg counting, egg hatchability and survival of offspring to day x.

4.4 AMPHIBIANS

Amphibians have a world-wide distribution, although this class of animals is concentrated in the tropics. The salamanders are found primarily in the northern temperate zone. While standard tests have not been developed, some testing of the effects of pesticides (Cooke, 1972, 1973) and pH changes (Pough, 1976; Saber and Dunson, 1978) on embryonic and larval stages of amphibians has been carried out.

Anurans (e.g. frogs and toads) have been used in laboratories for a long time for experiments including reproduction studies, and there are standardized systems for testing human pregnancy (genus *Xenopus*). The breeding biology of anurans has a wide diversity, and there are many different procedures for maintaining the moisture essential for their eggs. For many species the eggs are easily collected and may be studied in various respects. The tadpoles are likewise easy to raise up to and beyond metamorphosis. Anurans are, in nature, exposed to contaminants present in water or air; although not a deliberate target of pesticides, several cases of mortality due to pesticide use are known.

Many anurans are easy to propagate and raise. Species of the genera *Rana* and *Xenopus* have the advantage of having been bred and widely used in laboratory experiments (NAS, 1974).

Species of the Urodela order such as newts and salamanders are present in large areas of the world, and some species of the genus *Ambystoma* are used for a variety of laboratory experiments. Their developmental biology is well known. They are easy to handle and their developmental mechanics and fine structure have been studied in detail. The effect of pH in combination with temperature on *A. maculatum* and *A. jeffersonianum* has been studied. Species of genus *Ambystoma* should be useful for developing test methods.

4.4.1 Test Methods

There are no standardized methods for amphibians. In some cases methods have been worked out for *Rana temporaria* and *Bufo bufo* and have been used to study the effect of DDT and its metabolites on anuran eggs (Cooke, 1972). *Rana, Xenopus* and *Ambystoma* species are fairly easily bred and reach maturity fast enough to allow complete-life-cycle testing. Partial-life-cycle and early-life-history tests are very easily carried out and, in principle, testing guidelines for fish eggs or gametes to the point of metamorphosis could be used. Parental exposure is likewise possible, though protocols have not yet been worked out in a standardized way.

For complete-life-cycle tests, the exposure is most likely to be successful in water. The exposure should start from adults (sexual maturity) and continue until the first pairing after metamorphosis in the second generation.

For partial-life-cycle tests, adults should be exposed via food, water or by injection, and the number of eggs and percentage of fertile eggs determined; embryonic development, percentage of eggs hatching and survival to metamorphosis should be monitored. With respect to early-life-history tests, methods similar to standard fish tests could be used. For amphibians, early life history should also include the metamorphosis and the postmetamorphic stage because they are typical for the group. A proposed test is the inhibition of spawning as described for fish. Test end-points would include delay in maturation, inhibition of spawning and reduction in the number of eggs produced per female.

4.5 CONCLUSIONS AND RECOMMENDATIONS

(1) For both birds and fish there are good toxicological test methods but details are still lacking in many cases. Systematic application of these tests and comparison of results using a variety of pollutants are needed.

(2) Some studies of cytogenetic effects of pollutants have been carried out for both fish and birds but not fully evaluated. Cytogenetic methods should be developed and critically assessed. The desirability of incorporating such tests into standard toxicological procedures should be considered.

(3) Field techniques for assessing the effects of pollutants on birds are well advanced. Such techniques should be improved and further developed for fish.

(4) Multigeneration studies for possible built-up of resistance and for cumulative effects should be included into standard tests for birds and fish because increasing damage has been observed in the second and third generations of some species.

(5) The relationship between short-term tests and complete-life-cycle tests should be investigated.

(6) The relevance of reproductive toxicity tests performed on selected species to the survival of populations should be studied.

(7) Testing for the effects of chemicals on reptiles and amphibians is in its infancy. Test procedures should be developed for representative species of these two classes. A freshwater turtle, a lizard, two species of anurans and one species of urodeles are proposed.

4.6 REFERENCES

APHA, AWWA and WPCF (1981). Bioassay procedures for fish (Tentative). In *Standard Methods for the Examination of Water and Waste water*, 15th Edn, pp. 723–743. Prepared and jointly published by the American Public Health Association, American Water Works Association and Water Pollution Control Federation. American Public Health Association, Washington, DC.

ASTM (1981). *Standard Practice for Conducting Toxicity Tests with the Early Life Stages of Fishes* (4th draft), 53 pages. American Society for Testing and Materials, Philadelphia.

Billard, R. (1978a). Effets des alcools gras sur la fécondation et les gamètes de la truite arc-en-ciel. *Bull. Fr. Piscic.* **271**, 3–8.

Billard, R. (1978b). Effect of heat pollution and organo-chlorinated pesticides on fish reproduction. In *Final Reports on Research Sponsored under the First Environmental Research Programme (Indirect Action)*, pp. 265–267. Commission of the European Communities, Brussels.

Billard, R., Cazin, J. C., Dequidt, J., Erb, F. and Colein (1978). Toxicité du pryalène 3010 sur les ovules et les spermatozoides de la truite arc-en-ciel avant et pendant l'insemination. *Bull. Fr. Piscic.* **270**, 238–249.

Bloom, H. D., Perlmutter, A. and Seeley, R. J. (1978). Effect of a sublethal concentration of zinc on an aggregating pheromone system in the zebrafish *Brachydanio rerio* (Hamilton-Buchanan). *Environ. Pollut.* **17**, 127–132.

Bloom, S. E. (1978). Chick embryos for detecting environmental mutagens. In Hollaender, A. and de Serres, F. J. (Eds.) *Chemical Mutagens*, Vol. 5, pp. 203–232. Plenum Press, New York, London.

Bloom, S. E., Povar, G. and Peakall, D. B. (1972). Chromosome preparation from the avian allantoic sac. *Stain Technol.* **47**, 123–127.

Compbell, H. W. and Busack, S. D. (1979). Laboratory maintenance. In Harless, M. and Morlock, H. (Eds.) *Turtles, Perspectives and Research*, pp. 109–126. Wiley & Sons, Chichester, New York, Brisbane, Toronto.

Carnio, J. S. and McQueen, D. J. (1973). Adverse effects of 15 ppm of p, p'-DDT on three generations of Japanese quail. *Can. J. Zool.* **51**, 1307–1312.

Cavanaugh, K. P. and Holmes, W. N. (1982). Effects of ingested petroleum on plasma levels of ovarian steroid hormones in photo-stimulated mallard ducks (*Anas platyrhynchus*). *Arch. Environ. Contam. Toxicol.* **11**, 503–508.

Cole, C. J. and Townsend, C. R. (1977). Parthenogenetic reptiles: new subjects for laboratory research. *Experientia (Basel)* **33**, 285–289.

Conney, A. H. and Klutch, A. (1963). Increased activity of androgen hydroxylases in liver microsomes of rats pretreated with phenobartital and other drugs. *J. biol. Chem.* **238**, 1611–1617.

Cooke, A. S. (1972). The effects of DDT, dieldrin and 2, 4-D on amphibian spawn and tadpoles. *Environ. Pollut.* **3**, 51–68.

Cooke, A. S. (1973). Response of *Rana temporaria* tadpoles to chronic doses of p, p'-DDT. *Copeia* **4**, 647–652.

Curtis, L. R. and Beyers, R. J. (1978). Inhibition of oviposition in the teleost *Oryzias latipes*, induced by subacute kepone exposure. *Comp. Biochem. Physiol.* **C 66**, 15–16.

Donaldson, E. M. (1981). The pituitary-interrenal axis as an indicator of stress in fish. In Pickering, A. D. (Ed.) *Stress and Fish*, pp. 11–47. Academic Press, New York, San Francisco, London.

Dunachie, J. F. and Fletcher, W. W. (1969). An investigation of the toxicity of insecticides to birds' eggs using the egg injection technique. *Ann. appl. Biol.* **64**, 409–423.

Enderson, J. H. and Berger, D. D. (1970). Pesticides: eggshell thinning and lowered production of young in prairie falcons. *BioScience* **20**, 355–356.

Ewert, M. A. (1979). The embryo and its egg: development and natural history. In Harless, M. and Morlock, H. (Eds.) *Turtles, Perspectives and Research*, pp. 109–126. John Wiley & Sons, Chichester, New York, Brisbane, Toronto.

Freeman, N. C., Uthe, J. F. and Sangalang, G. (1980). The use of steroid hormone metabolism studies in assessing the sublethal effects of marine pollution. *Rapp. P.-V. Réun. Cons. Int. Explor. Mer* **179**, 16–22.

Gilman, A. P., Hallett, D. J., Fox, G. A., Allan, L. J., Learning, D. J. and Peakall, D. B. (1978). Effects of injected organochlorines on naturally incubated herring gull eggs. *J. Wildl. Manage.* **42**, 484–493.

Hansen, D. J. (1969). Avoidance of pesticides by untrained sheepshead minnows. *Trans. Am. Fish. Soc.* **98**, 426–429.

Hara, T. J. (1979). An electrophysiological test for neurotoxicity in fish. In Scherer, E. (Ed.) *Toxicity Tests for Freshwater Organisms*. Can. Spec. Publ. Fish. Aquat. Sci. No. 44, 46–56.

Heinz, G. H. (1979). Methylmercury: reproductive and behavioural effects of three generations of mallard ducks. *J. Wildl. Manage.* **43**, 394–401.

Höglund, L. B. (1953). A new method for studying the reactions of fishes in gradients of chemical and other agents. *Oikos* **3**, 247–267.

Holmes, W. N. and Gorsline, J. (1981). Effects on some environmental pollutants on the adrenal cortex. Symposium on Adrenal Steroid Biosynthesis. In Cummings, I. A., Funder, J. W. and Mendelsohn, F. A. O. (Eds.) *Proceedings of the VIth International Congress of Endocrinology, Melbourne, Australia*, pp. 311–314. Australian Academy of Science, Canberra.

Kaplan, H. M. (1974). Reptiles in laboratory animal science. In Melby, E. C. Jr. and Altman, N. H. (Eds.) *Handbook of Laboratory Animal Science*, Vol. I, pp. 285–417. CRC Press, Cleveland, Ohio.

Kihlström, J. E., Laudberg, C. and Halth, L. (1971). Number of eggs and young produced by zebrafish (*Brachydanio rerio*, Ham.-Buch.) spawning in water containing small amounts of phenylmercuric acetate. *Environ. Res.* **4**, 355–359.

Laale, H. W. (1977). The biology and use of zebrafish *Brachydanio rerio* in fisheries research. A literature review. *J. Fish Biol.* **10**, 121–173.

Lehrman, D. S. (1964). The reproductive behaviour of ring doves. *Sci. Am.* **211**, 48–54.

Licht, P. (1971). Regulation of the annual cycle by photoperiod and temperature in the lizard, *Anolis carolinensis*. *Ecology* **52**, 40–252.

Lillie, W. R., Harrison, S. E., Macdonald, W. A. and Klaverkamp, J. E. (1979). The use of the zebrafish (*Brachydanio*) in whole life-cycle tests. In Scherer, E. (Ed.) *Toxicity Tests for Freshwater Organisms*. Can. Spec. Publ. Fish. Aquat. Sci., No. 44, 104–111.

Longcore, J. R. and Stendell, R. C. (1977). Shell thinning and reproductive impairment in black ducks after cessation of DDE dosage. *Archs Environ. Contam. Toxicol.* **6**, 293–304.

Longwell, A. C. and Hughes, J. B. (1980). Cytologic, cytogenetic, and developmental state of Atlantic mackerel eggs from sea surface waters of the New York bight, and prospects for biological effects monitoring with ichthyoplankton. *Rapp. P.-V. Réun. Cons. Int. Explor. Mer* **179**, 275–291.

Macek, K. J. and Sleight, B. H., III (1977). Utility of toxicity tests with embryos and fry of fish in evaluating hazards associated with the chronic toxicity of chemicals to fishes. In Mayer, F. L. and Hamelink, J. L. (Eds.) *Aquatic Toxicology and Hazard Evaluation*, ASTM STP 634, pp. 137–146, American Society for Testing and Materials, Washington, DC.

Mathews, J. G., Favor, J. B. and Crenshaw, J. W. (1978). Dominant lethal effects of triethylenemelamine in the guppy *Poecilia reticulata*. *Mutat. Res.* **54**, 149–157.

McArthur, M. L. B. (1980). *The Effects of p, p'-DDE, PCBs, Mirex and Photomirex on the Reproductive Behaviour and Success of Ring Doves and Related Physiological Responses.* M.Sc. Thesis, University of Ottawa, Canada.

McKim, J. M. (1977). Evaluation of tests with early life stages of fish for predicting long-term toxicity. *J. Fish. Res. Board Can.* **34**, 1148–1154.

McLane, M. A. R. and Hall, L. C. (1972). DDE thins screech owl eggshells. *Bull. Environ. Contam. Toxicol.* **8**, 65–68.

McLaughlin, J., Jr., Marliac, J.-P., Verret, M. H., Mutchler, M. E. and Fitzhugh, O. G. (1963). The injection of chemicals into the yolk sac of fertile eggs prior to incubation as a toxicity test. *Toxic. appl. Pharmac.* **5**, 760–771.

NAS (1974). *Amphibians. Guideline for the Breeding, Care, and Management of*

Laboratory Animals. A report of the Subcommittee on Amphibian Standards, Committee on Standards, Institute of Laboratory Animal Resources, National Research Council, National Academy of Sciences, Washington, DC.

Osborn, D. and Harris, M. P. (1979). A procedure for implanting a slow release formulation of an environmental pollutant into a free-living animal. *Environ. Pollut.* **19**, 139–144.

Peakall, D. B., Fox, G. A., Gilman, A. P., Hallett, D. J. and Norstrom, R. J. (1980). Reproductive success of herring gulls as an indicator of Great Lakes Water quality. In Afghan, B. K. and Mackay, D. (Eds.) *Hydrocarbons and Halogenated Hydrocarbons in the Aquatic Environment*, pp. 337–344. Plenum Press, New York and London.

Peakall, D. B., Lincer, J. L. and Bloom, S. E. (1972). Embryonic mortality and chromosomal alterations caused by Aroclor 1254 in ring doves. *Environ. Health Perspect.* **1**, 103–104.

Peakall, D. B. and Peakall, M. L. (1973). Effect of a polychlorinated biphenyl on the reproduction of artificially and naturally incubated dove eggs. *J. appl. Ecol.* **10**, 363–868.

Peakall, D. B., Tremblay, Jr., Kinter, W. B. and Miller, D. S. (1981). Endocrine dysfunction in seabirds caused by ingested oil. *Environ. Res.* **24**, 6–14.

Pierson, K. B. (1981). Effects of chronic zinc exposure on the growth, sexual maturity, reproduction and bioaccumulation of the guppy, *Poecilia reticulata*. *Can. J. Fish. Aquat. Sci.* **38**, 23–31.

Porter, R. D. and Wiemeyer, S. H. (1969). Dieldrin and DDT: effects of sparrow hawk eggshells and reproduction. *Science* (*Washington, DC*) **165**, 199–200.

Pough, F. G. (1976). Acid precipitation and embryonic mortality of spotted salamanders, *Ambystoma maculatum, Science* (*Washington, DC*) **192**, 68–70.

Powell, G. V. N. and Gray, D. C. (1980). Dosing free-living nestling starlings with an organophosphate pesticide Famphur. *J. Wildl. Manage.* **44**, 918–921.

Ruby, S. M., Aczel, J. and Craig, G. R. (1977). The effects of depressed pH on oogenesis in flagfish *Jordanella floridae*. *Water Res.* **11**, 757–762.

Ruby, S. M., Aczel, J. and Craig, G. R. (1978). The effects of depressed pH on spermatogenesis in flagfish *Jordanella floridae*. *Water Res.* **12**, 621–626.

Saber, P. A. and Dunson, W. A. (1978). Toxocity of bog water to embryonic and larval anuran amphibians. *J. exp. Zool.* **204**, 33–42.

Sangalang, G. B. and Freeman, H. C. (1974). Effects of sublethal cadmium on maturation and testosterone and 11-ketotestosterone production *in vivo* in book trout. *Biol. Reprod.* **11**, 429–435.

Sangalang, G. B. and O'Halloran, M. J. (1973). Adverse effects of cadmium on brook trout testis and on *in vitro* testicular androgen synthesis. *Biol. Reprod.* **9**, 394–403.

Scherer, E. and Nowak, S. (1973). Apparatus for recording avoidance movements of fish. *J. Fish. Res. Board Can.* **30**, 1594–1596.

Singh, H. and Singh, T. P. (1980). Effect of two pesticides on ovarian ^{32}P uptake and gonadotropin concentration during different phases of annual reproductive cycle in the freshwater catfish, *Heteropneustes fossilis* (Bloch). *Environ. Res.* **22**, 190–200.

Sivarajah, K., Franklin, C. S. and Williams, W. P. (1978). The effects of polychlorinated biphenyls on plasma steroid levels and hepatic microsomal enzymes in fish. *J. Fish Biol.* **13**, 401–410.

Smith, W. E. (1973). A cyprinodontid fish *Jordanella floridae* as a laboratory animal for rapid chronic bioassays. *J. Fish. Res. Board Can,* **30**, 329–330.

Sprague, J. B. (1964). Avoidance of copper-zinc solutions by young salmon in the laboratory. *J. Water Pollut. Control Fedn* **36**, 990–1004.

Stoss, F. W. and Haines, T. A. (1979). The effects of toluene on embryos and fry of the

Japanese medaka *Oryzias latipes* with a proposal for rapid determination of maximum acceptable toxicant concentration. *Environ. Pollut.* **20**, 139–148.

Weseloh, D. V., Mineau, P. and Hallett, D. J. (1979). Organochlorine contaminants and trends in reproduction in Great Lakes herring gulls, 1974–1978. In *Trans. North Amer. Wildl. Nat. Resour. Conf.* **44**, 543–557.

Wiemeyer, S. N., Spitzer, P. R., Krant, W. C., Lamont, T. G. and Cromartie, E. (1975). Effects of environmental pollutants on Connecticut and Maryland ospreys. *J. Wildl. Manage.* **39**, 124–139.

Methods for Assessing the Effects of Chemicals on Reproductive Functions
Edited by V. B. Vouk and P. J. Sheehan
© 1983 SCOPE

5 *Invertebrates**

The invertebrate phyla constitute an extraordinarily diverse variety of organisms, ranging from the simple sponges to complex arthropods such as insects, and occupying every habitat: marine, freshwater, terrestrial and aerial. They are also extraordinarily numerous, constituting by far the majority of described animal species. For example, the class Insecta alone represents more than 90% of the known species of animals. In terms of total numbers they are equally impressive: there are estimated to be 300,000 individual insects alive for every man, woman and child on earth.

But it is not simply their numbers which render invertebrates important to man, although their dominance alone is sufficient to warrent our attention. Invertebrates play a critical role in several components of our ecosystem. Coral reefs owe their existence to Cnidaria. Nematodes are an important component of our soil fauna. Crustaceans play an important role in aquatic and marine food chains. Among the polychaete worms, a dominant group of intertidal and subtidal bottom communities, some species may serve as important indicators of pollution. Pulmonate snails and insects serve as intermediate hosts of some of the most important diseases of man and his domestic animals such as schistosomiasis, malaria and sleeping sickness. Invertebrates serve as food for humans and pollinate our plants. At the same time other invertebrates destroy our crops and reduce the quality of our life. Invertebrates thus represent an important component of all ecosystems of our planet, and interact both directly and indirectly with man, affecting both his health and the renewable resources upon which his existence depends. Thus, the effects of chemicals on invertebrate reproduction is of vital interest for human welfare.

In this report reproduction is defined as those processes which contribute in a direct way to the production of viable offspring. It is recognized that many developmental processes might be regarded as contributing in an indirect way to reproduction, in the sense that all physiological and developmental processes are directed ultimately towards reproduction or survival for reproduction. However, the Workgroup elected to be more restrictive and has concentrated on those processes which impinge directly on the production, release, and bringing together of the gametes in order to produce a viable offspring capable of

* This section was prepared by a Workgroup chaired by V. Landa. The rapporteur was K. G. Davey, and members were Bertil Åkesson, D. R. Dixon, B. V. Leone and Oscar Ravera.

development towards the adult reproducing form. As has been made clear elsewhere in this report, our knowledge of these processes is rudimentary for many taxa. This lack of knowledge should not be mistaken for simplicity; as research proceeds, it is becoming clear that reproductive processes in many invertebrate taxa are comparable in complexity to those in vertebrates.

In seeking to identify organisms from among the myriad of forms which offer themselves to be used as potential test species, two sorts of criteria apply. On the one hand are minimum essential characteristics which such organisms must, in the short term, display:

(1) The organism must reproduce in such a way that it is possible to obtain, as a minimum requirement, a quantitative description of the production of viable offspring.
(2) The organism should be representative of the community or ecosystem under scrutiny.
(3) The organism should be capable of being reared in the laboratory conveniently and inexpensively.

On the other hand, there are some desirable characteristics which such a test organism should be capable, in the long run, of displaying:

(1) There should be a rather complete description of the reproductive process at all levels. At the very least, there should exist the capability for obtaining this information.
(2) There should be some confidence that the response of the selected organism is in some way predictive of the response of that and other related organisms in the field.
(3) The food source used in rearing the organisms in the laboratory should preferably not itself be alive. The potential interaction of a living food source with the introduced chemical will complicate the interpretation of any results obtained.

The strict observance of even the minimum criteria for adoption of a test organism imposes severe limits on the number of organisms available for selection. Because there is no prospect for easy cultivation in the laboratory or because they play a limited or cryptic role in the ecosystem, Porifera and the protochordates are eliminated from consideration. Parasitic forms will not be considered, and Echinodermata will be dealt with as a special case.

5.1 FIELD STUDIES AND ANALYSES OF FIELD-COLLECTED MATERIAL

Given the difficulty of cultivating many of the ecologically significant species in the laboratory, methods for assessing reproductive function in the field assume a particular importance. Such studies are especially valuable where a comparison is made between a polluted environment and one in which pollution is minimal or absent, or where the study is conducted along a pollution gradient.

Because the general field of reproductive physiology of invertebrates is underdeveloped compared with that of most vertebrate taxa, tests for the assessment of reproductive function will have to rely on morphological or histological criteria. Biochemical assays are still over the horizon. Even in insects, where the endocrinology of reproduction is perhaps best understood, and where more than ten different hormones are envisaged as impinging upon the reproductive process, only three hormones have been fully characterized, and a reliable radioimmunoassay exists for only one of them. In those organisms in which a vitellogenin appears in the blood, a quantitative estimate of that protein, obtained perhaps by an immunoassay, might yield a good index of the reproductive function of the organism.

It is important that histological assessments be quantified. This can take a number of forms, such as the percentage of individuals in which the gonads can be assigned to various accepted growth stages. A more rigorous approach has been referred to elsewhere (Dixon, 1983, this volume). By using a Weibel test grid superimposed on randomly selected sections, an estimate of the volume fraction occupied by various tissue components in the gonad of *Mytilus edulis* can be derived, and can be used as a numerical index of reproductive function. This technique, which is relatively rapid and susceptible to considerable automation by various commercially available image analysers, deserves to be elaborated upon and standardized with a view to a more general adoption.

Histological examination of insect gonads has also been widely used in a variety of ways as an index of reproductive function. For example, extensive studies on the effects of chemosterilants during the last 20 years have involved histological characterization of lesions in the gonads, other reproductive organs and embryos. However, no standardized, quantifiable set of tests has emerged as a candidate for possible adoption.

Cages of particular invertebrate species, placed in polluted and unpolluted natural environments or along a pollution gradient might provide quantitative information about reproductive function in a quasi-natural environment free of the effects of competition and predation (Reish and Barnard, 1960). Similarly, enclosures have been used to conduct quantitative studies on manageable portions of an ecosystem which can be manipulated in various ways (Kerrison *et al.*, 1980).

5.2 LABORATORY STUDIES

Laboratory studies will, in the interest of standardization and because relatively few species are available in the laboratory, be confined to only a handful of species. Inevitably, some species may come to be considered as 'model species' for a taxon or a habitat. There are dangers in such a situation and it is important to be clear about the predictive value of such studies. When a chemical has been shown to have an effect on reproduction of a species in a laboratory culture, the only fact about which we can be certain is that the chemical affects that species in the laboratory. There is a relatively high degree of probability that a similar effect would be noted in that species in the field, but the reliability of such a prediction will decrease with the complexity of the ecosystem in which the species exists naturally and with the taxonomic distance of potential target species from the test species. Compromises are probably acceptable when a chemical with a pronounced effect is involved. However, when such tests are used as screens by industry or regulatory agencies, the meaning of a marginal effect or the absence of an effect becomes important. Few scientists would be willing to say that the absence of an effect on, for example, *Daphnia* predicts with a high degree of certainty that lobsters or terrestrial isopods, let alone annelids, will be unaffected.

These considerations imply that several test organisms from each of the major taxa would be desirable. While many of the invertebrate phyla are predominantly marine dwellers, several of these phyla also contain freshwater or terrestrial members, and it will be important to identify potentially useful species.

The conditions of the test require some general consideration. Under ideal conditions in a laboratory monoculture, test organisms are not subject to the same physiological and environmental stress as are wild populations. In the interests of uniformity, non-stressed animals are probably preferred, but the possibility of parallel or subsidiary tests using stressed animals needs to be considered.

The method of application of the chemical may require special attention. For marine and aquatic organisms the chemical need only be dissolved or suspended in the medium, and its concentration maintained. The concentration of the chemical may be maintained by a flow-through system or by more or less frequent additions. In such a situation, the organism may acquire the chemical not only through its surface, but also via the food. For terrestrial organisms the method of application is more complex. The chemical may be mixed with the food or coated on the surface of the container in which the organisms are reared. Where a single non-chronic exposure is acceptable, a single application to the surface or an injection may be appropriate. Application is further complicated when a larval form inhabits a distinctly different niche from the adult form, as with many insects and sedentary marine invertebrates.

Many variables could be measured in the laboratory. However, given our definition of reproduction and the relatively underdeveloped state of the field, the basic variable to be measured should be the number of viable offspring produced. Where the mode of action of a particular toxicant becomes important, the reasons for alteration in the basic rate of reproduction can be sought by examining the various organizational and functional levels as pointed out elsewhere (Davey *et al.*, 1983, this volume). Uniform methods for making such diagnoses do not yet exist, and the potential availability of such methods will vary from taxon to taxon. In a few instances, when selected components of the reproductive process can be studied in the laboratory, it may be necessary to use species which are readily available but not capable of being reared in the laboratory. These will be mentioned in the following discussion of the major taxa.

5.2.1 Platyhelminthes

Although the free-living flatworms such as the turbellarians are easily raised in the laboratory, and although we know something of their reproductive physiology, it is not recommended that this group be given a high priority at this time, on two grounds. First, the group is not regarded as occupying an important position in ecological terms. Second, there are some practical difficulties to be faced. Turbellarians are carnivores and frequently cannibalize one another. Given that they reproduce by fissiparity, this represents a major potential complication. In addition, they may refuse to eat contaminated food, resulting in a cessation of reproduction and a reversal of growth.

5.2.2 Cnidaria

Colonial hydroids such as *Eirene viridula* (Karbe, 1972) and *Campanularia flexuosa* (Stebbing, 1976, 1980) have been used as laboratory test organisms and are among the most sensitive. Effects on colony growth rates and proportion of gonozooids of the total colony members can be easily quantified. In *C. flexuosa*, gonozooid formation increased at contaminant concentrations often as low as $0.1 \mu g/1$ (Stebbing, 1980).

5.2.3 Aschelminthes

Samoiloff *et al.* (1980) developed a procedure for assessing the effects of chemicals on the development of and the mutation rate in the nematode *Panagrellus redivivus*. Although the assay as presently outlined does not specifically measure reproduction as defined here, the method would require only minor modifications in order to be able to assess the effects of chemicals on numbers of young produced. However, we know little about the basic facts of reproduction, so that further analysis would not be possible for the present.

Another aschelminth, the parthenogenic freshwater gastrotrich *Lepidodermella squammata*, has been used in a novel approach to the question of chronic toxicity testing. In effect, using single organisms, Hummon and Hummon (1975) and Faucon and Hummon (1976) have constructed life tables. Such an approach is very time consuming but generates a great deal of data.

5.2.4 Annelida

5.2.4.1 Polychaeta

Representatives from several important polychaete families (*Capitella capitata, Neanthes arenaceodentata, Ophryotrocha*) are already recognized as suitable test organisms. Whereas the effects of pollution on offspring numbers and viability are the primary concern in the present context, it is now possible to quantify most stages in reproduction, i.e. gametogenesis, egg and sperm abnormalities, fertilization, fertility, fecundity, developmental abnormalities, larval mortality and recruitment. Åkesson (1983, this volume) reports several case studies which indicate that the 'no toxic effect levels' (Hooftman and Wink, 1980) for various reproductive stages in the group are two to three orders of magnitude below the recognized 96-hour LC_{50} levels. This emphasizes the sensitivity of response associated with this type of approach. The tests can be performed over a single reproductive cycle or extended to include several generations. Semelparous species (reproducing only once in their lifetime) are less suitable than are the iteroparous species (breeding several times each lifetime) for long-term tests where the individuals are subject to prolonged exposures. In the case of the latter species, the experimental conditions can be extended so that the results can be analysed by life-table techniques, and thus provide a connection to population dynamics and, consequently, to the field situation. Alternatively, specific aspects of the reproductive cycle of some species may be used for studying the action of chemicals and its consequences.

One recent development has been the introduction of a new test species of polychaetes, the serpulid *Pomatoceros triqueter* (Dixon, 1981), whose embryos are excellent material for cytogenetic toxicity testing. The cells of the embryos are large and contain chromosomes which are less condensed and, consequently, larger than at any other stage in the organism's development. *Pomatoceros* has a karyotype consisting of 24 metacentric and submetacentric chromosomes. It is a broadcast spawner producing large numbers of gametes without the marked seasonality which is generally associated with gametogenesis in other groups. These features together with the worm's tolerance of aquarium conditions ensure a continuous supply of gametes for artificial fertilization to provide suitable embryonic material for cytogenetic and toxicological investigations. Aspects of the ecology and physiology of *Pomatoceros*—its sedentary filter-feeding habit, wide local (eurybathic) and geographical distributions, and the ability to withstand significant reductions in salinity—enhance the utility of this species for environmental monitoring.

A few asexually reproducing polychaetes are now available as test organisms. *Ctenodrilus serratus* has been used by Reish and his collaborators (Reish, 1978; Reish and Carr, 1978). A new dorvilleid species was recommended by Åkesson (1980) who also described those features pertinent to its selection for toxicity studies. An important feature was the ability to synchronize the reproductive states and the developmental and physiological conditions of clonal populations of this species by simple laboratory manipulation.

5.2.4.2 *Oligochaeta*

The oligochaetes, because of their burrowing habit, are in general less suitable for laboratory studies of chemical toxicity. However, a few species need to be identified as possible test organisms in view of the importance of the group both in the soil and in aquatic, freshwater and estuarine environments. These are: the terrestrial marine worm, *Eisenia foetida*, which is already maintained in large numbers in laboratory cultures (e.g. Dales, 1978); the white worm, *Enchytraeus*, now raised commercially as a fish food, and the freshwater blood worm, *Tubifex* sp. for use in aquatic studies.

5.2.5 Arthropoda

5.2.5.1 *Crustacea*

This is a diverse class within the phylum Arthropoda, occupying prominent positions in marine, freshwater, and, to a lesser degree, soil environments. In particular Crustacea occupy important positions in food chains in marine and freshwater environments, and of course the decapods are economically important in commerce.

The OECD (1981) guidelines for testing the effects of chemicals on the familiar *Daphnia magna* are excellent and may serve as a model for the development of similar guidelines for other organisms. In particular, these procedures should prove satisfactory in tests involving other small crustacea, such as harpacticoid copepods, thus extending the range of tests to include marine crustaceans.

Terrestrial isopods such as *Oniscus* are important components of the soil fauna, and can be reared in the laboratory (Steel, 1980). It would be useful to develop tests involving these organisms, especially since some of the facts of reproduction are now becoming known.

Because they have an extremely long generation time, there is little point in considering the decapods as potential test organisms at this time. However, in the crab *Pachygrapsas crassipes*, exposure to environmental chemicals destroyed mating behaviour (Kittredge *et al.*, 1974). It is possible that this might form the basis for a quantitative assay, but this should not have a high priority.

5.2.5.2 *Insecta*

The class Insecta presents us with an embarrassment of riches by comparison with the other taxa in this section. Many species are routinely cultured in the laboratory and some have been the subject of acute toxicity tests. Almost all of these represent potential test organisms which fulfil most of the minimum requirements outlined in the introduction. In addition, for several species, the basic facts of the morphology, physiology and endocrinology of the reproductive system, particularly as they apply to the female, are becoming known. It should be possible, therefore, to analyse the physiological changes and their morphological consequences involved in disturbances caused by chemicals.

There are, however, some special considerations. In some orders, the larvae tend to occupy habitats which are quite different from those of the adult. Gametogenesis at least is not limited to the adult stage, and is frequently complete by the end of the pupal stage. Insects are generally quite conservative in terms of the physiological controls which are imposed on reproduction, so that it is possible to make some generalizations which apply to the broad majority of insects. Nevertheless, there are signs that some of the Diptera may have a set of endocrine controls which differs markedly from that of other insects. While a good deal is known about the female, less is known about the male. Finally, there is no single species in which all of the phenomena impinging on reproduction have been adequately described. These considerations suggest that a number of test species should be developed. Such species are listed together with their advantages and disadvantages. It is important to point out that while no tests exist which specifically focus on reproduction, the many studies on the effects of chemosterilants on the insect gonad and embryogenesis provide a good basis for further studies (Landa, 1983, this volume).

Musca domestica, the common housefly, is probably the insect of choice for basic screening of the effects of chemicals on reproductive processes. It is easily raised, genetically defined strains are available, and it has been widely used in toxicological studies. In addition, the physiology and histology of the development of the gonads is well known.

Pyrrhocoris apterus, a hemipteran which feeds on the seeds of the lime tree, *Tilia europaea*, and which can be easily reared in the laboratory, has been widely used in studies on reproduction (see Landa, 1983, this volume). This insect provides an example of a phytophagous species in which the development of the ovary is well known. In addition, its embryology is well known and sex determination occurs later than in other insects.

Rhodnius prolixus, another hemipteran, feeds on blood and is a vector of Chagas' disease. It has been widely used in studies on reproduction for over 50 years and it is easily maintained in the laboratory. Although *Rhodnius* has a long life cycle (at least 15 weeks), it has some special advantages. A great deal is known about the reproductive endocrinology of the female and it is the only insect for which there is information about the endocrinology of testis development and the physiology of semen transfer. Moreover, egg production can be highly quantified (Davey, 1980).

Aedes aegypti is chosen not only as an example of an insect of health importance, but also as a representative of aquatic insects. Moreover, genetically defined strains exist and the World Health Organization has guidelines for toxicity testing on larvae and adults (WHO, 1975). These advantages outweigh the disadvantages of the need for a blood meal in order to produce eggs.

As a representative of lower insects the cockroach, *Leucophaea maderae*, has been selected. Although its developmental cycle is relatively long, a very great deal is known about reproductive processes in the female (Engelmann, 1980; Tobe, 1980).

Other insects are also available. Lepidoptera such as *Spodoptera littoralis* and stored product beetles such as *Dermestes* or *Trogoderma* have been widely used in assessing the damage from chemosterilants.

Few if any of the insects mentioned above could be regarded as occupying a central position in their biological community. They have been chosen primarily because of the ease with which they can be reared and the knowledge which is available about their reproductive function. A long-term objective includes the identification and development of insect models which will serve as more effective ecological indicators.

5.2.6 Mollusca

The bivalve molluscs are the marine species which have received the most attention. Many are of economic importance as food organisms for man or his food species, while being dominant both numerically and in terms of biomass in aquatic communities. A large body of information exists concerning all aspects of the biology of the family Mytilidae (Bayne, 1976).

Mytilus edulis, the blue mussel and near relatives, has been selected as a test organism for a number of pollution-oriented, international programmes of research including 'Mussel Watch', in which the ability to bioaccumulate xenobiotic compounds in their tissues is being exploited for chemical monitoring of the marine environment (Bayne, 1976; Goldberg, 1978). Selection was based on the recognition of its important role in marine food chains, coupled with a filter-feeding habit, capacity for bioaccumulating toxic agents from seawater, world-wide distribution and convenient size for experimentation. An additional advantage of these organisms is their physiological tolerance of reduced salinity, which is expressed in their wide natural distribution that extends from brackish environments to oceanic conditions. Consequently, a great deal is known about bivalve molluscs, probably more than for any other group of marine invertebrates. Marine mussels have proven reproductive sensitivity to sublethal chemical perturbations in their environment, which becomes expressed at different stages in their development at different levels of functional and cellular organization (Dixon, 1983, this volume).

In contrast, gastropods are generally less well understood with respect to the effects of chemicals on reproductive function. In the marine environment, our knowledge is restricted to some particular aspects of the reproductive process in a very few species. Those that have been studied do indicate, however, that some present research methods are likely to develop into useful tests for application both in the laboratory and in field monitoring. This applies particularly to the embryonic development of *Littorina saxatilis* in relation to a pollution exposure model referred to in the paper by D. R. Dixon (1983, this volume).

More is known about the freshwater gastropod species and particularly such pulmonates as *Lymnaea stagnalis, Physa acuta and Biomphalaria glabrata* (Ravera, 1977). Advantages of this group include: easy and inexpensive rearing in the laboratory of large numbers through a large number of generations; high fertility; year-round reproduction; mean life span of about 2 years; high hatching rate; rapid sexual maturity (3–4 weeks following hatching); and hermaphroditism with male and female sex cells in the same gland (ovotestis) (each receives the same treatment). Other advantages include their well-known reproductive physiology; the possibility of using either natural or artificial conditions for reproduction and development; and well-documented embryonic development which closely parallels that described for *Littorina*, although in these freshwater forms the development occurs outside the adult in an egg capsule which is laid near the food source.

As mentioned above, freshwater snails include a number of important disease vectors. *Biomphalaria glabrata* should be mentioned here in particular since this is the intermediate host for the organism *Schistosoma*.

Regarding sensitivity to pollutants, studies have shown that the reproduction of freshwater gastropods is extremely sensitive to a variety of chemical agents including heavy metals and detergents (Mariani, 1977; Ravera, 1977). Several test methods relating to reproductive function are available. These include histological changes in the gonad, fecundity (expressed both as egg numbers and viability) and fertility. One final advantage of this class appears to be the relative insensitivity of their reproductive function to natural stressors such as reduced oxygen tension and high organic levels.

5.2.7 Echinodermata

It is very difficult to raise echinoderms in the laboratory, and this phylum would normally not be considered further. However, the gametes of sea urchins are easily obtained and have been widely used in studies of the physiology and biochemistry of spermatozoa, of fertilization and of early development. There have been some excellent studies of the effect of toxicants on the gamete (Davey *et al.*, 1983, this volume). Because these studies may have some general applicability in terms of screening, it is important that a standardized test be established. Because no one species of sea urchins is distributed throughout the world, several species will have to be used.

5.3 CONCLUSIONS AND RECOMMENDATIONS

(1) Except for some arthropods (Crustacea and Insecta), nematodes and a marine annelid, there are no procedures available at this time which would be suitable for adoption as rapid and cost-effective assays of reproductive function in any invertebrate phylum.

(2) Because of their important role in ecosystems, there is a particularly urgent need for the development of assays of reproductive function in the following groups: marine Cnidaria, soil organisms (annelids and arthropods) and gastropod molluscs.

(3) The development of standard assays capable of assessing reproductive function of invertebrates in the field should be given some priority.

(4) The development of reliable and adequate assays is impeded by the scarcity of detailed information on all aspects of reproductive function in invertebrates. More basic research in this area is urgently required.

5.4 REFERENCES

Åkesson, B. (1980). The use of certain polychaetes in bioassay studies, *Rapp. P. V. Réun. Cons. Int. Explor. Mer.* **179**, 305–321.

Bayne, B. L. (Ed.) (1976). *Marine Mussels: Their Ecology and Physiology* (International Biological Programme Ser., No. 10), 506 pages. Cambridge University Press, Cambridge, London, New York, Melbourne.

Dales, R. P. (1978). Basis of graft rejection in earthworms *Lumibricus terrestris* and *Eisernia foetida*. *Invertebr. Path.* **32**, 264–277.

Davey, K. G. (1980). The physiology of reproduction in *Rhodnius* and some other insects: some questions. In Locke, M. and Smith, D. S. (Eds.) *Insect Biology in the Future*, pp. 325–344. Academic Press, New York.

Dixon, D. R. (1981). *Pomotoceros triqueter* (L.), a test system for environmental mutagenesis. In Bayne, B. L. (Ed.) *The Effects of Stress and Pollution on Marine Animals*. Praeger Publishers, New York.

Engelmann, F. (1980). Endocrine control of vitellogenin synthesis. In Smith, D. C. and Locke, M. (Eds.) *Insect Biology in the Future*, pp. 311–324. Academic Press, New York, San Francisco, London.

Faucon, A. S. and Hummon, W. D. (1976). Effects of mine acid on the longevity and reproductive rate of the Gastrotricha *Lepidodermella squammata* (Dujardin). *Hydrobiologia* **50**, 265–269.

Goldberg, E. D. (1978). The mussel watch. *Environ. Conserv.* **5**, 1–25.

Hooftman, R. N. and Wink, G. J. (1980). The determination of toxic effects of pollutants with the marine polychaete worm *Ophryotrocha diadema*. *Ecotoxicol. Environ. Saf.* **1**, 252–262.

Hummon, W. D. and Hummon, W. R. (1975). Use of life table data in tolerance experiments. *Cah. Biol. Mar.* **16**, 743–749.

Karbe, L. (1972). Marine Hydroiden als Testorganismen zur Prüfung der Toxizität von Abwasserstoffen: die Wirkung von Schwermetallen auf Kolonien von *Eirene viridula*. *Mar. Biol. (Berlin)* **12**, 316–328.

Kerrison, P. H., Sprocati, A. R., Ravera, O. and Amantini, L. (1980). Effects of cadmium on an aquatic community using artificial enclosures. *Environ. Technol. Letters* **1**, 169–176.

Kittredge, J. S., Takahashi, F. T. and Sarinana, F. (1974). Bioassays indicative of some sublethal effects of oil pollution. *Proceedings, MTS 10th Ann. Conf.*, pp. 891–897.

Mariani, M. (1977). *Effeti letali e subletali d'alcuni metalli (Al, Ni, Cu, In, Cd, Hg, Pb) su adulti e embrioni di* Biomphalaria glabrata *e* Lymneaea stagniedis. Thesis, University of Milan.

OECD (1981). *Guidelines for the Testing of Chemicals*, 700 pages. Organization of Economic Cooperation and Development, Paris.

Ravera, O. (1977). Effects of heavy metals (cadmium, copper, chromium and lead) on a freshwater snail *Biomphalaria glabrata* (Gastropoda, Prosobranchia). *Malacologia* **16(1)**, 231–236.

Reish, D. J. (1978). The effects of heavy metals on polychaetous annelids. *Rev. Int. Océanogr. Méd.* **49**, 99–104.

Reish, D. J. and Barnard, J. L. (1960). Field toxicity tests in marine waters utilizing the polychaetous annelid *Capitella capitata* (Fabricius). *Pac. Naturalist* **1(21–22)**, 1–8.

Reish, D. J. and Carr, K. S. (1978). The effect of heavy metals on the survival, reproduction, development, and life cycle for two species of polychaetous annelids. *Mar. Pollut. Bull.* **9(1)**, 24–27.

Samoiloff, M. R., Schulz, S., Jordan, Y., Dernch, K. and Arnett, E. (1980). A rapid, simple long-term toxicity assay for aquatic contaminants using the nematode *Panagrellus redivivus. Can. J. Fish. Aquat. Sci.* **27**, 1167–1174.

Stebbing, A. R. D. (1976). The effects of low metal levels on a clonal hydroid. *J. Mar. Biol. Ass. U.K.* **56**, 977–994.

Stebbing, A. R. D. (1980). The biological measurement of water quality. *Rapp. P.-V. Réun. Cons. Int. Explor. Mer.* **179**, 310–314.

Steel, C. G. H. (1980). Mechanism of coordination between moulting and reproduction in terrestrial isopod crustacea. *Biol. Bull. (Woods Hole, Mass.)* **159**, 206–218.

Tobe, S. S. (1980). Regulation of the corpora allata in adult female insects. In Locke, M. and Smith, D. C. (Eds.) *Insect Biology in the Future*, pp. 345–368. Academic Press, New York, San Francisco, London.

WHO (1975) *Manual on Practical Entomology in Malaria, Part II. Methods and Techniques*, World Health Organisation, Geneva.

Methods for Assessing the Effects of Chemicals on Reproductive Functions
Edited by V. B. Vouk and P. J. Sheehan
© 1983 SCOPE

6 Higher Plants, Algae and Microorganisms*

A superficial review may reveal some features common to higher plants, algae and microorganisms, such as photosynthesis, but fundamentally there are so many major differences between these groups that this section of the report had to be divided into two separate parts:

(1) higher plants, and
(2) microorganisms, including algae.

As a consequence little discussion is devoted to macroscopic algae, attention being directed principally towards the unicellular members of this large group of organisms.

6.1 HIGHER PLANTS

The term 'higher plants' includes more than 150,000 species in the division Spermatophyta which constitute a major part of the earth's visible vegetation in the form of trees, shrubs and herbs, and contains a major portion of the species used for human food, fibre and forestry products. Reproduction in higher plants, defined in an evolutionary or ecological sense, is the number of reproducing descendants generated by a species either sexually or asexually. This broad definition is necessary because higher plant species differ greatly in the length of life cycle, and chemicals introduced at any stage of their life cycle can ultimately alter reproduction.

The selection and development of accurate and meaningful tests require an understanding of the diversity of higher plant species, the diverse biological effects known to be produced by a large number of chemicals, the species–chemicals interactions, and the effects of the environment on both the species and the chemical. Differences between and within species in morphological, physiological and genetic characteristics and the environmental influences on the expression of these characteristics alter the response to a chemical. A wide range of organic and inorganic chemicals is known to change plant growth, development and reproduction, and their effects are modified by numerous environmental factors. At this degree of complexity, the development of such multitiered

---

* This section was prepared by a Workgroup chaired by J. H. Slater. Members were Arne Jensen (rapporteur) and Paul L. Pfahler.

assays as are used to predict the mutagenicity and carcinogenicity of chemical compounds to human subjects is not feasible for plants (Epler *et al.*, 1978; Heath, 1978). These rapid assays are based on the apparently correct assumption that any chemical that will induce mutations and/or chromosomal damage in certain microbes or mice will induce similar effects in humans. In higher plants, possible effects of chemical pollutants include mutations and chromosomal damage and a wide array of morphological and physiological alterations which depend on species and environmental factors and can ultimately alter reproduction. *In vitro* tests involving isolated enzyme systems or organelles, single cell cultures and selected plant tissues—which are of particular value when a quantitative measure of a specific response such as inhibition of growth, photosynthesis or respiration is required—are severely limited in their predictive value for intact, integrated plant systems since a far too narrow definition of biological activity of chemicals is often imposed (Saggers, 1976). Little is known about the relationship between *in vitro* and *in vivo* plant responses and, as a result, the predictive value of *in vitro* tests—which may be useful for the solution of certain specific problems—is uncertain.

At such a level of complexity with respect to diversity of species, chemicals and environments, the selection of an 'ideal' test with adequate predictability (defined as the ability of test results gathered from a few species to predict accurately the effect of chemicals on most if not all higher plant species), reproducibility (defined as the ability to duplicate the results which, in the case of higher plants, requires sufficient control of species variability and of environmental conditions), and sensitivity (defined as the ability to distinguish small differences in response between species and chemicals) is indeed difficult. In essence, the 'ideal' test would have to incorporate an impractically large number of species grown in a very large number of 'normal' environments and exposed to an indeterminate number of complex chemicals at all stages of their life cycle. The *in vivo* tests presented here do not attain or even closely approach this high standard but are the best available at this time. Further development and refinement are necessary to attain more desirable levels of predictability, reproducibility and sensitivity.

6.1.1 Test Methods

6.1.1.1 *Stage 1: From Seed Germination to the Reproductive Phase*

In vivo standardized tests which involve a broad range of annual herbaceous species of interest to agriculture and forestry are available for routine screening of a large number of highly purified chemicals for potential use as herbicides and/or plant growth regulators (Saggers, 1976). These tests are essentially lethality tests, but a graded quantitative response can be obtained by measuring the size of progeny produced by the species. The tests at the early stages of the life cycle are conducted under controlled environmental conditions to increase reproducibility. The tests at later stages of the life cycle must generally be conducted under field conditions, which decrease reproducibility. In general, the species for these tests are selected for their adaptability to these types of test, so that they can be propagated and grown under normal laboratory and field conditions without highly specialized professional personnel. These tests are routinely used for agricultural chemicals and can be accepted at the present time. Their predictability ranges from excellent to good depending on the number and diversity of species selected; their reproducibility is excellent under controlled environmental conditions at the early stages of the life cycle and good under field conditions; their sensitivity is unknown.

6.1.1.2 *Stage 2: Sporogenesis*

No standardized tests for sampling a broad range of species and environments are available for studying either megasporogenesis or microsporogenesis. *In vivo* tests involving a limited range of species and environments have been developed to study the effects of chemicals on microsporogenesis (Nelson and Rossman, 1958; Kaul and Singh, 1967; Hanna 1977). These *in vivo* tests are conducted in controlled environments or under field conditions and are quantitative using the seed number as the variable measured. In general, the species selection for these studies is limited to self-pollinated or cross-pollinated plants expressing hybrid vigour which have agricultural or forestry significance. These species can, therefore, be grown under normal laboratory and field conditions without highly specialized professional personnel. Predictability of such tests is severely limited because of the narrow range of species involved, but the reproducibility is excellent under controlled environmental conditions and good under field conditions. The sensitivity is unknown.

6.1.1.3 *Stage 3: From Mature Gametes to Mature Seeds*

No standardized tests applicable to a broad spectrum of species and environments are available. A small number of *in vivo* tests involving a limited range of species and environments are available to examine the pollination process in general, pollination control, pollen germination and tube growth, fertilization and seed development (Balatkova and Tupy, 1972; Schwartz and Osterman, 1976; Church and Williams, 1977; Kroh *et al.*, 1979). Test-tube fertilization (Balatkova and Tupy, 1972) has great potential if the predictability could be improved by increasing the number and diversity of species studied. For these *in vivo* tests, the species have been selected on the basis of their particular adaptability to the study rather than their economic significance. Obviously, most of the species selected could be grown under normal laboratory and field conditions without highly specialized professional personnel. The predictability is severely limited because of the narrow range of species involved. The reproducibility is excellent under controlled environmental conditions, and good under field conditions. The sensitivity is unknown.

6.2 ALGAE AND MICROORGANISMS

Before discussing the methods for assessing the effects of chemicals on the reproductive capabilities of these groups of organisms, it is necessary to state clearly two major considerations which affect the approaches that can be adopted.

First, it is important to recognize that the Protista and the algae represent a complete spectrum of nutritional and metabolic types found in the biosphere. Thus, among the members of these groups are heterotrophs (chemo-organo-trophs), phototrophs, including photoautotrophs and photo-organotrophs, chemoautotrophs, including chemolithotrophs and chemo-organotrophs, obligate aerobes, obligate anaerobes, facultative aerobes and other specialized groups with respect to their carbon and/or energy metabolism. Furthermore, within these groups there may be vast differences in the capacity to metabolize known natural organic compounds. These groups represent a plethora of different, and in many cases unique, metabolic mechanisms with substantial differences in their potential susceptibility to the same chemical.

Accordingly, in considering the effects of chemicals on the reproductive processes of microorganisms and algae, care has to be taken to ensure that an appropriate organism is tested for a given compound. To quote the example used by Slater (1983, this volume), the assessment of a compound known specifically to inhibit nitrogen fixation can be tested only with an organism able to fix nitrogen. Conversely, if the target of the chemical is unknown there are serious difficulties in selecting a test organism. Rationalizations will have to be made by a judicious selection of putatively appropriate organisms, but care must be taken not to underestimate possible effects on organisms not yet tested.

Second, it is necessary to define the reproductive function of microorganisms and algae, since in terms of mechanism this function is substantially different from most other groups of organisms considered in this workshop. Many algae and 'higher' microorganisms, especially those with cells of the eukaryotic type, frequently exhibit life cycles with sexual reproductive stages (e.g. microscopic red algae) and simple vegetative growth cycles (see Jensen, 1983, this volume). Much less is known about complex life-cycle modifications, particularly with respect to establishing and maintaining these modified life-cycle stages in the laboratory. Thus, most toxicity studies have been undertaken on vegetative cells growing by a mechanism of cell size increase followed by division into daughter cells. Many microorganisms, particularly those with a prokaryotic cell form, do not exhibit any morphological differentiation and reproduce simply by division of a parent cell into two or more daughter cells. Thus, cell growth and division, i.e. the cell cycle, represent the reproductive sequence, which transmits genetic information from one generation to the next. By and large the growth of a microbial population is a measure of its reproductive potential. Thus, within the terms of reference of this workshop, the assessment of the effects of a chemical on reproductive function may be measured in terms of its effect on the growth of a microbial or algal population. This is in fact one of the few ways in which it is possible to treat in a meaningful manner these vastly diverse organisms as a unified group.

6.2.1 Approaches to Testing for Effects on Reproduction

There are two basic approaches to the analysis of the effects of chemicals on microbes and algae (see Jensen, 1983; Slater, 1983; this volume).

First, test procedures, whether in the laboratory or in the field, need to demonstrate a statistically valid difference in response between the treated and untreated populations in terms of their growth potential. For pure culture systems the responses may be neutral, growth stimulatory, growth depressive (i.e. reduced rates of growth; growth inhibition but maintenance of viability; formation of resting structures such as spores) or lethal (resulting in cell death). There may be different sequences of these basic processes (e.g. growth depression leading to cell death) and their timing may be useful in characterizing the types of test chemicals under consideration. For mixed-culture systems the same basic responses may be monitored. In addition, differential effects on the component species of the mixture can be observed, which provide potentially valuable information on the specific target of the chemical (i.e. one metabolic type or one particular species may be a specific target for the test chemical). Such differential effects of chemicals will result in changes in the composition and/or diversity (e.g. loss of highly susceptible species) of the community. This general approach will provide information which may be extrapolated to natural habitats. In general terms, this first category of test procedures could be adequate, at least for initial screening and ranking of chemicals to assess the desirability of using a particular compound. Again in general terms, this approach has been adopted as the basis of most regulatory guidelines and directives.

Second, where possible, test procedures should identify specific cellular targets. Major processes such as photosynthesis, nitrification, denitrification, respiratory activity, carbon dioxide evolution, methanogenesis and many others may be screened for effects. These test procedures ought to be considered within the first tier of assessment tests since they are of major importance for the function of an ecosystem. Associated with these overall tests, attempts should be made to pinpoint the effect at the biochemical level, a procedure which may lead to the development of specific assays based, for example, on particular enzymes. Such tests have been developed for dehydrogenases, nitrogenases and various catabolic enzymes, but more detailed work on test development is required.

6.2.2 Choice of Organisms

A primary requirement for developing laboratory tests is the choice of the growth system and the type of organism to be used. The preceding section has indicated the nature of the problem of choosing organisms. Standard organisms covering all the possible metabolic modes cannot be recommended since much depends on the nature of the chemical under test. Furthermore, the use of type organisms or standard organisms may induce a false sense of security in that consideration of the possible effects on other organisms may be reduced if not excluded.

Standard algal cultures and standard bacterial strains have been recommended by recourse to national and international culture collections. There is clearly a value in using standard strains in terms of data comparison between laboratories and different test programmes. However, there are dangers in using a limited number of standard organisms. The organism may not have the required characteristics and alternative strains or species from either culture collections or newly isolated organisms must be considred. There are arguments against the use of single organisms (pure cultures), and test procedures using defined or undefined natural mixed cultures must be employed (e.g. OECD 1981); activated sludge systems and river die-away tests using, in both cases, undefined mixed-culture inocula).

Whichever organism or organisms are selected for the test systems, the same experimental techniques should be used for growth and population analyses in order to facilitate comparison of the results.

6.2.3 Methods of Growth

Laboratory test procedures require populations of microorganisms and algae grown under defined conditions, so that the treated and untreated populations can be compared. Differences in growth response may be quantified in terms of various characteristics which the growing cultures may, but need not, have. Thus a primary requisite in devising test procedures is to devise an appropriate growth system.

6.2.4 Growth Media and Physicochemical Conditions

The initial consideration must be to select an appropriate growth medium. For most test procedures a complete medium which supports the organism's growth is required. However, there may be occasions (e.g. testing growth promoting substances, such as vitamins) when an incomplete medium which is supplemented with varying amounts of the growth promoting substance is required. But, in general, most test procedures are aimed at detecting deleterious effects on organisms initially requiring complete media.

The range of media available both commercially or constructed for specific organisms is extensive. Where possible standard media ought to be used since this facilitates comparisons between tests and between laboratories; one should at least use recognized formulations of undefined, complex media. The selection of appropriate media must reflect the nature of the organisms to be cultured. It is, however, imperative that the media used are defined or described accurately, since the microbial and algal form, function, activity and chemical make-up are highly dependent on the growth conditions and nutrient composition. It is imperative that these are reported accurately, since in many cases comparison of the effects of chemicals cannot be undertaken between different tests and different laboratories if major variations are induced by differences in the composition of growth media. Similar restrictions must be applied to aeration, pH, temperature and other conditions used. Frequently these conditions are not adequately standardized, controlled or reported.

6.2.5 Growth Systems

6.2.5.1 *Systems Using Solidified Media*

A standard Petri dish technique is used with growth media normally solidified with agar. The technique may be adapted to include the test chemical at varying concentrations and to allow measurement of the effects in terms of concentrations that inhibit the growth and, perhaps, in terms of modifications of the colony and of individual cell morphology.

The system may be modified along the agar plate–well bioassay system producing inhibition zones in a lawn of microbes or algae. Standard calculations and statistical procedures exist to estimate variables such as potency and minimum inhibitory concentrations.

The system can be used to determine the development of the rate of resistance to a chemical, the rate of mutation and rate of survival in the presence of a compound. Similarly, the procedure can be used to select populations able to metabolize the compound, a particularly important factor in determining the rate of and/or potential for removal of a toxic chemical from the environment. Finally, this growth system is the basis for determining viable cell counts.

The technique is cheap, simple to handle, requires relatively low levels of technical competence, is reproducible and provides a powerful, quantitative assessment procedure.

6.2.5.2 *Closed (Batch) Culture Systems Using Liquid Media*

These systems include tube cultures (a known, usually small volume of a medium in a test tube); bottle cultures (especially for natural populations and natural nutrient sources); and flask cultures (usually conical flasks containing a known culture volume). The common feature of these systems is that they are closed (i.e.

there is no addition or subtraction of nutrients once the growth has started). The organisms grow at their maximum rate over a limited period and there is a characteristic sequence of transitory growth phases. Frequently, in comparison with microbial and algal growth in natural environments, these characteristics are inappropriate. Chemicals may be tested and the response monitored in a fashion similar to that for plate cultures. Methods for growth assessment are described in section 6.2.6.

This is often the method of choice despite various limitations, since it is cheap, reliable, technically simple to operate and may be replicated easily. It has the potential to provide data in screening procedures, an important consideration for any evaluation program.

6.2.5.3 *Continuous-Flow Culture Systems Using Liquid Media*

Many different continuous-flow culture systems, essentially based on chemostat or turbidostat principles, have been developed. There are some important features of these systems which are advantageous compared with closed culture procedures, including the capacity to examine growth rates at a range of submaximal values; growth under different substrate-limited conditions; growth at different population densities; and the growth of stable, interacting microbial populations. All these features represent important environmental characteristics and enable the effects of chemicals to be assayed under physiological conditions which cannot be achieved in plate or closed-culture systems.

The disadvantages are that these techniques require relatively complex equipment and more technical competence. The growth systems are more elaborate and costly. These features normally preclude the use of continuous-flow culture systems in screening programmes. However, they are strongly recommended as important methods of choice for second-tier analysis of chemicals identified as potential problems by the first-tier screening tests. Furthermore, continuous culture systems must be used to examine the effects on microbial communities grown in laboratory environments.

6.2.5.4 *Cage (Dialysis) Culture*

This technique, which was originally developed for bacteria and later adapted for algal cultures, allows the test medium to be more or less continuously renewed without losing the test organisms, thereby securing constant nutrient levels and stable doses of the chemicals to be tested. It also makes it possible to carry out the bioassay *in situ*, whether this is a host organism of reasonable size or a natural habitat. The cage technique is also one of the few systems which allows test organisms to exert extensively their ability to accumulate chemicals from dilute solution. Its relevance to environmental problems is also promising. Despite all these potential advantages, experience with this method is limited. There is still a need for standardization of techniques and conditions. The method can be regarded as an intermediate stage between laboratory and field experiments.

6.2.6 Methods for Assessing Algal and Microbial Growth

There are numerous methods for assessing growth. In many instances the selected method is probably immaterial as long as valid comparisons between control and treated samples can be made. However, interlaboratory comparisons require a uniform approach, and attempts ought to be made to refer the assessment method to a standard measure, namely the dry weight biomass of the organism.

The reliability of conversion factors used must be demonstrated. The major problem which is not universally recognized is that many cellular components and, indeed, basic characteristics such as organism size are highly dependent on the growth environment (Jensen, 1983; Slater, 1983; this volume). In many instances comparison of toxicity data is not feasible because of gross discrepancies between measurements of the same variable. Similarly, comparisons between control and treated populations require that non-specific chemical effects (e.g. simple changes in growth rate) are accounted for.

The following variables have been used to measure population numbers and/or density (biomass), and have been extensively described and discussed by Jones (1979):

(1) dry weight determinations by centrifugation or membrane filtering;
(2) turbidity or absorbance measurements;
(3) biomass determinations by correlation with a species cellular component including protein, DNA, RNA, lipid, lipopolysaccharide (LPS method), chlorophyll a, ATP, and total organic carbon;
(4) total cell number estimates by microscopic haemocytometer counting chamber methods or electronic particle counters, e.g. Coulter counter; and
(5) viable cell number estimates by dilution methods and recovery on solidified medium, i.e. plate counts on slide cultures, fluorescent antibody labelling, and immunofluorescent flow cytometry in conjunction with particle counting.
(6) Under certain circumstances there may be value in estimating the effects of chemicals on overall population characteristics which are related to growth, such as oxygen consumption. These methods include biological oxygen demand (BOD) assays and carbon dioxide fixation rates for photosynthetic organisms.

6.3 CONCLUSIONS AND RECOMMENDATIONS

(1) Well established methods exist which are suitable for analysis of the effects of chemicals on algal and microbial vegetative reproduction. They are highly

quantitative and applicable to routine laboratory-based testing that enables the characterization and ranking of a wide range of chemicals. By and large, the methods are simple, inexpensive and amenable to statistical analysis. Also, they are directly relevant to the problem of the interaction between the chemical and the organisms, i.e. the test systems may be made to reflect accurately situations likely to occur in the natural environment provided the chemical reaches the cell in the active form. Standardization of test procedures for systematic evaluation and ranking of the effects of chemicals on microbial and algal reproduction recommended.

(2) Notwithstanding the success and usefulness of these procedures, further attention must be given to devising appropriate test systems, to improve their predictive value with regard to the effects of chemicals in natural ecosystems. This must include parallel studies in a number of laboratories in order to develop reproducible procedures which model the effect of interphases, species diversity, physical and chemical heterogeneity (i.e. light–dark regimens; concentration gradients; temperature profiles), diurnal rhythms and interactions between organisms.

(3) There is a limited number of test organisms available from culture collections; this facilitates comparison. For a limited number of purposes reference organisms may be applicable but the diversity of microorganisms as a group must be borne in mind. The test procedures are generally based on organisms which are readily cultivated. These organisms represent a small fraction of the existing microflora, and, since differential effects of chemical action may be expected, this is a major problem. Efforts must be encouraged to establish in the laboratory some organisms with complex life cycles in order to evaluate the effects of chemicals on the complete reproduction cycle of these species. Similarly, it would be desirable to encourage work aimed at a controlled cultivation of organisms which cannot be currently grown in the laboratory.

(4) Although laboratory test procedures are adequate for predicting the immediate or direct effects of a chemical on a given organism, the ecological effects which may arise as a result of the initial chemical/organism interaction by and large will not be observed or quantitated in simple test systems. The test systems tend to be gross simplifications of conditions usually prevailing in natural habitats. They do not, normally, reflect the heterogeneity of natural habitats, transient phenomena, natural rhythmic cycles or interphases. Thus the chemical, physical and biological interactions may modify the effect of the chemical, a consequence which cannot be detected by standard test procedures. This problem may be partially resolved by using mixed culture systems, continuous culture systems, microcosms and, particularly, field studies. Such test programmes are often not simple or easy to mount, and they are expensive.

(5) It is recommended that attention be given to providing a limited number of test chemicals which can be used to examine the validity of both the developed and proposed tests, with particular attention focused on their sensitivity and

reproducibility between laboratories. A consequence of this recommendation is that an international organization needs to take responsibility for the coordination of this activity.

6.4 REFERENCES

Balatkova, V. and Tupy, J. (1972). Test-tube fertilization in *Nicotiana tabacum* by means of an artificial pollen tube culture. *Biol. Plant. (Prague)* **10**, 266–270.

Church, R. M. and Williams, R. R. (1977). The toxicity to apple pollen of several fungicides, as demonstrated by *in vivo* and *in vitro* techniques. *J. Hortic. Sci.* **52**, 429–436.

Epler, J. L., Larimer, F. W., Rao, T. K., Nix, C. E. and Ho, T. (1978). Energy-related pollutants in the environment: use of short-term tests for mutagenicity in the isolation and identification of biohazards. *Environ. Health Perspect.* **27**, 11–20.

Hanna, W. W. (1977). Effect of DPX 3778 on anther dehiscence in pearl millet. *Crop Sci.* **17**, 965–967.

Heath, C. W. Jr, (1978). Environmental pollutants and the epidemiology of cancer. *Environ. Health Perspect.* **27**, 7–10.

Jones, J. G. (1979). A guide to methods for estimating microbial numbers and biomass in freshwater. *Freshwater Biol. Ass. Sci. Publ. No. 39.*

Kaul, C. L. and Singh, S. P. (1967). Effects of certain growth retardants on growth, flowering, and pollen viability in fenugreek (*Trigonella foenum-graecum* L.). *Indian J. Plant Physiol.* **10**, 54–61.

Kroh, M., Gorissen, M. H. and Pfahler, P. L. (1979). Ultrastructural studies on styles and pollen tubes of *Zea mays* L.: general survey on pollen tube growth *in vivo*. *Acta Bot. Neerl.* **28**, 513–518.

Nelson, P. and Rossman, E. C. (1958). Chemical induction of male sterility in inbred lines of maize by the use of gibberellins. *Science (Washington, DC)* **127**, 1500–1501.

OECD (1981). *Guidelines for Testing of Chemicals*, 700 pages. Organization for Economic Cooperation and Development, Paris.

Saggers, D. T. (1976). The search for new herbicides. In Andus, L. J. (Ed.) *Herbicides: Physiology, Biochemistry, Ecology*, Vol. 2, pp. 447–473. Academic Press, New York, San Francisco, London.

Schwartz, D. and Osterman, J. (1976). A pollen selection system for alcohol-dehydrogenase-negative mutants in plants. *Genetics* **83**, 63–65.

Methods for Assessing the Effects of Chemicals on Reproductive Functions
Edited by V. B. Vouk and P. J. Sheehan
© 1983 SCOPE

ANNEX

General Aspects of Test Procedures in Reproduction Toxicology*

INTRODUCTION

The response of a biological system to a chemical stimulus is related to the toxicity of the test material, the dose level, the duration of exposure and the route of administration. Reproduction toxicology is particularly concerned with developmental stages (embryonic, fetal, lactational and pubertal) and gonadal cyclic or maturational activities. The absorption, distribution, biotransformation and elimination of administered substances must be taken into account when interpreting observed effects. Different sections of this annex must be considered, therefore, within the framework of all the available toxicological knowledge developed in relation to any test material. In addition, uniformly stringent test requirements are necessary for all chemicals. An equally important premise in developing cost-effective information is that the effort expended on testing a chemical for safety have some semblance to the true upper limit of the potential for harm of a given compound. This concept has been referred to as the 'principle of commensurate effort' and has also been used as a means of making testing requirements more cost effective.

An important consideration in the selection of appropriate reproduction tests is the intended use of the results. In general, test data are generated for three major purposes:

(1) new product screening;
(2) regulatory approval of new products; and
(3) safety review of chemicals already used and present in the human environment.

The many types of products to be tested include food additives, agricultural chemicals, pesticides, pharmaceuticals, cosmetics, environmental contaminants and industrial chemicals. Sometimes the intended use of the chemical also influences the selection of tests. Thus, the selection of tests in a given test programme depends on exposure, observed toxicity, purpose of testing and the intended use of the chemical.

* Extract from the report of the Workgroup on female reproductive function of mammals.

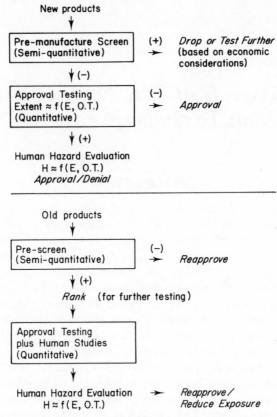

Figure 1A   Testing of new and old products E, exposure level; O.T., observed toxicity; H, human hazard

TEST VALIDATION

In order that a reproduction toxicology test be selected for use in an evaluation programme, it should be valid for the assessment of risk to reproduction by meeting the following criteria.

(1) It should be reproducible in a single species.
(2) The results in one species of experimental animals should be reproducible and predictive of results in one or more additional species of experimental animals.
(3) The results in experimental animals should be predictive of a human effect.
(4) The results in experimental animals should allow quantitative assessment of risk to human reproductive function.

The first criterion is simple to assess through repeated testing and interlaboratory comparisons. The second is more difficult to achieve in reproduction studies because of interspecies differences in reproduction systems (even among mammals) and in absorption, distribution, biotransformation and excretion of different compounds.

Even more difficult, and often impossible, is the validation of a test for human subjects. Direct epidemiological studies of effects on reproduction often cannot be carried out because human exposure has not occurred and cannot be achieved experimentally. Even when exposure has occurred, estimates of exposure dose are usually very difficult or impossible to make.

A possible approach to this problem would be to develop an understanding of the effects of chemical agent(s) at the cellular level and to demonstrate similar effects in human biopsied or cultured materials. This would be subject to the qualification that variations may occur in absorption or metabolism of the substance before it acts at the cellular level.

The demonstration that a test performed on an animal model system is predictive of human effects in a number of situations, where this is testable, would provide the best possible qualitative validation of any test to be used for human risk assessment.

The most important criterion required for quantitative validation of any test to be used for risk assessment is that the positive test result shows dose response. Cause–effect is most clearly established in situations where response (the number of individuals in an exposed population showing the effect) is positively correlated with dose. Because estimation of dose is difficult to accomplish in human populations, there are very few reliably determined human dose–response relationships for chemicals.

THE CHOICE OF TESTS

The choice of testing procedures depends on the purpose of testing. The most common purposes are outlined below.

Pre-manufacture Screening of New Products

The characteristics of the tests that are selected for this type of screening are in general as follows:

(1) end-points are semi-quantitative;
(2) the test should be convenient for screening large numbers of compounds;
(3) the tests should predict the biological hazard potential;
(4) tests should be rapid, cost effective and reproducible;
(5) negative responses in a test should indicate a low probability of effects occurring for the end-point measured;

(6) the test battery should cover as many reproduction variables as possible;
(7) test data are generated for 'in house' evaluation;
(8) human exposure associated with testing should be minimal; and
(9) metabolic considerations should be included.

Testing of New Products for Regulatory Approval

Characteristics of tests selected for this purpose are as follows:

(1) tests must be quantitative and it should be possible to extrapolate the results to human subjects;
(2) test designs must cover the anticipated exposure as well as a wide range of other exposure levels;
(3) where possible, routes of exposure should reflect anticipated or actual human exposure patterns;
(4) tests should be cost effective and reproducible; and
(5) test designs and data analyses must include metabolic considerations.

Safety Review of Chemicals in the Environment

Characteristics of tests selected for this purpose include the following:

(1) rapid or short-term screening procedures should be such that testing results can be used in priority ranking; and
(2) human studies can also be included for these compounds. The types of human studies may involve identification of populations at risk, followed by retrospective or prospective epidemiological studies and clinical monitoring of identified populations.

EXAMPLES OF TESTS ASSOCIATED WITH THE IDENTIFIED TEST AREAS

Proposed New Product Screens

These tests should be primarily short-term, inexpensive, and should have at least semi-quantitative reproductive function end-points. Examples are:

(1) fertility tests (see section 2.1.2);
(2) preimplantation development (see section 2.3.1);
(3) *in vitro* test for embryotoxicity (see section 2.3.3.2); and
(4) possible non-mammalian test systems (future development).

Approval of New Substances

These tests are discussed in section 2.1 on integrated reproduction function studies, including:

(1) multigeneration studies;
(2) fertility studies;
(3) *in vivo* tests for selective embryotoxicity; and
(4) peri- and postnatal studies (see sections 2.3.3.4 on parturition and 2.3.3.5 on lactation).

Safety Review of Chemicals Already Present in the Human Environment

Tests for this purpose involve both screening procedures and regulatory tests described above as well as screening of effects on human reproductive function and epidemiological studies of exposed populations.

PART B

CONTRIBUTED CHAPTERS

Methods for Assessing the Effects of Chemicals on Reproductive Functions
Edited by V. B. Vouk and P. J. Sheehan
© 1983 SCOPE

Adverse Effects of Environmental Agents on Mammalian Female Reproduction

W. LeRoy Heinrichs and Merrit Gadallah

1 INTRODUCTION

Twenty years have elapsed since Rachel Carson's *Silent Spring* called public attention to the adverse effects of environmental chemicals on avian reproduction in the Clear Lake region of Northern California. Decimation of the songbird population attributable to pesticide chemicals was soon confirmed in other avian species such as kestrels, peregrine falcons, and ospreys. Government, industry and public reaction to rapidly accumulating data has led to curtailment of the industrial manufacture and agricultural dissemination of some pesticides such as DDT. While the reproductive physiology of birds may be particularly vulnerable to the toxicity of such weakly oestrogenic chemicals, adverse effects were also observed in laboratory experiments with mammalian species and in humans following acute accidental exposure. The adverse effects of chronic exposure of women have been much more difficult to identify.

2 PRINCIPLES OF EXPOSURE

Reproduction shares with mutagenesis, teratogenesis and carcinogenesis some of the same attributes of biological injury. Usually the severity of a public health risk is directly proportional to the type and extent of potential damage that results from exposure to a chemical. Assessments of minimal risks remain controversial because of inadequate criteria and data. The risk is maximal when entire populations of biota are exposed to xenobiotic agents in concentrations that produce critical or significant injury in all groups and individuals, whether mature, immature or unborn. Most of our experience concerns lesser amounts of damage which has appeared in a limited number of species that have become exposed through accidental or unrecognized contact, either acutely or chronically. The risk of an adverse effect from involuntary exposure of a given species, i.e., mink, or Baltic seals, is related to the type and mode of transmission of the chemical, the position of the species in the food chain, the biological characteristics of the species, the evolutionary stability (or susceptibility) of the species, and the time in the reproductive cycle that exposure occurs. The important factors that determine a widespread adverse outcome are:

(1) specificity (chemical and/or biological) of the agent;
(2) dose and duration of exposure;
(3) route of exposure;
(4) time of exposure in relation to the reproductive event of interest.

These factors are common for the disparate outcomes of mutagenesis, teratogenesis, carcinogenesis and reproductive toxicity. Although mutagenesis and teratogenesis may be subcomponents of reproductive failure, the reproductive system has unique mechanisms of a physiological nature that separate it from those pathological processes. The unique factors influencing adverse outcomes of reproductive functions include:

(5) state of somatic development;
(6) state of sexual maturation (reproductive capacity);
(7) state of functional activity (sexual and reproductive performance).

The clinical pathological manifestations of chemical injury of the processes of development, maturation and function may be produced at any age in the fetus, the infant or child, or in the young or older adult. Somatic growth disturbance of the fetus often continues to be evident years later, as may the onset of injury during infancy or childhood. The earlier the injury occurs during development, the greater the deviations from normal potential growth. An excellent example demonstrating this principle is the effect of cigarette smoking on reducing human fetal growth by 150–200 g (term birth weight). The normal growth potential of smokers' progeny is not reached by adolescence and is probably reduced permanently. In contrast, the postpubertal onset of smoking does not produce inhibition of somatic development but advances reproductive senescence (menopause). Thus the stage of somatic development at the time of the exposure determines in part the type of injury produced.

Similarly, the stage of sexual maturation determines the consequences of exposure, particularly to the many agonists or antagonists of hormone action that exist among environmental chemicals. For example, an oestrogen agonist such as the family of polychlorinated biphenyls (PCBs) may alter the masculine differentiation of the male fetus, may induce precocious puberty in girls or produce menstrual disturbances with anovulation and infertility in postpubertal females, or oligospermia in adult males. Hypervitaminosis A or heavy metal exposure may produce similar deficits. The clinical response inducible in the reproductive system is therefore greatly dependent upon the state of sexual maturation at the time of exposure. The anatomical and functional integrity of the reproductive system may be described as *reproductive capacity*. It is sometimes designated in statistical descriptions as a population index: the total number of women between the ages of 15 and 45 years. This estimates the number of women who have the capacity to reproduce if they chose to seek the opportunity. This group of women usually constitutes approximately one-half of the women in an average population. This statistic assumes 100% fertility, which is of course an overestimate of at least 10% (those infertile).

Finally, the state of the functional activity of the reproductive system must be considered in assessments of adverse effects. In contrast to males in which failure of sexual performance (impotence) may limit fertility, sexual interest (libido) rather than sexual performance is much more likely to be adversely affected in females. The most sensitive end-point for injury is the ovulatory process. The earliest postconceptional injury that may become evident is 'subclinical' abortion, detectable only by observing a temporary appearance of plasma chorionic gonadotropin in association with a 'long cycle'. This newly recognized clinical entity remains to be associated with exposure to environmental chemicals. Even the cytogenetics have yet to be described. In contrast, clinical abortion has been associated with environmental chemical exposure to PCBs; however, the specific mechanism(s) is unknown. Maternal endocrine factors, placentation errors or teratological defects could account for that loss. Further, inhibition of lactogenesis or galactopoiesis could only be evident in the puerperal woman whose exposure may have begun during pregnancy (as with an acute PCB exposure) or in the puerperium as may result from initiation of oral contraception. The population statistic used to describe the set of women who are actively reproducing is the fertility rate or index: the number of conceptions annually per 1000 women in the 15–45 year age group. Within this group are those women demonstrating adversely affected *reproductive performance* such as second trimester abortions, stillbirths and newborn deaths. Ironically, women having spontaneous or voluntary abortions are not included in the fertility index. No systematic assessment has been developed to describe the set of sexually active or impotent men, or women with infertility or involuntary lactation failure.

3 MECHANISMS OF REPRODUCTIVE TOXICITY

Xenobiotic agents may produce biological injury in the chemical form in which they are absorbed (direct acting) or they may through bioactivation be transformed after absorption from inactive to active agents (indirect acting). Direct acting agents are often hormone agonists or antagonists having chemical structures similar to endogenous compounds (i.e. oestrogens) or they include compounds having chemical reactivities that interfere with physiological processes (i.e. alkylating agents, heavy metals, etc.). The more subtle reproductive toxicity of many direct-acting chemicals probably has been overlooked at low exposures because of their more obvious mutagenic, teratogenetic or carcinogenic properties.

Indirect-acting reproductive toxins produce their injury through bioactivation of inert or weakly reactive compounds to those having significant chemical activity. Such chemical products may have either agonistic or antagonistic properties. The major metabolic pathways responsible for activation and detoxication of xenobiotics are contained in hepatic and gonadal enzymes and include a variety of cytochrome P-450 dependent microsomal monooxygenases, deacylases, and transferases which conjugate a variety of non-polar substrates with sulphate, glucuronide and glutathione moieties. The balance between the activation and detoxication of foreign substances may be significantly upset by the selective induction or inhibition of some of these enzyme pathways. Perhaps most importantly, the balance of the peripheral metabolism of endogenous substrates (i.e., steroid hormones, bilirubin, thyroxine) may be disturbed by the altered activities of enzymes resulting from exposure to xenobiotics. Such metabolic changes may alter the intricate feedback loops between the CNS and gonads upon which reproductive function depends. These mechanisms are discussed in greater detail in two excellent reviews of the subject (Lee and Dixon, 1978; Mattison, 1981).

4 REPRODUCTIVE PROCESSES SUBJECT TO CHEMICAL INJURY

The various processes in the reproductive cycle of higher mammals which are subject to chemical injury are illustrated in Figure 1. Differences in the anatomy and the endocrinological regulation of the reproductive system cause

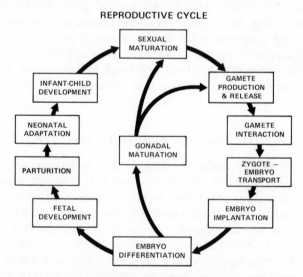

Figure 1. Reproductive processes subject to chemical injury. The inter-relationships between reproduction and mutagenesis, teratogenesis and carcinogenesis are indicated (after Mattison, 1981)

certain of the components of the reproductive cycle to be more vulnerable to injury. For example, the rapid metabolic activity of spermatogonia seems to make the production of sperm particularly vulnerable to injury by various drugs and environmentally acquired chemicals (Hunt *et al.*, 1979). Similarly, the profound inhibitory effect of vasoactive drugs on tumescence of the male copulatory organ is a sex-specific response not shared with females (Hunt *et al.*, 1979; Anonymous Consultants, 1980).

The complexity of the reproductive process makes this system particularly susceptible to chemical injury. The rapid cell division rates of spermatogonia and the recurring ovarian cycle are processes subject to injury from both acute and chronic exposures. These types of exposure are the primary objectives of routine toxicological testing. The three-generation test for toxicological injury of reproduction in rats represents a substantial although incomplete approach to defining defects among the various reproductive processes. Unfortunately, subtle latent injuries such as chronic anoestrus and premature ovarian senescence are not identified by this method because it utilizes only young animals (Friberg and Cederlöf, 1978; Wright, 1978).

5 ADVERSE REPRODUCTION EFFECTS

5.1 Reproduction Capacity (Females)

In women or in female animals, ovulatory defects have been observed or produced with DES, DDT, PCBs, chlordane, heptachlor, aldrin and hexachlorobenzene; all are halogenated hydrocarbons. The polycyclic hydrocarbons inhaled in cigarette smoke are thought to decrease the age of spontaneous menopause in women. Alkylating agents and Imuran are known to produce oocyte death and to produce premature menopause. In experimental animals, DES, PCBs and DDT given during the perinatal period have produced chronic anoestrus in female progeny (Hunt *et al.*, 1979; Longo, 1980; Mattison, 1981).

5.2 Reproductive Performance (Females)

5.2.1 *Sexual Dysfunction*

Little is known about any predictable inhibitory effects of xenobiotics or drugs on sexual secretions or orgasmic responses of women. Nevertheless monoamine oxidase inhibitors, sedative drugs, cannibus, heroin, methadone and alcohol have been suggested to disturb libido and perhaps, orgasmic responsivity (Bell and Trethowan, 1961; Gossop *et al*; 1974; Anonymous Consultants, 1980). Since the sexual activity of subhuman primates and of other mammals is tightly linked to ovulation, discrepancies between reproductive capacity and sexual performance, are difficult to model or to study of humans except in women.

5.2.2   *Abortion–Embryotoxicity*

Reproductive failure short of recognizable conceptions has not been studied adequately, although estimates are that 15% of potential conceptions fail because of defective ova and another 15% fail from faulty placentation (McKusick, 1978). The observation that the abortuses of smoking women have normal chromosomes suggests that implantation or placentation failures are responsible for such losses (Kline *et al.*, 1977). Current estimates are that at least 40% of conceptuses that successfully implant, as evident by plasma human chorionic gonadotrophin or by clinical abortions with histological confirmation, terminate in abortion (Roberts and Lowe, 1975). Approximately 50% of the clinically apparent conceptuses are genetically abnormal with unbalanced chromosome defects; others have balanced chromosome abnormalities or point to mutations that become evident subsequently if pregnancy continues (Boué and Boué, 1978).

Retrospective data indicate that exposure to anaesthetic gases, of either women or their male partners, results in a significantly increased abortion rate. Of the potential agents, nitrous oxide (N_2O) has been shown in humans and rats to be associated with abortion or embryotoxicity (Cohen *et al.*, 1980). Smoking cigarettes or moderate or excessive alcohol ingestion by women (but not the male partner) is related to a significantly higher rate of abortions, particularly of second trimester losses (Kline *et al.*, 1977; Himmelberger *et al.*, 1978; Harlap and Shiono, 1980). Embryotoxic effects of 2, 4, 5-T (2, 4, 5-trichlorophenoxy-acetic acid), a herbicide thought to have produced abortion in a population of Oregon women (Office of Pesticide Programs, 1979), have not been confirmed. Some species of laboratory animals (mice) have shown teratogenic responses to this compound (Courtney *et al.*, 1970); however, others (rats, rabbits) are not affected (Emerson *et al.*, 1971). Dioxin contamination of the herbicide may have produced the damage (Clegg, 1971). It was not possible to link the exposure of the Vietnamese to this herbicide with the occurrence of abortion, stillbirth or fetal malformations (National Research Council, 1974).

The polychlorinated biphenyls (PCBs) have been shown to produce stillborn or 'cola-coloured' babies (Miller, 1971; DHEW, 1978). Some halogenated hydrocarbons have oestrogenic properties, but no specific mechanisms of their reproductive toxicity have been elucidated. Sows fed Aroclor 1242 (one of the PCBs) at 20 p.p.m. during gestation farrowed fewer liveborn and had increased numbers of mummified fetuses (Hansen *et al.*, 1975). Rabbits, mink and rhesus monkeys seem to be particularly sensitive to PCBs during pregnancy with abortion resulting from 5–25 p.p.m. in the diet; mice and rats were affected at higher levels, but tended to produce neonatal loss rather than abortion (resorption sites) (Villenueve *et al.*, 1971; DHEW, 1978).

Bromine analogue, of PCBs, polybrominated biphenyls (PBBs), led to an increased incidence of stillbirths in cattle in Michigan which ingested the chemical as a food contaminant (Jackson and Halbert, 1974). A few human pregnancies involving women with large body burdens of PBBs delivered without recognized complications (DHEW, 1978).

Adverse embryotoxic effects of organochlorinated pesticides including DDT, Kepone, chlordane, mirex, DBCP and heptachlor have not been clearly identified in women, although effects on spermatogenesis have been well documented. Prematurely delivered infants had higher concentrations of DDE than infants delivered at term (O'Leary *et al.*, 1970; Gossop *et al.*, 1974). The latter observation in women is supported by studies indicating that when California sea lions were pupping prematurely, the mothers and their pups had two- to eightfold increases in tissue residues of organochlorine pesticides and polychlorinated biphenyls (DeLong *et al.*, 1973). The adverse effects of organochlorine pesticides have been documented in mice (Keplinger *et al.*, 1968; Lundberg and Kihlström, 1973) and beagle dogs (Deichmann *et al.*, 1971) but no embryotoxic effect was found in rats (Wrenn *et al.*, 1971a), ewes (Wrenn *et al.*, 1971b) or cattle (Maclin and Ribelin, 1971). Endrin and Kepone also reduced litter numbers and newborn weights (Good and Ware, 1969; Harr *et al.*, 1970) but dieldrin reduced only newborn weights. These observations emphasize the importance of specificity of the agents and species differences in reproductive toxicology.

The above limited description focuses only on the early components of the reproductive cycle. Space does not permit here an adequate enumeration of the many hundreds of agents which can be implicated in reproductive failure. No attempt has been made to include the body of teratological knowledge. One may safely speculate that *early* gestational injury, even prior to organogenesis, is the most commonly affected component, although deficits in fetal growth from unknown causes seem to clinicians to be increasingly frequent. Subsequent postnatal developmental and behavioural disorders in relation to a hostile intrauterine environment or transfer of chemicals via lactation are only beginning to be studied and catalogued. Perinatal and childhood deaths or carcinogenesis as consequences of embryonic–fetal differentiation and development is an old concept that is coming of age. Much more astute observation and experimental testing will be necessary to establish safety guidelines for avoiding chemical injury to human reproduction.

6 REFERENCES

Anonymous Consultants (1980). Drugs that cause sexual dysfunction. *The Medical Letter* **22**, 108.

Bell, D. S. and Trethowan, W. H. (1961). Amphetamine addiction and disturbed sexuality. *Archs gen. Psychiat* **4**, 74–78.

Boué, A. and Boué, J. (1978). Chromosomal anomalies associated with fetal malformation. In Scrimgeour, J. B. (Ed.) *Towards the Prevention of Fetal Malformations*. Edinburgh University Press, Edinburgh.

Clegg, D. J. (1971). Embryotoxicity of chemical contaminants of foods. *Food Cosmet. Toxical.* **9**, 195–205.

Cohen, E. N., Brown, B. W., Wu, M. L., Whitcher, C. E., Brodsky, J. B., Gift, H. C., Greenfield, W., Jones, T. W. and Driscoll, E. J. (1980). Occupational disease in dentistry and chronic exposure to trace anesthetic gases. *J. Am. dent. Ass.* **101**, 21–31.

Courtney, K. D., Gaylor, D. W., Hogan, M. D., Falk, H. L., Bates, R. R. and Mitchell, I. (1970). Teratogenic evaluation of 2, 4, 5-T. *Science (Washington, DC)* **168**, 864–866.

Deichmann, W. B., MacDonald, W. E., Beasley, A. G. and Cubit, D. (1971) Subnormal reproduction in beagle dogs induced by DDT and aldrin. *Indust. Med. Surg.* **40(2)**, 10–20.

DeLong, R. L., Gilmartin, W. G. and Simpson, J. G. (1973). Premature births in California sea lions: association with high organochlorine pollutant residue levels. *Science (Washington, DC)* **181**, 1168–1170.

DHEW (1978). Final Report of the Subcommittee on the Health Effects of Polychlorinated Biphenyls and Polybrominated Biphenyls of the DHEW Committee to Coordinate Toxicology and Related Programs, July 1976. *Environ. Health Perspect.* **24**, 129–132.

Emerson, J. L., Thompson, D. J., Strebing, R. J., Gerbig, C. G. and Robinson, V. B. (1971). Teratogenic studies on 2, 4, 5-trichlorophenoxyacetic acid in the rat and rabbit. *Food Cosmet. Toxicol.* **9**, 395–404.

Friberg, L. and Cederlöf, R. (1978). Late effects of air pollution with special reference to lung cancer. *Environ. Health Perspect.* **22**, 45–66.

Good, E. E. and Ware, G. W. (1969). Effects of insecticides on reproduction in the laboratory mouse. IV. Endrin and dieldrin. *Toxicol. appl. Pharmacol.* **14**, 201–203.

Gossop, M. R., Stern, R. and Connell, P. H. (1974). Drug dependence and sexual dysfunction: a comparison of intravenous users of narcotics and oral users of amphetamines. *Br. J. Psychiat.* **124**, 431–434.

Hansen, L. G., Byerly, C. S., Metcalf, R. L. and Bevill, R. F. (1975). Effect of a polychlorinated biphenyl mixture on swine reproduction and tissue residues. *Am. J. vet. Res.* **36**, 23–26.

Harlap, S. and Shiono, P. H. (1980). Alcohol, smoking, and incidence of spontaneous abortions in the first and second trimester. *Lancet* **ii**, 173–176.

Harr, J. R., Claeys, R. R., Bone, J. F. and McCorcle, T. W. (1970). Dieldrin toxicosis: rat reproduction. *Am. J. vet. Res.* **31**, 181–189.

Himmelberger, D. V., Brown, B. W. Jr. and Cohen, E. N. (1978). Cigarette smoking during pregnancy and the occurrence of spontaneous abortion and congenital abnormality. *Am. J. Epidemiol.* **108**, 470–479.

Hunt, V. R., Manson, J. M. and Lucas-Wallace, K. (1979). The chemical environment. In Hunt, V. (Ed.) *Work and the Health of Women*, pp. 97–142. CRC Press, Inc., Boca Raton, Florida.

Jackson, R. F. and Halbert, F. L. (1974). A toxic syndrome associated with feeding of polybrominated biphenyl-contaminated protein concentrate to dairy cattle. *J. Am. vet. Med. Ass.* **165**, 437–439.

Keplinger, M. L., Deichmann, W. B. and Sala, F. (1968). Effects of combinations of pesticides on reproduction in mice. In Deichmann, W. B. (Ed.) *Pesticides Symposia*, pp. 125–138. Halo and Ass., Miami, Florida.

Kline, J., Stein, Z. A., Susser, M. and Warburton, D. (1977). Smoking: a risk factor for spontaneous abortion. *New. Engl. J. Med.* **297**, 793–796.

Lee, I. P. and Dixon, R. L. (1978). Factors influencing reproduction and genetic toxic effects on male gonads. *Environ. Health Perspect.* **24**, 117–127.

Longo, L. D. (1980). Environmental pollution and pregnancy: risks and uncertainties for the fetus and infant. *Am. J. Obstet. Gynecol.* **137**, 162–173.

Lundberg, C. and Kihlström, J. E. (1973). DDT and the frequency of implanted ova in the mouse. *Bull. Environ. Contam. Toxicol.* **9**, 267–270.

Macklin, A. W. and Ribelin, W. E. (1971). The relation of pesticides to abortion in dairy cattle. *J. Am. vet. Med. Ass.* **159**, 1743–1748.

Mattison, D. R. (1981). The effects of biologically foreign compounds on reproduction. In Abdul-Karim, R. W. (Ed.) *Drugs in Pregnancy*, Ch. 4, Geo. F. Stickley, Philadelphia.

McKusick, V. (1978). *Mendelian Inheritance in Man*, 5th edn. The Johns Hopkins University Press, Baltimore, Maryland.

Miller, R. W. (1971). Cola-colored babies. Chlorobiphenyl poisoning in Japan. *Teratology* **4**, 211–212.

National Research Council (1974). *The Effects of Herbicides in South Vietnam. Part A: Summary and Conclusions*. Prepared by the Committee on the Effects of Herbicides in Vietnam. National Academy of Sciences, Washington, DC.

Office of Pesticide Programs (1979). *Preliminary Report of Assessment of a Field Investigation of 6-year Spontaneous Abortion Rate in Three Oregon Areas in Relation to Forest 245-T Spray Practices*. Environmental Protection Agency, Washington, DC.

O'Leary, J. A., Davies, J. E., Edmundson, W. F. and Feldman, M. (1970). Correlations of prematurity and DDE levels in fetal whole blood. *Am. J. Obstet. Gynecol.* **106**, 939.

Roberts, C. J. and Lowe, C. R. (1975). Where have all the conceptions gone? *Lancet* **i**, 498–499.

Villenueve, D. C., Grant, D. L., Khera, K., Clegg, D. J., Baar, H. and Phillips, W. E. J. (1971). The fetotoxicity of a polychlorinated biphenyl mixture (Aroclor 1254) in the rabbit and in the rat. *Environ. Physiol.* **1**, 67–71.

Wrenn, T. R., Weyant, J. R., Fries, G. F. and Bitman, J. (1971a) Effect of several dietary levels of o,p'-DDT on reproduction and lactation in the rat. *Bull. Environ. Contam. Toxicol.* **6**, 471–480.

Wrenn, T. R., Weyant, J. R., Fries, G. F. and Bitman, J. (1971b). Influence of dietary o,p'-DDT on reproduction and lactation of ewes. *J. anim. Sci.* **33**, 1288–1292.

Wright, P. L. (1978). Test procedures to evaluate effects of chemical exposure on fertility and reproduction. *Environ. Health Perspect.* **24**, 39–43.

Methods for Assessing the Effects of Chemicals on Reproductive Functions
Edited V. B. Vouk and P. J. Sheehan
© 1983 SCOPE

Adverse Effects of Chemicals on Male Reproductive Function in Mammals

THADDEUS MANN and CECILIA LUTWAK-MANN

1 INTRODUCTION

The two topics relating to male infertility caused by chemicals, namely:

(1) the effects of pharmacological and other chemical agents on the testis, male accessory organs, ejaculation and spermatozoa, and
(2) the criteria used in the evaluation of changes produced by these agents,

are described and discussed below in a general manner only. A more detailed account of current research aimed at solving the complex mechanisms which underlie the action of antifertility agents, and the means of quantitatively appraising the adverse effects, can be found in our recent monograph on *Male Reproductive Function and Semen. Themes and Trends in Physiology, Biochemistry and Investigative Andrology* (Mann and Lutwak-Mann, 1981) and in several review articles dealing with specific groups of chemicals (Thomas, 1975; Neumann *et al.*, 1976; Gomes, 1977; Lucier *et al.*, 1977; Thomas *et al.*, 1977; Patanelli, 1978; Dixon and Lee, 1980; Dougherty *et al.*, 1980; Davies, 1980; Amann, 1981).

2 EFFECTS ON TESTIS, ACCESSORY ORGANS, EJACULATION AND SPERMATOZOA

2.1 Hallucinogens, Opiates, Amphetamines, Cocaine and Alcohol

Sexual inadequacy has long been known to drive men to hallucinogens and psychodelic drugs, in hopes that they can thereby enhance their libido and sexual gratification. But it is equally recognized that addiction to substances such as the opiates, leads to an opposite effect, that is, an actual decrease in sexual desire and performance. On this subject there is a fast growing literature, and apart from opiates many other hallucinogenic agents, such as LSD (D-lysergic acid diethylamide), mescaline, psilocybin, cannabis derivatives and 'ayahuasca' among others, have been receiving increasing attention (Mann, 1968, 1970; Emboden, 1979). We have as yet much to learn about the mechanisms underlying the action of all these hallucinogens; concerning the last-mentioned 'ayahuasca' (*Banisteria caapi*), its hallucinogenic properties are supposedly derived from the presence of harmine and harmaline which by inhibiting monoamine oxidase, can lead to the accumulation of endogenously synthesized biogenic amines, such as epinephrine and norepinephrine. A direct inhibitory effect on monoamine oxidase is also at the basis of the action of some other potent pharmacological agents, and in particular certain psychopharmaceuticals such as phenelzine; by inhibiting monoamine oxidase, this drug interferes with the normal metabolism of biogenic amines, such as norepinephrine, dopamine, tryptamine and serotonin (5-hydroxytryptamine).

As in the case of narocotics and hallucinogens, there is evidence for the existence of a relationship between amphetamine dependence and sexual inadequacy (real or imaginary) in men. Though occasionally they stimulate libido, on the whole, amphetamine compounds tend to reduce the standard of the mating performance, and in this respect there is some, though admittedly not close, similarity between amphetamines and cocaine. The latter often enhances male sexual desire but at the same time reduces sexual power. It is important to bear in mind that men as well as animals exhibit a wide range of individual responses to drugs such as amphetamine, cocaine and morphine. This particularly applies to the action of these agents on the ejaculatory process. For example, in mice the extent to which morphine depresses contractions of the vas deferens and thereby inhibits the ejaculatory process is strain dependent; less morphine is required to suppress the contractions of the deferent duct in the TO, than in the C57/BL strain (Henderson and Hughes, 1976).

Excessive alcohol consumption by men is frequently associated with failure to achieve or maintain erection and a generally reduced sexual performance. The impotence pattern in the alcoholics has long been recognized by physicians and laymen, and it has been frequently expressed in the literature, as for example, in Macbeth, Act II, Scene III, where the porter thus answers Macduff's enquiry about the effect of 'drink': 'Lechery, sir, it provokes and it unprovokes; it provokes the desire, but it takes away the performance.' Animals don't seem to differ in this respect from man, and experiments on male rats inhaling alcohol or ether vapours have demonstrated clearly that erection, ejaculation and copulatory behaviour are all adversely affected. Moreover, there are indications that the deleterious effects express themselves in a reduced survival rate of progeny; in mice, progeny number and survival rate were shown to be distinctly lower in litters sired by ethanol-treated males than in controls (Badr and Badr, 1975; Anderson *et al.*, 1978). A respectable amount of work has also been done on effects of alcohol on testosterone clearance; consumption of alcohol by men elevates the metabolic clearance rate of testosterone, concomitantly with increased activity of the enzymatic system responsible for the aromatization of testosterone to oestrogen; hence the increased risk of gynaecomastia (Gordon *et al.*, 1976). Testicular atrophy and a high percentage of sperm abnormalities in semen are another frequently encountered findings in chronic alcoholics (Van Thiel *et al.*, 1979).

2.2 Industrial Chemicals

Among substances which influence adversely testicular function and the output of spermatozoa in semen, industrial and therapeutic chemicals rank high in importance. Many of them produce germinal aplasia, oligospermia, azoospermia and also a decrease in testosterone formation; they are furthermore responsible for failure of erection, ejaculatory disturbances and other symptoms of deficient male reproductive function.

Industrial chemicals with such properties include a wide range of insecticides, herbicides, fumigants and other pesticides, flame retardants and petrol additives. Some of them affect the testes and male accessory organs directly, some influence the metabolism of other organs as well, and as regards failure of erection and ejaculation, which has been reported for instance in agricultural workers handling herbicides and pesticides, these chemicals act on the parasympathetic and sympathetic nervous system and thereby influence the mechanism of central nervous transmission. Organochlorine and organobromine compounds constitute a particularly serious hazard to the male on account of their antifertility, mutagenic, carcinogenic and in some instances, oestrogenic properties, aggravated by easy absorption through the skin and accumulation in tissues. Polychorinated biphenyls (PCB) which are employed in the manufacture of plastics, lubricants and flame-retardant synthetic fibres, quickly penetrate the workers' protective clothing. High permeability of the skin and storage capacity in the tissues (fat in particular) are also characteristic of polybrominated biphenyls (PBBs), about which much has been heard since the Michigan incident in 1973 (Chen, 1979) when several thousand pounds of PBBs, inadvertently mixed into livestock feed, caused the death of large numbers of farm animals. An even more tragic event occurred in Italy, in 1976, when 'dioxin', another toxic chlorine compound, was accidentally discharged from the trichlorophenol reactor over a large populated area in Seveso, causing much hardship to adults and children, and necessitating prolonged large-scale evacuation of this region.

Arrest of spermatogenesis and severe degenerative changes in the testes are characteristic of the effects produced by a number of other chlorine and bromine organic industrial chemicals in men and animals. In this category are dibromochloropropane (soil fumigant against nematodes), dibromopropanol (the mutagenic derivative of Tris-BP) and dibromoethane (a petrol additive and a fumigant used in controlling grain insects and for disinfecting seed, tobacco and food in storage). Similarly dangerous are insecticides such ad DDT (dichlorodiphenyl trichloroethane), and herbicides such as the defoliant trichlorophenoxyacetic acid. Many other substances have also gained much attention in recent years as potential antifertility and mutagenic agents. Of special concern are in this respect Tris-BP (*tris*[2, 3-dibromopropyl]phosphate) and the chemically closely related *tris*[dichloropropyl]phosphate, since flame retardants speedily penetrate the skin of the human scrotum.

As regards insecticides, several organophosphorus compounds belonging to this group have been shown to be powerful inhibitors of choline esterase; and parathion, the extremely toxic phosphothioate analogue, was shown to be an effective inhibitor of testosterone metabolism in the liver. Testicular atrophy and in some instances involution of the male accessory organs have been observed in animals after the application of a good many other industrial chemicals, notably carbamate insecticides which inhibit choline esterase, paraquat and ethylene oxide cyclic tetramer (endowed with chelating properties).

2.3 Chemotherapeutic Drugs

Pronounced antifertility properties attributable to either spermatogenic failure or inhibition of steroidogenesis in the testis, are typical of a wide range of chemotherapeutic drugs. Niridazole, the schistosomicidal drug is a strong suppressor of the meiotic division of the spermatocytes. Cyclophosphamide, the cytostatic drug used effectively in the treatment of lymphoma, acute lymphocytic leukaemia and nephrotic syndrome, frequently produces germinal aplasia and azoospermia in patients on immunosuppressive therapy, especially when used in combination with other cytostatic agents. Cimetidine, which is widely used in the treatment of peptic ulcer disease, acts both as antiandrogen and antispermatogenic agent; it lowers the output of spermatozoa in the human ejaculate and in some cases produces impotence and gynaecomastia; in male rats it inhibits competitively the binding of dihydrotestosterone to cytoplasmic receptors in the ventral prostate and seminal vesicle.

2.4 Psychopharmaceuticals

Among the antipsychotic, antianxiety and antidepressant drugs belonging to this group and available for the treatment of emotional disorders, there are several that affect male reproductive function. Thioridazine and chlorpromazine have been reported to interfere with ejaculation, to weaken erection and delay ejaculation in men. Reserpine, another antipsychotic drug, inhibits ejaculation, though by no means consistently. Men treated with reserpine frequently complain of loss of libido, and some also exhibit feminization symptoms, probably due to changes in the neuroendocrine activity of the brain (the hypothalamus in particular) and interference with the biosynthesis, storage and release of biogenic amines. As regards the antianxiety and antidepressant agents, failure of ejaculation has been described in men treated with chlordiazepoxide;

some of the hydrazide derivatives have also been shown to possess antiejaculatory properties.

2.5 Antispermatogenic, Antiandrogenic and Spermicidal Agents

Broadly speaking, antispermatogenic agents fall into three groups, namely those acting on the mitotic, meiotic and postmeiotic stage of sperm development, but on close examination some of these substances affect several stages, pending on dosage and conditions of teatment. Colchicine acts mainly on mitosis, whereas two-phase sterility is typical of certain alkylating agents such as tretamine (2, 4, 6-triethyleneiminotriazine). Nitrofurane derivatives ingested by mice or rats inhibit predominantly the primary spermatocyte stage of spermatogenesis, but they can also destroy spermatogonia. Nitropyrroles are capable of interfering with the primary spermatocyte stage and the spermatid transformation.

Testosterone itself, notwithstanding the fact that it is a normal product of the testis and essential for spermatogenesis and function of the male accessory organs, when administered in suitable doses, can successfully suppress spermatogenesis and thereby produce oligospermia or temporary azoospermia. It is because of this antispermatogenic activity that testosterone, along with certain other steroids such as danazol or various progestational steroids, has been considered for use as a male contraceptive (Patanelli, 1978). These suppressive effects on the testis are, however, not the result of a direct interaction with the testis, but the outcome of inhibitory influence on the gonadotrophic function of the pituitary gland. The same is true of certain oestrogens, steroidal and nonsteroidal (e.g. diethylstilboestrol) which act mainly *via* the pituitary gland. In this respect, however, there are notable exceptions, and oestrogens in particular can produce inhibitory effects by acting on the testis directly. The antispermatogenic action of methallibure is mediated by the pituitary gland, and the same applies to certain siloxanes and chlormadinone, as well as the new synthetic agonists of the hypothalamic gonadotropin-releasing hormone, which when injected in suitable doses over a period of several weeks, strongly inhibit spermatogenesis.

Quite distinct from the pituitary-mediated mechanism of action exerted by testosterone and other steroids on the testis, is the mode of action of the so-called antiandrogens. Cyproterone acetate, methylnortestosterone and other antiandrogens act at the level of target organs, be it the testis, prostate, seminal vesicle or other organs. Their principal action depends on competing with testosterone and dihydrotestosterone for androgen receptors. By blocking access to testosterone and dihydrotestosterone, the antiandrogens prevent the Sertoli cells in the testis from forming normal secretory products such as the androgen-binding protein, and they prevent the male accessory organs from carrying out their normal secretory function, expressed in the formation of fructose, citric acid and other chemical constituents of the seminal plasma.

Concerning the mechanism of action of drugs which interact directly with spermatozoa, distinction must be drawn between substances which, when acting on spermatozoa *in vitro*, immobilize them reversibly, that is temporarily, and can therefore be designated as spermiostatic, and other agents, more properly called spermicidal, which incapacitate the spermatozoa permanently (Mann, 1958, 1964). Enzyme inhibitors, such as sodium fluoride, are on the whole spermiostatic, provided that their contact with the sperm cell is not a prolonged one; when fluoride is removed from the spermatozoa in good time, motility recovers. Many thiol reagents and most detergents, on the other hand, particularly when applied in high concentrations, are spermicidal in the full sense of the term; the structural and biochemical changes which they induce, such as disruption of the sperm plasmalemma or the leakage of intracellular enzymes and coenzymes, cannot be reversed. But in some instances the adverse effects of these substances can be prevented by advanced application of certain protective agents. Thus, for example, the antiperoxidant factor which we detected in the seminal plasma, effectively protects the spermatozoa from the lethal effects of unsaturated fatty acid peroxides (Jones *et al.*, 1979; Mann *et al.*, 1980), and sulphhydryl-containing substances such as reduced glutathione, cysteine or ergothioneine can protect the spermatozoa from the spermicidal effect of certain heavy metals.

Among heavy metals, copper and mercury (inorganic and organically bound) have strong spermicidal properties. Systemically introduced cadmium also constitutes a hazard to testicular function as clearly demonstrated by Pařizek (1956, 1960), but the available evidence favours the view that the destructive influence of cadmium on the seminiferous epithelium is caused primarily by ischaemia and necrotic changes due to interference with testicular vascularization and breakdown of the blood–testis barrier. In line with this concept are some observations on the countereffects of selenium which protects the testis from the injurious effects of cadmium. Apart from the seminiferous tubules and spermatogenesis, cadmium damages also the interstitial tissue; in the hamster, a single injection of 1 mg $CdCl_2$ produces a marked reduction in the content of testosterone, dihydrotestosterone and other steroids in both the testis and the blood (Lau *et al.*, 1978).

Of the many other substances with either antispermatogenic or spermicidal properties, two have received exceptional attention in recent years. One is gossypol and the other α-chlorohydrin. As a result of extensive clinical trials, conducted mainly in China, gossypol, a disesquiterpene aldehydic constituent of cottonseed oil, has been recommended in that country as a male antifertility agent; after 20 mg/day, orally given for 2 months, most men had a sperm count below 4 million/ml or showed necrospermia. The mechanism of the anti-spermatogenic action of gossypol and the various general side effects resulting from its ingestion, are still under investigation; gossypol is also known to immobilize human spermatozoa *in vitro*, but at concentration levels (5–40 mg/ml) which are far in excess of doses effective *in vivo* (Waller *et al.*, 1981). Chlorohydrin acts on the spermatozoa primarily in the epididymis, as shown by experiments on rats; the toxicity of chlorohydrin precludes its testing in man. Two enzymatic reactions in the spermatozoa seem to be specially sensitive to chlorohydrin; one involving glycerol kinase, and the other glyceraldehyde-3-phosphate dehydrogenase. Other competitive inhibitors of sperm enzymes include a variety of antimetabolites, such as deoxyglucose and chlorinated sugars.

3 METHODOLOGICAL CRITERIA IN THE APPRAISAL OF DAMAGE INDUCED BY CHEMICALS IN THE MALE REPRODUCTIVE TRACT AND SEMEN

3.1 The *in Vitro* Fertilization Test

The ultimate test of male fertility is the ability of the spermatozoon to fertilize the egg cell and to produce healthy offspring. The quickest way to assess the fertilizing ability of the spermatozoon under laboratory conditions is to perform the fertilization test *in vitro*. This procedure is now extensively utilized in investigations with the gametes of laboratory animals, and it has been suggested that it may form a basis for exploring the effect of drugs that interfere with the process of sperm penetration and fertilization. For example, fertilization of a freshly procured mouse egg with zona pellucida intact, by a mouse spermatozoon, can be inhibited (*in vitro*) in a dose-dependent fashion by some cholinomimetic agents (Florman and Storey, 1981). However, a test of this kind could hardly be routinely applied to human eggs, not merely because they are not readily available, but also because their use for laboratory experiments may conflict with ethical views. It is noteworthy that *in vitro* human spermatozoa are capable of fusing with the vitelline membrane of zona-denuded hamster eggs and are subsequently capable of undergoing decondensation, and this observation gave rise to the suggestion that hamster eggs could be used for assaying the fertilizing potential of human spermatozoa (Barros *et al.*, 1979); zona-free eggs of the hamster also fuse with spermatozoa of other animals, e.g. those of the guinea pig and boar, the latter being able to fuse only after they have undergone the acrosome reaction, which is a normal prerequisite of fertilization (Imai *et al.*, 1980).

So far, the reproducibility of the hamster-egg *in vitro* test as a method of assaying fertility in individual men has been investigated only on a small scale (Bentwood *et al.*, 1981), but its clinical practicability for drug screening certainly deserves further exploration.

3.2 Evaluation of Testicular Function

Testicular biopsy is not free of hazards. None the less, histological analysis of tissue specimens obtained by this method has been recognized for some time as a helpful procedure for diagnosing spermatogenic failure and assessing the extent of damage inflicted upon the testis by antispermatogenic agents. The quantifiable histological techniques involving light microscopy are now being supplemented by electron microscopic assays. In addition, as a result of the perfection of chemical methods of androgen analysis (radioimmunoassay in particular), testicular biopsy specimens are increasingly used for determinations of testosterone and other testicular steroids, and also for exploring the ability of the testicular tissue to synthesize testosterone *in vitro* from added labelled precursors. Another frequently employed method of assessing the endocrine function of the testis, and the androgenic status of the male as a whole, depends on measuring testosterone in blood plasma. However, in view of the large fluctuations in the blood testosterone level of man and animals, sporadic analyses of blood plasma are of little value, since the results are strongly influenced by the episodic, circadian and seasonal variations in the pattern of testosterone release by the testis, also by the age of the individual, schedule of blood sampling, the amount of luteinizing hormone available to the testis around the time of blood sampling, and nutritional and environmental factors (the phototropic stimuli in particular). An additional factor that must be carefully considered in evaluating the results of androgen analysis in blood is that under normal conditions only a small proportion of testosterone is in a free, that is, active form, and the major part is protein bound.

A variety of testis-specific proteins and enzymes has been described in man and animals, and their appearance in the normally developing prepubescent testis has been shown to coincide with specific stages of spermatogenesis, that is, the appearance of primary spermatocytes, secondary spermatocytes, spermatids and testicular spermatozoa (still immotile and infertile). Enzymes in this category are the testis-specific LDH-X isozyme of lactate dehdrogenase, acid phosphatase, esterase, sorbitol dehydrogenase and various glycosidases, peptidases and proteases. These findings gave rise to the idea that enzymes of this kind could be used as biochemical markers or 'fingerprints' of particular steps in the spermatogenic process, not merely in the normal testis, but also in gonads with abnormal spermatogenesis. It remains to be seen how far enzymatic fingerprinting, along with other methods, such as histochemical and autoradiographic techniques, can be developed for assessing the adverse effects of chemicals on spermatogenesis.

For the moment, direct examination of the ejaculated semen provides the simplest and most reliable means of assessing the degree of damage inflicted by an antispermatogenic agent on testicular gametogenic function. The volume of the ejaculate, the concentration and total number of spermatozoa in that ejaculate, the relative proportion of motile and immotile spermatozoa and the ratio between live and dead sperm cells (assessed by live–dead differential staining procedures), the degree of motility (assessed microscopically or by physical means), and the type and percentage of abnormal spermatozoa, along with related tests such as the cervical mucus penetration and postcoital tests, offer the best chance of evaluating the effects of drugs on gametogenic function, provided of course, that several factors are taken into account. Time interval since the previous emission of semen, frequency of ejaculation, microbial contamination of semen, and the method by means of which semen has been collected and stored prior to examination, all these and other factors have to be considered in the appraisal of semen quality. Above all, whilst considering the adverse effect of a drug on spermatogenesis, one must bear in mind the fact that the injury to the testis might have occurred as long as 2 months prior to the time of semen collection and examination, in view of the period of time required for completion of spermatogenesis in the testis and sperm passage (and maturation) in the epididymis.

It is possible that in the future hormone analyses in ejaculated semen will become part of the routine examination of semen for assessing defects in the androgenic status of the male. Testosterone, dihydrotestosterone, follicle-stimulating hormone, luteinizing hormone, a chorionic-gonadotrophin-like hormone, prolactin, these and other hormones occur in the seminal plasma of man and animals (for recent literature see Eiler and Graves, 1981; Mann and Lutwak-Mann, 1981; p. 135, this paper).

3.3 Evaluation of the Functional State of Male Accessory Organs

When semen is collected by the split-ejaculate method, it is frequently possible to obtain several fractions of the ejaculate, originating in different and distinct parts of the male reproductive tract, such as the epididymis, seminal vesicle, prostate, Cowper's gland and urethral glands. In man, the determination of the activity of acid phosphatase and the concentration of citric acid and zinc provides a sensitive criterion of the prostatic secretory activity, whilst that of fructose, lactoferrin and prostaglandins, among other substances, can serve as a criterion for assessing the secretory output of the seminal vesicles. Carnitine and glycerylphosphorylcholine are sometimes used for determining the contribution of the epididymal secretion, but in man the usefulness of glycerylphosphoryl-choline as an indicator of the epididymal secretory function is limited by the occurrence of this substance also in the seminal vesicle secretion.

The secretory output of male accessory glands of reproduction and consequently the composition of the seminal plasma are both strictly dependent upon androgenic stimuli emanating from the testis, and therefore, chemical analysis of either whole semen or even more so, of a split ejaculate, can be used for diagnosing effects of androgen deficiency on male reproductive function in a number of species, amongst them the bull, boar, stallion, rabbit and deer. Chemical analyses of semen and seminal fractions can also serve to diagnose degenerative changes in distinct parts of the male reproductive tract, such as inborn occlusion of the ejaculatory duct and deferent duct in cases of cystic fibrosis. Chemical methods of semen analyses also help to express in a quantitative manner the effects of drugs on the output of individual male accessory glands of reproduction, as demonstrated for example, by the investigations of the action of pilocarpine and atropine (Mann and Lutwak-Mann, 1976).

3.4 Drug-induced Disturbances in the Ejaculatory Process

Earlier on in our paper, examples were given of drugs which influence adversely erection and ejaculation. Underlying this pathology are probably faults in the autonomous nervous mechanism which controls the contractile pattern of the male reproductive tract. Normally, ejaculation is initiated by strong contraction, probably starting in the ductuli efferentes of the testis, and quickly spreading along the entire length of the tract, when first the prostate, next the ampullae and finally the seminal vesicles contract in an orderly fashion, thus predetermining the chemical character of the various seminal fractions which constitute the split ejaculate. In man, the secretion of Littré's (urethral) and Cowper's (bulbourethral) glands precedes the ejection of the prostatic secretion, which is then followed by the spermatozoa and finally, the seminal vesicle secretion. Chemical analysis of the seminal fractions by the split-ejaculate method enables one to decide whether the ejaculatory pattern is normal, slightly upset or seriously disturbed. In extreme cases of ejaculatory sterility, semen is ejaculated into the bladder, and this state of retrograde ejaculation is best diagnosed by urine analysis; collection of spermatozoa from urine is sometimes useful in connection with artificial insemination.

Ejaculation disturbances are also encountered in animals, as for example, in the stallion, in which ejaculation is a fairly prolonged process, enabling one to collect several distinct seminal fractions. Combined analyses of citric acid (coming from the seminal vesicles) and ergothioneine (a secretory product of the large ampullary glands) in split ejaculates of stallions with ejaculatory disturbances have shown that in some such animals the citric acid appears in the ejaculate before instead of after the spermatozoa and ergothioneine (Mann, 1975).

3.5 Passage of Chemicals into Semen

Alcohol, salicylates and sulphonamides, to name but a few, pass after ingestion into human and animal semen. The same is true of ampicillin, erythromycin and other antibiotics, but it is possible that in some studies leading to the detection of drugs in semen insufficient care may have been exercised to exclude contamination of semen by traces of urine. Tetracycline and thalidomide together with its metabolites, also readily find their way into semen; having passed into the semen, thalidomide becomes firmly attached to the spermatozoa (Lutwak-Mann *et al.*, 1967).

Methadone, phenytoin, valproic acid, tranexamic acid, urea and selenite provide further examples of substances capable of passing into semen. A recent addition to this list is *tris*[dichloropropyl]phosphate, above-mentioned as one of the flame retardants with mutagenic and antifertility properties (Hudec *et al.*, 1981). Detection of unusual chemicals in semen is made easier nowadays by the perfection of sensitive chemical methods. Compounds that may have escaped detection, even by gas chromatography–mass spectrometry, can now be screened in human and animal seminal plasma by more sophisticated means. Negative-chemical-ionization mass spectral screening used in the detection of *tris*[dichloropropyl]phosphate in extracts of human seminal plasma, provides a good example of the advantages that modern analytical techniques offer in investigations of drug passage into the semen.

4 CONCLUDING REMARKS

As this brief survey indicates, the information available to date on the mechanisms underlying the adverse effects of chemicals on male reproductive function is patchy and in need of more thorough documentation. Equally, the methodological criteria for appraising the damage induced by chemicals in the male reproductive tract and semen are too few and imperfect. These particular aspects of andrological pharmacology and toxicology, while still underdeveloped, represent an eminently attractive area for future research.

5 REFERENCES

Amann, R. P. (1981). A critical review of methods for evaluation of spermatogenesis for seminal characteristics. *J. Androl.* **2**, 37–58.

Anderson, R. A., Beyler, S. A. and Zaneveld, L. J. D. (1978). Alterations of male reproduction induced by chronic ingestion of ethanol: development of an animal model. *Fertil. Steril.* **30**, 103–105.

Badr, F. M. and Badr, R. S. (1975). Induction of dominant lethal mutations in male mice by ethyl alcohol. *Nature (London)* **253**, 134–136.

Barros, C., Gonzalez, J., Herrera, E. and Bustos-Obregon, E. (1979). Human sperm penetration into zona-free hamster oocytes as a test to evaluate the sperm fertilizing ability. *Andrologia* **11**, 197–210.

Bentwood, B. J., Rogers, J. and McCarville, C. (1981). Variation of human fertilization using the *in vitro* fertilization assay. *J. Androl.* **2**, 8.

Chen, E. (1979). *PBB: An American Tragedy*. Prentice-Hall, Englewood Cliffs, New Jersey.

Davies, A. G. (1980). Effects of hormones, drugs and chemicals on testicular function. *Eden Press Annual Research Reviews: Endocrinology*, Vol. 1, pp. 1–276. Eden Press, Westmount, Quebec, Canada.

Dixon, R. L. and Lee, I. P. (1980). Pharmacokinetic and adaptation factors in testicular toxicity. *Fedn Proc.* **39**, 66.

Dougherty, R. C., Whitaker, M. J., Tang, S-Y, Bottcher, R., Keller, M. and Kuehl, D. W. (1980). Sperm density and toxic substances: a potential key to environmental health hazards. In McKinney, J. D. (Ed.) *The Chemistry of Environmental Agents as Potential Human Hazards*, pp. 263–278. Ann Arbor Science Publishers, Inc., Ann Arbor, Michigan.

Eiler, H. and Graves, C. N. (1981). Nature of the clearance of exogenous testosterone and progesterone in ejaculated bovine semen. *J. Androl.* **2**, 205–210.

Emboden, W. (1979). *Narcotic Plants, Hallucinogens, Stimulants, Inebriants and Hypnotics, their Origin and Uses*, 202 pages. Collier Books (Division of Macmillan Publishing Co., Inc.), New York.

Florman, H. M. and Storey, B. T. (1981). Cholinomimetic agents as inhibitors of mouse fertilization *in vitro*: indications of a different approach to male fertility regulation. *J. Androl.* **2**, 12.

Gomes, W. R. (1977). Pharmacological agents and male fertility. In Johnson, A. D., and Gomes, W. R. (Eds.) *The Testis*, Vol. 4, pp. 605–627. Academic Press, Inc., New York.

Gordon, G. G., Altman, K., Southren, L., Rubin, E. and Lieber, C. S. (1976). Effect of alcohol (ethanol) administration on sex-hormone metabolism in normal men. *New Engl. J. Med.* **295**, 795–797.

Henderson, G. and Hughes, J. (1976). The effects of morphine on the release of noradrenaline from the mouse vas deferens. *Br. J. Pharmacol.* **57**, 551–557.

Hudec, T., Thean, J., Kuehl, D. and Dougherty, R. C. (1981). *Tris*(dichloropropyl)phosphate, a mutagenic flame retardant: frequent occurrence in human seminal plasma. *Science (Washington, DC)* **211**, 951–952.

Imai, H., Niva, K. and Iritani, A. (1980). Ultrastructural observations of boar spermatozoa penetrating zona-free hamster eggs. *Biol. Reprod.* **23**, 481–486.

Jones, R., Mann, T. and Sherins, R. J. (1979). Peroxidative breakdown of phospholipids in human spermatozoa, spermicidal properties of fatty acid peroxides, and protective action of seminal plasma. *Fertil. Steril.* **31**, 531–537.

Lau, I. F., Saksena, S. K., Dahlgren, L. and Chang, M. C. (1978). Steroids in the blood serum and testes of cadmium chloride treated hamsters. *Biol. Reprod.* **19**, 886–889.

Lucier, G. W., Lee, J. P. and Dixon, R. L. (1977). Effects of environmental agents on male reproduction. In Johnson, A. D. and Gomes, W. R. (Eds.) *The Testis*, Vol. 4, pp. 577–603. Academic Press, Inc., New York.

Lutwak-Mann, C., Schmid, K. and Keberle, H. (1967). Thalidomide in rabbit semen. *Nature (London)* **214**, 1018–1020.

Mann, T. (1958). Biochemical basis of spermicidal activity. *Proc. Soc. Study Fertil.* **9**, 3–27.

Mann, T. (1964). *The Biochemistry of Semen and of the Male Reproductive Tract*, 493 pages. Methuen & Co., Ltd, London, and John Wiley & Sons, Inc., New York.

Mann, T. (1968). Effects of pharmacological agents on male sexual functions. *J. Reprod. Fertil., Suppl.* **4**, 101–114.

Mann, T. (1970). Reproduction: sex, drugs and ethics. *Impact Sci. Soc.* (Engl. ed.), **20**, 255–265.

Mann, T. (1975). Biochemistry of stallion semen. *J. Reprod. Fertil. Suppl.* **23**, 47–52.

Mann, T. and Lutwak-Mann C. (1976). Evaluation of the functional state of male accessory glands by the analysis of seminal plasma. *Andrologia* **8**, 237–242.

Mann, T., Jones, R. and Sherins, R. (1980). Oxygen damage, lipid peroxidation, and motility of spermatozoa. In Steinberger, A. and Steinberger, E. (Eds.) *Testicular Development, Structure and Function*, pp. 497–501. Raven Press, Inc., New York.

Neumann, F., Diallo, F. A., Hasan, S. H., Schenck, B. and Traore, I. (1976). The influence of pharmaceutical compounds on male fertility. *Andrologia* **8**, 203–235.

Pařizek, J. (1956). Effect of cadmium salts on testicular tissue. *Nature* (*London*) **177**, 1036–1037.

Pařizek, J. (1960). Sterilization of the male by cadmium salts. *J. Reprod. Fertil.* **1**, 294–309.

Patanelli, D. J. (Ed.) (1978). *Hormonal Control of Male Fertility*, 420 pages. US Department of Health, Education, and Welfare Publication No. NIH-78-1097.

Thomas, J. A. (1975). Effects of pesticides on reproduction. In Thomas, J. A. and Singhal, R. L. (Eds.) *Molecular Mechanisms of Gonadal Hormone Action*, pp. 205–223. University Park Press, Baltimore, London, Tokyo.

Thomas, J. A., Shahid-Salles, K. S. and Donovan, M. P. (1977). Effects of narcotics on the reproductive system. In Thomas, J. A. and Singhal, R. L. (Eds.) *Regulatory Mechanisms Affecting Gonadal Hormone Action*, pp. 169–195. University Park Press, Baltimore, London, Tokyo.

Van Thiel, D. H., Gavaler, J. S., Cobb, C. F., Sherins, R. J. and Lester, R. (1979). Alcohol-induced testicular atrophy in the adult male rat. *Endocrinology* **105**, 888–895.

Waller, D. P., Cameron, S. M. and Zaneveld, L. J. D. (1981). Spermicidal effect of gossypol in an *in vitro* animal model for vaginal contraceptives. *J. Androl.* **2**, 32.

Methods for Assessing the Effects of Chemicals on Reproductive Functions
Edited by V. B. Vouk and P. J. Sheehan
© 1983 SCOPE

Laboratory Aspects of Reproductive Toxicology

ROBERT L. DIXON

1 INTRODUCTION

There is an increasing concern that gonadal effects of environmental chemicals are having ecological consequences as well as effects on human reproduction. Scientific and public attention has recently been focused on such agents as dibromochloropropane (DBCP), Kepone, TRIS, as well as the phenoxyacid components of the herbicide Agent Orange and its 'dioxin' contaminant (Dixon, and Hall, 1982; CEQ, 1981). Suggestions have been made that the average sperm count has decreased, and that the percentage of men whose sperm counts fall below a level generally associated with optimal fertility has increased (Dougherty et al., 1981).

Although the primary focus of attention is usually the effects of environmental agents on the testis, it is appropriate to recall that the final indicator of testicular function is the number of viable sperm ejaculated, and that semen represents the contributions of the epididymides and accessory sex glands as well as the testis (Amann, 1981; Dixon, 1981a; Mann and Lutwak-Mann, 1981).

Thus, this paper will consider the spectrum of biological processes which contribute to the ejaculation of high quality semen and the effects of environmental agents on them. These include:

(1) the hypothalamo–pituitary–gonadal axis;
(2) the testicular interstitial compartment and steroidogenesis;
(3) the blood–testis barrier;
(4) the seminiferous tubules and spermatogenesis;
(5) the efferent ducts;
(6) the epididymides;
(7) formation and composition of semen; and
(8) erection and ejaculation.

2 HYPOTHALAMO–PITUITARY–GONADAL AXIS

Follicle-stimulating hormone (FSH) and luteinizing hormone (LH/ICSH) are glycoproteins released from the basophilic cells of the pituitary. Central

149

regulation of the pituitary is mediated by the hypothalamus communicating via a specialized vascular system called the hypophyseal portal system. Hypothalamic neuroendocrine neurons are present in the arcuate and other nuclei of the median eminence. These neurons secrete specific releasing or release-inhibiting factors into the hypophyseal portal system. These hormones are carried in the blood of the portal system to the cells of the adenohypophysis where they act on their target cells to stimulate or inhibit the release of FSH or ICSH. Follicle-stimulating hormone-releasing hormone (FSH-RH) and luteinizing hormone-releasing hormone (LH-RH) have been isolated and appear to be identical (Amann, 1981).

This sensitive and complex system presents a number of targets by which environmental chemicals may produce an altered function. However, few examples of toxic effects are well documented despite the great variety of drugs known to exert significant effects.

3 THE TESTIS

The testis can be divided into two major compartments: the interstitial space and the seminiferous tubules. These compartments have different embryological origins, unique cell populations, and distinct functions. The major products of the interstitial space are androgens secreted by the Leydig cells; the major products of the seminiferous tubules are the male gametes which arise from the spermatogonial stem cells. Both compartments are closely inter-related with the pituitary and hypothalamus.

3.1 The Interstitial Compartment and Steroidogenesis

The Leydig cells are the main site of testosterone synthesis and are closely associated with the blood vessels and the lymphatic space of the testis. This inter-relationship facilitates the transport of testosterone from the Leydig cells into the tubules.

ICSH stimulates steroidogenesis, in part, by increasing the hydrolysis of cholesterol esters to free cholesterol which is subsequently taken up by the mitochondria. Cholesterol is probably the source of all testicular steroid hormones. Large doses of testosterone maintain spermatogenesis in adult male hypophysectomized rats, hence the effect of LH on spermatogenesis is assumed to be mediated, in large part, through the stimulation of testosterone production.

3.2 Role of Testosterone in Sexual Development

The fetal testes synthesize large amounts of androgens which subsequently play a critical role in the differentiation of the gonads and secondary sex characteristics. The initial critical period for testosterone production is gestational days 14–17 in the rat and weeks 4–6 in the human.

Knowledge of the dynamics of testosterone production and cellular inter-actions are important prerequisites to the understanding of which chemicals might affect sexual differentiation. In the synthesis of testosterone from pregnenolone, the rate-limiting enzyme is the microsomal 3β-hydroxysteroid dehydrogenase which oxidizes the A ring hydroxyl of the steroid precursors. Free testosterone is transformed to a more active hormone, 5α-dihydrotestosterone (DHT), by 5α-reductase in the target tissue. To initiate their actions, both testosterone and DHT must be bound to specific cytoplasmic receptor proteins that permit translocation to the nucleus. Subsequent nuclear interactions initiate DNA synthesis and RNA directed synthesis of androgen-dependent proteins. Blocking or interrupting this process during any one of its steps during the initial critical period of gestation could deter the androgen's action and allow complete or partial expression of the innate female programme.

Because androgen synthesis by the fetal testis dictates changes in the Mullerian and Wolffian duct systems which account for the phenotypical male sexual differentiation, factors which alter the synthesis or actions of these androgens might have important toxicological consequences. Under the influence of a Mullerian inhibiting factor (MIF), the Mullerian ducts begin to regress shortly after testicular differentiation. Males with dysgenetic testes fail to produce MIH, thus, Mullerian ducts persist and female internal genitalia are formed.

The epididymides, vas deferens, seminal vesicle and ejaculatory duct are derived from the Wolffian elements and are under control of testosterone. Testosterone also controls the differentiation of the urethra and prostate gland which are derived from the urogenital sinus as well as the development of the scrotum and penis.

Any factor which would reduce the ability of testosterone to be synthesized, activated, enter the cell, and/or affect the cell nucleus' ability to regulate the synthesis of androgen-dependent proteins would have a potential to alter sexual differentiation. A variety of endogenous and exogenous chemicals are capable of exerting a testosterone-depriving action on the developing systems. Targets of action include the feedback regulation of gonadotropin secretion, gonadotropin effectiveness, testosterone and dihydrotestosterone synthesis, plasma binding, as well as cytoplasmic receptors and nuclear binding. The end result of such chemical effects is a chemical castration. However, no systematic attempt has been made to survey environmental chemicals for their ability to act by the mechanisms described (Dixon, 1982).

3.3 The Blood–Testis Barrier

The blood–testis barrier (BTB) functionally separates the interstitial space from the seminiferous tubules. Physiological evidence for the existence of the blood–testis barrier was first reported by Setchell *et al.* (1969). They de-monstrated that immunoglobulins and iodinated albumin, inulin, and some small molecules were excluded from the seminiferous tubules by the BTB. Dym and Fawcett (1970), studying the distribution of a low molecular weight protein, horseradish peroxidases, and the lanthanum ion in the testis, suggested that the primary permeability barrier for the seminiferous tubules was the surrounding layers of myoid cells. Where these layers were breached, specialized Sertoli-cell-to-Sertoli-cell junctions within the seminiferous epithelium constituted a secondary cellular barrier.

To quantify the functional BTB, we investigated some of the physicochemical parameters governing the movement of chemicals and drugs across the BTB into the male rat testis (Okumura *et al.*, 1975). In these studies, the permeability of non-electrolytes with varying molecular sizes and of barbiturates, sulphonamides and salicylic acid with varying partition coefficients and pK_a values was determined. The movement of the non-electrolytes indicated that the permeability of compounds across the BTB depends on their molecular size. Apparently, molecules smaller than 3.6 Å (e.g., water, urea) can be transported readily across the BTB, while larger molecules such as galactose and inulin cannot.

Permeability studies of drugs with varying lipid solubilities, such as thiopentone, pentobarbitone, barbitone, sulphamethoxypyridazine, sulphanilamide, sulphaguanidine, and salicylic acid, demonstrated that such drugs do not attain rete testis concentrations greater than plasma and that the transport processes appear to be exponential with time. Transport rate constants for all drugs studied plotted as straight lines; the rates of entry into the rete testis fluid were proportional to the concentration gradient in accordance with Fick's law. Transfer rate constants derived from the slopes of the seven test chemicals demonstrated good correlation between their respective lipid solubilities and membrane penetrabilities, suggesting that the rate-limiting factor for transport of these compounds across the BTB is the lipid solubility of chemicals at physiological pH. The permeability characteristics of the BTB appeared to be generally similar to those of membranes which limit penetration of foreign chemicals into the central nervous system, gastrointestinal tract, mammary gland, and aqueous humour.

The ability of the BTB to control the entry of chemicals into the seminiferous tubules is affected by a number of physiological, chemical and pathological factors (Dixon, 1981b). It has been reported that the BTB in newborn animals may be immature and less effective than at puberty; the BTB might also become less efficient as testicular function wanes in later life. Heating of ram testes increased the transfer rate of various ions and other chemicals, and exposure to ionizing radiation might be expected to have similar effects. Cadmium has also been reported to alter the permeability of the BTB. However, these changes appear to be associated more with entry to the rete testis than the seminiferous tubules. Thus, a number of factors are known and others can be suggested which could alter the function of the BTB and result in altered penetration of foreign chemicals to the germ cells, thus creating an unnatural chemical environment for the maturing sperm.

3.4 The Seminiferous Tubules and Spermatogenesis

The major cell types of the seminiferous tubules are the various spermatogenic cells and the Sertoli cells (Burger and de Kretser, 1981). The Sertoli cells appear to be the host cells for the developing germ cells. Sertoli cells or spermatogonia line the tubule with other germinal cells either situated between adjacent pairs of Sertoli cells or embedded in the luminal margin of the Sertoli cell cytoplasm. Specialized junctions form where adjacent Sertoli cells meet. These junctions divide the extracellular space inside the tubule into a basal compartment between the Sertoli cells and spermatogonia and an adluminal compartment between the Sertoli cells and the spermatocytes and spermatids.

The Sertoli cells perform an essential role in spermatogenesis by controlling the immediate environment around the spermatocytes and spermatids. The Sertoli cells may also play a role in the genetic induction of testicular differentiation because a testis-determining gene on the Y chromosome apparently determines gonadal sex and converts the indifferent gonad into a testis. There is increasing experimental evidence that plasma membrane protein, known as H-Y antigen, is this testis-determining gene product. The Sertoli cells also secrete fluid, synthesize androgen binding protein (ABP) and produce inhibin which is involved in the feedback regulation with the pituitary. It is probable that many chemicals which affect spermatogenesis act via an effect on the Sertoli cells rather than directly on the germ cell.

Spermatogonia cell mitosis takes place in the basal compartment, and the spermatogonia, preleptotene and leptotene spermatocytes are observed there. At the end of the leptotene phase of meiosis, the primary spermatocytes pass between the Sertoli cells and enter the adluminal compartment where the zygotene spermatocytes continue to develop through the pachytene and diplotene phases of mitosis and then divide meiotically to form secondary spermatocytes.

Thus, shortly after completing DNA synthesis, the developing gametes leave the basal compartment, traverse the blood–testis barrier, and enter the adluminal compartment. Sequestered behind the blood–testis barrier, the developing germ cells experience a unique chemical environment which is apparently essential for the completion of meiosis and spermatogenesis.

The primary role of the seminiferous tubules is spermatogenesis, the production of sperm. However, the sperm mature in the proximal epididymis and fertile sperm are stored in the distal epididymis. Spermatogenesis represents the total series of cellular transformations that allow spermatogonia to differentiate into sperm while retaining the spermatogonial reserve.

In the common laboratory animals, numerous spermatogonia in a particular area of the seminiferous tubules divide synchronously and the cohorts of cells which result differentiate in unison. Because intracellular bridges persist between the cytoplasm of the germinal cells after the nuclei divide, adjacent histological cross-sections through the seminiferous tubules appear different. Detailed analyses have defined as many as 14 different cellular association stages in the rat. Each cellular association contains four or five types or layers of germ cells associated in a specific pattern. The complete series of cellular associations is termed the cycle of the seminiferous epithelium. In contrast to laboratory animals, only a few adjacent cohorts of germ cells develop synchronously in man and the cellular patterns are much less distinct. Degeneration of potential germ cells contributes to this phenomenon.

Two classes of spermatogonia are present in the seminiferous tubules. The first, spermatogonia A, does not enter the normal process of spermatogenesis but continually divides by mitosis. The other class, spermatogonia B, also proliferates by mitosis but gives rise to cohorts of increasingly differentiated spermatogenic cells. The end product of this cellular differentiation is sperm.

The relative duration of each stage of spermatogenesis can be estimated histologically or with tritiated thymidine pulse labelling. The seminiferous tubule cycle ranges from 8 to 16 days depending on species. However, for each species it is quite constant and unaffected by sexual activity. The duration of spermatogenesis is the interval between the time when stem spermatogonia become committed to produce a cohort of spermatids and the time of the release of the resulting sperm from the germinal epithelium. The duration of spermatogenesis equals about 4.5 cycles of the seminiferous epithelium. Thus, each cycle of mature spermatids released from the germinal epithelium originates from spermatogonia committed to differentiation approximately 4.5 cycles earlier. Because cohorts of developing germ cells in different regions within the tubules complete spermatogenesis at different times, sperm are continuously released from the germinal epithelium.

The regularity of spermatogenesis allows one to define the spermatogenic cell stages affected by chemicals and suggests mechanisms of toxicity. Various drugs and environmental chemicals can produce specific lesions that result in the degeneration of all germ cells at the point of attack and eventually eliminate those more advanced forms which would have differentiated from the affected cells. In order to discover such effects, we routinely develop fertility profiles by serially mating males following chemical treatment (Lee and Dixon, 1972). Treated male rodents are housed with females at 4–5-day intervals. The number of fertile males is determined by pregnant females. Females are considered pregnant if there are four or more viable fetuses. The mean litter size for 100 control animals was 9.5 with a standard deviation of 1.9. Therefore, less than four fetuses is more than three standard deviations from the control mean. The percentage of fertile males is plotted for each breeding period after chemical treatment. The cell types represented at various times after chemical treatment are well known.

Serial mating assesses the biological functionality of sperm and produces fertility patterns which are inversely related in time to the phase of spermatogenesis damaged by the test chemical. For instance, chemical effects on spermatozoa appear first and those due to interference with spermatogonia appear last. The successful application of this method depends upon the fact that in rodents spermatogenesis and elimination of spermatozoa proceed continously without regard to frequency of mating. Thus, the relationship between a chemical's effect on fertility and the type of spermatogenic stage affected by the chemical can be readily demonstrated. Without knowing anything about the chemical producing a particular fertility profile, one can easily identify the cells affected. Because unique biochemical events are associated with various spermatogenic stages, mechanisms of action, such as DNA inhibition or mitotic arrest can be predicted.

To assess testicular function in either the laboratory or clinic, a longitudinal study is preferred. Many important parameters are relatively easy to determine. Testicular size and/or weight can be correlated with sperm production. Daily sperm production can also be estimated from daily sperm output. The simplest laboratory approach to determine sperm production is to homogenize a weighed sample of testicular parenchyma (or epididymis) with the appropriate media using a Waring blender. Particulate matter is solubilized and the highly condensed and cross-linked nucleoprotein of the elongated spermatid makes the nucleus resistant to homogenization. Homogenization-resistant spermatid nuclei provide an estimate of spermatids in the testis (Amann, 1981).

It must be recalled, however, that the number of sperm in the ejaculate will have been influenced by many factors: age, season, testicular size, ejaculation frequency or interval since the preceding ejaculation, and the degree of sexual arousal. Sperm production is far less efficient in humans than in laboratory or domestic mammals. In addition, more than 10% of human males have an abnormally low sperm production. This difference in sperm production between laboratory animals and man might account for the concern surrounding the use of laboratory animals as reliable predictors of chemicals affecting man.

3.5 Biotransformation of Exogenous Chemicals

A number of investigators have reported on the capability of the seminiferous tubules to biotransform exogenous chemicals. This has been an area of particular interest at the NIEHS where Mukhtar *et al.* (1978a, b) have determined the differential distribution of aryl hydrocarbon hydroxylase (AHH), epoxide hydrase (EH), glutathione *S*-transferase (GSH-ST) and cytochrome P-450 content in interstitial and spermatogenic cells in the seminiferous tubules and have compared levels of enzyme activity in the testes with the liver.

Appreciable activities of both mixed-function oxidases and epoxide-degrading enzymes, as well as cytochrome P-450, were found in testicular tissue. Glutathione *S*-transferase activity was relatively high. The distribution of these enzymes and cytochrome P-450 in the interstitial and germ cell compartments indicates that AHH activity and cytochrome P-450 content of microsomes from the interstitial cells was nearly two-fold greater than that in the tubules. In contrast, the specific activities of the detoxication enzymes, EH and GSH-ST, in tubules were twice that in the interstitial cells.

Although AHH activity in interstitial cell microsomes was only 5% of that of hepatic microsomes, its close proximity to the germ cells may be important for enzyme-activated chemicals. Therefore, factors affecting induction of AHH, EH, GSH-ST, and cytochrome P-450 probably play a significant role in germ cell toxicity, 2,3,7,8-Tetrachlorodibenzo-*p*-dioxin (TCDD) significantly induces both testicular and prostatic AHH activity and cytochrome P-448. AHH activity induced by TCDD in rat testis and prostate gland was 2 and 150 times that of its controls, respectively. Thus, exposure to environmental chemicals can induce significant levels of activating enzyme systems in male testis as well as in the prostate gland (Dixon and Lee, 1980a).

The metabolism of benzo(a)pyrene by isolated perfused testis and testicular homogenate has recently been compared (Dixon and Lee, 1980b). The cell-free *in vitro* system metabolized benzo(a)pyrene at a much greater rate than the perfused testis and produced a different spectrum of metabolites. The perfused organ system may better reflect the metabolic capabilities of the whole organ and intact animal than do cell-free preparations because the complex biological organization of tissues, cell types, and enzymes involved in testicular metabolism are retained.

3.6 Unscheduled DNA Synthesis

Our laboratory and others, have also been interested in the capacity of spermatogenic cells to repair DNA damaged as a consequence of exposure to environmental chemicals (Dixon and Lee, 1980a). It has been shown that both physical (ultraviolet and X-ray radiation) and chemical agents can cause damage to DNA molecules. Damage inflicted on the DNA templates, unless repaired, may interfere with transcription or replication and result in lethal mutations (cell death), mutations which result in transformed cells, or genetic mutations. Testis of mouse strains differ in their ability to repair DNA damage.

We have used the velocity sedimentation cell separation technique to identify spermatogenic cells capable of unscheduled DNA synthesis. To study unscheduled DNA synthesis after methyl methanesulphonate (MMS) treatment, male mice were first treated with varying doses of MMS (16.3, 32.5 and 65 mg/kg), followed 2 hours later by the intratesticular administration of ^{3}H-thymidine 1 hour before sacrifice. Spermatogenic cell types were then isolated.

Control mice receiving saline followed by intratesticular injection of ^{3}H-thymidine showed a single peak of radioactivity which identified spermatogonial cells passing through S-phase. In contrast, the radioactive profiles obtained after

MMS treatment demonstrated that thymidine incorporation now occurred not only in the spermatogonia but also in the leptotene, zygotene, pachytene, and diplotene cells in decreasing order. Normally no DNA synthesis occurs in these premeiotic cells; therefore, the thymidine incorporation in untreated cells is very low. These studies suggest that non-S-phase spermatogonial cells were also induced to undergo unscheduled DNA synthesis. In contrast, no thymidine radioactivity was present in spermatids or sperm (spermiogenic cells). Therefore, spermiogenic cells appear unable to repair DNA damage and, thus, are more vulnerable to the effects of monofunctional alkylating agents such as MMS.

A modified alkaline sucrose density gradient technique was used to determine the dose–response relationship for MMS-induced DNA single-strand breaks and the time-response for subsequent repair. Male mice were treated intraperitoneally with tritium-labelled thymidine three times daily for 5 days prior to MMS treatment. The mice were treated with MMS at doses of 22.5, 45, and 90 mg/kg, and killed 1 hour later. The DNA from spermatogenic cells was fractionated and gently layered on the alkaline detergent surface of the gradient. Single-strand DNA breaks were analysed. Results of these experiments suggested that repair of DNA single-strand breaks induced by MMS in spermatogenic cells appear to be dose and time dependent and that the DNA repair systems might be saturated at high test doeses or with repeated exposures to toxic chemicals (Dixon and Lee, 1980a). Overwhelming the repair system could result in a larger number of affected cells and increased toxicity. Thus, the DNA repair system is another protective mechanism with regard to toxic effects of environmental chemicals, as well as a sensitive indicator of toxicity.

4 THE EFFERENT DUCTS

The rete testis fluid conveys sperm from the testes into the epididymides and is relatively easily obtained in laboratory species. As already mentioned, the accumulation of chemicals in the rete testis relative to constant unbound plasma concentrations has been used to estimate the permeability of the blood–testis barrier for selected chemicals. The rete testis fluid normally contains inhibin, androgen binding protein (ABP), transferrin, γ-glutamyltransferase, myoinositol, steroids, amino acids and various enzymes. However, only ABP and inhibin appear to be specific products of the seminiferous tubules and reflect the function of the germinal epithelium (or Sertoli cells). More research is needed to define markers of seminiferous tubule activity and to develop sensitive and specific assays to measure them.

5 EPIDIDYMIS

The initial and intermediate segments of the epididymis, the caput and corpus, are involved in sperm maturation. The terminal segment, the cauda, serves as a storage organ for fertile sperm in many species. Resorption and metabolism of components entering the epididymis in rete testis fluid, secretion by the epithelium, sperm maturation, and maintenance of sperm fertility are important functions of the epididymis and, perhaps, targets for toxicity.

About one-half of the sperm in the epididymis are in the cauda. About one-half of the number of sperm in the paired caudae and ductuli are available for ejaculation. Sperm available for ejaculation are restored rapidly following successive ejaculation if daily sperm production is large relative to sperm reserves in the caudae. If the rate of ejaculation depletes the epididymal reserve, daily sperm output then reflects daily sperm production.

Animals with a large reserve of sperm can successfully breed more females in a short interval. In males ejaculating regularly, the number of sperm in the caudae and vas deferens is reduced relative to the number found in a male that has not ejaculated during the previous week.

From the epididymides, seminal fluid moves into the vas deferens where glandular secretions are added. Semen is a complex mixture of products of the testis, epididymides, ductuli deferentia and ampullae, prostate gland, vesicular glands, bulbourethral glands, and in some species, the urethral glands. Thus, chemically altered function of any of these secretory organs can alter seminal characteristics. Semen characteristics are also influenced by season, age, interval since previous ejaculation, methods for inducing ejaculation and collecting semen, and the laboratory procedures used for evaluation.

6 SEMEN

Semen can be collected from rabbits and other laboratory animals by electro-ejaculation or artificial vagina. However, such procedures are not commonly used for rodents. Human semen is, of course, collected by masturbation or in a condom following sexual intercourse. With few exceptions, chemically induced alterations of the biochemical composition of semen do not reflect testicular function but rather the functionality and relative contributions of the epididymides and accessory sex glands. The standard components of a semen analysis include semen volume, viscosity, liquefaction, and number, morphology, and motility of the sperm. These methods were recently carefully described in a comprehensive monograph (Belsey *et al.*, 1980).

A change in the volume will most likely reflect an altered secretory function of the prostate or the seminal vesicles. Biochemical markers of the seminal fluid such as acid phosphatase, citric acid, zinc, and magnesium are specific secretory products from the prostate. Most of the liquefying enzymes also originate from the prostate. Fructose and prostaglandins are secreted from the seminal vesicles.

Compartmental analyses have been used to determine the relative contribution of the epididymides and the accessory sex glands to the ejaculate. Unique markers, produced only by a single organ, are sought. Such analyses would allow evaluation of the function of the epididymis and of each accessory sex gland, as well as the germinal epithelium. However, components produced exclusively by a single organ and suitable for use as markers are rare.

Sperm density is the most common parameter in studies on the possible effects of drugs or chemical compounds on the male reproductive system. However, the number of sperm potentially available for ejaculation, expressed as a function of daily sperm production or the average number of sperm per ejaculate, differs greatly among species. Even within a single species, sperm density varies greatly and changes daily for a single individual.

Sperm concentrations are usually determined microscopically by counting all sperm in a known suspension of diluted semen with a cytometer. Light transmission measured spectrophotometrically through an appropriately diluted aliquot of the ejaculate has also been used.

Because the acrosome is critical in the penetration of the ovum by the sperm, approaches for evaluating the normalcy of the acrosome have been developed. In normal sperm, the acrosome closely adheres to the nucleus and an apical ridge can be clearly visualized in many species. In abnormal sperm, acrosome irregularities include swelling and vesiculations.

Evaluation of sperm morphology provides information on testicular function and also aids in predicting fertilizing potential. However, these methods are subjective with large variations between laboratories and technicians. The problem is especially difficult with human sperm because of the great variability and high percentage of abnormal sperm usually found in the ejaculate.

Sperm motility is routinely analysed and represents an important indicator of function. To be meaningful the motility assessment must include three factors: the mean progressive motility, the per cent motile spermatozoa, and the time after ejaculation. The percentage of motile sperm is a widely used test of sperm quality. Proper dilution of sperm and careful temperature control is essential (Amann, 1981).

Major improvements in semen analysis could be made by:

(1) more accurate determination of sperm concentrations;
(2) routine determination of the total number of sperm per ejaculate;
(3) more precise determination of the percentage of progressively motile sperm;
(4) more critical evaluation of sperm morphology by using a phase-contrast or differential interference contrast microscope for careful examination of wet preparations as well as stained smears.

Functional parameters that would be reliable predictors of chemical and environmental factors affecting the male reproductive system and male fertility. These include sperm motility and survival in seminal plasma; motility in cervical mucus; resistance to physical stress; metabolism; resistance to sodium dodecyl sulphate (SDS); zinc uptake; and release of enzymes, proteins and lipids. Prostatic dysfunction and perhaps other factors decrease the resistance of human spermatozoa to stress factors like gravitational force during centrifugation, dilution and low temperature (Amann, 1981; Belsey *et al.*, 1980). Release of enzymes, specific proteins, and phospholipids by bull, ram, and boar spermatozoa may also be functional parameters related to fertility. The relevance of physiological and biochemical research in relation to semen properties and fertility was recently reviewed (Mann and Lutwak-Mann, 1981).

7 PATERNALLY RELATED BIRTH DEFECTS

Reproductive problems and increased incidences of birth defects in their children reported by Vietnam veterans exposed to Agent Orange have focused attention upon paternal chemical exposure and perinatal outcome. This rather controversial area has been reviewed recently by Soyka and Joffe (1980) and Strobino *et al.* (1978). Laboratory studies have demonstrated that certain drugs and chemicals affect the progeny of male animals which were dosed before mating. Although there are few systematic studies of the effects of paternal drug exposure on offspring in humans, associations have been reported for lead, narcotics, caffeine, ethanol, anticonvulsants, anaesthetic gases and smoking, tobacco.

8 ERECTION AND LIBIDO

Because laboratory and clinical studies are rare, little is known concerning the effects of chemicals on libido, erection or ejaculation. The primary complaint of lost or decreased libido in male patients, in the absence of severe organic disease or advanced age, is most often dependent upon emotional or psychological disturbances. However, drugs may definitely play a role and occupational or environmental chemical exposure might also be the culprits (Woods, 1979). Impotence, the failure to obtain or sustain an erection, is rarely of endocrine origin. Attaining an erection depends upon complex neurological and circulatory pathways. The parasympathetic nervous system is primarily involved in the erection process; the sympathetic nervous system plays a major role in ejaculation. Thus, drugs and environmental chemicals affecting the autonomic nervous system may result in substantial reproductive dysfunction.

9 SUMMARY

Male reproductive effectiveness represents a number of inter-related organs and tissues which are carefully controlled by hormonal as well as other factors. Each process in the sequence of events is a potential target for toxic environmental and occupational chemicals. In addition, pharmacokinetic, adaptive, and homoeostatic mechanisms each play an important role in chemically induced testicular toxicity, decreased fertility and reduced fecundity. Current laboratory methods for detecting chemicals which affect reproductive processes are relatively crude and inexact. They do not extrapolate well to humans, nor do they provide reliable estimates of risk associated with chemical exposure. Clinical methods are only slightly better. A great deal more effort must be devoted to understanding the cellular and molecular processes which underlie reproduction, to determining how chemicals perturb them and to knowing the effects of such perturbation, and to estimate the potential human health hazards associated with exposure to chemicals which exhibit such effects.

10. REFERENCES

Amann, R. P. (1981). A critical review of methods for evaluation of spermatogenesis from seminal characteristics. *J. Androl.* **2**, 37–58.

Belsey, M. A., Eliasson, R., Gallegos, A. J., Moghissi, K. S., Paulsen, C. A. and Prasad, M. R. N. (1980). *Laboratory Manual for the Examination of Human Semen and Semen–Cervical Mucus Interaction*. Press Concern, Singapore.

Burger, H. and de Kretser, D. (Eds.) (1981). *Comprehensive Endocrinology: The Testis*. Raven Press, New York.

CEQ (Council on Environmental Quality) (1981). *Chemical Hazards to Human Reproduction*. US Government Printing Office, Washington, DC.

Dixon, R. L. and Hall, J. L. (1982). Reproductive toxicology. In Hayes, A. W. (Ed.) *Principles and Methods of Toxicology*, pp. 107–140, Raven Press, New York.

Dixon, R. L. (Ed.) (1981a). *Reproductive Toxicology Workshop: Workshop Recommendations*. National Toxicology Program/National Institute of Environmental Health Sciences. Research Triangle Park, NC.

Dixon, R. L. (1982). Environmental factors affecting development of reproductive systems. *Fund. appl. Toxicol.* **2**, 5–12.

Dixon, R. L. (1981b). The role of pharmacokinetic, adaptive and homeostatic factors in testicular toxicity and risk assessment. In Richmond, C. R., Walsh, P. J. and Copenhaver, E. D. (Eds.) *Proceedings of the Third Life Sciences Symposium on Risk Analysis*, pp. 196–212, Franklin Institute Press, Philadelphia, Pennsylvania.

Dixon, R. L. and Lee, I. P. (1980a). Pharmacokinetic and adaptation factors in testicular toxicity. *Feds Proc.* **39**, 66–72.

Dixon, R. L. and Lee, I. P. (1980b). Metabolism of benzo(a)pyrene by isolated perfused testis and testicular homogenate. *Life Sci.* **27**, 2439–2444.

Dougherty, R. C., Whitaker, M. J., Tang, S.-Y., Bottcher, R., Keller, M. and Kuehl, D. W. (1981). Sperm density and toxic substances: a potential key to environmental health hazards. In McKinney, J. D. (Ed.) *Environmental Health Chemistry: The Chemistry of Environmental Agents as Potential Human Hazards*, pp. 263–278. Ann Arbor Science Publishers, Inc., Ann Arbor, Michigan.

Dym, M. and Fawcett, D. W. (1970). The blood–testis barrier in the rat and the physiological compartmentation of the seminiferous epithelium. *Biol. Reprod.* **3**, 300–326.

Lee, I. P. and Dixon, R. L. (1972). Antineoplastic drug effects on spermatogenesis studied by velocity sedimentation cell separation. *Toxic. appl. Pharmac.* **23**, 20–41.

Mann, T. and Lutwak-Mann, C. (1981). *Male Reproductive Function and Semen: Themes and Trends in Physiology, Biochemistry and Investigative Andrology*. Springer-Verlag, New York.

Mukhtar, H., Lee, I. P., Foureman, G. L. and Bend, J. R. (1978a). Epoxide metabolizing enzyme activities in rat testis: postnatal development and relative activity in interstitial and spermatogenic cell compartments. *Chem. Biol. Interact.* **22**, 153–165.

Mukhtar, H., Philpot, R. M., Lee, I. P. and Bend, J. R. (1978b). Developmental aspects of epoxide-metabolizing enzyme activities in adrenals, ovaries, and testes of the rat. In Mahlum, D., Sikov, U., Hackett, P. and Andrew, F. (Eds.) *Developmental Toxicology of Energy-Related Pollutants*, pp. 89–104. US Department of Energy, Technical Information Center.

Okumura, K., Lee, I. P. and Dixon, R. L. (1975). Permeability of selected drugs and chemicals across the blood–testis barrier of the rat. *J. Pharmac. exp. Ther.* **194**, 89–95.

Setchell, B. P., Voglmayr, J. K. and Waites, G. M. H. (1969). A blood–testis barrier restricting passage from blood lymph into rete testis fluid but not into lymph. *J. Physiol. (London)* **200**, 73–85.

Soyka, L. F. and Joffe, J. M. (1980). Male mediated drug effects on offspring. In Schwarz, R. H. and Yaffe, S. J. (Eds.) *Drug and Chemical Risks to the Fetus and Newborn*, pp. 49–66. Alan R. Liss, Inc., New York.

Strobino, B. R., Kline, J. and Stein Z. (1978). Chemical and physical exposure of parents: effects on human reproduction and offspring. *Early Hum. Dev.* **1**, 371–399.

Woods, J. S. (1979). Drug affects on human sexual behavior. In Woods, N. F. (Ed.) *Human Sexuality in Health and Illness*, 2nd edn, pp. 364–382. C. V. Mosby Company, St. Louis.

Methods for Assessing the Effects of Chemicals on Reproductive Functions
Edited by V. B. Vouk and P. J. Sheehan
© 1983 SCOPE

Effects of Chemicals on Reproductive Function

I. V. SANOCKIJ

1 INTRODUCTION

In view of a steadily increasing number of abnormal pregnancies, childless marriages and congenital developmental defects observed during the recent years, toxicologists have to improve their capability of predicting possible effects of environmental chemicals on reproductive function. The effects on reproductive function should be considered together with other long-term effects—carcinogenic, genetic and immunological—which many chemicals are capable of inducing when absorbed into the body even in very small quantities. Sometimes there is a long latent period before such effects become apparent.

Clinical observations have demonstrated a growing number of disturbances in the menstrual cycle among female workers in some industries, notably in the chemical industry. Such pathological changes frequently occur without the loss of working ability and may not be included in the routine medical records.

Sanitary standards for the majority of industrial chemicals previously tested were established without considering possible long-term effects. A convincing documentation has accumulated in the meantime which provides evidence for selective toxicity of many chemicals, and a number of already adopted hygiene regulations have therefore been revised in the Soviet Union and in the member countries of the Council of Mutual Economic Assistance (CMEA). When establishing sanitary standards for chemicals in the environment, it is now mandatory to take into account the possible long-term effects.

Disturbances of reproductive function may result from injuries in the testes and ovaries, from pathological changes in their control systems and from some diseases of the urogenital tract which impair sexual processes. These impairments may become manifest as disturbances in the individual components of the integrated reproductive cycle, such as libido, erection, ejaculation and orgasm. For example, the impairment of ejaculation—even its complete disappearance—following an experimental exposure to 3% solution of hexachlorophene, proved to be related to fibrosis of the prostate (Gellert et al., 1978).

Evaluation of the effects of psychogenic factors is now considered obligatory in clinical investigations. It is well known that neuroses with marked emotional disturbances may have a depressive effect on sexual behaviour, on spermatogenesis (Krištal and Sergienko, 1977; Vasilčenko *et al.*, 1977; Sanockij *et al.*, 1980a,b), and on reproductive capacity in general. For instance, occupational exposure to vinyl chloride may result in symptoms of asthenia, and may initiate sexual disturbances; a man with a weak sexual constitution may have a lower libido if he is asthenic. Thus some industrial chemicals may have an indirect effect on reproductive function by way of their action on the nervous, endocrine and other systems.

In view of this, an important task of toxicology is to determine whether the effect of a chemical agent on reproductive function is specific (selective) or not. Such toxicological studies can be successfully performed in experiments on laboratory animals (Sanockij, 1976; 1979).

2 AN OUTLINE OF METHODOLOGY FOR EVALUATING THE EFFECTS OF CHEMICALS ON REPRODUCTIVE FUNCTION

Systematic evaluation of the effects of chemicals on reproductive function should consider the following.

(1) Gonadotoxicity (see Figure 1):
  (a) effects on the testes and on the control of their function, and
  (b) effects on the ovaries and on the control of their function.
(2) Effects on the embryo, fetus and 'mother–embryo/fetus' system (see Figure 2):
  (a) embryotoxicity,
  (b) teratogenicity,
  (c) effects on the placenta and uterus, and on the control of their function.

Genetic effects, although conceptually a part of reproductive toxicology, are considered separately (see Figure 3).

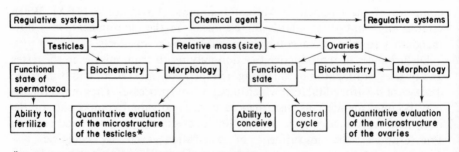

Evaluation of the index of spermatogenesis is not obligatory.

Figure 1   Scheme for investigating gonadotoxic effects

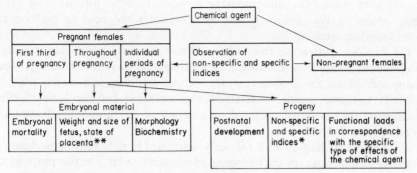

*Special attention should be paid to behavioural and biochemical tests.
**Examination of the placenta is not obligatory, but data on the permeability of placenta substantially improve the quality of information.

Figure 2 Scheme for investigating embryotropic effects

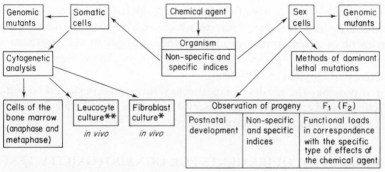

* Not obligatory
** When examining working persons for substances which are already in use in industry (hygienic evaluation of MAC).

Figure 3 Scheme for investigating mutagenic effects of industrial chemicals

3 BASIC PRINCIPLES

Design of experiments in preventive toxicology involves some fundamental principles, the neglect of which may diminish the value of the work performed and make the interpretation of the results difficult. These basic principles are as follows:

(1) A system of functional, morphological and biochemical indices of effects should be used. Results obtained by using only one type of indices cannot be subject to exhaustive interpretation.

(2) Similarity in chemical structure or biological activity to other substances

known to be mutagenic, embryotoxic or gonadotoxic either directly or by way of their effects on the control mechanisms indicates the need to perform the corresponding studies.

(3) Particular attention should be paid to substances which demonstrate a pronounced ability to accumulate in the organism, and to substances with which many individuals are in contact either occupationally or in everyday life.

(4) It is indispensable to establish the threshold for the harmful effect considered (Lim_{sp}) based on the determination of the minimum effective and subthreshold doses.

(5) The risk of long-term effects can be estimated by determining the degree of selectivity (specificity) or the biological effects considered. For this purpose, the threshold for the effects on the specific function under study (Lim_{sp}) is compared with the threshold for the effect on the organism as a whole as indicated by indices of overall (integrated) toxicity (Lim_{int}). The degree of selectivity (specificity) of the effect is then determined by calculating the 'zone of specific effect' defined as $Z_{sp} = Lim_{int}/Lim_{sp}$; $Z_{sp} > 1$ indicates a selective (specific) effect on the function under study.

The threshold for a harmful effect is considered to be the smallest concentration (or dose), the exposure to which—under specific conditions of the experiment or observation—produces either changes in the organism which exceed the limits of physiological adaptation, or latent, temporarily compensated pathological conditions.

(6) If possible, the results of experimental investigation should be compared with clinical and epidemiological observations. This provides a reliable basis for setting up or correcting sanitary standards.

4 MINIMUM REQUIREMENTS FOR GONADOTOXICITY TESTING

The condition and function of the testes can be evaluated by quantitatively assessing the morphology of spermatogenic epithelium and by examining the functional state of spermatozoa (Fomenko, 1975).

The morphometric assessment can be carried out by estimating:

(1) the spermatogenesis index as determined by a method proposed by Fogg and Cowing (1951) (not obligatory);
(2) the relative number of tubules with desquamated spermatogenic epithelium;
(3) the average number of normal spermatogonia;
(4) the relative number of tubules with cells in the 12th stage of meiosis.

The functional state of spermatozoa is examined by:

(1) observing the character and duration of their movement;
(2) estimating the relative number of live spermatozoa;
(3) determining the concentration of spermatozoa in the tail of epididymis;

(4) estimating the relative number of degenerated forms of spermatozoa;
(5) determining the osmotic and acid resistance.

The control of testicular function can be evaluated by:

(1) determining the levels of gonadotropins in blood serum;
(2) determining the level of testosterone in blood plasma.

The clinical examination of male reproductive function includes the evaluation of the state of neurohormonal, psychological, erectional and ejaculatory components of the sexual cycle by using methods of structural analysis of sexual disturbances (Vasilčenko, 1977).

The examination of the ejaculate comprises the following variables:

(1) volume;
(2) colour;
(3) period of liquefaction;
(4) viscosity;
(5) sperm concentration (number per ml);
(6) total number of spermatozoa in the ejaculate;
(7) relative number of live spermatozoa;
(8) percentage of morphologically altered forms; and
(9) pH of the ejaculate.

The biochemical investigations include the determination of testosterone level in blood plasma, the amount of fructose in the ejaculate and the activity of hyaluronidase in the heads of spermatozoa.

The examination of ovaries comprises the determination of their weight and quantitative evaluation of their microstructures (Mandl and Zuckerman, 1951a,b,c, 1952) including:

(1) primordial follicles and follicles with one layer of granulosa cells;
(2) follicles with two or more layers of granulosa cells;
(3) Graafian follicles;
(4) corpora lutea;
(5) total number of generated forms.

When evaluating the control of ovarian function in the preliminary experiment, the gonadotropic function of the pituitary gland should be examined.

5 EMBRYOTOXICITY

The exposure to chemicals during pregnancy can result in various abnormalities in the development of embryo which can be provisionally classified as being the results of:

(1) *teratogenicity* when histomorphological, biochemical, functional and other abnormalities—sometimes incompatible with life—of organ and system functions of the embryo occur; these abnormalities can become manifest in the postnatal development;

(2) *embryotoxicity* when intrauterine death or reduced size and weight of embryos occur but the tissues are normally differentiated.

As a rule, when the doses or concentrations of different chemical substances are small a, weak embryotoxicity is observed. Teratogenicity is also rare at exposures to low concentrations of chemicals. Nevertheless, some specific embryotoxic substances (for example, chloroprene) may be teratogenic even when administered at low concentrations during specific days of pregnancy (Sanockij and Sal' nikova, 1979).

The correlation between teratogenicity, the stage of embryogenesis and the duration of exposure is particularly significant. In our own studies of chloroprene, predinsolone, vinyl chloride and other substances we were able to establish an important fact, i.e. that for some chemicals the relative embryotoxicity is higher when the exposure during specific periods of embryogenesis is compared to the total exposure during pregnancy. We consider this typical for substances which have a specific embryotoxic action. Undoubtedly, this question needs further study since it is of practical importance for recommending the work regimen of pregnant women in the chemical industry.

In some cases embryotoxicity can be related to the transfer of the chemical through the placenta. Direct and indirect methods may be used for studying the degree of placental permeability to chemical substances. The direct methods consist in determining the amount of substance transferred through the placenta and its distribution in embryonic tissues. For example, the determination of N,N'-dimethylformamide (DMFA) in the embryonic tissues, placenta and liver of a mother showed that the inhalation exposure to DMFA even at the maximum allowable concentration and at minimum chronic effects levels (Lim_{ch}) leads to the accumulation of the chemical in embryonal tissues.

The change of placental permeability with the stage of pregnancy and with the concentration (dose) of the chemical is an important problem. As demonstrated by Dr. Sivočalova in 1975, the placental permeability can be used for determining the threshold for adverse effects of tetracycline and other substances.

Apart from using a direct measurement of the transfer of chemicals through the placenta, the permeability can be estimated by means of test substances such as ^{139}I, ^{35}S and others. The combination of the direct and indirect methods enables a better understanding of the degree of permeability of placental barrier to foreign substances and normal metabolites.

Evaluation of disturbances of compensatory mechanisms of maternal and fetal organisms plays an important role in determining the selectivity of embryotoxic effects of chemicals. For example, during inhalation exposure to DMFA, the cardiac function of the fetus of experimental animals exposed to hypoxia at the intermediate and late stages of pregnancy was damaged; at the same time the functional state of the uterus was not impaired. This fact confirms the selective action of DMFA on the fetus. Similar data were obtained when the embryotoxic action of tertiary butyl hydroperoxide was investigated.

Taking into account the interconnection between the organs of the mother and the fetus, it is necessary to examine thoroughly those organs of the fetus and offspring which were injured to a larger degree in their mothers. In an experiment with hydrogen chloride, it was established that regardless of the stage of pregnancy the most serious alterations take place in the lungs and kidneys of experimental animals. The alterations in the fetuses and offspring followed the 'organ to organ' relationship; the degree of damage depended on the degree of injury of the same organs in their mothers.

6 MINIMUM REQUIREMENTS FOR EMBRYOTOXICITY AND TERATOGENICITY TESTING

Methods for evaluating embryotoxicity include the determination of:

(1) preimplantation losses;
(2) postimplantation losses;
(3) total embryonal mortality.

Methods for evaluating teratogenicity comprise:

(1) analysis of the pathology of internal organs by Wilson's microanatomical method;
(2) analysis of the cardiovascular pathology according to Staples' method.

Evaluation of the health status of the offspring:

(1) postnatal loss (coefficients of survival and lactation);
(2) evaluation of the functional state of individual organs and systems of the offspring;
(3) application of functional loads.

The application of methodological approaches mentioned above was validated by testing several dozens of chemicals. This provided an opportunity to elaborate the main criteria for the evaluation of long-term effects of the industrial chemicals and establishing limits for their concentration in the environment.

7 CONCLUSIONS

The methods described represent only the minimum testing requirements sufficient for solving some practical tasks, such as sanitary standardization of toxic chemicals in the air, soil, food and some other environmental components;

determination of the degree of toxicity of chemicals; and the prediction of related long-term effects.

This list of methods should not be considered dogmatically. New methods are being developed, and as the amount of information they provide, the difficulties in their use and their reliability are evaluated, they gradually supplement or replace currently used methods.

The author is grateful to Dr. V. I. Gluščenko for his assistance in the preparation of this paper.

8. REFERENCES

Fogg, L. C. and Cowing, R. F. (1951). The changes in cell morphology and histochemistry of the testis following irradiation and their relation to other induced testicular changes. *Cancer Res.* **11**, 23–28.

Fomenko, V. N. (1975). Long-term effects of exposure to toxic substances. In *Methods used in the U.S.S.R. for Establishing Biologically Safe Levels of Toxic Substances*, pp. 75–85. World Health Organization, Geneva.

Gellert, R. J., Wallace, C. A., Wiesmeier, E. M. and Shuman, R. M. (1978). Topical exposure of neonates to hexachlorophene: long-standing effects on mating behaviour and prostatic development in rats. *Toxic. appl. Pharmac.* **43**, 339–349.

Krištal, V. V. and Sergienko, L. V. (1977). The influence of psychogenic factors on spermatogenesis. In *Diagnosis and Treatment of Nervous System Diseases and Problems of Organizing Psychoneurological Care in Railway Transport Systems*, pp. 86–87. Harkov (in Russian).

Mandl, A. M. and Zuckerman, S. (1951a). The effect of destruction of the germinal epithelium on the number of oocytes. *J. Endocrinol.* **7**, 103–111.

Mandl, A. M. and Zuckerman, S. (1951b). The relation of age to numbers of oocytes. *J. Endocrinol.* **7**, 190–193.

Mandl, A. M. and Zuckerman, S. (1951c). Changes in ovarian structure following the injection of carbolic acid into the ovarian burse. *J. Endocrinol.* **7**, 227–234.

Mandl, A. M. and Zuckerman, S. (1952). Cyclical changes in the number of medium and large follicles in the adult rat ovary. *J. Endocrinol.* **8**, 341–346.

Sanockij, I. V. Paškova, G. A. and Fomenko, V. N. The extrapolation of animal data to humans for effects of chemicals on reproduction. In Plasunov, A. K. and Paškova, G. A. (Eds.). *Fundamental Problems of Long-term Consequences of Industrial Poisons*, pp. 21–27, Moscow (In Russian).

Sanockij, I. V. (1979). In Fomenko, V. N. (Ed.) *Long-term Consequences of the Effects of Chemicals on the Organism*. Medicina, Moscow (in Russian).

Sanockij, I. V. and Sal'nikova, L. S. (1979). Embriotropic action of environmental chemicals. In *Ecological Forecasting*, pp. 236–260. Nauka, Moscow (in Russian).

Sanockij, I. V., Davtjan, R. M. and Gluščenko, V. I. (1980a). A study of reproductive function in men exposed to some chemicals. *Gig. Truda Prof. Zabol.* **5**, 28–32 (in Russian).

Sanockij, I. V., Fomenko, V. B. and Grodeckaja, N. S. (1980b). Substantiation of methodological approaches to the evaluation of late consequences of exposure to chemical compounds. *J. Hyg. Epidemiol. Microbiol. Immunol.* **24(3)**, 338–345.

Vasilčenko, G. S. (1977). *General Sexual Pathology*. Medicina, Moscow (in Russian).

Methods for Assessing the Effects of Chemicals on Reproductive Functions
Edited by V. B. Vouk and P. J. Sheehan
© 1983 SCOPE

Effects of Chemicals on Reproductive Functions of Mammals: Mechanisms of Cell Injury and Adaptive Responses

LINDA R. WUDL and MICHAEL I. SHERMAN

1 INTRODUCTION

It is a relatively simple matter to assess cell injury in unicellular organisms in response to adverse chemicals: measurements of rates of macromolecular synthesis will indicate whether basic metabolic processes and proliferative capacities have been affected and simple viability tests can be used to monitor survival. On the other hand, the effects of chemical insult upon mammals, as on other multicellular organisms, can be substantially more difficult to analyse because of the large number of variables that are introduced. Even within a single species, detrimental chemicals might have a severe effect upon some individuals but not upon others because of size, age or sex differences. Various cell types might by virtue of their nature or location be differentially susceptible. In higher animals, adverse effects and even death can result from exposure to chemicals even if these agents do not kill cells directly; it is sufficient merely to interfere with the specialized functions of any of a number of cell types involved in the regulation of neural, circulatory, hormonal or immunological processes. Secondary and long-term effects in response to chemical injury make it difficult to pinpoint the initial site or sites of action of the adverse chemical.

At the molecular level, chemicals can cause damage in numerous ways including interference with normal metabolic processes, disruption of cellular architecture, induction of mutations and prevention of cell division.

The reproductive process in mammals is perhaps substantially more susceptible to disruption by detrimental chemicals than one might expect based solely upon anatomical considerations. It is likely that the rapid proliferation rates of germ cells and embryonic cells at various stages of their development are responsible for the observed sensitivity. Although infertility in males exposed to damaging chemicals is usually transient, females have less likelihood of recovering reproductive function if they are exposed to the same chemicals at particular developmental periods (see section 4). Exposure of pregnant females

171

to appropriate doses of many chemicals can lead to abortion; alternatively, offspring might survive albeit in a weakened or abnormal condition. If a pregnant female is exposed to chemical insult at a critical period during pregnancy, the resulting offspring might initially appear to be unaffected but might later be found to be abnormal with respect to growth rate, behaviour or fertility (e.g. McLachlan, 1977; Felton *et al*, 1978; Snow and Tam, 1979).

In attempting to elucidate mechanisms of chemical injury to the reproductive system, one must consider effects at the tissue, cellular and molecular levels. Well-established *in vivo* techniques and some newer and promising *in vitro* tests have been designed specifically for studying gross effects on the reproductive system. These procedures are discussed below and detailed in accompanying papers. Investigations of chemical insult at the cellular and molecular levels are generally carried out *in vitro* and are similar to procedures commonly used to study the behaviour of other cells in response to environmental change. Finally, related studies can be undertaken to learn how cells in the reproductive system can under certain conditions recover from, or escape lasting damage following exposure to, detrimental chemicals.

2 MECHANISMS OF CELL INJURY: MOLECULAR CONSIDERATIONS

Since normal cellular function involves the interdependent and coordinated activities of several classes of macromolecules (DNA, RNA, enzymes, structural proteins), disruption at any of a number of levels can have widespread effects upon overall cellular integrity. Chemicals can cause cell injury directly by disrupting membrane structure, which could lead to a loss of cellular integrity as well as the inability to take up essential nutrients. Alternatively, the flow of genetic information could be interrupted by chemicals that block the normal synthesis, processing or interaction of RNAs necessary for the translation of structural proteins and enzymes, or that act at the level of translation *per se*. Some chemicals can be equally injurious to the cell, by disrupting intermediary metabolism, or the production, acquisition, translocation and/or utilization of enzyme precursors, substrates and cofactors. Finally, in rapidly proliferating cells such as those involved in reproduction, mutagens and agents that interfere with replication or mitosis can have profound effects upon ultimate cellular and tissue integrity and function.

In general terms, macromolecules can be prevented from functioning normally, and thereby have a detrimental effect upon cellular well-being, if their structure or activity is adversely affected. We shall first consider ways in which chemicals can disrupt the function of macromolecules by interfering with their structure; subsequently, we shall describe means by which chemicals can interrupt normal macromolecular function without directly causing structural alterations.

When attempting to elucidate mechanisms by which chemicals cause cell injury and reproductive damage, it is important to bear in mind that a chemical to which an animal has been exposed might not be inherently harmful. Chemicals which are actually essential for the survival of an individual or drugs with proven therapeutic benefits can be deleterious if administered to an individual in excessive dosages (see, e.g., Hurley, 1977). Furthermore, since many xenobiotic chemicals are non-polar, the organism attempts to facilitate excretion of such chemicals by first making them more polar and subsequently conjugating them to a hydrophilic moiety such as glucuronic acid, sulphate, acetate, etc. (see Dutton, 1978). Often the polar intermediate metabolite is, or is converted to, a highly reactive species capable of disrupting cellular integrity by binding covalently to macromolecules or by initiating free radical chain reactions. One group of enzymes responsible for the formation of such reactive compounds is the microsome-bound, cytochrome P-450-dependent, mixed-function oxidase system.

Although the liver appears to be the main clearing house for foreign compounds, mixed-function oxidases have also been detected in lung, kidney, spleen, skin fibroblasts, intestine, embryo, placenta and other tissues (Atlas *et al.*, 1977; Schenkman *et al.*, 1977). The site of metabolic activation/detoxication of a given compound will, therefore, depend on its portal of entry and its tissue distribution. Activities vary widely from tissue to tissue and with the species, age and sex of the animal. Accordingly, generalizations cannot be made regarding the potential damage to a given tissue or animal from exposure to a xenobiotic which is susceptible to metabolic activation. Furthermore, an active intermediate may pose a hazard to tissues or organs themselves incapable of metabolic activation. This would depend on such physicochemical parameters as half-life, accessibility to and reaction rates with cellular substituents and lipid/water partition coefficient of the unconjugated or reactive species. Absence or inhibition of the conjugation reaction or depletion of the endogenous hydrophilic substrate could also increase the threat of damage to all tissues.

Since this paper is concerned primarily with the mechanisms by which chemically reactive and biologically active compounds damage cells, we shall in many cases consider general classes of compounds, their activities and consequences rather than providing a survey of xenobiotics and their metabolic fates.

2.1 Structural Alterations

Xenobiotic chemicals or environmental pollutants are often characterized by a multiplicity of possible chemical interactions with biological macromolecules. In most cases the cytotoxic or teratogenic effects of such reactive compounds can be attributed to more than one such interaction, while mutagenic and carcinogenic effects of xenobiotics are, with few exceptions, the result of chemical reactions or interactions with DNA. Nucleic acid structure can be altered in a number of ways, all of which can severely affect function. Nucleotide analogues can be incorporated into DNA or RNA causing chain termination, a potentially lethal event, or resulting in intact but defective nucleic acid (see Kornberg, 1980). Some base analogues can also exert cytotoxic effects by causing DNA damage which leads to strand breaks and even chromosome breakage. For example, 5-bromodeoxyuridine (BrdU) can act as a simple base analogue and cause point mutations by mispairing , but it can also be photoactivated to form dimers more readily than its analogue, thymidine (Kornberg, 1980).

Some oligopeptide antibiotics like Netropsin and distamycin A form stable complexes with DNA via hydrogen bonding and electrostatic interactions, resulting in inhibition of DNA and RNA synthesis (Kornberg, 1980). Other non-covalent interactions with DNA are achieved by a class of polycyclic planar compounds called intercalating agents. Compounds such as acridine form stable complexes by inserting between stacked bases in the double helix. The resulting loss of structural integrity can be mutagenic, teratogenic and/or cytotoxic. Actinomycin D exerts cytotoxic effects by intercalating into the DNA molecule and forming a hydrogen bond between its cyclic peptide portion and guanine resulting in a stable complex which distorts the DNA sufficiently to inhibit RNA and DNA synthesis (Sobell, 1973). Many planar polycyclic compounds also have alkylating side chains, or are metabolically activated to reactive species, and are therefore capable of interacting with DNA covalently and perhaps which some stereoselectivity.

Divalent cations are important in all aspects of cellular function. Fidelity of DNA replication can be altered by chelating the metal ions necessary for DNA polymerase activity (magnesium and zinc) or by substitution with metals such as cadmium (Springgate *et al.*, 1973) or beryllium (Sirover and Loeb, 1976). Compounds which chelate metal cations could also interfere with DNA structure by removing some of the phosphate counterions. Lead has been shown to cause hydrolysis of RNA and nucleoside triphosphates (Rosenthal *et al.*, 1966; Farkas, 1968). Other cytotoxic effects of metal ions and chelators will be discussed below.

From the standpoint of environmentally related teratogenesis, carcinogenesis, mutagenesis and toxicity, the greatest hazards are those compounds which are, or are metabolically converted to, electrophilically reactive species. Such compounds can alter DNA, RNA, protein and lipid with devastating effects on cellular integrity and function. Alkylating agents bind covalently to DNA at the O^6 or N^7 of guanine, N^3 of adenine and to a lesser degree N^1 of adenine, O^2 and N^3 of cytosine, and O^4 and O^2 of thymine (Sun and Singer, 1975; Beranek *et al.*, 1980). Alkylation of DNA can result in chromosome damage, intragenic mutation or inhibition of synthesis (Brooks, 1977). DNA structure can also be affected by protein–DNA and lipid–DNA cross-linking. In some cases, alkylation of protein could have direct effects on DNA structure. For example, alkylation of the cysteine-rich DNA binding protein(s) could destabilize sperm chromatin and make the DNA subject to shear stress at fertilization. RNA alkylation, unless quite extensive or involved in DNA cross-linking, would have less significance upon the ultimate fate of the cell than DNA alkylation.

The effects of DNA alkylation, e.g. the extent of mutagenesis and carcinogenesis, can vary among species and from tissue to tissue in a given organism. Since the differences do not lie in the double helical structure of DNA or with the chemical reaction *per se*, the physiological state of the cell must influence these processes. Adaptive responses, such as xenobiotic metabolism and DNA repair, will be discussed below (section 4) but it should be kept in mind that both influence susceptibility of cells to alkylating agents. Although the patterns of base alkylation in DNA depend on the specific alkylating agent, the extent of alkylation damage to DNA exposed to a given dose of a chemical might depend on whether or not the DNA is 'active'. For example, replicating, transcriptionally active and bridge (non-nucleosomal) DNA are thought to be most susceptible to alkylation (Bartholomew *et al.*, 1980). Alkylation is most detrimental at sites which are damaged at replication or which are not repaired prior to replication (Berman *et al.*, 1978). With some alkylating agents preferential binding to mitochondrial DNA has been demonstrated, probably reflecting the lipophilic nature of those agents (Wunderlich *et al.*, 1970; Allen and Coombs, 1980; Backer and Weinstein, 1980).

Alterations in protein structure can lead to mutation, teratogenesis and/or cytotoxicity. Such alterations can be divided into two classes: those affecting specific enzymes and resulting in interference with their function, and those which can affect all proteins indiscriminately. We have already mentioned how certain metal ions can alter fidelity of DNA replication by interfering with DNA polymerase activity. Mercury, cadmium and lead all have a strong affinity for phosphates, sulphhydryl and imidazole groups of proteins, purines, pteridines and porphyrins. Thus, they are capable of inhibiting enzymes, binding to and affecting conformation of nucleic acids and disrupting pathways of oxidative phosphorylation (Vallee and Ulmer, 1972). Lead interferes with haem synthesis and causes zinc to be substituted for iron, thus specifically reducing haemoglobin function as well as that of other haem proteins (Eisinger, 1978). Lead ion binds to sulphhydryl groups of proteins (Vallee and Ulmer, 1972), leading to enzyme inactivation and alkyllead has been shown to adversely affect mitochondrial membrane ion transport and inhibit oxidative phosphorylation (Skilleter, 1975). Cadmium can affect a number of cellular processes with resulting cytotoxic effects observed in many tissues and organs including testis, placenta and embryo (Flick *et al.*, 1971). In addition to its inhibitory effects on zinc metalloenzymes, cadmium has been shown to exert direct effects on both synthesis and degradation of cytochrome P-450 enzymes while at the same time causing reduction in substrate binding (Schnell, 1980), thus decreasing both the total amount of enzyme and its effectiveness. Mercury has been shown to affect membrane stability, permeability and function. Mercury poisoning is probably due to loss of mitochondrial function as a result of disruption of ion transport (Tyson and Southard, 1980).

Environmentally related metal toxicity is an important consideration. Of equal concern is the problem of toxicity caused by environmental pollutants which bind metals. Carbon monoxide and chemicals in cigarette smoke can bind metal ions, thereby inhibiting essential enzyme functions (Petering and Petering, 1980). Although the lung is the primary target of such cytotoxic effects, the loss of haem can have effects on all tissues.

Collagen has received much attention in recent years as an important target protein for environmentally induced lung and liver damage as well as teratogenic effects. Increased collagen synthesis causing lung and liver fibrosis appears to be related to increased levels of superoxide, a product of oxidative metabolism (Hussain and Bhatnagar, 1979). Perhaps more pertinent to reproductive function is the fact that certain environmental pollutants and drugs can interfere with secondary modifications of collagen which are critical for generating its proper physical characteristics. Hydroxylation of proline is one such modification. Prolyl hydroxylase can be inhibited by drugs such as aspirin and thalidomide and by mercury salts and methyl mercury. Zinc and nickel also inhibit prolyl hydroxylase as do iron chelating agents. (Aspirin may exert its inhibitory effects by chelating iron required for enzyme function.) Lysyl hydroxylase and lysyl oxidase are also required for collagen processing and are subject to a variety of inhibitory agents. All such agents which interfere with collagen formation and function are teratogenic (Bhatnagar *et al.*, 1980).

Chemicals which affect proteins indiscriminately include amino acid analogues and reagents which react with the nucleophilic groups of proteins, peptides and amino acids. As is the case with RNA, alkylation of proteins, unless quite extensive or restricted to that macromolecule, would be of less consequence than reactions of the same alkylating agents with DNA. Exceptions would be chemicals which are metabolically activated by microsomal enzymes to such highly reactive species that they never reach the DNA. However, as will be discussed below, lipid probably provides a more critical target for such electrophilic reactants. Damaging effects of protein alkylation could result from cross-linking. For example, cross-linking of proteins on the cell surface could affect membrane fluidity (Edidin, 1972) as well as cell surface recognition functions which are implicated in fertilization (Vacquier and Moy, 1977) development and differentiation (Rutter, 1980). Protein–DNA cross-linking is probably less cytotoxic or mutagenic than DNA–DNA cross-linking as evidenced by the effects of *trans*-Pt(II) diamminedichloride which induces primarily protein–DNA cross-linking (Fornace, 1980).

Membrane lipids have been the focus of attention for many researchers interested in the toxic effects of environmental pollutants. Extensive lipid peroxidation leading to auto-oxidation chain reactions is inevitably cytotoxic. In addition, lipids can be involved in cross-linking to DNA and protein with bifunctional alkylating agents; lipid peroxides, as well as epoxides formed as byproducts in lipid peroxidation–autooxidation reactions, are also alkylating agents (Hogberg, 1977; Sevanian *et al.*, 1980).

Membrane auto-oxidation is a self-perpetuating chain reaction initiated by free radicals and resulting in destruction of membrane integrity and function (Svingen and Aust, 1980). An example of such a reaction caused by a xenobiotic is seen in the case of exposure to carbon tetrachloride (Recknagel, 1967). This compound is metabolized in the liver (and other tissues) to a carbon free radical which subsequently generates oxygen free radicals. These in turn initiate formation of lipid peroxides in polyunsaturated fatty acids. Carbon free radicals are also generated in the oxidative metabolism of polycyclic aromatic hydrocarbons. Metabolic activation of some nitrogen-containing carcinogens, such as nitrosopiperidine, produces oxygen radicals directly (Autor *et al.*, 1980). Since normal cellular oxygen metabolism produces oxygen free radicals, the cell has several protective mechanisms which will be discussed later in this paper. Cytotoxic effects due to free radical production are the result of saturation of the cells' ability to inhibit or repair damage (Svingen and Aust, 1980). Most organic free radical intermediates are extremely reactive and probably do not escape the site of formation (Recknagel *et al.*, 1977). Therefore, even weak teratogenic effects of a compound such as carbon tetrachloride provide indirect evidence for the ability of the embryo to oxidatively metabolize such xenobiotics (Harbison, 1978). Cytotoxicity due to membrane oxidation is probably a result of a combination of events including loss of mitochondrial function, release of lysosomal enzymes and disruption of nuclear membrane function resulting in inhibition of replication (Autor *et al.*, 1980; Svingen and Aust, 1980).

2.2 Functional Alterations

In general, the chemicals in this category act as antimetabolites or cellular poisons. In large part, the agents to be discussed are natural products of microorganisms. It should not be inferred that this is the only class of chemicals which act by these mechanisms. Rather, these agents have been studied extensively because of their potential value as tools for the elucidation of mechanisms by which macromolecules normally function. Thus, the objective here is to point out in general ways how a chemical agent can cause cell injury by disrupting metabolism. With this information in mind, it might subsequently be easier to determine the mechanisms by which other xenobiotic chemicals act.

In some cases, the action of an antimetabolite seems to be at a single level; it is thus relatively easy to deduce its primary target. As an example, aphidicolin, a tetracyclic diterpenoid produced by *Cephalosporium aphidicola*, seems to act specifically at the level of DNA replication by inhibiting DNA polymerase activity, and in particular DNA ploymerase α (Kornberg, 1980). Among specific inhibitors of RNA synthesis, α-amanitin, a bicyclic polypeptide mushroom toxin, interferes with RNA polymerase II (the enzyme responsible for messenger RNA biosynthesis) at low concentrations and RNA polymerase III (the enzyme involved in transfer and 5S RNA production) at much higher concentrations (Lindell *et al.*, 1970; Weinmann and Roeder, 1974). Because protein synthesis is a complex event involving many macromolecular factors, there are several levels at which inhibitors can specifically interrupt the production of proteins (e.g. binding of messenger RNA or transfer RNA, initiation, elongation or termination of the protein). (For a consideration of some specific protein synthesis inhibitors, see Ritter, 1977.) Tunicamycin, an aminoglycoside antibiotic, appears to act primarily at the level of inhibition of protein glycosylation (Takatsuki *et al.*, 1971; Tkacz and Lampen, 1975). This effect can, in unknown ways, cause death of rapidly proliferating cells (Olden *et al.*, 1979), including those of early embryos (Atienza-Samols *et al.*, 1980). Finally, other chemicals such as digitalis and ouabain can exert their adverse effects at the level of plasma membrane transport, by inhibiting Na^+, K^+-ATPase activity (Schultz and Zalusky, 1965; Skou, 1965).

Unlike the antimetabolites described above, other agents can interfere with normal cell function at several levels, making it difficult to determine the activity which is primarily responsible for cell injury. For example, several nucleotide analogues (e.g. 6-mercaptopurine, 8-azaguanine and 6-azauridine) interfere with nucleotide biosynthesis by competitive inhibition and can thus interrupt both RNA and DNA production (Kornberg, 1980). Other chemicals can affect quite different cellular processes: for example, 6-diazo-5-oxo-L-norleucine, a glutamine analogue produced by *Streptomyces*, can inhibit nucleic acid synthesis (Langen, 1975) as well as protein glycosylation and glycosaminoglycan formation (Telser *et al.*, 1965), since glutamine serves as a precursor of purine synthesis and, in certain proteins, as an acceptor residue for oligosaccharide side chains. Enzyme cofactor analogues can also have widespread effects: for example, methotrexate, aminopterin and other inhibitors of folate (dihydrofolate) reductase can lead to reduced availability of purine nucleotides, thymidylic acid and methionine, thereby affecting DNA, RNA and protein synthesis (Calabresi and Parks, 1980). The nicotinamide analogue, 6-aminonicotinamide, can be incorporated to form non-functional NAD-like and NADP-like cofactors, with profound adverse effects upon glycolysis, respiration, electron transport and undoubtedly other enzyme systems requiring these cofactors (Ritter, 1977).

The distinction between chemicals that act by altering structure and those that function in other ways becomes particularly clouded when one considers that some antimetabolites can have both properties. As an example, BrdU can competitively inhibit ribonucleotide reductase activity (Meuth and Green, 1974) but can also be incorporated into DNA where it can, through structural alteration of the genetic material, interfere with expression of selected genes (Rutter *et al.*, 1973).

In the above discussion, we have considered how chemicals adversely influence cell metabolism at single or multiple sites. Some of these agents exert their effects on virtually all cell types whereas others, particularly those which act upon DNA synthesis, are most disruptive of rapidly proliferating cells. Cells of the reproductive system would likely be susceptible to virtually all of the above agents, at least during times of rapid division. Other chemicals might be targeted more specifically to reproductive cells because of the nature and function of the latter. For example, germ cells and embryonic cells might be especially sensitive to agents which cause imbalance of gonadal hormones, which promote growth of particular cells types at the expense of others, or which interfere with cellular recognition and interaction. It is presently difficult to distinguish between primary and secondary sites of action of agents operating in these ways because several different cell types might be involved: as one of many examples, it is not always clear whether chemicals which inhibit implantation do so by directly altering the state of maternal cells, embryonic cells or both. Our limitations in understanding how such agents act adversely upon germ cells and embryonic cells are further restricted by our uncertainty of the molecular mechanisms involved in the development and differentiation of such cells.

3 ASSESSMENT OF CELL INJURY AND EFFECTS ON REPRODUCTIVE FUNCTION

3.1 Molecular Considerations

Before assessing cell injury at the molecular level, one must use classical techniques of pathology to determine target tissues, target cells within the tissue, and target organelles within the cell. Given a suspected target, biochemical and analytical chemistry techniques may then be used, for example, to assess particular functions or enzyme activities, to measure the products of lipid auto-oxidation, or to determine whether or not a chemical has bound covalently to cellular macromolecules. Correlation of the results of such studies with the underlying mechanism(s) of cytotoxicity of a given compound is generally difficult, if not impossible, since as mentioned above, multiple effects are often seen and are probably contributing factors. In most instances we must be content to use gross evaluation of cell and target tissue damage as criteria when screening for detrimental chemicals. On the other hand, chemical action at the DNA level can be assessed easily and routinely by direct molecular analyses or by mutagenesis testing. Since compounds which alter DNA structure or function can exert a negative influence upon all phases of reproduction by causing cell death or inducing mutations, routine analyses of DNA as a potential target for chemically induced damage *are* warranted.

In addition to measuring direct covalent binding of chemicals to DNA, routine screening procedures for DNA damage include:

(1) measurement of DNA repair as indicated by unscheduled DNA synthesis (Cleaver, 1975);
(2) measurement of alkali labile sites (apurinic or apyrimidinic sites), DNA–DNA, DNA–RNA or DNA–protein cross-linking, and single- or double-strand breaks in DNA by alkaline elution under varying conditions (Kohn, 1979);
(3) *in vitro* or *in vivo* mutagenesis (point mutations, chromosome aberrations, or sister chromatid exchange (Perry, 1980) in model systems;
(4) assays for heritable mutagenesis in a mammal, indicating germ cell susceptibility to the chemical (mammalian specific locus test, Russell, 1951 and heritable translocation test, Leonard, 1973); and
(5) assays for *in utero* sensitivity to DNA damaging agents by sister chromatid exchange, chromosome aberrations or induced point mutations (mammalian spot test, Fahrig, 1975 and Russell, 1978).

Since whole mammal testing is expensive and time consuming, much information can be gained by determining:

(1) the covalent interaction of a chemical with the DNA of a model system;
(2) mutagenic effects in that model system;
(3) the amount of chemical actually found bound to target tissue DNA; and finally
(4) correlation of the dose of chemicals bound to the target tissue with the dose required for a mutagenic response in the model system (Lee, 1976).

This latter method of obtaining a quantitative evaluation of the mutagenic potential of a xenobiotic is a valuable tool provided that the compound in question or its metabolite binds covalently to DNA and provided that the same metabolic intermediate is produced in the target tissue as in the model system.

Cytogenetic or sister chromatid exchange (SCE) analyses can be used to assess the effects upon male or female germ cells as well as embryos of parental exposure to agents which have the potential to damage DNA. Cytogenetic examination of the pronuclei in fertilized eggs before cleavage will indicate whether prior DNA damage had occurred in the germ cells (Brewen *et al.*, 1975; Brewen and Payne, 1976). Similar analyses can be carried out on embryos following exposure of the mother to the test chemical. Finally, comparison of the latter analyses with those of embryos exposed to the chemical *in vitro* will indicate the role, if any, of the mother in activation and transport of the potentially toxic agent (Allen *et al.*, 1981).

SCE studies can be carried out *in vitro*, following *in vitro* or *in vivo* exposure to a test substance, by incubating cells or embryos in the presence of BrdU. After a period of time appropriate to achieve incorporation of the base analogue into DNA during two rounds of replication (24–30 hours), Colcemid is added and mitotic figures are stained with Hoechst 33258 and the preparations exposed to u.v. light (Galloway *et al.*, 1980). The resultant 'harlequin chromosomes' are scored for SCE. *In vivo* studies can be performed by exposing midgestation rodent females to the test chemical simultaneously with intravenous infusion of BrdU (Kram *et al.*, 1979), implantation with a BrdU tablet (Allen *et al.*, 1981), or similar techniques. Such methodologies are still in the experimental stages but will undoubtedly provide advantages over the more classical techniques presently in use. For example, measurements of fetal wastage at midgestation as a result of chromosome damage due to chemical exposure of either parent (mammalian dominant lethal assay, Generoso, 1969) is very expensive, time consuming and insensitive. An *in vitro* dominant lethal assay, in which preimplantation and peri-implantation embryos are screened for normal morphological development (Goldstein *et al.*, 1978; Bürki and Sheridan, 1978; Pedersen and Goldstein, 1979), is perhaps less time consuming and costly. However, direct cytogenetic analysis would give a far more direct and accurate assessment of clastogenic effects on DNA (Brewen *et al.*, 1975). SCE occurs by mechanisms as yet unknown but correlates well with mutagenic effects of chemicals (Perry, 1980). It is a very sensitive, reproducible and inexpensive procedure capable of detecting various classes of mutagens. Higher order genetic screening (e.g mouse specific locus test) is beyond the scope of this paper but is the only method now available for determining whether or not a chemical is capable of causing heritable gene mutations ('point mutations') in a mammal.

Caution must be exercised before one extrapolates to humans the detrimental effects on reproductive function (or lack thereof) of a xenobiotic chemical in an animal model system. For example, studies of the oxidative metabolism of xenobiotics in various mammals have shown that chemicals can be metabolized differently even in closely related species: for instance, coumarin can be hydroxylated at the 3, 4, 5, 6, 7, and 8 positions. Liver microsomal enzymes in the mouse are capable of producing 3-, 5-, 6-, 7-, and 8-OH coumarin, whereas the rat produces only 3-, 6- and 8-OH coumarin, and in human liver microsomes only 7-hydroxylating activity is detectable (Wudl and Wood, in preparation). Such differences in metabolism of a given compound could lead to differences in chemical reactivity and thus to differences in biological activity. Therefore, comparative metabolism studies should be considered as part of any battery of biological tests.

3.2 Biological Effects on Embryo

Accessibility and sensitivity are critical factors influencing the susceptibility of embryos to chemical damage. Both of these factors can differ among species and at different stages of embryogenesis. This is not surprising since parameters such as duration of embryogenesis and type of placentation can vary dramatically. Also, embryonic structure changes profoundly during gestation.

Many principles established in teratological studies are also pertinent to reproductive toxicology. It is usually the case that a chemical which is teratogenic within a given concentration range is embryotoxic at greater doses (see Wilson, 1977). Some chemicals, however, can be embryotoxic without showing an intermediate dosage range in which they are teratogenic. Usually, such chemicals (e.g. inhibitors of protein synthesis and certain inhibitors of nucleic acid synthesis, (Chaube and Murphy, 1968)) interrupt processes which are indispensible and critical for generalized cell integrity (Wilson, 1977). Of course, in order for a chemical to be recognizable as an embryotoxic agent of this sort, the conceptus must be significantly more sensitive to it than is the mother.

It is well established that embryos are most susceptible to teratogenic chemicals during organogenesis and histogenesis. Probably for this reason as much as for any other, investigators have tended to ignore the pre- and peri-implantation embryo in studies with xenobiotic chemicals (with the exception of experimentation aimed at the development of contraceptives). It would appear from the relatively few studies that have been done (e.g. Adams *et al.*, 1961) that potential teratogens administered prior to organogenesis either kill the embryo or are without effect. Both accessibility and sensitivity are likely to be involved in this all-or-none situation. There are two reasons why potentially harmful chemicals might fail to reach their targets in the early embryo. First, the plasma membrane of the early preimplantation embryo has not developed some of the sophisticated transport functions characteristic of membranes from later embryonic and adult cells (e.g. Borland and Tasca, 1974, 1975); thus harmful chemicals which are not able to penetrate cell membranes by passive means are less likely to be detrimental to the embryo at these early stages than subsequently. Also, prior to implantation, chemicals can only reach the embryo via genital tract fluids. Although this might in some cases have a protective effect upon the embryo, there is evidence that mitomycin C, a potent mutagen which is teratogenic and/or embryotoxic during organogenesis (Shepard, 1973), can induce sister chromatid exchanges in pre- as well as postimplantation embryos (Wudl and Roy, unpublished).

During preimplantation and peri-implantation stages, the mammalian embryo undergoes important developmental and metabolic changes. Although such alterations are overtly less obvious than those occurring during organogenesis, they could have profound effects upon sensitivity to chemical agents. For example, following fertilization, rates of biosynthetic processes in mammalian embryos are slow and, at least in rodent embryos, much of the informational RNA and protein synthesizing apparatus is preformed (see Sherman and Schindler, in press). Thus the very early embryo appears to be relatively refractory to inhibitors of RNA and protein synthesis. On the other hand, inhibitors of DNA synthesis and agents which interrupt cell division are generally harmful (see Sherman, 1979). Also, intermediary metabolism is primitive in early embryonic cells and development of cleaving embryos is easily blocked by deprivation of, or interference with the use of, essential metabolites (Biggers and Stern, 1973).

As the embryo progresses through the morula and blastocyst stages, biosynthetic rates and rates of cell division increase dramatically. There are also notable changes in membrane function and cell interaction (Sherman, 1979). *In vitro* studies suggest that at this time the embryo becomes unusually sensitive to a wide array of antimetabolites, including those which affect DNA, RNA and protein synthesis as well as cytoskeletal structure and protein glycosylation (Sherman, 1979).

It is during the peri-implantation stages (late blastocyst to early egg-cylinder) that various cell types in the embryo become distinguishable. As embryogenesis proceeds, cells become differentially susceptible to chemical damage. Cells which have undergone differentiative changes are usually more resistant to generalized chemical insult than cells which are undifferentiated or especially those which are undergoing critical transformations in the process of differentiation (Atienza and Sherman, 1975; Rowinski *et al.*, 1975). This principle of differential sensitivity of cells to perturbation as the embryo develops appears to persist throughout organogenesis and helps to explain the common observation that teratogens which disrupt critical metabolic processes can affect a particular tissue on one day of gestation but have a completely different target when administered one or two days earlier or later (Wilson, 1977). The different end result of exposure of peri-implantation *vs* later embryos to harmful chemicals, i.e. embryolethality *vs* teratogenicity, is probably due to the combination of smaller cell numbers and lower cell diversity prior to, as opposed to during, organogenesis (see section 4).

Finally, some consideration should be given to implantation and placentation. It appears that with implantation the conceptus becomes more intimately involved with the maternal organism and more susceptible to maternal imbalances, particularly hormonal ones. Perhaps one of the most striking illustrations in support of this view is the observation in rodents that disruption of ovarian steroid hormone production prior to implantation prevents embryos from implanting but does not result in embryo mortality, at least for several days; on the other hand, such interference with hormonal levels during or after implantation results in prompt abortion or resorption (see Sherman and Wudl, 1976). Since there is no convincing evidence that maternal steroid hormones act *directly* upon implanting and early postimplantation rodent embryos (Sherman and Wudl, 1976), the inference is that disruptive chemicals can have adverse effects upon embryogenesis *indirectly* by altering the uterine milieu.

It is now apparent that the placenta is not so effective a chemical barrier as it was once thought to be (Wilson, 1977). However, because of its structural and metabolic properties, the placenta undoubtedly influences the rate at which, and the degree to which, chemicals reach the fetus. Furthermore, the placental membranes *per se* might serve as specific targets for some chemicals causing embryotoxicity (e.g. Lloyd *et al.*, 1968) or they might convert xenobiotic chemicals to reactive species (e.g. Juchau, 1971; Pelkonen *et al.*, 1971).

Therefore, in the assessment of mechanisms by which chemicals might cause embryotoxicity, the possible role of the placenta either as the agent for transmission or production of the deleterious agent, or as its direct target, should not be ignored.

In view of the above discussion, it is clear that attempts to elucidate mechanisms by which chemicals cause injury to embryos at the cellular or organismal level should include studies at several developmental stages: prior to implantation, during organogenesis and shortly before parturition. It is also worth noting again that objectives in setting up regimens for screening chemicals for embryotoxicity are not always the same as those concerned with mechanism. In screening for harmful chemicals, *in vivo* studies play a major role; it is likely that the primary value of *in vitro* systems, even as they continue to become increasingly effective and informative through improved technology, will be that of preliminary or supplemental testing. On the other hand, *in vitro* systems are often more amenable than *in vivo* studies to investigations of the mechanisms of action of toxic chemicals in the embryo. Some advantages are:

(1) the relative ease of determining dose–response relationships since embryos can be treated individually or in groups of equal size, thus eliminating variables such as maternal differences and differences in litter size;
(2) Convenience and economy in labelling or prelabelling cultured embryos or embryonic cells with radioactive macromolecular precursors, enzyme substrates or the test chemicals *per se*;
(3) reduced problems of accessibility of the chemical to the embryo; and
(4) the ability to monitor embryos continuously for their biochemical and morphological responses to toxic chemicals.

Historically, limitations in mammalian embryo culture techniques precluded *in vitro* toxicity studies. However, in recent years rodent embryo culture procedures have improved dramatically with respect to fidelity and consistency of development. For example, it is now possible to fertilize eggs *in vitro* (Bedford, 1971), to achieve development from cleavage stages to peri-implantation stages and beyond (Hsu, 1978) and through several phases of organogenesis (New, 1978), all at rates and frequencies approaching those *in vivo*. Recent refinements to existing *in vitro* techniques, such as the use of uterine monolayers for studying implantation (Sherman, 1978), the coupling of a microsomal activation system with whole embryo culture (Fantel *et al.*, 1979; Kitchin *et al.*, 1981) and the culturing of embryos in the serum of animals exposed to potentially toxic chemicals (Sadler, 1980) to some extent reintroduce maternal effects into the system. *In vivo* analyses do, however, have some value in studies on mechanisms of action of toxic chemicals and they should be used as appropriate adjuncts to *in vitro* investigations. *In vivo* experimentation is particularly important for determination of the effects of chemicals on placental structure and function since satisfactory *in vitro* systems with this complex tissue are limited.

Several parameters can be monitored to assess toxic effects upon embryos at various developmental stages. Cell death can be monitored directly by gross examination and by histological analysis. It is difficult to quantitate cell death by these techniques; such quantitative estimates might not be necessary when screening chemicals for toxicity but might be more important in studies of mechanisms. Snow (1976) has determined tissue and cell volumes as well as cell numbers of the germ layers of mouse egg-cylinder stage embryos. This knowledge makes it possible to estimate cell number when tissue or embryo volume is known (Snow and Tam, 1979). It is not yet clear whether this relationship can be reliably extrapolated to other stages of embryogenesis.

In lieu of cell number, one can assess effects of chemicals upon embryonic integrity by measuring macromolecular content or the net rates at which macromolecules are synthesized in the presence *vs* the absence of the perturbant. In this regard, DNA measurements are probably most closely rated to cell number. With new analytical microtechniques (e.g. Boer, 1975) it is possible to measure DNA contents of individual rodent embryos during late stages of organogenesis (e.g., Kitchin *et al.*, 1981). Protein microfluorescence analysis is also possible using the fluorescamine reagent (Bohlen *et al.*, 1973); with appropriate microfluorometry equipment, protein contents of individual mouse embryos can be determined at early postimplantation stages (Sellens *et al.*, 1981).

Measurements of rates of macromolecular synthesis using radioactive precursors can serve as another useful indicator of cellular integrity in cultured embryos. Such measurements might be complicated by alterations in endogenous pool size, a parameter which is difficult to correct for on a routine basis. Another potentially serious limitation, especially for *in vivo* studies or culture experiments involving embryos of relatively large size, is accessibility to labelled precursor. Nevertheless, useful comparative data might be obtained, particularly at very early stages of development when it is not possible to routinely measure absolute nucleic acid or protein contents without pooling embryos. Other criteria that can be used to measure ill effects of chemicals upon embryos developing *in vitro* are oxygen consumption (Shepard *et al.*, 1970), rate of glucose metabolism and levels of several enzymes (e.g. Tanimura and Shepard, 1970; Sanyal, 1980).

Finally, in testing chemicals which might exert their detrimental effects through DNA damage or mutagenesis, techniques for measuring SCE are particularly useful. Procedures have been developed for the detection of SCE which should be applicable to embryos in culture at virtually all stages of development (e.g. Galloway *et al.*, 1980; Wudl and Roy, unpublished observations). Similar analyses can also be carried out on midgestation rodent embryos developing *in vivo* (Kram *et al.*, 1979; Allen *et al.*, 1981).

As mentioned above, patterns of embryogenesis can vary dramatically from one mammal to the next. This is of concern in the choice of appropriate *in vivo* animal models for the screening of potentially toxic chemicals. For *in vitro* studies on the mechanisms by which harmful chemicals exert their adverse effects, the choice of animal model is primarily restricted to rodents at this time. However, this should not be a great disadvantage: it is likely that a knowledge of the ways in which toxic chemicals interfere at the molecular and cellular levels with rodent embryos will provide pertinent information regarding effects upon the human embryo.

3.3 Biological Effects on Germ Cells

Assessment of detrimental effects of chemicals on both the male and female reproductive systems will be discussed in detail in other papers (Mann; Kerr and de Kretser; Mattison and Ross, this volume). In addition to assessing the physiological states of reproductive tissues, direct observations of male and female germ cells, and, in some cases, biochemical analyses, can be informative. Gross evaluation of loss of reproductive function (sterility) is the most obvious starting point for assessment of injury to male and female germ cells. For example, sperm function can be studied by *in vitro* fertilization (Bedford, 1971). Sperm count, morphology and motility have long been used as methods for determining the cause of sterility. At the molecular level, DNA is the target macromolecule most accessible to analysis, by measuring direct covalent binding of foreign chemicals, structural alterations, DNA repair, or mutation.

Oocyte damage can be assessed directly by the oocyte depletion assay of Felton and co-workers (Dobson *et al.*, 1978; Felton *et al.*, 1978). After treating immature female mice with a test compound, ovaries are fixed and thin sectioned. Selected sections are stained and oocytes counted. This assay has been shown to be quite sensitive for detecting reproductive damage caused by exposure to polycyclic aromatic hydrocarbons or to radiation.

4 ADAPTIVE RESPONSES TO CELL INJURY

To this point we have considered ways in which reproductive processes can be disrupted by exposure of the individual to detrimental chemicals. The extent to which the various components of the reproductive system have been affected can be assessed by a variety of *in vivo* and *in vitro* tests, as described above and in other presentations. However, it is often the case that by the use of such tests aimed specifically at detecting toxic effects we are looking at *the net result* of the response to the chemical insult. That is, one is observing the difference between the damage caused and the ability of cells, tissues and/or organs to respond to the damage and to repair it. Thus, at one extreme the cells under study might be able to respond to a chemical challenge so rapidly and effectively that by routine screening it is not possible to determine whether adaptation had occurred or whether the harmful chemical had in fact failed to reach the cells under study. At the other extreme, exposure to the chemical might be at such an overwhelming dosage that attempts at repair are ineffectual. Accordingly, characterization of adaptive and repair processes requires studies aimed specifically at detection of these phenomena; consideration must be given to the use of appropriate dosages of the potentially harmful chemical in such investigations.

We have maintained that in order to elucidate mechanisms by which chemicals interfere with reproductive processes it is necessary to examine the problem at molecular, cellular and tissue levels. A similar situation applies to the response to chemical inteference: the reproductive system can escape serious or permanent damage if the adverse effect can be neutralized at the molecular level or if cells which remain viable after the chemical insult can be recruited in adequate numbers to replace those that are lost.

4.1 Molecular Considerations

4.1.1 *DNA Repair*

Although DNA repair mechanisms have been studied most extensively in prokaryotic cells, more recent studies have shown that eukaryotic cells have the capability to repair DNA damage by both excision repair (Cleaver, 1975) and postreplication repair (Lehman, 1972) mechanisms. The latter mechanism has been called 'error-prone repair' and is thought to contribute significantly to the mutagenic effects of radiation and chemicals. Although inducible repair systems exist in bacteria, there is limited evidence that such a system exists in higher organisms (Samson and Schwartz, 1980). In the mouse and human excision repair, as measured by unscheduled DNA synthesis (see section 4.4), occurs in spermatogonial cells and early spermatids but not in later stages of maturation (Chandley and Kofman-Alfaro, 1971; Kofman-Alfaro and Chandley, 1971; Sega, 1974). This accounts for the increased sensitivity of later stages to chemical mutagenesis by alkylating agents (Sega, 1974). Brandriff and Pedersen (1981) have recently shown that radiation-damaged spermatozoan DNA can be repaired in the egg following fertilization. Excision repair has also been demonstrated in resting, growing and mature oocytes (Masui and Pedersen, 1975; Pedersen and Mangia, 1978), as well as pre- and postimplantation embryos (Pedersen and Cleaver, 1975). There is also some evidence that early preimplantation mouse embryos are capable of postreplication repair (Eibs and Spielmann, 1977).

4.1.2 *Membrane: protection and repair mechanisms*

Unless damage to membranes is so extensive that protective and repair mechanisms are ineffective, cells are capable of repairing, and thus recovering from, the effects of lipid peroxidation (Svingen and Aust, 1980). Peroxidation of membrane lipid by free radicals can be blocked by free radical scavengers such as vitamin E, cholesterol, ascorbic acid, glutathione, NADH and NADPH (Dybing *et al.*, 1977; Autor *et al.*, 1980; Mustafa *et al.*, 1980; Svingen and Aust, 1980). Enzymatic protection from peroxides and free radicals is provided by catalase, peroxidase, superoxide dismutase and glutathione peroxidase, an inducible enzyme which reduces organic peroxides (Dybing *et al.*, 1977; Autor *et al.*, 1980; Mustafa *et al.*, 1980; Svingen and Aust, 1980). In the lung, it has been shown that ozone induces enzymes capable of replenishing non-protein sulph-hydryl compounds: glutathione reductase, disulphide reductase and glutathione-disulphide transhydrogenase (Mustafa *et al.*, 1980). After carbon tetrachloride damage to hepatocytes *in vitro*, mitochondrial integrity and function can be restored by replacement of both the damaged lipid (through excision and replacement of the oxidized fatty acid moieties) and the proteins lost through membrane leakage (by synthesis of new proteins) (Brabec *et al.*, 1980).

4.1.3 *Protection from Metal Toxicity*

In addition to the capability of normal cellular constituents to bind metals (e.g. glutathione which binds Pb^{2+}, Cd^{2+}, Hg^{2+} and Cu^{2+}) (Vallee and Ulmer, 1972), liver and kidney have been shown to possess a cadmium-inducible chelator called metallothionein (Vallee and Ulmer, 1972; Shaihk and Smith, 1976).

4.1.4 *Metabolism/Detoxication*

Although we have pointed out earlier (section 2) that microsomal mixed function oxidases can activate relatively innocuous chemicals into potentially damaging ones, it is important to bear in mind that the same enzyme systems can promote excretion of toxic chemicals. Studies of rat and mouse cytochrome P-450 enzymes indicate there are at least a dozen enzymes with similar activities and overlapping substrate specificities and responses to inducers. Non-cytochrome P-450 activities involved in xenobiotic metabolism, such as epoxide hydrase, UDP-glucuronyltransferase, sulphotransferase, reductases and non-microsomal oxidases to name a few, are also critical elements in the detoxication process.

There is only limited information concerning xenobiotic metabolism in reproductive tissues. Components of the microsomal mixed function oxidase system have been detected in human fetal liver, fetal adrenal gland and placenta (Juchau, 1971; Pelkonen *et al.*, 1971; Berry *et al.*, 1977; Pelkonen, 1977).

Galloway *et al.* (1980) used SCE to demonstrate that mouse embryos at early postimplantation stages, and possibly preimplantation stages as well, can activate benzo(a)pyrene. This approach is more sensitive than direct analysis, and the results indicate that the early mouse embryo contains at least some mixed function microsomal oxidase activity and thus the potential for detoxication of chemicals. The embryonic enzyme system also appears to be inducible, as is the case in adults (Galloway *et al.*, 1980). It should, however, be noted that cultured eleventh day rat embryos appear incapable of activating cyclophosphamide to its teratogenic and embryotoxic state(s) whereas the addition to the cultures of rat liver microsome preparations achieves activation (Fantel *et al.*, 1979; Kitchin *et al.*, 1981). Therefore, there is either species difference in the time at which mixed function microsomal oxidases are active during embryogenesis or the embryos do not acquire all oxidase activities or induction mechanisms simultaneously.

Conjugation reactions (glucuronidations, sulphation, acetylation), which render xenobiotic chemicals more polar and thus more susceptible to excretion, appear to be substantially less prevalent in conceptuses than in the adult. According to Dutton (1978), the enzymes responsible for these conjugation reactions are probably present in fetal tissues since they are required for normal metabolic processes. However, evidence of acetylation of xenobiotic chemicals by prenatal tissues is limited to conjugation of *p*-aminobenzoate (but not isoniazid) by the placenta; no data were described to suggest that fetal sulphotransferases could conjugate xenobiotic chemicals; and although there is some indication that fetal tissues (probably liver) possess glucuronidating enzymes and are capable of carrying out glucuronidation, activities are low compared to adult tissues and the enzymes do not appear to be inducible until birth (Dutton, 1978).

4.2 The Embryo

The degree to which an embryo can adapt to chemical damage at the cellular level depends upon how effectively it can compensate for cell loss. In other words, the *regulative capacity* of the embryo is of critical importance. As indicated in a thoughtful consideration of size regulation by Snow *et al.* (1981), this capacity is not necessarily the same among mammals; it is not fixed throughout gestation and different organs do not compensate for cell loss at the same rate or to the same degree. It is possible to obtain viable young from a single blastomere of a two-cell mouse embryo, of a four-cell sheep embryo or of an eight-cell rabbit embryo (see Snow *et al.*, 1981). Tarkowski (1959) reported that embryos developing from a single blastomere from the two-cell stage developed morphologically at a normal rate but failed to regulate for size until the eleventh or twelfth day of pregnancy (although N. Lewis and J. Rossant, personal communication) have recently observed evidence for a transient 'catch-up' period in size on the seventh day of pregnancy after which experimental embryos fall behind controls once again). On the basis of such observations it is reasonable to assume that the embryo might be able to compensate successfully for destruction of a substantial proportion of its cells due to chemical insult. In fact, there is some support for this assumption (see below) although the situation is complicated by other factors which must be considered. For example, studies on manipulated preimplantation mouse embryos have indicated that at least eight cells are required at the time of blastocoele formation in order for one cell or more to become completely enclosed by others during subsequent development; failing this, the structure will take shape of a 'trophectodermal vesicle' which will form only trophoblast cells when transplanted to foster mothers (reviewed by Sherman, 1981). Thus, the preimplantation embryo will be unable to adapt to any perturbation which reduces cell number below the critical level required to produce one or more enclosed cells by the morulla stage.

Relatively few investigations on size regulation have been carried out in which postimplantation embryos were perturbed. A notable exception is the study by Snow and Tam (1979). These investigators observed that embryos from pregnant mice treated with 4–6 mg/kg mitomycin C on the seventh day of pregnancy showed a reduction in cell number relative to untreated controls of almost 90% in 24 hours. Yet by the eleventh day of gestation, the majority of the embryos, although somewhat smaller than controls, had not only survived but appeared to possess a perfectly normal morphology! Normal-size litters were born from the mitomycin C-treated mice. Although many of the pups were runted, sterile, or died prior to weaning, this is, nevertheless, a remarkable demonstration of the compensatory properties of the early postimplantation embryo. On the other hand, microsurgical experiments by Snow and Tam (personal communication) indicate that embryos cannot regulate for ablation of discrete blocks of tissue at the egg-cylinder stage. Taken together with the mitomycin C results, it is reasonable to assume that the early postimplantation embryo can compensate for substantial cell loss only if the remaining cells contain representatives of each of the essential stem populations.

Perturbation studies similar to those of Snow and Tam (1979) have not yet been carried out on embryos undergoing organogenesis. However, it is likely from the teratogenic action of many chemical treatments at these stages that the regulative capacity of the embryos has been altered: cells now appear to be so compartmentalized that they have differential sensitivities at different times. At any given stage, chemicals will interfere with the normal structure and/or function of cells which are most vulnerable. Cells from different stem populations, while they themselves are refractory to damage, might be too far committed to other developmental pathways to compensate for injuries to cells in other populations. Differential sensitivity, as mentioned above, might depend upon whether or not the cells are in a critical stage along their developmental pathway and/or their proliferative rate. Consistent with this view is the finding by Snow *et al.* (1981) that following the aforementioned mitomycin C treatments, cells from the different stem populations (e.g. neural cells, somites, germ cells) 'up-regulate' to reach normal numbers at their own independent, characteristic rates. In a sense, then, compartmentalization of cell populations during organogenesis has allowed the embryo to adapt to moderate chemical insult by sacrificing only a limited proportion of cells at any one time.

4.3 Germ Cells

Fertility can be severely compromised by exposure to chemicals or radiation. However, there is evidence that the female and male reproductive systems are capable of responding to chemical, as well as radiation, insult at some stages. At the primordial germ cell stages, adaptation appears to be primarily by repopulation. Snow *et al.* (1981) have demonstrated that embryos have approximately one-tenth of the normal number of primordial germ cells on the ninth gestation day following exposure to mitomycin C on the seventh or eighth gestation day. However, the numbers of these cells increase relative to controls so that they reach about half the normal value by the eleventh day of gestation and proliferate at the same rate as controls thereafter (Snow *et al.*, 1981). When viable offspring were tested for fertility it was found that more than half of the males and 9 of 11 females were fertile (Snow and Tam, 1979). These results suggest that early germ cells can in some way reverse the effects of severe depletion; repopulation apparently plays a role. Similar observations of germ cell refractivity have been made in studies with ionizing raditation (Brent, 1977).

Recent studies by Dobson *et al.* (1978) and by Felton *et al.* (1978) indicate that as they develop, oocytes have periods of marked sensitivity to chemicals and radiation. Studies with squirrel monkeys and mice indicate that severe oocyte depletion ultimately arises from both types of perturbation late in pregnancy. Mouse oocytes are particularly sensitive to alkylating agents and radiation within the first three weeks of birth and then become increasingly refractory beyond 20 days of age (Brent, 1977; Dobson *et al.*, 1978). The reason for this acquired resistance is not clear since cell division is already arrested in primordial oocytes of early postnatal animals and yet these cells are remarkably sensitive to perturbation. It is, perhaps, a reflection of developmental differences between juvenile *vs* adult oocytes that explains their differing sensitivity, as might be the case for embryonic cells in general (see section 4.2).

Whatever the reason for differential sensitivity to damaging agents, the loss of oocytes (primordial, immature or mature) cannot be compensated for by repopulation. Loss of male germ cells at the various stages of spermatogenesis can result in transient sterility with recovery of function after repopulation, provided that stem cells have survived. For example, treatment of male mice with the alkylating agent ethylnitrosourea causes sterility for a period of 13 weeks followed by recovery of fertility (Russell *et al.*, 1979).

Although many xenobiotic chemicals which require metabolic activation have been shown to be mutagenic or cytotoxic to both male and female germ cells, the site of activation could be elsewhere. In fact, molecular and genetic studies have revealed that murine oocytes possess little if any mixed-function microsomal oxidase activity (Dobson *et al.*, 1978; Felton *et al.*, 1978). However, Lee and Dixon (1978) have reported that oxidative metabolism occurs in seminiferous tubules and interstitial cellular compartments of the testis.

4.4 Methods of Assessment

Procedures have been described for measuring repair of DNA in spermatogenic cells (Chandley and Kofman-Alfaro, 1971; Kofman-Alfaro and Chandley, 1971), oocytes (Masui and Pedersen, 1975; Pedersen and Mangia, 1978) and early embryos (Pederson and Cleaver, 1975). In general, cells exposed to the test chemical *in vitro* are subsequently incubated with ^{3}H-thymidine for 1–2 hours. The cells are mounted on slides and prepared for autoradiography. A comparison of frequency of nuclear labelling in treated *vs* unexposed cells indicates whether unscheduled DNA synthesis has occurred. The presence of microsomal mixed-function oxidase activities can be monitored in embryonic cells and germ cells either by direct measurement or by indirect methods such as that described by Galloway *et al.* (1980) (see section 3.1).

To determine the ability of primordial germ cells to repopulate after chemical insult, these cells can be stained relatively specifically for alkaline phosphatase (Mintz, 1957); cells from other tissues can be karyotyped to reveal the sex of the embryo. At present, oocyte numbers must be estimated from representative histological sections through the ovary (Dobson *et al.*, 1978). Extended fertility testing of adult mice will reveal the ability of more developed germ cells to survive adverse chemical treatment. Embryo integrity can be measured morphological or biochemically as described in section 3.2. Before it can be concluded that germ cells or embryos have adapted to chemical damage by repopulation it must be demonstrated that there was a transient period during which the treated animals were infertile or the embryos were overtly abnormal.

5 REFERENCES

Adams, C. E., Hay, M. F. and Lutwak-Mann, C. (1961). The action of various agents upon the rabbit embryo. *J. Embryol. exp. Morphol.* **9**, 468–491.

Allen, J. A. and Coombs, M. M. (1980). Covalent binding of polycyclic aromatic compounds to mitochondrial and nuclear DNA. *Nature (London)* **287**, 244–245.

Allen, J. W., El-Nahass, E., Sanyal, M. K., Dunn, R. L., Gladen, B. and Dixon, R. L. (1981). Sister chromatid exchange analyses in rodent maternal, embryonic, and extraembryonic tissues: transplacental and direct mutagen exposures. *Mutat. Res.* **80**, 297–311.

Atienza, S. B. and Sherman, M. I. (1975). Effects of bromodeoxyuridine, cytosine arabinoside and Colcemid upon *in vitro* development of mouse blastocysts. *J. Embryol. exp. Morphol.* **34**, 467–484.

Atienza-Samols, S. B., Pine, P. R. and Sherman, M. I. (1980). Effects of tunicamycin upon glycoprotein synthesis and development of early mouse embryos. *Devel. Biol.* **79**, 19–32.

Atlas, S. A., Boobis, A. R., Felton, J. S., Thorgiersson, S. S. and Nebert, D. W. (1977). Ontogenetic expression of polycyclic aromatic compound-inducible monooxygenase activities and forms of cytochrome P-450 in rabbit. *J. biol. Chem.* **252**, 4712–4721.

Autor, A. P., McLennan, G. and Fox, A. W. (1980). Oxygen free radicals generated by dihydrofumarate and ionizing radiation: cytotoxic effect on isolated pulmonary macrophages. In Bhatnagar, R. S. (Ed.) *Molecular Basis of Environmental Toxicity*, pp. 51–68. Ann Arbor Science Publishers, Inc., Ann Arbor, Michigan.

Backer, J. M. and Weinstein, I. B. (1980). Mitochondrial DNA is a major cellular target for a dihydrodiol-epoxide derivative of benzo(a)pyrene. *Science* (*Washington, DC*) **209**, 297–299.

Bartholomew, J. C., Gamper, H. B. and Yokota, H. A. (1980). Chemical carcinogenesis and the physiological state of the cell. In Bhatnagar, R. S. (Ed.) *Molecular Basis of Environmental Toxicity*, pp. 293–327. Ann Arbor Science Publishers, Inc., Ann Arbor, Michigan.

Bedford, J. M. (1971). Techniques and criteria used in the study of fertilization. In Daniel, J. C. (Ed.) *Methods in Mammalian Embryology*, pp. 37–63. W. H. Freeman, San Francisco.

Beranek, D. T., Weis, C. C. and Swenson, D. H. (1980). A comprehensive quantitative analysis of methylated and ethylated DNA using high pressure liquid chromatography. *Carcinogenesis* (*London*) **1**, 595–606.

Berman, J. J., Tong, C. and Williams, G. M. (1978). Enhancement of mutagenesis during cell replication of cultured liver epithelial cells. *Cancer Lett.* **4**, 277–283.

Berry, D. L., Zachariah, P. K., Slaga, T. J. and Juchau, M. R. (1977). Analysis of the biotransformation of benzo(a)pyrene in human fetal and placental tissues with high-pressure liquid chromatography. *Eur. J. Cancer* **13**, 667–675.

Bhatnagar, R. S., Hussain, M. Z. and Lee S. D. (1980). The role of collagen as a primary molecular site of environmental injury. In Bhatnagar, R. S. (Ed.) *Molecular Basis of Environmental Toxicity*, pp. 531–558. Ann Arbor Science Publishers, Inc., Ann Arbor, Michigan.

Biggers, J. D. and Stern, S. (1973). Metabolism of the preimplantation mammalian embryo. *Adv. Reprod. Physiol.* **6**, 1–59.

Boer, G. J. (1975). A simplified microassay of DNA and RNA using ethidium bromide. *Anal. Biochem.* **65**, 225–231.

Bohlen, P., Stein, S., Dairman, W. and Udenfriend, S. (1973). Fluorimetric assay of proteins in the nanogram range. *Archs Biochem. Biophys.* **155**, 213–220.

Borland, R. M. and Tasca, R. J. (1974). Activation of a Na^+-dependent amino acid transport system in preimplantation mouse embryos. *Devel. Biol.* **36**, 169–182.

Borland, R. M. and Tasca, R. J. (1975). Na^+-dependent amino acid transport in preimplantation mouse embryos. *Deveel. Biol.* **46**, 192–201.

Brabec, M. J., Dolci, E. D. and Bernstein, I. A. (1980). Restoration of hepatic mito-chondria following chemically induced damage. In Bhatnagar, R. S. (Ed.) *Molecular Basis of Environmental Toxicity*, pp. 135–149. Ann Arbor Science Publishers, Inc., Ann Arbor, Michigan.

Brandriff, B. and Pedersen, R. A. (1981). Repair of the ultraviolet-irradiated male genome in fertilized mouse eggs. *Science* (*Washington, DC*) **211**, 1431–1432.

Brent, R. L. (1977). Radiations and other physical agents. In Wilson, J. G. and Fraser, R. C. (Eds.) *Handbook of Teratology*, Vol. 1, pp. 153–224. Plenum Press, New York.

Brewen, J. G. and Payne, H. S. (1976). Studies on chemically induced dominant lethality. II. Cytogenetic studies on MMS-induced dominant lethality in maturing dictyate mouse oocytes. *Mutat. Res.* **37**, 77–82.

Brewen, J. G., Payne, H. S., Jones, K. P. and Preston, R. J. (1975). Studies on chemically induced dominant lethality. I. The cytogenetic basis of MMS-induced dominant lethality in post-meiotic male germ cells. *Mutat. Res.* **33**, 239–250.

Brooks, P. (1977). Role of covalent binding in carcinogenicity. In Jollow, D. J., Kocsis, J. J., Snyder, R. and Vainio, H. (Eds.) *Biological Reactive Intermediates*, pp. 470–480. Plenum Press, New York.

Bürki, K., and Sheridan, W. (1978). Expression of TEM-induced damage to postmeiotic stages of spermatogenesis of the mouse during early embryogenesis. I. Investigations with *in vitro* embryo culture. *Mutat. Res.* **49**, 259–268.

Calabresi, P. and Parks, R. E. (1980). Antiproliferative agents and drugs used for immunosuppression. In Gilman, A. D., Goodman, L. S. and Gilman, A. (Eds.) and Mayer, S. E. and Malman, K. S. (Assoc. Eds.) *Goodman and Gilman's The Pharmacological Basis of Therapeutics*, 6th edn, pp. 1254–1307. Macmillan Publishing Co., New York, Collien Macmillan Canada Ltd and Baillière Tindall, London.

Chandley, A. C. and Kofman-Alfaro, S. (1971). 'Unscheduled' DNA synthesis in human germ cells following UV irradiation. *Exp. Cell Res.* **69**, 45–48.

Chaube, S. and Murphy, M. L. (1968). The teratogenic effects of the recent drugs active in cancer chemotherapy. In Woollam, D. H. M. (Ed.) *Advances in Teratology*, Vol. 3, pp. 181–237. Academic Press, New York.

Cleaver, J. E. (1975). Methods for studying repair of DNA damaged by physical and chemical carcinogens. *Methods Cancer Res.* **11**, 123–165.

Dobson, R. L., Koehler, C. G., Felton, J. S., Kwan, T. C., Wuebbles, B. J. and Jones, D. C. L. (1978). Vulnerability of female germ cells in developing mice and monkeys to tritium, gamma rays, and polycyclic aromatic hydrocarbons. In Mahlum, D. D., Sikov, M. R., Hackett, P. L. and Andrews, F. D. (Eds.) *Developmental Toxicology in Energy-Related Pollutants*, pp. 1–14, D.O.E. Symposium Series 47.

Dutton, G. J. (1978). Developmental aspects of drug conjugation, with special reference to glucuronidation. *A. Rev. Pharmac. Toxicol.* **18**, 17–35.

Dybing, E., Mitchell, J. R., Nelson, S. D. and Gillette, J. R. (1977). Metabolic activation of methyldopa by cytochrome P450-generated superoxide anion. In Jollow, D. J., Kocsis, J. J., Snyder, R. and Vainio, H. (Eds.) *Biological Reactive Intermediates*, pp. 167–172. Plenum Press, New York.

Edidin, M. (1972). Aspects of plasma membrane fluidity. In Fox, C. F. (Ed.) *Membrane Research*, pp. 15–25. Academic Press, New York.

Eibs, H.-G. and Spielmann, H. (1977). Differential sensitivity of preimplantation mouse embryos to UV irradiation *in vitro* and evidence for postreplication repair. *Radiat. Res.* **71**, 367–376.

Eisinger, J. (1978). Biochemistry and measurement of environmental lead intoxication. *Quart. Rev. Biophys.* **11**, 439–466.

Fahrig, R. (1975). A mammalian spot test: induction of genetic alterations in pigment cells of mouse embryos with X rays and chemical mutagens. *Mol. Gen. Genet.* **138**, 309–314.

Fantel, A. G., Greenaway, J. C., Juchau, M. R. and Shepard, T. H. (1979). Teratogenic bioactivation of cyclophosphamide *in vitro*. *Life Sci.* **25**, 67–72.

Farkas, W. R. (1968). Depolymerization of ribonucleic acid by plumbous ion. *Biochim. biophys. Acta* **155**, 401–409.

Felton, J. S., Kwan, T. C., Wuebbles, B. J. and Dobson, R. L. (1978). Genetic differences in polycyclic-aromatic-hydrocarbon metabolism and their effects on oocyte killing in developing mice. In Mahlum, D. D., Sikov, M. R., Hackett, P. L. and Andrews, F. D. (Eds.) *Developmental Toxicology of Energy-Related Pollutants*, pp. 15–26. D.O.E. Symposium Series 47.

Flick, D. F., Kraybill, H. G. and Dimitroff, J. M. (1971). Toxic effects of cadmium, a review. *Environ. Res.* **4**, 71–81.

Fornace, A. J. (1980). Malignant transformation by the DNA-protein crosslinking agent trans-Pt [Pt (H) diammine dichloride]. *Proc. Am. Ass. Cancer Res.* **21**, 118.

Galloway, S. M., Perry, P. E., Meneses, J., Nebert, D. W. and Pedersen, R. A. (1980). Cultured mouse embryos metabolize benzo(a)pyrene during early gestation: genetic differences detectable by sister chromatid exchange. *Proc. natn Acad. Sci. U.S.A.* **77**, 3524–3528.

Generoso, W. M. (1969). Chemical induction of dominant lethals in female mice. *Genetics* **61**, 461–470.

Goldstein, L. S., Meneses, J., and Pedersen, R. A. (1978). Dose response relationship for X-ray induced dominant lethal mutations detected in mouse embryos *in vitro*. *Mutat. Res.* **51**, 55–59.

Harbison, R. D. (1978). Chemical-biological reactions common to teratogenesis and mutagenesis. *Environ. Health Perspect.* **24**, 87–100.

Hogberg, J. (1977). Regulation and effects of lipid peroxidation in isolated hepatocytes. In Jollow, D. J., Kocsis, J. J., Snyder, R. and Vainio, H. (Eds.) *Biological Reactive Intermediates*, pp. 401–414. Plenum Press, New York.

Hsu, Y.-C. (1978). *In vitro* development of whole mouse embryos beyond the implantation stage. In Daniel, J. C. (Ed.) *Methods in Mammalian Reproduction*, pp. 229–245. Academic Press, New York.

Hurley, L. S. (1977). Nutritional deficiencies and excesses. In Wilson, H. G. and Fraser, F. C. (Eds.) *Handbook of Teratology*, Vol. 1, pp. 261–308. Plenum Press, New York.

Hussain, M. Z. and Bhatnagar, R. S. (1979). Involvement of superoxide in paraquat induced enhancement of lung collagen synthesis in organ culture. *Biochem. Biophys. Res. Commun.* **89**, 71–76.

Juchau, M. R. (1971). Human placental hydroxylation of 3, 4-benzpyrene during early gestation and at term. *Toxic. appl. Pharmac.* **18**, 665–675.

Kitchin, K. T., Schmid, B. T. and Sanyal, M. K. (1981). Teratogenicity of cyclophosphamide in a coupled microsomal activating/embryo culture system. *Biochem. Pharmac.* **30**, 59–64.

Kofman-Alfaro, S. and Chandley, A. C. (1971). Radiation-initiated DNA synthesis in spermatogenic cells of the mouse. *Exp. Cell Res.* **69**, 33–44.

Kohn, K. W. (1979), DNA as a target in cancer chemotherapy: measurement of macromolecular DNA damage produced in mammalian cells by anticancer agents and carcinogens. *Methods Cancer Res.* **16**, 291–345.

Kornberg, A. (1980). *DNA Replication*. W. H. Freeman, San Francisco.

Kram, D., Bynum, G. D., Senula, G. C. and Schneider, E. L. (1979). *In utero* sister chromatid exchange analysis for detection of transplacental mutagens. *Nature (London)* **279**, 531.

Langen, P. (1975). *Antimetabolites of Nucleic Acid Metabolism*. Gordon and Breach, New York.

Lee, I. P. and Dixon, R. L. (1978). Factors influencing reproduction and genetic toxic effects on male gonads. *Environ. Health Perspect.* **24**, 117–127.

Lee, W. R. (1976). Molecular dosimetry of chemical mutagens. Detection of molecular dose to its germ line. *Mutat. Res.* **38**, 311–316.

Lehman, A. R. (1972). Post-replication repair of ultraviolet irradiated mammalian cells. *J. molec. Biol.* **66**, 319–337.

Leonard, A. (1973). Observations on meiotic chromosomes of the male mouse as a test of the potential mutagenicity of chemicals in mammals. In Hollaender, A. (Ed.) *Chemical Mutagens: Principles and Methods for Their Detection*, Vol. 3, pp. 21–56. Plenum Press, New York.

Lindell, T., Weinberg, F., Morris, P., Roeder, R. and Rutter, W. (1970). Specific inhibition of nuclear RNA polymerase II by α-amanitin. *Science (Washington, DC)* **170**, 447–449.

Lloyd, J. B., Bede, F., Griffiths, A. and Parry, L. M. (1968). The mechanism of action of acid diazo dyes. In Campbell, P. N. (Ed.) *The Interactions of Drugs and Subcellular Components on Animal Cells*, pp. 171–202. Churchill, London.

Masui, Y. and Pedersen, R. A. (1975). Ultraviolet light-induced unscheduled DNA synthesis in mouse oocytes during meiotic maturation. *Nature (London)* **257**, 705–706.

McLachlan, J. A. (1977). Prenatal exposure to diethylstilbestrol in mice: toxicological studies. *J. Toxicol. environ. Health* **2**, 527–537.

Meuth, M. and Green, H. (1974). Induction of a deoxycytidineless state in cultured mammalian cells by bromodeoxyuridine. *Cell* **2**, 109–112.

Mintz, B. (1957). Embryological development of primordial germ-cells in the mouse: influence of a new mutation, Wj. *J. Embryol. exp. Morphol.* **5**, 396–403.

Mustafa, M. G., Faeder, E. J. and Lee, S. D. (1980). Biochemical basis of pulmonary response to ozone and nitrogen dioxide injury. In Bhatnagar, R. S. (Ed.) *Molecular Basis of Environmental Toxicity*, pp. 151–172. Ann Arbor Science Publishers, Inc., Ann Arbor, Michigan.

New, D. A. T. (1978). Whole embryo culture of mammalian embryos during organogenesis. *Biol. Rev.* **53**, 81–122.

Olden, K., Pratt, R. M. and Yamada, K. M. (1979). Selective toxicity of tunicamycin for transformed cells. *Int. J. Cancer* **24**, 60–66.

Pedersen, R. A. and Cleaver, J. E. (1975). Repair of UV damage to DNA of implantation-stage mouse embryos *in vitro*. *Exp. Cell Res.* **95**, 247–253.

Pedersen, R. A. and Mangia, F. (1978). Ultraviolet-light-induced unscheduled DNA synthesis by resting and growing mouse oocytes. *Mutat. Res.* **49**, 425–429.

Pelkonen, O. (1977). Formation of toxic intermediates in fetal tissues. In Dollow, D. J., Kocsis, J. J., Snyder, R. and Vainio, H. (Eds.) *Biological Reactive Intermediates*, pp. 148–159. Plenum Press, New York.

Pelkonen, O., Arvela, P. and Karki, N. T. (1971). 3, 4-Benzpyrene and *N*-methylaniline metabolizing enzymes in immature foetus and placenta. *Acta pharmac. tox.* **30**, 385–392.

Perry, P. E. (1980). Chemical mutagens and sister chromatid exchange. In de Serres, F. J. and Hollaender, A. (Eds.) *Chemical Mutagens: Principles and Methods for Their Detection*, pp. 1–39. Plenum Press, New York.

Petering, D. H. and Petering, H. G. (1980). A molecular basis for metal toxicity. In Bhatnagar, R. S. (Ed.) *Molecular Basis of Environmental Toxicity*, pp. 449–474. Ann Arbor Science Publishers, Inc., Ann Arbor, Michigan.

Recknagel, R. O. (1967). Carbon tetrachloride hepatotoxicity. *Pharmacol. Rev.* **19**, 145–208.

Recknagel, R. O., Glende, E. A. Jr. and Hruszkewycz, A. M. (1977). New data supporting an obligatory role for lipid peroxidation in carbon tetrachloride-induced loss of aminopyrine demethylase, cytochrome P-450, and glucose-6-phosphatase. In Jollow, D. J., Kocsis, J. J., Snyder, R. and Vainio, H. (Eds.) *Biological Reactive Intermediates*, pp. 417–428. Plenum Press, New York.

Ritter, E. J. (1977). Altered biosynthesis. In Wilson, J. G. and Fraser, F. C. (Eds.) *Handbook of Teratology*, Vol. 2, pp. 99–116. Plenum Press, New York.

Rosenthal, A. S., Moses, H. L., Beaver, D. L. and Schuffman, S. S. (1966). Lead ion and phosphatase histochemistry. I. Nonenzymatic hydrolysis of nucleoside phosphates by lead ion. *J. Histochem. Cytochem.* **14**, 698–701.

Rowinski, J., Solter, D. and Koprowski, H. (1975). Mouse embryo development *in vitro*: effects of inhibitors of RNA and protein synthesis on blastocyst and post-blastocyst embryos. *J. exp. Zool.* **192**, 133–142.

Russell, L. B. (1978). Somatic cells as indicators of germinal mutations in the mouse. *Environ. Health Perspect.* **24**, 113–116.

Russell, W. L. (1951). X-ray induced mutations in mice. *Cold Spring Harbor Symp. Quant. Biol.* **16**, 327–336.

Russell, W. L., Kelly, E. M., Hunsicker, P. R., Bangham, J. W., Maddux, S. C. and Phipps, E. L. (1979). Specific-locus test shows ethylnitrosurea to be the most potent mutagen in the mouse. *Proc. natn Acad. Sci. U.S.A.* **76**, 5818–5819.

Rutter, W. J. (1980). Control of cellular differentiation: overview. *Ann. N. Y. Acad. Sci.* **339**, 263–264.

Rutter, W. J., Pictet, R. L. and Morris, P. W. (1973). Toward developmental mechanisms of developmental processes. *A. Rev. Biochem.* **42**, 601–646.

Sadler, T. W. (1980). Effects of maternal diabetes on early embryogenesis. *Teratology* **21**, 339–347.

Samson, L. and Schwartz, J. L. (1980). Evidence for an adaptive DNA repair pathway in CHO and human skin fibroblast cell lines. *Nature (London)* **287**, 861–863.

Sanyal, M. K. (1980). Development of the rat conceptus *in vitro* and associated changes in components of culture medium. *J. Embryol. exp. Morphol.* **58**, 1–12.

Schenkman, J. B., Robie, K. M. and Jansson, I. (1977). Aryl hydrocarbon hydroxylase: induction. In Jollow, D. J., Kocsis, J. J., Snyder, R. and Vainio, H. (Eds.) *Biological Reactive Intermediates*, pp. 83–95. Plenum Press, New York.

Schnell, R. C. (1980). Cadmium-induced inhibition of hepatic xenobiotic transformation. In Bhatnagar, R. S. (Ed.) *Molecular Basis of Environmental Toxicity*, pp. 403–417. Ann Arbor Science Publishers, Inc., Ann Arbor, Michigan.

Schultz, S. G. and Zalusky, R. (1965). Interactions between sodium transport and active amino acid transport in isolated rabbit ileum. *Nature (London)* **205**, 292–294.

Sega, G. A. (1974). Unscheduled DNA synthesis in the germ cells of male mice exposed *in vivo* to the chemical mutagen ethyl methanesulfonate. *Proc. natn Acad. U.S.A.* **71**, 4955–4959.

Sellens, M. H., Stein, S. and Sherman, M. I. (1981). Protein and free amino acid content in preimplantation mouse embryos and in blastocysts under various culture conditions. *J. Reprod. Fertil.* **61**, 307–315.

Sevanian, A., Mead, J. F. and Stein, R. F. (1980). Lipid epoxidation in the lung: major isolable products of lipid autoxidation *in vivo*. In Bhatnagar, R. S. (Ed.) *Molecular Basis of Environmental Toxicity*, pp. 213–228. Ann Arbor Science Publishers, Inc., Ann Arbor, Michigan.

Shaihk, Z. A. and Smith, J. C. (1976). The biosynthesis of metallothionein in rat liver and kidney after administration of cadmium. *Chem. Biol. Interact.* **15**, 327–336.

Shepard, T. H. (1973). *Catalog of Teratogenic Agents*. The Johns Hopkins University Press, Baltimore, Maryland.

Shepard, T. H., Tanimura, T. and Robkin, M. A. (1970). Energy metabolism in early mammalian embryos. *Devel. Biol. Suppl.* **4**, 42–58.

Sherman, M. I. (1978). Implantation of mouse blastocysts *in vitro*. In Daniel, J. C. (Ed.) *Methods in Mammalian Reproduction*, pp. 247–257. Academic Press, New York.

Sherman, M. I. (1979). Developmental biochemistry of preimplantation mammalian embryos. *A. Rev. Biochem.* **48**, 443–470.

Sherman, M. I. (1981). Control of cell fate during early mouse embryogenesis. In Jagiello, G. and Vogel, H. J. (Eds.) *Bioregulators of Reproduction*, pp. 559–576. Academic Press, New York.

Sherman, M. I. and Schindler, J. (in press). Control of gene expression during early mammalian embryogenesis. In Siddiqui, M.A.Q. (Ed.) *Control of Embryonic Gene Expression*, CRC press, Boca Raton, Florida.

Sherman, M. I. and Wudl, L. R. (1976). The implanting mouse blastocyst. In Poste, G. and Nicolson, G. L. (Eds.) *The Cell Surface in Animal Embryogenesis and Development*, pp. 81–125. North-Holland, Amsterdam.

Sirover, M. A. and Loeb, L. A. (1976). Metal-induced infidelity during DNA synthesis. *Proc. natn Acad. Sci. U.S.A.* **73**, 2331–2335.

Skilleter, D. N. (1975). The decrease of mitochondrial substrate uptake by trialkyltin and trialkyllead compounds in chloride media and its relevance to inhibition of oxidative phosphorylation. *Biochem. J.* **146**, 465–471.

Skou, J. C. (1965). Enzymatic basis for active transport of Na^+ and K^+ across cell membranes. *Physiol. Rev.* **45**, 596–617.

Snow, M. H. L. (1976). Embryo growth during the immediate postimplantation period. In Elliott, K. and O'Connor, M. (Eds.) *Embryogenesis in Mammals*, pp. 53–70. Elsevier, Amsterdam.

Snow, M. H. L. and Tam, P. P. L. (1979). Is compensatory growth a complicating factor in mouse teratology? *Nature (London)* **279**, 555–557.

Snow, M. H. L., Tam, P. P. L. and McLaren, A. (1981). On the control and regulation of size and morphogenesis in mammalian embryos. In Subtelny, S. and Abbott, U.K. (Eds.) *Levels of Genetic Control in Development*. Alan Liss, New York.

Sobell, H. M. (1973). The stereochemistry of actinomycin binding to DNA and its implications in molecular biology. *Prog. Nucleic Acid Res.* **13**, 153–190.

Springgate, C. F., Mildvan, A. S., Abramson, R., Engle, J. L. and Loeb, L. A. (1973). *Escherichia coli* deoxyribonucleic acid polymerase I, a zinc metalloenzyme: nuclear quadrupolar relaxation studies of the role of bound zinc. *J. biol. Chem.* **248**, 5987–5993.

Sun, L. and Singer, B. (1975). The specificity of different classes of ethylating agents toward various sites of HeLa cell DNA *in vivo* and *in vitro*. *Biochemistry* **14**, 1795–1802.

Svingen, B. A. and Aust, S. D. (1980). The mechanism of NADPH-dependent and O_2^- dependent lipid peroxidation. In Bhatnagar, R. S. (Ed.) *Molecular Basis of Environmental Toxicity*, pp. 69–110. Ann Arbor Science Publishers, Inc., Ann Arbor, Michigan.

Takatsuki, A., Arima, A. and Tamura, G. (1971). Tunicamycin, a new antibiotic. *J. Antibiot. (Tokyo)* **24**, 215–233.

Tanimura, T. and Shepard, T. H. (1970). Glucose metabolism by rat embryos *in vitro*. *Proc. Soc. exp. Biol. Med.* **135**, 51–54.

Tarkowski, A. K. (1959). Experimental studies on regulation in the development of isolated blastomeres of mouse eggs. *Acta Theriol.* **3**, 191–267.

Telser, A., Robinson, H. C. and Dorfman, A. (1965). The biosynthesis of chondroitin-sulfate protein complex. *Proc. natn Acad. Sci. U.S.A.* **54**, 912–919.

Tkacz, J. S. and Lampen, J. O. (1975). Tunicamycin inhibition of polyisoprenol N-acetylglucosaminyl pyrophosphate formation of calf liver microsomes. *Biochem. Biophys. Res. Commun.* **65**, 248–257.

Tyson, C. A. and Southard, J. H. (1980). Low-affinity Ca^{2+} transport in heart mitochondria induced by mercurials. In Bhatnagar, R. S. (Ed.) *Molecular Basis of Environmental Toxicity*, pp. 429–447. Ann Arbor Science Publishers, Inc., Ann Arbor, Michigan.

Vacquier, V. D. and Moy, G. S. (1977). Isolation of bindin: the protein responsible for adhesion of sperm to sea urchin eggs. *Proc. natn Acad. Sci. U.S.A.* **74**, 2456–2460.

Vallee, B. L. and Ulmer, D. D. (1972). Biochemical effects of mercury, cadmium and lead. *A. Rev. Biochem.* **41**, 91–128.

Weinmann, R. and Roeder, R. G. (1974). Role of DNA-dependent RNA polymerase III in the transcription of the tRNA and 5S RNA genes. *Proc. natn Acad Sci. U.S.A.* **71**, 1790–1794.

Wilson, J. G. (1977). Current status of teratology. In Wilson, J. G. and Fraser, F. C. (Eds.) *Handbook of Teratology*, Vol. 1, pp. 47–74. Plenum Press, New York.

Wunderlich, V., Schutt, M., Bottger, M. and Graffi, A. (1970). Preferential alkylation of mitochondrial deoxyribonucleic acid by *N*-methyl-*N*-nitrosourea. *Biochem. J.* **118**, 99–109.

Methods for Assessing the Effects of Chemicals on Reproductive Functions
Edited by V. B. Vouk and P. J. Sheehan
© 1983 SCOPE

Epidemiological Approach To Human Reproductive Failure Assessment

DOROTHY WARBURTON, ZENA STEIN and JENNIE KLINE

1 INTRODUCTION

The most direct method of assessing the effects of chemical exposures on human reproduction is to look in human populations for an association between the exposure and the frequency of end-points indicating reproductive failure or dysfunction. That such an epidemiological approach is not simple, quick, inexpensive or without pitfalls is attested to by the widespread attempts to find laboratory methods which can accurately predict human reproductive performance. These laboratory methods have the advantages, not immediately available from an epidemiological approach, of providing clues to the mechanisms involved and demonstrating potential hazards before actual human populations are allowed to be exposed. However, the validity of any laboratory approach must ultimately depend on a proven relationship between the laboratory end-point and human population risks. The uncertainties which arise when this kind of evidence is not available are well illustrated by:

(1) the problem in extrapolating from animal data on teratogenesis to the human situation; and
(2) the difficulties in interpreting the significance of induced somatic chromosomal aberrations in man.

The existence of great interspecific and intraspecific variability in susceptibility to teratogens (Cahen, 1966) makes the prediction of human risks from animal experiments very unreliable, as was well illustrated by thalidomide, which was not teratogenic in rats and mice. While chromosomal damage can clearly be induced both *in vitro* and *in vivo* by chemical exposures in man, the usefulness of such damage as a predictor of reproductive or other problems in the individual or in the population has yet to be established. These problems will not be solved until epidemiological studies confirm an association between the chromosomal effects observed in the laboratory and reproductive outcome.

This paper will attempt to describe the epidemiological approaches currently available for the investigation of human reproductive failure related to chemical

199

exposures. The special problems of experimental design and statistical analysis in this area will be pointed out, and suggestions made as to how improved methods of data recording and gathering could improve such studies in the future. This paper is based largely on methods available in the United States, with the understanding that our country often lags behind in systems of health care and vital statistics which facilitate epidemiological research. We will draw heavily on a document which was prepared for a Conference on the Evaluation of Human Populations Exposed to Potential Mutagenic and Reproductive Hazards, which was held in Washington, DC in January 1981, under the sponsorship of the

Table 1   Reproductive end-points to indicate reproductive dysfunction

Sexual dysfunction: decreased libido; impotence

Sperm abnormalities: decreased number; decreased motility; abnormal morphology

Subfecundity: abnormal gonads, ducts and external genitalia; abnormal pubertal development; infertility of male or female origin; amenorrhoea; anovulatory cycles; delay in conception.

Illness during pregnancy and parturition: toxaemia; haemorrhage

Early fetal loss (to 28 weeks)

Late fetal loss (after 28 weeks) and stillbirth ⎫

Intrapartum death   ⎬ Perinatal death

Death in first week   ⎭

Decreased birth weight

Change in gestational age at delivery: prematurity; postmaturity

Altered sex ratio

Multiple births

Birth defects, major and minor

Chromosome abnormalities in fetal deaths, at amniocentesis, in perinatal deaths, in livebirths

Infant death

Childhood morbidity

Childhood malignancies

Age at menopause

March of Dimes Birth Defects Foundation, the Center for Disease Control, the National Institute for Occupational Safety and Health, the National Institute for Environmental Health Sciences, and the Environmental Protection Agency. The document was prepared by a committee, chaired by Dorothy Warburton and Zena Stein, and consisting of L. Edmonds (CDC); M. Hatch (Columbia); J. Kline (Columbia); L. Holmes (Harvard); P. Shrout (Columbia); M. Weinstock (Columbia); D. Whorton (Berkeley); A. Wyrobek (Livermore).

2 REPRODUCTIVE END-POINTS

Table 1 lists end-points which might be useful for assessing human reproductive failure or dysfunction. Some of these were discussed in detail from the laboratory point of view in other papers at the present meeting. However, the questions of study design and analysis are equally relevant to the evaluation of these traits in a population.

The inter-relationships among these end-points are complex, and largely unexplored in man. In a few circumstances the type of adverse outcome which is most likely can be predicted from what is known about the mode of action of the chemical exposure; in other cases finding a particular reproductive outcome will rule out certain kinds of mechanisms of action, e.g., constitutional chromosome abnormalities cannot be the result of tubal disease. Table 2

Table 2   Relation of reproductive outcomes to environmental insults

Environmental insult	Mechanism of action of toxic substance	Observable outcome
Paternal toxin	Defective spermatogenesis	SP, I, nSA, aSA, BD
	Defective Wolffian duct system	SP, I
	Defective sexual performance	I
Maternal toxin (preconception)	Defective oogenesis	I, nSA, aSA, BD
	Defective Mullerian duct system	I, nSA, P
	Defective hormonal regulation	I, nSA, P
Maternal toxin (postconception)	Defective gestation–nutrition, hormones, placental function	I, nSA, SGA
	Defective parturition	P, PM
Mutagen (maternal or paternal exposure)	Defective gametes	SP, I, nSA, aSA, BD
Teratogen	Defective fetal anatomical development	I, nSA, BD
Fetal toxin	Defective fetal development	SGA, SD
Carcinogen	Transplacental carcinogenesis	CA

*I, infertility; nSA, karyotypically normal spontaneous abortion; aSA, aneuploid spontaneous abortion; P, prematurity; BD, birth defects (malformations); CA, cancer; SD, slow development; SGA, low birth weight for gestational age; PM, postmaturity; SP, abnormal semen.

attempts to relate the observable reproductive outcome to the mechanisms by which a chemical exposure might act. Many exposures might be expected to have multiple effects, e.g. infertility, fetal loss, birth defects, and decreased birth weight may all result from an agent which is toxic to embryos, but for which there is a difference in susceptibility of the mother and fetus, and in the timing of the exposures. Similarly an agent leading to meiotic abnormalities will result not only in offspring born at term with chromosome abnormalities, but also in infertility and fetal loss, depending upon the stage at which the chromosomal imbalance was lethal.

3 GENERAL PRINCIPLES OF EPIDEMIOLOGICAL INVESTIGATIONS

3.1 Definitions of Levels of Investigation

One may envision an epidemiological investigation of reproductive failure as arising from two kinds of situations, which we call a 'cluster' and an 'exposure'. A 'cluster' arises when a population appears to experience a rise in the frequency of some adverse reproductive outcome. Health authorities may be alerted by the community itself (e.g., a labour union), by alert physicians in the area, or by a monitoring system if such is in place. Examples would be the increase in phocomelia observed in Europe during the 1960s (Taussig, 1962), and the increase in spontaneous abortion reported in Oregon populations exposed to 2, 4, 5-T (USEPA, 1979). Here the supposed outcome is known; the task is to establish whether there are real grounds for considering that an increase has occurred, and if so, to attempt to find the exposure which might be involved.

An 'exposure' arises when a population is known or suspected to be exposed to a potentially hazardous agent. Examples would be the Seveso incident in Italy, and the Three Mile Island nuclear accident in the US. In this case the exposure is known, but the range of reproductive end-points which might be affected is not known.

In practice, the distinction between a cluster and an exposure may not always be possible, since the population experiencing a cluster may have already attributed this to a particular exposure. The response to such a situation may include several stages involving varying amounts of time, money and community involvement, which can be classified as follows. In level I studies the investigator looks only at readily accessible sources of data, there is little community contact, and the investigation can be carried out quickly. In level II studies full scale epidemiological investigations (case-control or cohort) are put in place, involving individual contact with the population, and the gathering of new data on exposures and outcomes. This may involve acquiring laboratory or interview data, or undertaking more extensive record searching than in level I. In level III studies longer term follow-up studies are undertaken of a population at risk, requiring the greatest investment of time and money.

3.2 Statistical Considerations

3.2.1 *The Concept of Statistical Power*

A consideration of statistical power is crucial to any investigation of the hazardous effects of chemical exposures. Power is a measure of the ability of a study to detect an effect, and is defined as $(1 - \beta)$ where β is the probability of falsely accepting the null hypothesis. Power depends upon the sample size, the size of the effect which is present, and the level of significance which is chosen, i.e. the probability of falsely rejecting the null hypothesis (Cohen, 1977). For a given study, then, one can calculate for a chosen value of power the magnitude of the effect which is likely to be detected. The negative results of a study which has demonstrated no statistically significant effect are best expressed in a 'power statement' of the form: 'This study has 95% power to detect a 3.5-fold increase in the rate of congenital anomalies', i.e., only 5% of the time a true effect of the given size would be missed by chance.

Experimentalists are more accustomed to thinking of minimizing their chances of falsely *rejecting* the null hypothesis, and may be rigorous in requiring a significance level of 0.01 before considering the experiment to have disproved the null hypothesis. However, when the investigation attempts to establish whether there is a harmful effect of an environmental hazard on human reproduction, it may be more important to minimize the chances of missing a significant effect. An exposed population may not be content to remain in an area where an investigation showed no significant effect, if there is still a one in five chance that a three-fold increase in reproductive problems has occurred. In the following sections, methods of experimental design and analysis will be considered largely from the stand point of maximizing the power of the investigation.

3.2.2 *Sample Size*

Increasing the sample size is the simplest way to increase the power of an investigation. However, studies of environmental exposures are often limited in this respect by the small size of the exposed population. This is particularly true when considering reproductive effects, which will affect only a part of the group at any one time. For example, although there may be 1000 exposed workers at a chemical plant, only 100 pregnancies may occur during the relevant period of study. The power of the study can be somewhat increased by increasing the control group. The effective size of a comparison with unequal groups is equal to the harmonic mean of the two groups, i.e., $n = 2n_1 n_2/(n_1 + n_2)$. Increases beyond three-fold in the size of the control population compared to the exposed population are not worth the additional effort.

3.2.3 *Selecting the End-point*

The higher the frequency of an outcome in the unexposed population, the greater will be the power of the study when sample size is constant. It will take a very much larger sample to detect a doubling of a rare event than a frequent event. Table 3 illustrates this, giving the sample size necessary to detect an effect of a particular size for various reproductive end-points.

It will therefore be an advantage for the investigator to choose those reproductive end-points which are not only biologically relevant to the exposure but are most common. The observed frequency of a particular outcome can be maximized also by increasing the intensity of case-finding, or by restricting the investigation to a sample where a particular outcome is more frequent. Thus, chromosomal abnormalities are 100 times as common in spontaneous abortions as in live births, so that a possible increase in rates of non-disjunction might be studied in aborted fetuses rather than in live births.

3.2.4 *Significance Level*

Significance levels of 0.05 or 0.01 are commonly used in experimental situations. Since we will only reject the hypothesis of no association if the frequency of adverse reproductive outcomes is greater in an exposed than in an unexposed

Table 3   Relationship of power to end-point frequency

Endpoints	Frequency per 100	Unit	Sample size of two equal comparison groups	Increase in frequency detectable with 95% confidence
Major congenital			50	7.7-fold
malformations		Live births	100	5.3-fold
	3		250	3.3-fold
Stillbirths		Full term births	300	3.2-fold
Birth weight			50	4.6-fold
≤ 2500 grams	7	Live births	100	3.4-fold
			250	2.3-fold
			300	2.3-fold
Spontaneous			50	3.0-fold
abortion,		Pregnancies	100	2.4-fold
	15		250	1.8-fold
Infertility		Couples	300	1.7-fold

$\alpha = 0.10$, two-tailed.

population, we can validly use a one-tailed test. In some situations one might consider setting the significance level at 0.10, at least as a level to indicate a need for further investigation, since the undesirability of falsely concluding that no effect exists may outweigh the undesirability of falsely concluding than an effect does exist.

Whenever an investigation must explore a large number of possible associations between end-points and exposures, some of the hypotheses tested may show statistically significant results by chance alone. Thus if one tests for an increase in three adverse effects, with a 5% significance level, the chance that one of the three will have a statistically significant increase is greater than 5%. The appropriate adjustment is to use a significance level $= \alpha/k$ where α is the desired level of significance, and k is the number of hypotheses tested (Miller, 1966). The necessity for increasing the significance level in this kind of situation decreases the power of a study. It is always advisable to formulate specific hypotheses concerning the exposure to be examined or the type of reproductive outcome which can be reasonably expected to occur, since for these *a priori* hypotheses the significance level does not have to be adjusted.

3.2.5 *The Magnitude of the Effect*

The actual magnitude of the effect is of course not under the control of the investigator. However, the observed association will be greatest if all sources of variation irrelevant to the association are kept to a minimum. Misclassification of exposure or outcome adds noise to the system and thus decreases the observable association.

Precise data on exposures may be very difficult to ascertain. Real exposures are likely to involve multiple toxic agents such as those found at chemical dump sites, and the exposure may vary in time as well as in amount from individual to individual. Studies may be carried out some time after an actual exposure has occurred, so that current measures of exposure in air or water may be uninformative. Occupational exposures may provide better data, but must be subdivided according to which parent is exposed. Biological effects such as somatic chromosomal damage, increased sister chromatid exchanges, or other observables described at this meeting may provide measures of exposure, but this remains to be documented. A combination of laboratory measures of exposure and an epidemiological investigation of reproductive outcomes might provide the strongest approach to the problem of assessing reproductive hazards in human populations.

Misclassification of a reproductive outcome can be avoided by making the investigated outcome as specific as is possible from knowledge of the type and timing of the exposure. Thus if the frequency of conditions due to new gene mutations is to be investigated, one should exclude cases of single gene disorders born to known carrier parents, and cases of malformations largely believed to be the result of *in utero* positioning. Similarly, a paternal exposure is unlikely to act during gestation itself, although one can postulate mechanisms for such an effect, e.g. substances carried in the semen at intercourse, or on work clothing.

The observed effect size can be altered by confounding variables, i.e. variables which relate both to the reproductive outcome and the chance of exposure. The bias introduced in this way may lead to faulty conclusions, either positive or negative, about the existence of an association. As an example consider febrile illness during pregnancy, which might be associated both with an increased rate of fetal loss and the ingestion of particular drugs. A false association between the drugs and the fetal loss might then be inferred.

Statistical methods such as 'log-linear' regression for discrete data and multiple linear regression for continuous data will control for confounding variables and permit an estimation of interactions. One may also simply stratify the data for analysis according to relevant variables (e.g. smoking women *vs* non-smoking women) and use statistical techniques such as the Mantel–Haenszel procedure or Fisher's method to combine the evidence from several strata and test the consistency of an effect across strata.

3.2.6 *Use of Conceptions Rather than Parents as Unit of Study*

One way to increase the size of the sample is to consider individual conceptions as the unit of study rather than men or women, since each individual may have several conceptions in the time under study. The danger in this approach is that conceptions of the same individual are more similar than conceptions of different individuals, and this may result in undue weight being given to the characteristics of the individuals with the most conceptions, who may not be representative of the population. One must first estimate the degree of correlation among pregnancies of the same parent, and compare this with the correlation among pregnancies of different parents in the exposed and unexposed groups. If the differences are slight, than a considerable gain in power may be possible by using each conception as a different observation.

3.3 Level I Investigation: Use of Readily Accessible Data

A level I analysis will consist of a comparison of the observed frequencies of reproductive events with available baseline data, in order to decide whether a significant increase in an adverse outcome has occurred.

Only certain reproductive end-points routinely included in vital records or screening programmes will be available for this type of study. In most parts of the world these will consist of late fetal loss, birthrate, incidence of low birth weight and some congenital malformations. Newborn or prenatal screening programmes may also be used when available, the latter being especially valuable in providing an early warning of increases in some kinds of reproductive problems such as neural tube defects. In a 'cluster' situation level I studies can only be used if the end-point under suspicion is available in vital records. In 'exposure' situations a range of possible outcomes must be tested, and these might begin with those available for level I analysis.

In order to calculate the expected frequencies of the outcomes under study, one must define the population at risk, and then determine the baseline frequencies. For an exposure situation, the population may be defined by choosing a given geographical distance from the exposure source, or a given time period of exposure. For a cluster situation the problem is more difficult, and a political subdivision such as a city or county, with common vital statistics records, may be the most convenient way to define the population at risk.

Baseline frequencies may be established using data collected from the same population before the suspected exposure or cluster, if they are available. In their absence, state or national statistics may have to be used. Birth rates, infant mortality and low birth weight are all accurately recorded in the United States by the National Center for Health Statistics, and available for states and metropolitan areas in some years. Malformations are much less reliably recorded on birth and death certificates, but good baseline data on malformations may sometimes be available from special registries such as those kept in the United States by the Center for Disease Control malformation surveillance programmes (DHEW, 1979). It is important to compare malformation data only with data collected from a similar source because of the serious under-reporting of malformations in most record systems.

A level I investigation of a cluster of a particular outcome will also require an attempt to verify the reported cases through medical records, and a search for artefactual causes of an increase, such as changes in referral patterns, the introduction of a new diagnostic technique, or a change in definition of a variable. For example, the increase in congenital hypothyroidism originally reported at the site of the Three Mile Island nuclear accident was shown to be the result of the recent introduction of a newborn screening programme for this disease.

3.4 Level II Investigation: Epidemiological Field Studies

If a level I investigation leads to a clear-cut negative result, proceeding with further investigation may be unwarranted. However, such an investigation often lacks power to detect changes which might still be considered significant by the community, and it might then be considered wise to proceed with more extensive studies which would have greater power to detect an effect. Even if level I studies provided evidence for a positive effect, fuller investigations may be advisable to search for other end-points which might be affected. The decision as to when to proceed will be made only partly on scientific grounds; the degree of community concern and political considerations also play a large role.

The two basic experimental designs which can be used in an epidemiological investigation of an association between a hazardous exposure and reproductive failure are the *case-control* study and the *cohort* study. In a case-control study the frequency of an exposure is compared among those who experience the outcome in question (cases), and those who do not (controls). In a cohort study the frequency of a reproductive outcome is compared among those who are exposed to the potential hazard and those who are not exposed. A cohort study may be retrospective, i.e. consider those outcomes which have already taken place, or prospective, i.e. study future outcomes in an identified exposed and unexposed group. The advantages and disadvantages of case-control and cohort studies are discussed below with particular reference to studies of reproductive failure.

3.4.1 *Sample Size*

When the end-point to be studied is rare and the exposure relatively common, case-control studies will require a smaller sample size for the same power to detect a given effort than will cohort studies. The opposite is true when the exposure is rare and the end-point is relatively common. In general, cluster situations lend themselves to case-control studies, and exposure situations to cohort studies, but this is not necessarily true.

3.4.2 *Definition of Exposure*

In a case-control study the presence of the exposure may be determined by interview data, by place of work or residence, or by objective measures of exposure such as chemical analysis of body tissues or bioassays such as the incidence of chromosome or sperm abnormalities. The major disadvantage of case-control studies is that recall bias must be suspected whenever the major source of information on exposures comes from interview data. Recall bias refers to the fact that the case responses may be influenced by knowledge of the presence of an adverse reproductive outcome. Cases may over-report exposures, especially if publicity about the suspected exposure has already occurred, or cases may simply remember exposures more accurately than controls. Cases may also under-report exposures if these are associated with feelings of guilt (e.g. alcohol consumption). Validation of exposures by other methods (medical records or biochemical tests) for at least a part of the sample may indicate the extent of the problem. Another approach is to use several control groups, including one which has experienced another adverse outcome not likely to be the result of the same exposure as the one under investigation (e.g. Down's syndrome as a control for neural tube defects). The problem of recall bias will not be present in prospective cohort studies, since the outcome is not known when exposure status is determined. However, prospective studies have the disadvantage of being the most expensive and time consuming to carry out. Also bias may be introduced by the inevitable loss of patients to follow-up.

In a cohort study the presence of the exposure is used to define the comparison groups. This may be done by using groups with varying degrees of exposure, or by using only an unexposed comparison group. The relationship between exposures and reproduction is complex. To be effective an exposure may have to occur before fertilization (perhaps many years) or it may have to occur during gestation; it may act through the male parent or through the female parent, or both. Cohort studies have the disadvantage of requiring decisions about what range of exposure to include in the study before it begins: a case-control study can investigate a wider range of exposure situations.

3.4.3 *Definition of Reproductive Outcomes*

A cohort study will permit an investigation of a wider range of outcomes than a case-control study. Data on outcome may be obtained in a cohort study from interviews, from vital statistics or from hospital and physicians' records. Some data, such as that on infertility and early spontaneous abortions, will often not be available from any source except interviews. When medical records are used as sources of data on outcome, one must be careful to exclude biases caused by different patterns of hospital or physician use among the exposed and unexposed group.

In a retrospective cohort study, recall bias may lead to an overestimate of the effect of exposure, since the presence of the exposure may influence recall of adverse outcomes.

3.4.4 *Selection of Comparison Groups*

In a case-control study the case group and the control group must be chosen to have the same *a priori* probability of exposure. In a cohort study, the exposed and unexposed group must be chosen to have the same *a priori* probability of an adverse outcome. Thus the methods used to determine exposure status and reproductive outcome must be the same for the comparison groups. Also, variables known to be associated with both outcome and exposure must either be matched in the comparison groups or controlled in the analysis by stratification of the sample. Good data are often available concerning the important risk factors for the adverse reproductive outcomes under study, but the data are usually not so good concerning the association of these factors with particular exposures. These associations can be sought in the data, and then controlled in analysis. However, it may be advisable to match comparison groups for known risk factors for a particular outcome even if an association with exposure status is not known. For example, race, maternal age and social class are important risk factors for many reproductive outcomes which might best be controlled in the experimental design.

3.4.5 *Measures of Association*

In case-control studies the measurement of risk is the 'odds-ratio', i.e. the odds that an individual in the case group has been exposed, compared to a control. Thus an odds ratio of 2.1 for heavy drinking with spontaneous abortion means that in the population studied a woman experiencing a spontaneous abortion is 2.1 times more likely to drink heavily than is a woman experiencing a term delivery.

In a cohort study, the measurement of risk is the 'relative risk', i.e. the odds that an individual in the exposed group will experience a particular outcome, compared to an unexposed individual. Thus a relative risk of 2.1 for heavy drinking with spontaneous abortion means that in the population studied a woman who is a heavy drinker is 2.1 times more likely to experience a spontaneous abortion than is a woman who does not drink.

3.5 Level III: Long-Term Follow-Up Investigations

The reproductive effects of chemical hazards and the predictive value of laboratory and clinical observations could best be assessed by following up groups of individuals over their reproductive period. If carried out through continued personal contact with the subjects, such studies involve great amounts of time and effort from the investigators. The best example of such a study in the field of reproduction is the follow-up of the atomic bomb survivors and their offspring in Japan.

Any follow-up study is bound to include a considerable group of patients who are lost to follow-up, and it is important to consider biases which may be introduced if such a loss is not independent of outcome. For example, in a study of women ascertained in early pregnancy, those who have an early spontaneous abortion may not seek medical care of the abortion, and may not return to the prenatal clinic.

Long-term follow-up studies are greatly facilitated if record linking systems exist so that birth and death certificates, disease registries, etc. can be searched for a particular subject. Such facilities are rather poorly developed in the United States, but are much further advanced in Canada and in many European countries (Beebe, 1980). It is important that the essential information for record linking be recorded for subjects who have extensive laboratory studies of exposure, somatic damage or reproductive effects, so that the value of these tests in assessing long-term effects on reproduction can be evaluated in the future.

4 STUDIES OF PARTICULAR REPRODUCTIVE END-POINTS

4.1 Infertility

Infertility is a relatively difficult outcome to investigate epidemiologically. Nevertheless, this has been a reported outcome of 1, 2-dibromo-3-chloropropane (DBCP) exposures in men (Whorton *et al.*, 1977) and anaesthetic gases in women (Knill-Jones *et al.*, 1972). In come cases such as the exposure to DBCP the outcome was sufficiently dramatic to be recognized by the population itself.

Fertility may be measured very crudely by the number of births which occur to a given population over a particular period of time. If interview data are available in a level II study, one can use time taken to conceive during a period of unprotected intercourse as a measure of fertility. The first measure does not distinguish between actual failure of conception and loss of conceptions as spontaneous abortions. The second measure avoids this problem, except for those pregnancies which terminate so early as to be unrecognized.

Parental age, race, social class, religion and previous reproductive history are all important determinants of fertility which have to be taken into account in designing or analysing a study using this end-point. A case-control study using infertility as the adverse reproductive outcome might collect cases in an infertility clinic, and compare exposure rates with a control group.

While there are strong reasons for assuming that abnormalities of sperm count, morphology and motility may correlate with male infertility, only azoospermia or oligospermia can at the moment be considered equivalent to infertility in men.

4.2 Spontaneous Abortion

Spontaneous abortion is the most common event signifying reproductive dysfunction. About 15% of recognized pregnancies end in spontaneous abortion, defined here as termination of pregnancy at less than 28 weeks gestation. The incidence of early loss (before pregnancy is recognized by the first missed menses) is only beginning to be explored using the human chorionic gonadotropin (hCG) assays which can diagnose very early pregnancy. A recent study estimated the rate of such early loss to be about the same as that of recognized abortion (Miller *et al.*, 1980).

Data on spontaneous abortions can be obtained from several sources: vital certificate data, hospital records, physicians' records and interview data from the woman or her mate. Vital certificate data are likely to be very poor for pregnancies terminating under 20 weeks, which is the time when reporting of fetal deaths is usually mandated. Hospital and physician records will not contain information on those spontaneous abortions for which medical attention was not sought, which will tend to be those earliest in gestation. The pattern of use of medical services is likely to vary greatly between communities (e.g. rural *vs* urban) and between socioeconomic groups. In 40% of first trimester spontaneous abortions reported in interviews in a New York City study, no medical care was sought (J. Kline, personal communication). The most complete information on spontaneous abortions is likely to come from interviews with the women involved, although this kind of information is of course subject to recall bias, and errors in self-diagnosis. There is some evidence to suggest that maternal reports are reliable, in that they are generally compatible with data available on the obstetrical record (Kline *et al.*, 1978).

Known risk factors which should be considered in the analysis of spontaneous abortions are maternal age, previous spontaneous abortions, multiple previous induced abortions, social class, maternal smoking and maternal alcohol consumption.

An increase in the rate of spontaneous abortion has been suggested to occur after exposure to anaesthetic gases (Pharaoh *et al.*, 1977), after exposure to lead smelters (Nordström *et al.*, 1979a) and after paternal exposure to vinyl chloride (Infante *et al.*, 1976). None of these studies was rigorously controlled.

Spontaneous abortion will be most informative as an end-point for studies of environmental hazards when it is further classified according to gestation, pathological description and chromosomal status. Data on the latter two features will require special procedures for collection and examination of specimens, and for culturing fetal tissue for chromosomal analysis. About half of all first trimester abortions and about one-third of all spontaneous abortions up to 28 weeks are chromosomally abnormal (Warburton *et al.*, 1980). More than 90% of all chromosomally abnormal conceptions end in spontaneous abortion, so that if one is interested in identifying factors which increase the rate of chromosomal anomalies such as Down's syndrome at term, far fewer pregnancies need to be examined if spontaneous abortions rather than term births are used. In most exposed populations of moderate size there will be no chance of observing a significant increase in chromosomal anomalies at term, since it would require about 23,000 pregnancies to detect a doubling with 80% power. To detect the rise in the incidence of spontaneous abortion which would accompany a doubling in the frequency of chromosome anomalies, only about 900 pregnancies would have to be examined, and only about 200 abortuses karyo typed.

Of the chromosomally normal spontaneous abortions, about half are morphologically abnormal, either grossly so, suggesting a failure in very early development, or with focal abnormalities of the kind seen at term. Classification of specimens may thus provide information about the mechanisms involved in a rise in spontaneous abortion of chromosomally normal fetuses.

4.3 Congenital Malformations

Congenital malformations are much less common than low birth weight, infertility or spontaneous abortion. The usual estimates of the frequency of major malformations in term births is 2–3%. However, this is a reproductive outcome which is perceived by the families involved as very distressing, and it is the most costly in terms of health resources required to care for the children. It is also more easily visible to the population at large than the other end-points, and thus the one most likely to be reported as a cluster.

Since fetal malformations are about five times as common in spontaneous abortions as in live births, they are apparently selected against during gestation. Greater power to detect an increase in malformations would occur if aborted fetuses rather than live births were studied; however, the increased difficulties of ascertainment of material, and the lack of individuals trained in the examination of fetuses may outweigh this advantage.

The rarity of individual malformations usually makes it necessary to classify them in some way into meaningful groups. Classifying by the organ system involved is convenient, but does not generally achieve any aetiological separation. Classification into malformations due to chromosomal imbalance, malformations due to single mutant genes, malformations due to known environmental factors and those of mixed or unknown origin may be the most helpful. This will generally require more detailed information than is available in a level I analysis. Other useful methods of classification might involve grouping the malformations by the developmental stage when the anomaly originates, or by the embryological pathway which is disturbed. Information about the pathogenesis of most human malformation is too limited as yet to make this possible in most cases.

Increased rates of specific malformations have been definitively shown to result from maternal drug ingestions during pregnancy (e.g. thalidomide, anticonvulsants, warfarin), and some studies have suggested increases due to an environmental exposure such as anaesthetic gases or lead (Pharaoh *et al.*, 1977; Nordström *et al.*, 1979a, b). In general one might expect specific patterns of malformations, forming a syndrome, to occur as a result of *maternal exposure during gestation*, while rather diverse effects should occur from *genetic changes* induced by exposure of either parent before conception.

Malformations are generally recorded on birth certificates, in hospital records and, in some areas, in registries. However, there is usually a serious underreporting, at least in the United States. It is therefore important that the comparison groups in an epidemiological study of malformations derive their information by the same method of ascertainment. In a level II study examination of offspring by a trained dysmorphologist, preferably blind to exposure status of the patient, will provide the greatest ability to classify these by aetiology. Diagnostic laboratory studies such as chromosome studies may also be built into such a study. Registries of chromosomal abnormalities, at amniocentesis and in live birth, may provide good information on this class of birth defects in some areas (Hook, 1978; Prescott *et al.*, 1978).

The frequency and type of malformations are related to parental race, age and social class, as well as the sex and age of the offspring at examination. The frequency of detection of some anomalies will increase with the age of the subject (e.g. congenital heart disease) but the frequency of other anomalies which are lethal early in life (e.g. neural tube defects) will decrease. All these factors must be considered in the analysis as possibly confounding variables.

4.4 Birth Weight

Birth weight has many advantages for use as a measure of reproductive outcome. It is routinely recorded on birth certificates and hospital records in most parts of the world, and is thus amenable to level I analysis. When combined with an estimate of gestation, one can distinguish the babies small only because of prematurity from those small for gestational age. About 7% of American infants are less than 2500 grams at birth, and low birth weight is strongly associated with neonatal death rates, congenital malformations, developmental delay and chromosomal anomalies. It is also known to be a sensitive indicator of maternal exposures such as cigarette smoking. An increase in low birth weight infants is the best documented effect found at the Love Canal dump site (Vianna, 1980), and in areas close to lead smelters in Sweden (Nordström *et al.*, 1979a).

Maternal age, parity, and race are other known risk factors, which must be considered as possible confounding variables. Although birth weight may be classified into weight categories, or simply as low, normal and high for gestational age, the analysis will have more power if it is used as a continuous variable.

4.5 Childhood Cancer

Transplacental carcinogenesis, i.e. cancer caused by an environmental agent which crosses the placenta during pregnancy, may be considered an end-point indicating reproductive dysfunction. Childhood cancers are rare, but such effects may not be limited to cancer occurring in childhood. Theoretically any agent that can cause cancer in adults and is known to cross the placenta may cause cancer in the offspring. Since the latent period for carcinogenesis is often long, this may be a very difficult effect to detect, especially if the cancers which are induced are among the most common varieties. To date there are two known transplacental carcinogens in man, diethylstilboesterol (DES) (associated with vaginal cancer, Herbst *et al.*, 1977) and hydantoin (associated with neuroblastoma, Allen *et al.*, 1980). Both these are uncommon effects of exposure, but the rarity of the cancer in the case of DES, and the association with a syndrome of fetal defects known to be the result of a specific environmental agent in the case of hydantoin, enabled the detection of the effect.

Transplacental carcinogenesis can be investigated by case-control studies when a cluster of rare tumours is observed (as with DES). It could also be investigated prospectively in a cohort study when a substantial proportion of the population is exposed, by using identifying information from the children to match the data in tumour registries, or on death certificates.

5 CONCLUSIONS

The epidemiological approach to the study of environmental hazards is not less sophisticated than the laboratory approach. It requires careful planning, attention to statistical and methodological problems, trained personnel, and a clear understanding of the biology of the situation. Studies of reproductive dysfunction in exposed populations have special problems:

(1) there is a great variety of outcomes which might be affected;
(2) there are three possibly exposed persons in the reproductive unit—mother, father and offspring;
(3) populations involved are likely to be small;
(4) exposure status is difficult to define; and
(5) publicity surrounding the investigation may lead to biased reporting.

In this report we have tried to describe the nature of these problems and indicate ways in which they can be circumvented.

The ideal study would include laboratory methods for refining the information on outcome (e.g. sperm analysis, chromosomal analysis of aborted fetuses) and on exposures (e.g. biochemical tests, bioassays in man or other organisms). However, there is no substitute for the epidemiological approach to validate the predictive value of laboratory tests or results in experimental animals for human reproductive performance.

6 REFERENCES

Allen, R. W., Jr, Ogdon, B., Bentley, F. L. and Jung, A. L. (1980). Fetal hydantoin syndrome, neuroblastoma and hemorrhagic disease in a neonate. *J. Am. med. Ass.* **244**, 1464–1465.

Beebe, G. W. (1980). Record linkage systems—Canada vs. the United States. *Am. J. Publ. Health* **70**, 1246–1248.

Cahen, R. L. (1966). Experimental and clinical chemoteratogenesis. *Adv. Pharmacol.* **4**, 263–349.

Cohen, J. (1977). *Statistical Power Analysis for Behavioural Sciences.* Revised Edition, p. 188. Academic Press, New York, San Francisco, London.

DHEW (1979). *Congenital Malformations Surveillance Annual Summary 1978.* Center for Disease Control, Bureau of Epidemiology. U. S. Department of Health, Education and Welfare, Public Health Service, Atlanta.

Herbst, A. L., Cole, P., Colton, T., Robboy, S. J. and Scully, R. E. (1977). Age-incidence and risk of diethylstilbesterol-related clear cell adenocarcinoma of the vagina and cervix. *Am. J. Obstet. Gynec.* **128**, 43–50.

Hook, E. B. (1978). Monitoring human mutations and consideration of a dilemma posed by an apparent increase in one type of mutation rate. In Chung, C. (Ed.). *Genetic Epidemiology*, pp. 483–528. Academic Press, New York, San Francisco, London.

Infante, P. E., Wagoner, J. K., McMichael, A. J., Wexweiler, R. J. and Falk, H. (1976). Genetic risks of vinyl chloride. *Lancet* **i**, 734–735.

Kline, J., Shrout, P. E., Susser, M., Stein, Z. and Weiss, M. (1978). II. An epidemiological study of the role of gravidity in spontaneous abortion. *Early hum. Dev.* **1**, 345–356.

Knill-Jones, R. R., Newman, B. J. and Spence, A. A. (1972). Anaesthetic practice and pregnancy: controlled survey of women anesthetists in the United Kingdom. *Lancet* **i**, 1326–1328.

Miller, J. I., Williamson, E., Glue, J., Gordon, Y. B., Grudzinskes, J. B., and Sykes, A. (1980). Fetal loss after implantation. A prospective study. *Lancet* **2**, No. 8194, 554–556.

Miller, R. G. (1966). *Simultaneous Statistical Inference.* McGraw-Hill, New York.

Nordström, S., Beckman, L. and Nordenson, I. (1979a). Occupational and environmental risks in and around a smelter in northern Sweden. V. Spontaneous abortion among female employees and decreased birthweight in their offspring. *Hereditas* **90**, 291–296.

Nordström, S., Beckman, L., and Nordenson, I. (1979b) Occupational and environmental risks in and around a smelter in northern Sweden. VI. Congenital malformations. *Hereditas* **90**, 297–302.

Pharaoh, P. D., Alberman, E. and Doyle, P. (1977). Outcome of pregnancy among women working in anaesthetic practice. *Lancet* **i**, 34–36.

Prescott, G., Rivas, M., Shanbeck, L., Macfarlane, D., Wuandt, H., Breg, W., Lubs, H., Magenis, E., Summitt, R., Palmer, C., Hecht, F., Kimberling, W. and Clow, D. (1978). The interregional cytogenetic register system. *Birth Defects Original Article Series* **14(6C)**, 269–279.

Taussig, H. B. (1962). A study of the German outbreak of phocomelia. The thalidomide syndrome. *J. Am. med. Ass.* **180**, 1106–1114.

USEPA (1979). *Report of Assessment of a Field Investigation of Six-Year Spontaneous Abortion Rates in Three Oregon Areas in Relation to Forest 2, 4, 5-T Practices.* Environmental Protection Agency, Environmental Studies Program, Washington, DC.

Vianna, N. (1980). Adverse pregnancy outcomes—potential endpoints of human toxicity in the Love Canal. Preliminary results. In Porter, I. H. and Hook, E. B. (Eds.). *Human Embryonic and Fetal Death*, pp. 165–168. Academic Press, New York, San Francisco, London.

Warburton, D., Stein, Z., Kline, J. and Susser, M. (1980). Chromosome abnormalities in spontaneous abortion: data from the New York City study. In Porter, I. H. and Hook, E. B. (Eds.). *Human Embryonic and Fetal Death*, pp. 261–287. Academic Press, New York, San Francisco, London.

Whorton, D., Krauss, R. M., Marshall, S. and Milby, T. (1977). Infertility in male pesticide workers. *Lancet* **ii**, 1259–1261.

Methods for Assessing the Effects of Chemicals on Reproductive Functions
Edited by V. B. Vouk and P. J. Sheehan
© 1983 SCOPE

Laboratory Methods for Evaluating and Predicting Specific Reproductive Dysfunctions: Oogenesis and Ovulation

Donald R. Mattison and Griff T. Ross

1 INTRODUCTION

Normal female reproductive functioning requires the successful completion of an integrated series of events beginning with oogenesis, continuing through ovulation and corpus luteum function, gamete transport, endometrial development, implantation, embryonic development, parturition, and is completed with the sexual maturation of the newly formed individual (Figure 1). As most of these biological processes are complex, involving multiple levels of both local and systemic control, it would indeed be surprising to find them resistant to adverse xenobiotic effects. We now know that there are xenobiotic exposures (occupational, drug, or environmental) which can adversely alter many of the biological processes involved in both male and female reproduction (Newburgh, 1975; American College of Obstetricians and Gynecologists, 1976; Schardein, 1976; Lucier et al., 1977; Symposium on Target Organ Toxicity, 1978; Hunt, 1979; Heinrichs and Juchau, 1980; Shepard, 1980; Mattison, 1981a, b).

Prospective experimental demonstration that some xenobiotic agents adversely affect fertility in humans is neither ethically nor logistically practical. However, the occurrence of reproductive dysfunction as a side effect of certain drug therapies for affective disorders, seizure disorders, some infectious diseases, hypertension, neoplasms, and radiation therapy have provided indirect evidence that xenobiotics can temporarily or permanently adversely affect oocyte or follicle number, follicular growth or ovulation in women. Moreover, in many instances, effects on human reproduction might have been anticipated on the basis of responses to these agents in animal model systems where prospective scientifically valid experiments are feasible.

As in toxicology, in reproductive biology the physiological mechanisms involved are complex and species dependent. To assist the interaction between toxicologists and reproductive biologists we have provided several general

217

REPRODUCTIVE CYCLE

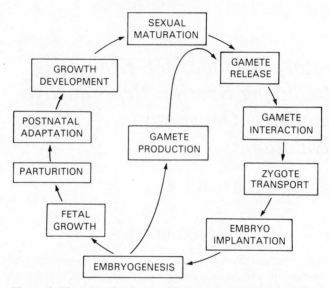

Figure 1 The reproductive cycle represents a general outline of the physiological processes necessary in most mammalian species for successful propagation. (From Mattison, 1981a with permission)

references dealing with reproductive biology (Van Tienhoven, 1968; Green, 1975; Zuckerman and Weir, 1977; Jones, 1978; Yen and Jaffe, 1978; Ross and Vande Wiele, 1981; Whittingham and Wood, 1981) and toxicology (Casarett and Doull, 1975). For similar reasons, several pertinent references on mutagenesis and carcinogenesis are also included (Goldstein *et al.*, 1974; Searle, 1976; Brooks, 1980; Gelboin, 1980), since agents affecting gametogenesis, or the gamete, are also potential mutagens and carcinogens. In most cases we will refer to recent books or reviews rather than the original articles. This provides economy in space and information retrieval, as well as a broader perspective for interested readers.

1.1 Physiological Considerations

Follicle complexes are the basic structural and functional components of mammalian ovaries, including human ovaries which will be described here. The cellular components of these structures consist of an oocyte and granulosa cells enclosed by a basal lamina which separates these cells from adjacent interstitial (thecal) cells, blood, and lymphatic vessels, and supportive stromal cells (Ross and Schreiber, 1978). The oocyte is the essential component of this complex, since follicles either fail to form until oocytes appear during fetal life or degenerate when oocytes are destroyed postnatally.

From the time that follicle complexes appear during fetal life until they disappear after the menopause, small aliquots of the extant population begin to grow. Some cells undergo hypertrophy (oocytes and thecal cells) while others undergo hyperplasia, hypertrophy, and functional differentiation. Prior to puberty, this growth terminates in follicular degeneration, called atresia and characterized by death and degeneration of oocytes and granulosa cells which are replaced by fibrous tissue, and by dedifferentiation of thecal cells (Peters *et al.*, 1976). After puberty, atresia persists but in addition, one follicle ovulates with extrusion of an oocyte followed by transformation of residual granulosa and interstitial cells into a corpus luteum during each menstrual cycle.

This sequence of events leading to ovulation depends upon pituitary secretion of adequate quantities of the gonadotropins: follicle-stimulating hormone (FSH) and luteinizing hormone (LH) (Figure 2). These hormones are secreted in pulses which reflect pulsatile secretion of at least one hypophysiotropic hormone, gonadotropin-releasing hormone (GnRH), by neuronal cells in the hypothalamus (Yen, 1978). The frequency and amplitude of these pulses are modulated by sex steroid hormones, oestrogens, androgens, and progesterones which act on pituitary cells to modulate responses to GnRH, and possibly on hypothalamic cells as well (Knobil, 1980). Within a cycle, changes in blood levels of these sex steroid hormones reflect the secretory activity of either the follicle destined to ovulate or of the corpus luteum which succeeds it.

Sex steroid hormones produced by follicle cells responding to gonadotropins act locally to mediate the stimulating effects of gonadotropins on follicle growth and atresia, in part by participating in the induction of membrane receptors for gonadotropins. Moreover, the hormonal composition of follicle fluid appears to be a reflection of whether a follicle ovulates or becomes atretic (McKnatty, 1978). Manipulation of the biological actions of both gonadotropins and steroid hormones in follicular fluid has been shown to influence numbers of follicles ovulating in response to endogenous or exogenous gonadotropins in rodents and sheep.

In addition to modulating gonadotropin secretion and mediating gonado-tropin effects on follicle growth, atresia, and ovulation, sex steroid hormones secreted by the dominant follicle or the corpus luteum coordinate the functions of epithelial cells in the gonaducts, uterus, cervix, and vagina to create an environment supporting gamete transport and fertilization, implantation of the zygote, and maintainance of early pregnancy in fertile cycles (Ross and Vande Wiele, 1981). Consequently, infertility may result when the function of any component of the hypothalamic–pituitary–ovary–genital axis is compromised. More dramatically, dysfunction may result in amenorrhoea, either primary or secondary.

The development and use of radioligand binding assays to measure

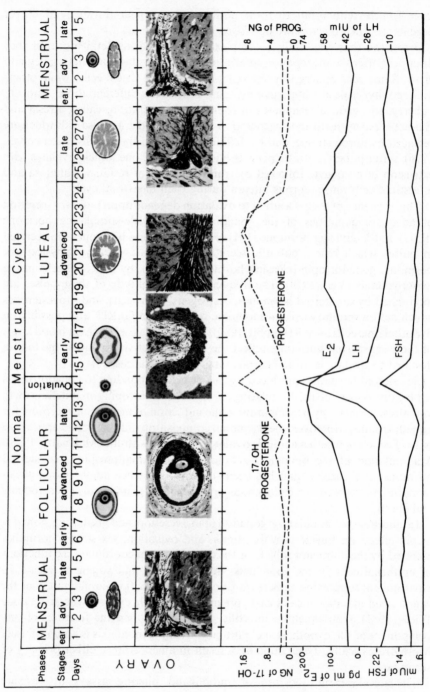

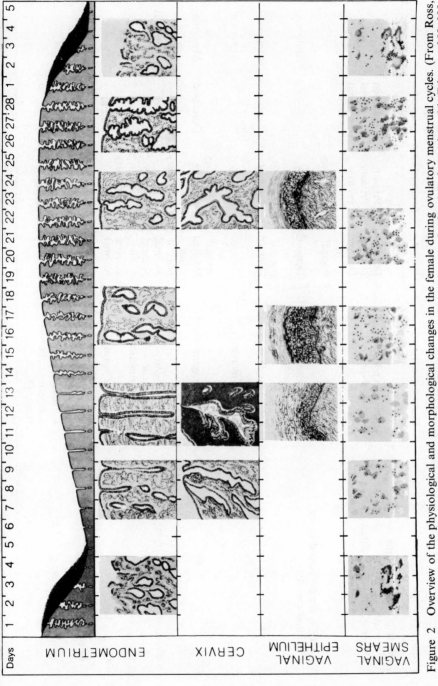

Figure 2 Overview of the physiological and morphological changes in the female during ovulatory menstrual cycles. (From Ross, G. T. and Vande Wiele, R. L. (1981). The ovaries. In Williams, R. H. (Ed.) *Textbook of Endocrinology* 6th Ed., pp. 355–399. Philadelphia, W. B. Saunders.)

Table 1   Clinical correlates of xenobiotic ovarian toxicity

Pathophysiologic basis	Human syndromes	Clinical features			
		Puberty	Amenorrhoea	Oocyte/follicle number	Follicle profile
Toxicity in the developing ovary					
Oogenesis	Turner's syndrome	Delayed	Primary	Decreased	—
Oogenesis or follicle differentiation	Gonadal dysgenesis	Delayed	Primary	Decreased	—
	Premature ovarian failure	Delayed or normal	Primary or secondary	Decreased	—
Toxicity in the developed ovary					
Follicular growth	Hypogonadotropic hypogonadism	Delayed or normal	Primary or secondary	—	Abnormal
	17α-Hydroxylase deficiency	Delayed	Primary	—	Abnormal
	'Resistant' ovaries	Delayed or normal	Primary or secondary	—	Abnormal
	Alkylating agent therapy	Delayed or normal	Primary or secondary	Decreased	Abnormal
Ovulation	Polycystic ovary	Normal	—	—	Abnormal
	Hypothalamic—pituitary dysfunction	Normal or delayed	Primary or secondary	—	—
Corpus luteum	Inadequate luteal phase	Normal	—	—	—
Oocyte or follicle	Premature ovarian failure (ionizing radiation, antitumour chemotherapy)	Normal or delayed	Primary or secondary	Decreased	—

gonadotropins and sex steroid hormones in blood specimens collected in both the basal state and following pharmacological perturbation has made it possible to determine the locus of the functional compromise (Yen and Jaffe, 1978). However, it should be pointed out that functional compromise at a given locus may be the final common pathway for expressing responses to a variety of insults including exposure to xenobiotic agents, such as drugs given as therapy for affective disorders, neoplasms or hypertension. Clues to these relationships have been obtained from drug surveillance studies or from long-term follow-up of patients surviving chemotherapy. Moreover, these dysfunctions may be anticipated when similar disorders are observed during preclinical testing of these agents in animals.

However, data describing frequencies of dysfunction at the various loci in human population are inadequate for monitoring secular trends in incidence. Indeed, such data have rarely been sought in drug surveillance studies. Moreover, most reproductive disorders are not 'reportable' diseases, the incidence of which is monitored by departments of public health. As a result, there are no adequate epidemiological data by which increased incidence of these disorders might be perceived among women inadvertently exposed to unsuspected toxins.

As noted above, the oocyte is essential for the structural and functional integrity of the follicle complex. In turn, functional integrity of the complex is essential for regulating hypothalamic, pituitary, and genital tract functions collectively required for reproduction to proceed normally. Any noxious agent then which injures and destroys oocytes or alternatively acts locally or systemically to interfere with follicle function might be expected to compromise reproduction. The reproductive consequences observed in certain experiments of nature in which follicles fail to form, are depleted prematurely or, though present in normal numbers fail to function normally, validate these predictions. The clinical and laboratory correlates of these aberrations, summarized in Table 1, provide the basis for our discussion of methods for testing for the adverse effects of chemicals on oogenesis and ovulation.

2 THE DEVELOPING OVARY

2.1 Oogenesis and Follicle Differentiation

2.1.1 *Primordial Germ Cells*

Oogenesis begins early in embryonic development with differentiation of the primordial germ cells (Zuckerman and Baker, 1977; Hardesty, 1978). Although this process is not well understood in mammals, extrapolation from submammalian species suggests the informational molecules (germinal determinants) present in the mature oocyte contain the information necessary for primordial germ cell differentiation and segregation from somatic cells.

GAMETE PRODUCTION
GAMETOGENESIS

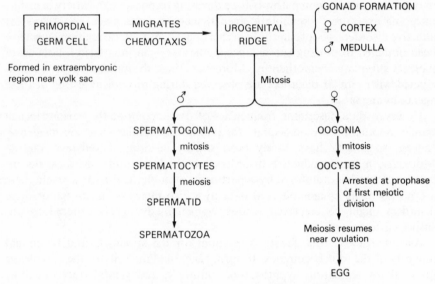

Figure 3   Gametogenesis in the male and female

The primordial germ cells do not form in the region of the presumptive gonad but rather differentiate extraembryonically in the wall of the yolk sac (Figure 3). Three mechanisms are used to bring primordial germ cells into the urogenital ridge:

(1) differential growth of tissue layers in the conceptus places primordial germ cells in the hindgut epithelium;
(2) the primordial germ cells then begin active 'amoeboid' movement toward the urogenital ridge;
(3) chemotactic factors elaborated by the urogenital ridge are responsible for the final step in population of the presumptive gonad.

During passive and active movement of the primordial germ cells into the urogenital ridge, mitoses of these cells occur, increasing their number to approximately 100–1000 in most mammalian species.

Identification of primordial germ cells is facilitated by virtue of their size, being larger than surrounding stromal cells, and distinctive nuclear staining pattern. Additionally, after differentiation, primordial germ cells acquire a marked alkaline phosphatase activity at the plasma membrane, making this a suitable stain for their identification. During passive movement and after taking up residence within the ovary, the primordial germs cells have a rounded or elipsoidal shape. During active movement pseudopodia can be identified. As the mammalian primordial germ cell is strongly dependent on surrounding stroma for metabolic support, frequent associations with stromal cells are seen both outside and inside the presumptive gonad.

Although factors altering mammalian primordial germ cell differentiation have not been shown to produce reproductive failure, destruction of the germinal determinants in submammalian species will produce sterility. Similarly, interruption of chemotactic signals or primordial germ cell access to the urgogenital ridge produces sterility.

The factors controlling primordial germ cell number are not known. Partial destruction of primordial germ cells increases the mitotic rate of the remaining cells, producing partial or complete repopulation of the gonad (Mandl, 1964; Felton *et al.*, 1978). Murine models with defects in primordial germ cell mitosis have also been identified and result in semi- or completely sterile offspring.

2.1.2 *Oogonia*

Oogonial differentiation and ovarian embryology are intimately interrelated (Haffen, 1977; Gondos, 1978; Merchant-Larios, 1978). Shortly after primordial germ cells are first seen in the germinal epithelium of the urogenital ridge, this coelomic epithelial layer begins to proliferate, sending cords of epithelial cells and primordial germ cells into the medullary region of the gonadal anlage (Figure 4). This intimate relationship with epithelial cells, and association with mesenchymal cells in the medulla appear responsible for oogonial differentiation.

The differentiation of oogonia from primordial germ cells is signalled by morphological, histological, and functional changes. Oogonial cells are rounder and appear metabolically less active than primordial germ cells. The oogonial cytoplasm appears less dense than primordial germ cells because of a decrease in organelles. Oogonia also lose the surface membrane alkaline phosphatase activity associated with primordial germ cells.

After oogonia are formed, they begin to proliferate in a manner unique to gonial cells—with multiple intercellular cytoplasmic bridges. Similar intercellular bridging, observed during spermatogonial proliferation, is thought to explain the simultaneous initiation and passage through spermatogenesis of a cohort of sperm cells. By analogy, oogonial bridges are thought to explain the synchronous meiosis and differentiation into oocytes of all oogonial cells in a nest. The cytoplasmic bridges persist until the formation of primordial follicles (folliculogenesis) separates the oocytes within a nest from their sister gametes.

Sex differences in the duration of gonial cell persistence gives rise to sex-related differences in reproductive toxicity. In male mammalian species spermatogonial cells persist throughout life (Figure 3). Adverse xenobiotic exposures which

I
CELL PROLIFERATION IN THE GENITAL RIDGES

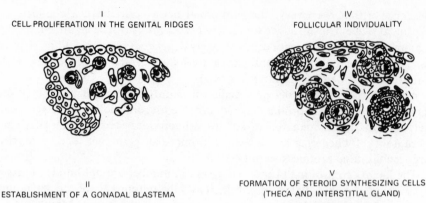

IV
FOLLICULAR INDIVIDUALITY

II
ESTABLISHMENT OF A GONADAL BLASTEMA

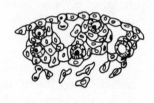

V
FORMATION OF STEROID SYNTHESIZING CELLS
(THECA AND INTERSTITIAL GLAND)

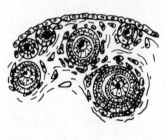

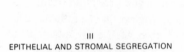

III
EPITHELIAL AND STROMAL SEGREGATION

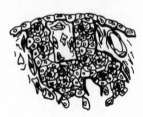

VI
ADULT OVARY
(CORPORA LUTEA, THECA AND INTERSTITIAL GLAND)

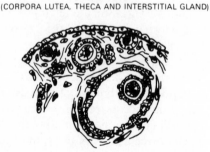

Figure 4   Mammalian ovarian development. The intimate association of germ cells, epithelial and mesenchymal cells is the prelude to oogonial differentiation. Oogonial proliferation proceeds after segregation of the epithelium and stroma. (Modified from Merchant-Larios (1978) with permission of the author)

destroy sperm cells or temporarily decrease spermatogonial cell number, will result in temporary sterility since the testis can be repopulated with sperm as long as functional spermatogonial cells persist. In most mammalian ovaries, however, oogonial cells do not persist beyond birth or the immediate neonatal period. This means that oocyte destruction or irreparable DNA damage (Masui and

Pederson, 1975; Pederson and Mangia, 1978; Generoso *et al.*, 1979) is permanent and may have important implications for germ cell mutagenesis and subsequent teratogenesis.

2.1.3 *Oocytes and Folliculogenesis*

During oogonial proliferation, nests of oogonia will stop dividing, replicate their DNA and enter meiosis (Block, 1952; Baker, 1975; Weir and Rowlands, 1977; Gondos, 1978; Peters, 1978; Tsafriri, 1978). This step differentiates oogonia from primary oocytes, which then enter a prefollicular stage. During oogonial proliferation and the prefollicular phase of oocyte formation, considerable numbers of oogonia and oocytes degenerate. Cessation of oogonial proliferation, formation of oocytes and degeneration of oogonia and oocytes act initially to slow the rate of increase and subsequently to decrease the number of germ cells in the ovary.

The temporal course of changes in germ cell number for the human ovary, shown in Figure 5, is similar to that observed in most mammalian species: a peak germ cell number occurring during gestation is followed by a rapid decrease which continues into the neonatal and peripubertal period, and is succeeded by a second, slower postpubertal decline in oocyte number that continues until

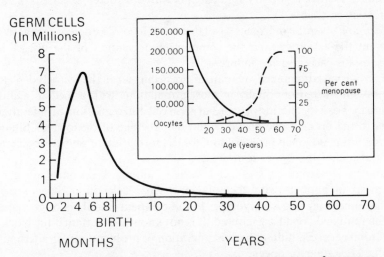

Figure 5 Ovarian germ cell population with respect to age, for women. Insert shows oocyte number and percentage of women postmenopausal in the second through sixth decades of life. (From Mattison, 1980 with permission)

oocytes disappear from the ovary. The initial rapid decline in oocyte number during the prefollicular stage of ovarian development is thought to be due to inadequate numbers of granulosa cells to enclose all oocytes in follicles, leading to the degeneration of those oocytes excluded from follicles. The second, slower decline in oocyte number with age represents oocyte loss predominantly due to recruitment of primordial follicles into the growing pool and subsequent atresia.

Meiosis or reduction division, which results in the formation of an ovum with a haploid composition of DNA, begins before birth in most mammals and then becomes arrested in prophase of the first meiotic division. As noted above, after oocytes enter meiosis they become surrounded by, and closely associated with, granulosa cells to form primordial follicles, and the cytoplasmic bridges that link oogonial cells disappear. The loss of the cytoplasmic bridges at this point is appropriate, as their function appears to be that of synchronizing the initiation of meiosis in nests of oogonial cells. Although the factors controlling the entry of oocytes into meiosis remain to be elucidated, Byskov (1976) has proposed that a substance she calls meiosis initiating factor, secreted by cells of the rete ovarii, is responsible for initiating the process.

2.2 Clinical Correlates of Ootoxicity in the Developing Ovary

In some instances it may be necessary to investigate human populations exposed to xenobiotic compounds thought to exert adverse effects on oogenesis, oocytes, or follicular differentiation. To assist in this type of investigation we will review the clinical syndromes observed in patients with disordered oogenesis or follicle differentiation (Table 1).

There are several syndromes available for which disordered oogenesis may represent the aetiology, and the common manifestation of the disease in all syndromes is early ovarian failure.

Although variations exist, ovarian failure occurs when the ovary is depleted of oocytes. This occurs normally in most populations with a median age of 50 (Figure 5). Toxicity altering primordial germ cell differentiation, proliferation, or access to the presumptive gonad might alter the age of menopause. Similarly, toxins altering oogonial proliferation, follicle formation or oocyte degeneration might also alter the age of menopause.

Turner's syndrome is a special variant among syndromes of gonadal dysgenesis in patients with the total or partial deletion of one of the sex chromosomes and a 45X karyotype. In these patients numbers of germ cells in the differentiated gonad are reduced. It is not known for certain if the block is in primordial germ cell differentiation, migration or proliferation, or alternatively, at some later stage in oogenesis.

The ultimate effect of the disease is premature ovarian failure with amenorrhoea (absence of menses), elevated serum levels of the gonadotropins, FSH and

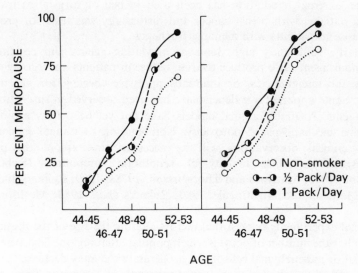

Figure 6   Age of menopause in women in the United States (left panel) and Europe (right panel) as a function of smoking habits. Data from Jick *et al.* (1977). (Figure reprinted from Mattison, 1981 b, with permission)

LH (see discussion of ovulation), and low levels of the ovarian steroid hormone (oestradiol). Other syndromes of gonadal dysgenesis occur in the absence of any evidence of chromosomal abnormalities, and some of these are familial.

A mouse model of this disease in which a genetic variant is associated with premature depletion of oocytes from the ovary may exist in the W mutants described by both Mintz and Russell (Ingram, 1962).

Premature ovarian failure is an idiopathic disease generally resulting from premature depletion of oocytes from the ovary. The serum levels of gonadotropins are elevated, and ovarian steroids are decreased. Earlier ovarian failure has been observed in smokers (Figure 6) suggesting that some cases with this condition may result from toxic environmental exposure (Jick *et al.*, 1977; Mattison and Thorgeirsson, 1978b; Mattison, 1981a,b). As the epidemiology of premature ovarian failure has never been explored, environmental or occupational factors cannot be excluded in the condition. Murine strain-dependent differences in the rate of oocyte loss have been observed (Jones and Krohn, 1961) paralleling familial forms of premature ovarian failure; however, these hereditary forms appear to be relatively uncommon.

In addition to these idiopathic syndromes of oocyte depletion, ample clinical evidence exists demonstrating sensitivity of the human ovary to ootoxic effects of ionizing radiation (Baker and Neal, 1977; Ash, 1980), alkylating agents and other antitumour drugs (Sieber and Adamson, 1975; Mattison *et al.*, 1981). For example, external irradiation has been used in lieu of surgical castration in treating patients with breast cancer and historically was used for producing menopause in patients with menometrorrhagia.

Similarly, sufficiently high doses of alkylating agents and certain other antitumour agents also produce ovarian failure in patients undergoing chemotherapy for malignancies, or immunosuppressive therapy for autoimmune disease. Some apparent age dependence has been observed in susceptibility to these agents. Available animal models have not yet been fully exploited to determine mechanisms of ootoxicity. Combination of animal models with human clinical observations will be necessary to explore the putative oogenesis/oocyte/follicle toxicity of xenobiotic compounds (Sieber and Adamson, 1975; Mattison and Thorgeirsson, 1978a, 1979; Reimers and Sluss, 1978; Mattison and Nightingale, 1980; Reimers et al., 1980; Mattison et al., 1981).

Animal experiments suggest that factors altering the size of the presumptive gonad alter the number of oocytes which populate that region. Toxins acting on epithelial or mesenchymal cells in the urogenital ridge may decrease the size of the gonad and thereby lower the age of spontaneous ovarian failure indirectly.

Recent evidence suggests that nutritional and metabolic disorders also effect ovarian development and provide a direct model of prenatal ovarian toxicity. Women with galactosaemia have a high incidence of premature ovarian failure (Kaufman et al., 1981). Premature ovarian failure in these women occurs even with early diagnosis and dietary restriction suggesting prenatal toxicity. Recent animal experimentation has also demonstrated that prenatal but not postnatal exposure to a high galactose diet can decrease oocyte number in rats (Chen et al., 1981). This data suggests that the adverse effect of galactose (or its metabolites) occurs during the development of the ovary.

2.3 Laboratory Assessment of Xenobiotic Effects on the Developing Ovary

2.3.1 *Primordial Germ Cells*

Early events in the differentiation of mammalian primordial germ cells are not presently amenable to experimental study since cells in these stages of differentiation cannot be identified. After alkaline phosphatase and some characteristic morphological features appear these cells may be quantitated. Cytoplasmic inclusions such as yolk, lipid or glycogen facilitate identification of primordial germ cells in some vertebrates.

Population of the presumptive gonad with primordial germ cells requires both passive and active motion, and the elaboration and recognition of chemotactic factors for direction, all of which may be vulnerable to adverse effects of xenobiotics.

Two general *in vivo* experimental approaches to the identification of xenobiotics which alter one or all of these processes seem feasible:

(1) differential mapping of primordial germ cell populations in control and treated embryos;
(2) selective treatment during specific stages of oogenesis followed by quantitative assessment of oocyte/follicle number at an appropriate time.

The second method has been used to explore the adverse reproductive effects of pre- and postnatal treatment with the purine analogues, azathioprine and 6-mercaptopurine (Reimers and Sluss, 1978; Reimers *et al.*, 1980; Mattison *et al.*, 1981), polycyclic aromatic hydrocarbons (Dobson *et al.*, 1978; Felton *et al.*, 1978), alkylating agents (Merchant-Larios, 1978), and ionizing radiation (Mandl, 1964; Dobson and Cooper, 1974; Baker, 1976; Dobson *et al.*, 1978).

Useful *in vitro* assay systems include:

(1) embryo culture techniques which minimize strain or species differences in the problems of distribution, metabolism and/or excretion of the xenobiotic in the pregnant female;
(2) urogenital ridge explant systems which might provide a useful assay system for studying agents affecting chemotaxis, primordial germ cell migration, and mitosis of primordial germ cells and oogonia.

Although these techniques have been used to explore basic issues in gonadal and gonaductal development with varying degrees of success, to our knowledge they have not been applied to reproductive toxicology. Further study of the applicability of these systems appears to be warranted.

2.3.2 *Oogonia and Oocytes*

After formation of oogonia, rapid proliferation of these stem cells occurs, and several classes of xenobiotic compounds (polycyclic aromatic hydrocarbons, alkylating agents) and ionizing radiation adversely affect these cells. In a typical *in vivo* assay, pregnant females are treated with the agents, and quantitative oocyte follicle counts are performed on ovaries of fetuses or offspring recovered at appropriate times after exposure.

In vitro techniques using primary ovarian culture may also be useful in understanding the mechanism of these toxicities. Cultures of dissociated ovarian cells may also prove useful for exploring xenobiotic effects on oocyte–granulosa cell interactions during follicle formation.

Differential follicle counts are useful for monitoring *in vivo* toxic effects on oocytes/follicles in the postnatal ovary. Age matching is important in these studies because of age-dependent differences in both ootoxicity and oocyte/follicle number. Comparison of prenatal and postnatal treatment may prove useful in differentiating adverse xenobiotic effects on oogenesis versus effects on mature oocyte/follicles, as previously mentioned.

3 THE DEVELOPED OVARY

3.1 Ovulation

Ovulation, like oogenesis and folliculogenesis, is a complex process requiring integration of, and appropriate response to, local and systemic signals (Knobil, 1974, 1980; Hutchinson and Sharp, 1977; Espey, 1978). Ovulation of a functionally mature oocyte requires follicular and oocyte growth, resumption of meiosis within the oocyte rupture of the follicle, and release of the oocyte. In addition to this complex sequence of events the ovary of the follicle destined to ovulate (dominant follicle) is also responsible for establishing the appropriate hormonal milieu for implantation and support of pregnancy if fertilization occurs (Figure 2).

3.1.1 *Preovulatory Follicle Growth and Rupture*

Most of the follicles in the ovary are those in the resting pool, the primordial follicles (Figure 7). These are the follicles formed during the process of folliculogenesis and consist of a primordial oocyte, several attenuated crescent-shaped granulosa cells, and a basement membrane. Although these follicles are traditionally termed 'resting follicles', there is ample evidence demonstrating their metabolic activity.

Following some as yet incompletely characterized signal primordial follicles begin to grow. Once follicles and oocytes have left the 'resting' pool and begin to grow, they continue this process until ovulation or degeneration (atresia) occurs (Peters *et al.*, 1976; Rowlands and Weir, 1977; Bjersing, 1978; Richards, 1978; Ross and Schreiber, 1978; Ross and Vande Wiele, 1981). In studies on follicular and oocyte growth in sexually mature rodents, the length of time necessary for a follicle and oocyte to reach full preovulatory maturation has been shown to be approximately 19 days in the mouse (Pederson and Peters, 1968; Pederson, 1970). These studies have also allowed the dynamics of follicular growth to be modeled (Faddy *et al.*, 1976). While there are virtually no kinetic studies on follicle growth in humans, an ovulatory follicle can be formed approximately 15 days after the initiation of gonadotropin therapy in hypogonadotropic women undergoing ovulation induction.

Preantral follicle growth occurs in the absence of gonadotropic stimulation albeit in limited numbers of follicles. Moreover, in rodent models, hypophysectomy has minimal effects on numbers of follicles beginning to mature. Once initiated, oestrogens stimulate and androgens inhibit granulosa cell proliferation and thus influence the rate of preantral follicle growth.

CLASSIFICATION SCHEME

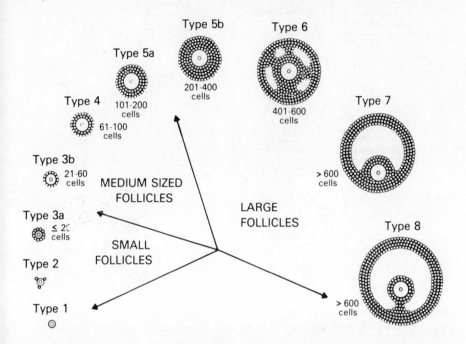

Classification of follicles into different types according to the number of granulosa cells in the largest cross-section of each follicle.

Figure 7   Classification scheme for oocytes and follicles in mouse ovaries (Pedersen and Peters, 1968). Similar schemes have been used to study follicular dynamics in the rodent ovary (Zuckerman and Mandl, 1950, 1952; Pedersen, 1970; Faddy *et al.*, 1976) and have been proposed for the human ovary (Peters *et al.*, 1976). The type 1 oocyte, without granulosa cells, does not exist following folliculogenesis in most mammalian species and is seldom seen after birth

Maturation of follicular complexes beyond preantral stages, that is, formation of a Graafian follicle, is dependent on FSH stimulation (Figures 2 and 8). Under control of FSH, multifocal accumulations of mucopolysaccharides become confluent to form a fluid-filled antrum (Zuckerman and Mandl, 1952). Increasing amounts of antral fluid contribute to the rapid preovulatory enlargement of the dominant follicle. In addition to plasma proteins with molecular weights less than 1×10^6 daltons, antral fluid contains peptide and steroid hormones in quantities which vary with respect to whether the follicle is destined to ovulate or degenerate. Antral fluid in dominant follicles destined to ovulate contains more oestrogens and progestogens, more FSH and LH, and less

GAMETE RELEASE

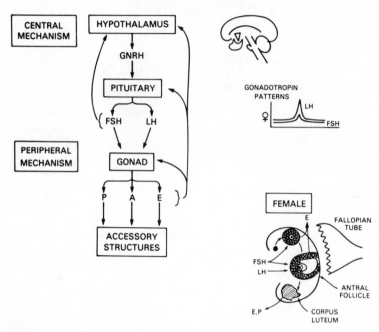

Figure 8   Interrelationships along the hypothalamic–pituitary–ovarian axis

prolactin than antral fluid from atretic follicles in which androgens are the dominant steroids, and FSH levels are undetectable.

In addition to stimulating antrum formation, FSH induces aromatase activity required for oestrogen synthesis and in conjunction with oestrogen induces membrane receptors for LH essential for postovulatory corpus luteum formation and function. After antrum formation the preovulatory follicle begins to grow rapidly and produces increasing quantities of oestrogens required to signal the preovulatory LH surge.

Within 24 hours following the LH surge, ultrastructural changes are initiated in the basal lamina, consistent with enzymatic degradation of the structural proteins, anticipating rupture a conical stigma forms and through this site, the oocyte–cumulus complex is extruded. As the remainder of the basal lamina degenerates, blood vessels and fibroblasts permeate the residual granulosa cells to form a corpus luteum in which thecal cells are also incorporated. During the luteal phase, changes in blood oestrogen and progestogen concentration reflect the rise and decline of secretory activity of the corpus luteum.

3.1.2 *Meiosis*

As noted above, the oocyte enters and becomes arrested in prophase of the first meiotic division prior to the formation of the follicle complexes (Baker, 1975; Tsafriri, 1978). Although factors involved in initiating arrest of meiosis are poorly understood, proteins found in follicular fluid are thought by some investigators to maintain it. It is not known if these proteins are also responsible for initiating the arrest of meiosis during oocyte differentiation, so that different factors may be responsible for the establishment and maintainance of meiotic arrest at different stages of follicular development. Cytoplasmic projections of granulosa cells which form gap junctions with the oocyte are required for maintainance of meiotic arrest once established.

After the LH surge, these junctions are altered and meiosis resumes in the oocyte. Around the time of ovulation the first polar body containing 2N DNA is extruded, giving rise to a secondary oocyte which enters a second, shorter arrest of meiosis. Sperm penetration of the secondary oocyte initiates the resumption of meiosis, resulting in extrusion of the second polar body containing N DNA, forming an ovum containing a haploid chromosome set and a male pronucleus with a haploid set, thus reconstituting the diploid complement in the zygote.

3.1.3 *Corpus Luteum*

Following the LH surge, changes in follicular morphology leading to release of the gamete complex are also essential for the formation of the corpus luteum. Breakdown of the basal lamina allows capillary penetration into the previously avascular follicle. Concomitant with these changes in follicular architecture, alterations occur in the morphology and function of the granulosa cells which differentiate into luteal cells whose major secretory product is progesterone.

The duration and quantity of progesterone secreted by the corpus luteum is crucial for fertility. Progesterone produced by luteal cells is essential for maintainance and modification of the endometrium as an epithelial, stromal and glandular structure suitable for implantation of the conceptus. In non-fertile cycles the corpus luteum produces increasing amounts of progesterone for a 10-day period following ovulation. At that point, maternal or intrinsic luteal factors which are poorly understood act to terminate the functional and morphological integrity of the corpus luteum. In some species, prostaglandins produced by the uterus have been identified as a luteolytic factor. However, in primates uterine production of prostaglandins plays no role in the control of the duration of corpus luteum life span.

In fertile cycles there is a finely balanced interplay between hormones produced by the implanted embryo supporting the continued functional existence of the corpus luteum and the luteolytic factors which act to terminate the functional existence of the corpus luteum. If the luteolytic factors act before the conceptus is able to rescue the corpus luteum, the duration of progesterone production will be less than normal (inadequate luteal phase), the endometrium is sloughed from the uterus less than 14 days after ovulation, and a preimplantation or early implanting embryo may be lost.

3.2 Clinical Correlates of Ootoxicity in the Developed Ovary

As inadvertent environmental, occupational, or drug exposure may impair follicular growth, ovulation corpus luteum function, or produce oocyte toxicity, we have summarized clinical syndromes associated with disorders of these processes (Table 1).

3.2.1 *Follicular Growth*

There are three syndromes and one form of follicle toxicity associated with each failure of normal progression in follicle growth. Although the full spectrum of clinical features associated with examples differs, the common manifestations of disordered follicular growth are similar, reflecting lack of production of oestrogen by the follicle complex.

Patients with hypogonadotropic hypogonadism have diminished production of the gonadotropins FSH and LH. As FSH is essential for preantral follicular growth and the formation of antral follicles, the extent of follicular development observed is minimal.

Antral follicles are the major source of oestradiol production necessary for pubertal development of the secondary sex characteristics. In the absence of follicular development before puberty, little endogeneous oestrogen is produced, and pubertal progression is delayed. These individuals have primary amenorrhoea with decreased gonadotropins and oestrogens.

If the hypothalamus or pituitary fails after puberty, the individual will have normal development of secondary sex characteristics, but will have secondary amenorrhoea. Again, the progression of follicle growth will be minimal, reflecting decreased levels of gonadotropins, and because follicle growth is not occurring, oestrogen production will also be decreased.

Patients with 17α-hydroxylase deficiency have a genetic enzymatic defect in oestrogen production. Inability to produce oestrogens blocks follicular growth, demonstrating that follicular growth in the presence of gonadotropin stimulation requires oestrogen production. These individuals have delayed puberty, primary amenorrhoea, and decreased ovarian size, with a minimal progression of follicle growth.

A small number of patients have been described with elevated bioactive gonadotropins, decreased oestrogens, delayed or normal puberty, and abnormal follicle profiles with many resting, but no growing follicles. The aetiology of this condition, termed 'resistant ovary', is unknown, but has been postulated to result from disordered or absent gonadotropin receptors, or ovarian defects in oestrogen production.

There is ample evidence indicating that alkylating agents like cyclophosphamide disrupt follicular growth. As these patients have elevated gonadotropins in the presence of low oestrogens, the toxicity is felt to reside in the ovary rather than the hypothalamus or pituitary. While on chronic alkylating agent therapy, these individuals have amenorrhoea with decreased oestrogens and are essentially postmenopausal. The ovary is small, and the follicle profile is abnormal, reflecting destruction of growing follicles. After cessation of alkylating agent therapy, if oocytes still remain within the ovary, cyclic ovarian function will resume with concomitant oestrogen production, decrease of gonadotropins to normal, menses, and fertility.

3.2.2 *Ovulation*

Sclerocystic or polycystic ovary syndrome is an ovarian disease associated with anovulation, infertility, hirsutism, and obesity. Patients with this disease have normal puberty, excessive hair growth beginning near puberty, and continuation of postmenorrhoeal menstrual irregularity beyond adolescence. The pathophysiology of the disease is thought to reflect excessive ovarian androgen production which stimulates hirsutism and also serves as substrate for peripheral conversion to oestrogen. The elevated levels of oestrogen feed back on the hypothalamus–pituitary and disrupt the normal gonadotropin release patterns leading to decreased circulating FSH and increased LH.

The ovaries of these individuals are enlarged with a smooth glistening capsule. There are multiple subcapsular, small follicular cysts with thecal cell hypertrophy responsible for the excessive androgen production.

An intriguing epidemiological study has suggested that exposure to halogenated aromatic hydrocarbon pesticides may be associated with this disease in humans. Strikingly parallel rodent experiments with halogenated hydrocarbons have also produced a disease similar to human polycystic ovary disease. It is not known if these effects are produced by alterations in the patterning (or imprinting) of ovarian monooxygenases or if it reflects a central (hypothalamic–pituitary) disturbance (Mattison, 1981a,b).

Disordered hypothalamic–pituitary function has been observed in several syndromes including amenorrhoea following oral contraceptive use, psychogenic amenorrhoea, prolactin-secreting tumours, isolated gonadotropin deficiency, etc. These syndromes are instructive because they may represent paradigms which may be useful in exploring putative reproductive toxins. In the hypothalamic–pituitary dysfunction associated with post-pill or idiopathic amenorrhoea, the levels of FSH, LH and prolactin are normal, and there is evidence of ovarian oestrogen production. In prolactin-secreting tumours and amenorrhoea–galactorrhoea syndromes, the levels of FSH, LH and prolactin are elevated. The role of prolactin in ovulation and ovarian function in primates, including humans, remains controversial (Pepperell, 1981).

In hypothalamic–pituitary failure there is no evidence of ovarian oestrogen production, and the gonadotropins are low. Circulating levels of prolactin may be elevated or normal.

3.2.3 *Corpus Luteum*

Patients with disorders of luteal function have inadequate progesterone secretion and abnormal endometrial transformation which are thought to lead to infertility or early pregnancy failure (DiZerega and Hodgen, 1981a,b). Careful study of hormone production by the follicle and corpus luteum during the menstrual cycle is necessary to demonstrate this disorder.

3.3 Laboratory Assessment of Xenobiotic Effects on the Developed Ovary

3.3.1 *Follicle Growth and Maturation*

Differential oocyte and follicle counts The laboratory assessment of the temporal determinants of follicle growth has previously only been determined in measuring development time (Pederson and Peters, 1968; Pederson, 1970; Faddy *et al.*, 1976). To our knowledge no studies have been done using these techniques to determine the effects of xenobiotics on follicular dynamics.

Xenobiotics impairing or stimulating follicle growth will alter the differential follicle composition of the ovary of treated animals. The assessment of follicle profiles requires serial sectioning of the ovary and follicle enumeration (Pederson and Peters, 1968). This method can also be used to evaluate toxins thought to destroy oocytes or follicles.

Dynamic assays to explore xenobiotic inhibition of follicular growth are directly approachable using standard gonadotropin and steroid hormone-stimulation techniques in intact (Greenwald, 1978) and hypophysectomized immature female rats (Hillier *et al.*, 1980).

Hormonal profiles The feedback loops between the hypothalamus–pituitary and ovary are accessible to evaluation via serum sampling and sensitive radioimmunoassays for gonadotropins and steroid hormones. Xenobiotics which directly or indirectly alter the rate of synthesis, secretion, distribution or excretion of these compounds would be expected to alter reproductive function in an individual so treated or exposed. Rodent experimentation has demonstrated that oestrus cycles are lengthened following acute exposure to xenobiotics which induce microsomal cytochrome P-450 dependent monooxygenases and/or transferases (Mattison, 1981a). Similarly, xenobiotics possessing steroid hormone agonist or antagonist properties would be expected to alter reproductive function by interrupting feedback loops. This accounts for alterations in fertility after exposure to environmental estrogens (McLachlan, 1980).

3.3.2 *Corpus Luteum*

Corpus luteum formation and function may be assessed indirectly by length and duration of progesterone production in pseudopregnant rodents or by decidual response of the endometrium of rodents. The decidual response has been demonstrated to be altered in rodents treated with nicotine, presumably in response to decreased progesterone production (Card and Mitchell, 1978).

The follicle is the precursor of the corpus luteum. Xenobiotics altering luteal function may exert their effect during the follicular phase of the cycle by impairing granulosa cell proliferation, during the periovulatory period by altering differentiation of granulosa cells, or capillary recruitment. These effects may be ascertained directly by measurement of follicle size, antrum size, granulosa cell number, corpus luteum size or progesterone secretion *in vitro*. Indirect assessment is possible by measuring circulating levels of oestrogens in the follicular phase or progestogens in the luteal phase of the cycle. To our knowledge, this system has not been explored to determine its validity in predicting xenobiotic luteal toxicity.

3.3.3 *Follicular Fluid*

Available information suggests that there is essentially no block in the access of blood-borne xenobiotics to the follicular fluid (McNatty, 1978). Although the follicle is surrounded by a basement membrane through which no capillaries penetrate during follicular development, the molecular weight cutoff for access to follicular fluid is approximately 1×10^6 daltons. Gap junctions between cumulus cells and oocytes provide an additional barrier. This relatively unfettered access to the oocyte may explain why certain xenobiotics have been demonstrated to produce adverse effects on meiosis.

3.3.4 *Oocyte Growth and Maturation*

As indicated above, xenobiotics have been demonstrated to alter meiosis and produce heritable translocations as a result of ootoxicity (Basler and Rohrburn, 1976; Russell and Mutter, 1980). This clearly represents an area which deserves much more research. It is especially important because of the role of meiosis in the genetics of reproduction. Impairment of hormonal control mechanisms

which produce infertility without altering the genetic mechanisms of reproduction offer no threat to the genetic integrity of a population. Xenobiotics
which produce meiotic errors, however, may have a profound effect on the genetic
integrity of a population.

It is not known if xenobiotics which alter meiosis produce dissociation of
oocyte and follicular maturation that might be ascertained by differential
measure of oocyte, follicle, or zona pellucida size. All of these parameters,
however, are easily accessible for investigation, Oocyte mRNA and proteins as
well as zonal proteins reflect the functional state of the gamete; measurement of
individual macromolecules or patterns of macromolecular synthesis in superovulated rodents may provide useful tools for characterizing xenobiotic effects
on the oocyte.

3.3.5 *Ovulation and Implantation*

Several assays, especially the dominant lethal assay utilized in genetic toxicology,
are directly applicable to the laboratory assessment of reproductive toxins.
Although the dominant lethal assay has been extensively used for male genetic
toxicology, it has not been widely used in assessing xenobiotic toxicity to the
female (Russell and Mutter, 1980). Extensions of the standard dominant lethal
assay including corpora lutea and implantation site counts might utilize uterine
flushing for oocyte or embryo counts, or ovarian sectioning and examination to
enumerate trapped oocytes.

Dynamic assays of ovulation are directly approachable using gonadotropin
stimulation and corpora lutea or ova counts.

3.3.6 *Fertility Assays*

Various animal fertility assays are available to explore reproductive toxins.
These assays include litter size, pregnancy intervals, total reproductive capacity,
and reproductive life span. (Mattison *et al.*, 1980).

4 CONCLUSIONS AND RECOMMENDATIONS

The complex of integrated physiological and cellular processes necessary for
oogenesis, follicle differentiation, follicle growth, ovulation, meiosis, and corpus
luteum function are potentially liable to xenobiotic interference at several levels.
In some instances evidence from humans, non-human primates, or subprimate
experimental animals has demonstrated xenobiotic toxicity to one or more of
these processes.

The clinical and laboratory assessments discussed have in certain cases been
adequate to identify and provide basic characterization of reproductive toxins.
Unfortunately, some of the suggested laboratory assessments have not been well

characterized and will require further evaluation. The clinical correlates discussed (Table 1) may provide the bridge between laboratory models and the identification of human reproductive toxins. It is reasonable to assume at the outset that a xenobiotic which produces reproductive toxicity in experimental animals will also be a reproductive toxin in humans. It is important, however, not to assume that the site of toxicity or the sensitivity will be similar. Species differences in the distribution and metabolism of xenobiotics as well as differences in reproductive physiology will determine the ultimate site and mechanism of action.

The importance of monitoring secular trends in the incidence of reproductive disorders in human and animal populations as it relates to recognizing adverse effects of xenobiotic exposure is worthy of special emphasis. Implementing these efforts does not require large initial outlays for research and development, since the technology required to accomplish these goals efficiently and effectively already exists. For populations in which health care delivery is either regional or nationally centralized, data gathering is simplified. These range from privately to state supported medical care plans which serve 'captive' populations for large periods of time.

The information we have summarized here has led us to the following conclusions and recommendations.

(1) Screening all potential toxicants in extant assay systems is impractical and prohibitively expensive.

(2) Research and development efforts should be directed toward acquiring less expensive and more efficient methods for assaying substances suspected of having adverse effects on oogenesis and ovulation in humans. The development of alternatives to the tedious methods currently available for counting and assessing morphology of follicles in serial sections is especially important.

(3) In contrast, maintaining surveillance over secular trends in the incidence of syndromes due to disorders of oogenesis or ovulation in humans, and feral and domestic animals would provide a practical method for monitoring for adverse effects of xenobiotic exposure. Similar surveillance systems have serendipitiously demonstrated that smoking is associated with secondary amenorrhoea (Petterson *et al.*, 1973; Vessey *et al.*, 1978), infertility (Tokuhata, 1968), and early menopause (Jick *et al.*, 1977; Mattison and Thorgeirsson, 1978b).

(4) Suggested adverse reproductive effects identified by large population surveillance can be studied in greater detail by comparing incidence of reproductive dysfunction in selected populations at risk (i.e. occupational, regional environmental, or drug exposure) with suitable control populations.

(5) Since such epidemiological data are not being collected presently, initiating data collection and analysis as soon as possible is desirable.

Progressive advancement toward these goals will provide a greater security to human reproduction from adverse reproductive effects of xenobiotics.

ACKNOWLEDGEMENT

We thank Mrs. Ollie S. Monger and Ms. Cecelia Kaiser for patience and perseverance in their superb preparation of this manuscript.

5 REFERENCES

American College of Obstetricians and Gynecologists (1976). *Guidelines on Pregnancy and Work*. Chicago, Illinois.

Ash, P. (1980). The influence of radiation on fertility in man. *Br. J. Radiol.* **53**, 271–278.

Baker, T. G. (1975). Oogenesis and ovarian development. In Balin, H. and Glasser, S. R. (Eds.) *Reproductive Biology*, pp. 398–437. Excerpta Medica, Amsterdam.

Baker, T. G. (1976). The effects of ionizing radiation on the mammalian ovary with particular reference to oogenesis. In Greep, R. O. and Astwork, E. B. (Eds.) *Handbook of Physiology. Endocrinology II*, Part I, pp. 349–361. American Physiological Society, Washington, DC.

Baker, T. G. and Neal, P. (1977). Action of ionizing radiations on the mammalian ovary. In Zuckerman, S. J. and Weir, B. J. (Eds.) *The Ovary*, 2nd edn, Vol. III, pp. 1–58. Academic Press, New York.

Basler, A. and Rohrburn, G. (1976). Chromosome aberrations in oocytes of NMRI mice and bone marrow cells of Chinese hamsters induced with 3, 4-benzpyrene. *Mutat. Res.* **38**, 327–332.

Bjersing, L. (1978). Maturation, morphology and endocrine function of the follicular wall in mammals. In Jones, R. E. (Ed.) *The Vertebrate Ovary: Comparative Biology and Evolution*, pp. 181–214. Plenum Press, New York.

Block, E. (1952). Quantitative morphological investigations of the follicular system in women. Variations at different ages. *Acta anat.* **14**, 108–112.

Brooks, P. (1980). Chemical carcinogenesis. *Br. med. J.* **36**, 1–104.

Byskov, A. G. and Saxon, L. (1976). Induction of meiosis in fetal mouse testis *in vitro, Develop. Biol.* **52**, 193–200.

Card, J. P. and Mitchell, J. A. (1978). The effects of nicotine administration on deciduoma induction in the rat. *Biol. Reprod.* **19**, 326–331.

Casarett, L. J. and Doull, J. (1975). *Toxicology: The Basic Science of Poisons*. Macmillan, New York.

Chen, Y. T., Mattison, D. R., Feigenbaum, L., Fukui, H. and Schulman, J. D. (1981). Reduction in oocyte number following prenatal exposure to a high galactose diet. *Pediatr. Res.* **15**, 642.

diZerega, G. S. and Hodgen, G. D. (1981a). Folliculogenesis in the primate ovarian cycle. *Endocrine Rev.* **2**, 27–49.

diZerega, G. S. and Hodgen, G. D. (1981b). Luteal phase dysfunction infertility: a sequel to abberrant folliculogenesis. *Fertil. Steril.* **35**, 489–499.

Dobson, P. L. and Cooper, M. F. (1974). Tritium toxicity: Effect of low-level 3HOH exposure on developing female germs cells in the mouse. *Radiat. Res.* **38**, 91–100.

Dobson, P. L., Koehler, C. G., Felton, J. S., Kwan, T. C., Wuebbles, B. J. and Jones, D. L. C. (1978). Vulnerability of female cells in developing mice and monkeys to tritium, gamma rays, and polycyclic aromatic hydrocarbons. In Mahlum, D. D., Sikov, M. R., Hackett, P. L. and Andrew, F. D. (Eds.) *Developmental Toxicology of Energy-Related Pollutants*. DOE Symposium Series 47, Conference 71017.

Espey, L. L. (1978). Ovulation. In Jones, R. E. (Ed.) *The Vertebrate Ovary: Comparative Biology and Evolution*, pp. 503–532. Plenum Press, New York.

Faddy, M. J., Jones, E. L. and Edwards, R. G. (1976). An analytical model for ovarian follicle dynamics. *J. exp. Zool.* **197**, 173–185.

Felton, J. S., Kwan, T. C., Wuebbles, B. J. and Dobson, R. L. (1978). Genetic differences in polycyclic-aromatic hydrocarbon metabolism and their effects on oocyte killing in developing mice. In Mahlum, D. D., Sikov, M. R., Hackett, P. L. and Andrews, F. D. (Eds.) *Developmental Toxicology of Energy-Related Pollutants*. DOE Symposium Series 47, Conference 771017.

Gelboin, H. V. (1980). Benzo(a)pyrene metabolism, activation, and carcinogenesis: role and regulation of mixed-function oxidases and related enzymes. *Physiol. Rev.* **60**, 1107–1166.

Generoso, W., Cain, K., Krishner, M. and Huff, S. W., (1979). Genetic lesions induced by chemicals in spermatozoa and spermatids of mice are repaired in the egg. *Proc. natn Acad. Sci. U.S.R.* **76**, 435–437.

Goldstein, A., Aronow, L. and Kalman, S. M. (1974). Chemical mutagenesis. In Goldstein, A., Aronow, L. and Kalman, S. M. (Eds.) *Principles of Drug Action. The Basis of Pharmacology*, pp. 623–666. John wiley, New York.

Gondos, B. (1978). Oogonia and oocytes in mammals. In Jones, R. E. (Ed.) *The Vertebrate Ovary: Comparative Biology and Evolution*, pp. 83–120. Plenum Press, New York.

Green, E. L. (1975). *The Biology of the Laboratory Mouse*. Dover Publications, New York.

Greenwald, G. S. (1978). Follicular activity in mammalian ovary. In Jones, R. E. (Ed.) *The Vertebrate Ovary: Comparative Biology and Evolution*, pp. 639–690. Plenum Press, New York.

Haffen, K. (1977). Sexual differentiation of the ovary. In Zuckerman, S. J. and Weir, B. J. (Eds.) *The Ovary*, 2nd edn, Vol. I, pp. 69–112. Academic Press, New York.

Hardesty, W. M. (1978). Primordial germ cells and the vertebrate germ line. In Jones, R. E. (Ed.) *The Vertebrate Ovary: Comparative Biology and Evolution*, pp. 1–45. Plenum Press, New York.

Heinrichs, W. L. and Juchau, M. R. (1980). Extrahepatic drug metabolism: the gonads. In Grum, T. E. (Ed.) *Extrahepatic Metabolism of Drugs and Other Foreign Compounds*, pp. 319–332. S. P. Medical and Scientific Books, New York.

Hillier, S. G., Zeleznik, A. J., Knazek, R. A. and Ross, G. T. (1980). Hormonal regulation of preovulatory follicle maturation in the rat. *J. Reprod. Fertil.* **60**, 219–229.

Hunt, V. R. (1979). *Work and the Health of Women*. CRC Press, Boca Raton, Florida.

Hutchinson, J. S. M. and Sharp, P. J. (1977). Hypothalamus–pituitary control of the ovary. In Zuckerman, S. J. and Weir, B. J. (Eds.) *The Ovary*, 2nd edn, Vol. III, pp. 227–304. Academic Press, New York.

Ingram, D. C. (1962). Atresia. In Zuckerman, S. (Ed.) *The Ovary*, 1st edn, Vol. I, pp. 247–273. Academic Press, New York.

Jick, H., Porter, J. and Morrison, A. S. (1977). Relation between smoking and age of natural menopause. *Lancet* **i**, 1354–1355.

Jones, E. C. and Krohn, P. L. (1961). The relationship between age, numbers of oocytes and fertility in virgin and multiparous mice. *J. Endocrinol.* **21**, 469–495.

Jones, R. E. (1978). *The Vertebrate Ovary: Comparative Biology and Evolution*. Plenum Press, New York.

Kaufman, F. R., Kogut, M. D., Donnel, G. N., Goebelsman, U., March, C. and Koch, R. (1981). Hypergonadotropic hypogonadism in female patients with galactosemia. *New Engl. J. Med.* **304**, 994–998.

Knobil, E. (1974). On the control of gonadotropin secretion in the rhesus monkey. *Recent Progr. Horm. Res.* **30**, 1–46.

Knobil, E. (1980). The neuroendocrine control of gonadotropin secretion in the rhesus monkey. *Recent Progr. Horm. Res.* **36**, 53–88.

Lucier, G. W., Lee, I. P. and Dixon, R. L. (1977). Effects of environmental agents on male reproduction. In Johnson, A. D. and Gomes, W. R. (Eds.) *The Testis*, Vol. III, pp. 557–628. Academic Press, New York.

Mandl, A. M. (1964). The radiosensitivity of germ cells. *Biol. Rev.* **39**, 288–371.

Masui, Y. and Pederson, R. (1975). Ultraviolet-light-induced DNA synthesis in mouse oocytes during meiotic maturation. *Nature (London)* **257**, 705–707.

Mattison, D. R. (1980). Oocyte destruction by xenobiotic compounds. *Contemp. Obstet. Gynecol.* **15**, 157–169.

Mattison, D. R. (1981a). The effects of biologically foreign compounds on reproduction. In Abdul-Karim, R. W. (Ed.) *Drugs during Pregnancy*, pp. 101–125, G. E. Stickley, Philadelphia.

Mattison, D. R. (1981b). Drugs, xenobiotics, and the adolescents. Implications for reproduction. In Soyka, L. F. and Redmond, G. P. (Eds.) *Drug Metabolism in the Immature Human*, pp. 129–143, Raven Press, New York.

Mattison, D. R., Chang, L., Thorgeirsson, S. S. and Shiromizu, K. (1981). The effects of cyclophosphamide, azathioprine, and 6-mercaptopurine on oocyte and follicle number in C57BL/6N mice. *Res. Comm. Chem. Pathol. Pharmacol.* **31**, 155–161.

Mattison, D. R. and Nightingale, M. S. (1980). The biochemical and genetic characteristics of murine ovarian aryl hydrocarbon (benzo(a)pyrene) hydroxylase activity and its relationship to primordial oocyte destruction by polycyclic aromatic hydrocarbon toxicology and applied pharmacology. *Toxic. appl. Pharmac.* **56**, 399–408.

Mattison, D. R. and Thorgeirsson, S. S. (1978a). Gonadal aryl hydrocarbon hydroxylase in rats and mice. *Cancer Res.* **38**, 1368–1373.

Mattison, D. R. and Thorgeirsson, S. S. (1978b). Smoking and industrial pollution, and their effects on menopause and ovarian cancer. *Lancet* **i**, 187–188.

Mattison, D. R. and Thorgeirsson, S. S. (1979). Ovarian aryl hydrocarbon hydroxylase activity and primordial oocyte toxicity of polycyclic aromatic hydrocarbons in mice. *Cancer Res.* **39**, 3471–3475.

Mattison, D. R., White, N. B. and Nightingale, M. S. (1980). The effect of benzo(a)pyrene on fertility, primordial oocyte number, and ovarian response to pregnant mare's serum gonadotropin. *Pediatr. Pharmacol.* **1**, 143–151.

McLachlan, J. A. (1980). *Estrogens in The Environment.* Elsevier North-Holland, New York.

McNatty, K. P. (1978). Follicular fluid. In Jones, R. E. (Ed.) *The Vertebrate Ovary: Comparative Biology and Evolution*, pp. 215–260. Plenum Press, New York.

Merchant-Larios, H. (1978). Ovarian differentiation. In Jones, R. E. (Ed.) *The Vertebrate Ovary: Comparative Biology and Evolution*, pp. 47–81. Plenum Press, New York.

Newburgh, R. W. (1975). Toxicology of the reproductive system. In Casarett, L. J. and Doull, J. (Eds.) *Toxicology, The Basic Science of Poisons*, pp. 261–274. Macmillan Publishing Company, New York.

Pederson, T. (1970). Follicle kinetics in the ovary of the cyclic mouse. *Acta endocrinol.* **64**, 304–323.

Pederson, R. and Mangia, F. (1978). Ultraviolet-light-induced unscheduled DNA synthesis by resting and growing mouse oocytes. *Mutat. Res.* **49**, 425–429.

Pederson, T. and Peters, H. (1968). Proposal for a classification of oocytes and follicles in the mouse ovary. *J. Reprod. Fertil.* **17**, 555–557.

Pepperell, R. J. (1981). Prolactin and reproduction. *Fertil. Steril.* **35**, 267–274.

Peters, H. (1978). Folliculogenesis in mammals. In Jones, R. E. (Ed.) *The Vertebrate Ovary: Comparative Biology and Evolution*, pp. 121–144. Plenum Press, New York.

Peters, H., Himelstein-Braw, R. and Faber, M. (1976). the normal development of the ovary in childhood. *Acta endocrinol.* **82**, 617–630.

Petterson, F., Fries, H. and Nillius, S. J. (1973). Epidemiology of secondary amenorrhoea I. Incidence and prevalence rates. *Am. J. Obstet. Gynec.* **117**, 80–86.

Reimers, T. J. and Sluss, P. M. (1978). 6-Mercaptopurine treatment of pregnant mice. Effects on second and third generations. *Science (Washington DC)* **201**, 65–67.

Reimers, T. J., Sluss, P. M., Goodwin, J. and Seidel, G. E. (1980). Bi-generational effects of 6-mercaptopurine on reproduction in mice. *Biol. Reprod.* **22**, 367–375.

Richards, J. S. (1978). Hormonal control of follicular growth and maturation in mammals. In Jones, R. E. (Ed.) *The Vertebrate Ovary: Comparative Biology and Evolution*, pp. 331–360. Plenum Press, New York.

Ross, G. T. and Schreiber, J. R. (1978). The Ovary. In Yen, S. S. C. and Jaffe, R. B. (Eds.) *Reproductive Endocrinology. Physiology, Pathophysiology, and Clinical Management*, pp. 63–79. W. B. Saunders Company, Philadelphia.

Ross, G. T. and Vande Wiele, R. L. (1981). The ovaries, and Frantz, A. G. The breasts. In Williams, R. H. (Ed.) *Textbook of Endocrinology*, 6th edn. W. B. Saunders Company, Philadelphia.

Rowlands, I. W. and Weir, B. J. (1977). The ovarian cycle in vertebrates. In Zuckerman, S. J. and Weir, B. J. (Eds.) *The Ovary*, 2nd edn, Vol. II, pp. 217–274. Academic Press, New York.

Russell, L. B. and Mutter, B. E. (1980). Whole mammal mutagenicity tests: Evaluation of five methods. *Mutat. Res.* **75**, 279–302.

Schardein, J. L. (1976). *Drugs as Teratogens*. CRC Press, Boca. Raton, Florida.

Searle, C. E. (1976). *Chemical Carcinogens*. ACS Monograph 173, American Chemical Society, Washington, DC.

Shepard, T. H. (1980). Catalog of Teratogenic Agents, 3rd edn. The John's Hopkins University Press, Baltimore, Maryland.

Sieber, S. M. and Adamson, R. H. (1975). Toxicity of antineoplastic agents in man: Chromosomal aberrations, antifertility effects, congenital malformations, and carcinogenic potential. *Adv. Cancer Res.* **22**, 57–155.

Symposium on Target Organ Toxicity (1978). Gonads (Reproductive and Genetic Toxicity). *Environ. Health Perspect.* **24**, 1–127.

Tokuhata, G. M. (1968). Smoking in relation to infertility and fetal loss. *Archs Environ. Health* **17**, 353–359.

Tsafriri, A. (1978). Oocyte maturation in mammals. In Jones, R. E. (Ed.) *The Vertebrate Ovary: Comparative Biology and Evolution*, pp. 409–442. Plenum Press, New York.

Van Tienhoven, A. (1968). *Reproductive Physiology of Vertebrates*. W. B. Saunders Company, Philadelphia.

Vessey, M. P., Wright, N. H., McPherson, K. and Wiggins, P. (1978). Fertility after stopping different methods of contraception. *Br. med. J.* **1**, 265–267.

Weir, B. J. and Rowlands, I. W. (1977). Ovulation and atresia. In Zuckerman, S. J. and Weir, B. J. (Eds.) *The Ovary*, 2nd edn, Vol. I, pp. 265–302. Academic Press, New York.

Whittingham, D. G. and Wood, M. J. (1981). Reproductive physiology. In Foster, H. L., Small, J. D. and Fox, J. G. (Eds.) *The Mouse in Biomedical Research*, Vol. 2, Academic Press, New York.

Yen, S. S. C. (1978). The human menstrual cycle (integrative function of the hypothalamic–pituitary–overian–endometrial axis). In Yen, S. S. C. and Jaffe, R. B. (Eds.) *Reproductive Endocrinology: Physiology, Pathophysiology and Clinical Management*, pp. 121–151. W. B. Saunders Company, Philadelphia.

Yen, S. S. C. and Jaffe, R. B. (1978). *Reproductive Endocrinology: Physiology, Pathophysiology and Clinical Management*. W. B. Saunders Company, Philadelphia.

Zuckerman, S. and Baker, T. G. (1977). The development of the ovary and the process of oogenesis. In Zuckerman, S. J. and Weir, B. J. (Eds.) *The Ovary*, 2nd edn, Vol. I, pp. 42–68. Academic Press, New York.

Zuckerman, S. and Mandl, A. M. (1950). The numbers of normal atretic ova in the mature rat. *J. Endocrinol.* **6**, 426–435.

Zuckerman, S. and Mandl, A. M. (1952). The growth of the oocyte and follicle in the adult rat. *J. Endocrinol.* **8**, 126–132.

Zuckerman, S. J. and Weir, B. J. (1977). *The Ovary*, 2nd edn, Vols. I, II and III. Academic Press, New York.

Methods for Assessing the Effects of Chemicals on Reproductive Functions
Edited by V. B. Vouk and P. J. Sheehan
© 1983 SCOPE

Techniques for Detecting and Evaluating Abnormalities in Testicular Function

Jeffrey B. Kerr and David M. de Kretser

1 INTRODUCTION

The adverse effects of chemical agents upon testicular function have often been assumed to interfere selectively with the process of spermatogenesis, with relatively little attention being directed to the functional integrity of the Sertoli cells and Leydig cells. Different agents act at different levels of the spermatogenic process. Some may cause damage to the mitotic or meiotic division process, while others may interfere with the differentiation of spermatids. Variation in the dose or length of exposure of the testis to a particular noxious chemical may produce widely different effects which result in damage to normal testicular function. There is increasing evidence to suggest that such substances do not simply cause selective damage to the spermatogenic process but also markedly alter the structural and biochemical properties of Sertoli cells and Leydig cells which in turn may profoundly affect the process of spermatogenesis.

It is recognized that chemicals suspected of causing damage to the testis may be assessed for their effects on sperm production by semen analysis obtained from ejaculation, and these methods are reviewed by other contributors to this Workshop.

The aim of this contribution is to focus attention on methods which have been developed to assess the effects of chemical agents which may damage the functional status of various components of the mammalian testis.

2 METHODS FOR MORPHOLOGICAL ASSESSMENT

2.1 Laboratory Species

The principal method presently available for detection of abnormalities of testicular function is the histological examination of the seminiferous epithelium and intertubular tissue using conventional cytological techniques of fixation, paraffin embedding and examination of sections 5–10 μm in thickness. The widespread acceptance of this simple method of evaluating spermatogenic function may lead to doubtful conclusions of the morphological integrity of the testis. Previously, it has been accepted that agents causing disruption of spermatogenesis may not alter the Sertoli cells or Leydig cells. However light microscopic examination of testicular tissues prepared by the above method may fail to reveal a number of structural alterations to the Sertoli cells or Leydig cells which accompany damage to the testis. This proposal has been substantiated from a number of studies of the functional status of the Sertoli cells and Leydig cells following exposure of the testis to noxious agents which suggest that these cells are rather sensitive to substances causing spermatogenic disruption.

Reliable morphological assessment of both compartments of the testis, the seminiferous epithelium and the intertubular tissue may be achieved with improved tissue preservation suitable for both light and electron microscopic analysis.

2.1.1 Selection of Fixative

Previously formalin has been widely chosen as a fixative for preservation of mammalian tissues but the resultant architecture of the testis fixed in formalin may display marked disruption of cellular elements chiefly as a result of shrinkage of the tissue, leaving many artefacts which may be indistinguishable from the structural alterations within the testis. Considerable improvement of tissue preservation is achieved with Bouins fixative (picric acid–formaldehyde–acetic acid) or buffered picric acid–formaldehyde (PAF), originally described by Stefanini *et al.* (1967) for fixation of ejaculated human spermatozoa. These fixatives are selected if the tissue is to be embedded in a medium applicable to light microscopic examination. The choice of fixative for ultrastructural analysis is chiefly determined by cost, ease of preparation and degree of preservation of cellular and subcellular organization, and mixtures of buffered aldehydes are presently used for optimal fixation of the testis.

Two fixatives commonly used for ultrastructural analysis of the testis are glutaraldehyde buffered in *s*-collidine as originally proposed by Bennett and Luft (1959) or buffered mixtures of glutaraldehyde and formaldehyde originally described by Karnovsky (1965) and later modified by Ito and Karnovsky (1968). Additional fixation of testicular tissues in buffered osmium tetroxide is now routinely used for preparation of tissues for electron microscopy.

2.1.2 Administration of Fixative

Wherever possible, optimal preservation of the testis should be achieved by a perfusion method in which the fixative is delivered via a cannula inserted into an artery leading to the testis, a method originally proposed by Christensen (1965). Blood is removed from the testicular vascular system by brief flushing with physiological saline followed by the fixative. Where possible, studies designed to evaluate changes in the form and structure of the testis should utilize perfusion-fixed material. Marked physical disruption accompanies the use of small or large pieces of excised testicular tissue obtained by biopsy, and immersion fixation of testicular fragments may result in unequal penetration of the fixative, thereby permitting morphological alterations to cellular and subcellular components. These structural modifications may be erroneously interpreted as a reflection of damage to the tissue by exogenous factors. A guide to the successful perfusion fixation of the testis requires that the saline solution should cause rapid blanching of the testis and after 15–30 minutes of administration of fixative, the testis should become hardened upon palpation (Forssmann *et al.*, 1977).

2.1.3 *Embedding Media*

The use of polymerizing resins as embedding media for tissues provides superior preservation of the fixed tissues compared to conventional paraffin. The major advantages of plastic resin sections of carefully fixed testicular tissues are lower distortion of cellular associations and considerably more information content due to the ability of such tissues to be cut at 0.25–1 μm as compared to sections cut from paraffin blocks, commonly 5–10 μm in thickness. For light microscopy, testis tissue may be fixed in Bouins or PAF and embedded in paraffin or acrylic ester, glycol methacrylate (Bennett *et al.*, 1976), the latter providing both superior resolution and a variety of histochemical reactions compared to paraffin embedding (Figures 1, 2). For electron microscopy, we recommend fixation in 3–5% glutaraldehyde buffered with 0.1 M *s*-collidine, pH 7.4 (Mori and Christensen, 1980) or cacodylate buffered mixtures of glutaraldehyde, formaldehyde and trinitrocresol (Kerr and de Kretser, 1975; Kerr *et al.*, 1979a, b). Fixed tissues are post-fixed in buffered osmium tetroxide and embedded in the epoxy resins Epon or Araldite for subsequent light or electron microscopic analysis (Figure 3).

2.1.4 *Tracer Studies*

The spermatogenic process is dependent upon continuous proliferation and differentiation of the germ cells and upon the functional status of the Sertoli cells, the latter providing a physiological compartmentalization of the seminiferous epithelium into basal and adluminal regions. Creation of these compartments is dependent upon intact inter-Sertoli cell-tight junctions which form the blood–testis barrier (Dym and Fawcett, 1970; Dym, 1973; Fawcett, 1975; Russell, 1978, 1980). Assessment of the integrity of the blood–testis barrier is performed by introducing electron-dense tracers into the medium used to fix the testis and observing their passage into the seminiferous epithelium. The intact blood–testis barrier provided by the inter-Sertoli junctions prevents penetration of the tracer into the adluminal compartment of the epithelium (Figure 4). The

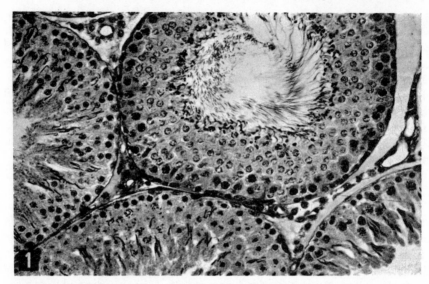

Figure 1   Light micrograph of normal rat testis fixed by perfusion with Bouin's fixative, embedded in paraffin, sectioned at 5 μm and stained with haematoxylin and eosin. Although spermatogenic activity is illustrated, detailed morphology of the germ cells, Sertoli cells and Leydig cells is not distinguishable

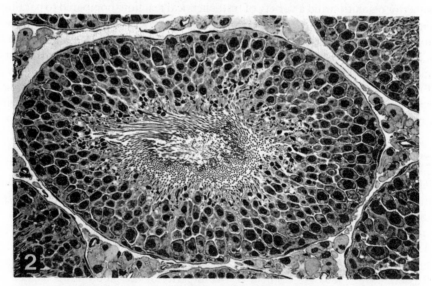

Figure 2   Light micrograph of normal rat testis fixed by perfusion with phosphate buffered picric acid–formaldehyde, embedded in glycol methacrylate, sectioned at 1 μm and stained with Lee's methylene-blue–basic-fuchsin method. Greater detail of the cellular elements within the seminiferous tubule and intertubular tissue is illustrated

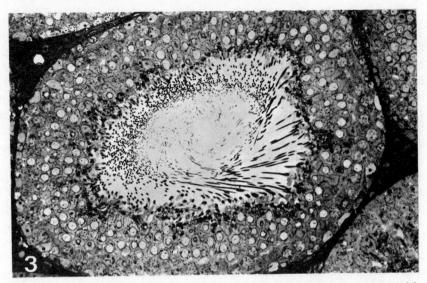

Figure 3 Light micrograph of normal rat testis fixed by perfusion with glutaraldehyde buffered in collidine, embedded in Epon–Araldite, sectioned at $0.5\,\mu$m and stained with toluidine blue. Cell associations within the seminiferous epithelium are maintained and preservation of the tissue is satisfactory for ultrastructural analysis

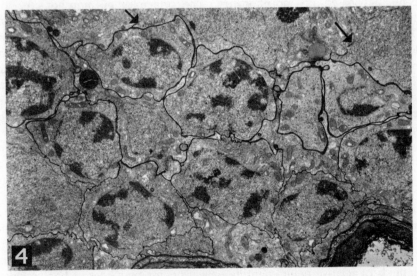

Figure 4 Electron micrograph of the basal aspect of seminiferous epithelium of normal 20-day-old rat testis. The division of the epithelium into two compartments with the aid of lanthanum which is prevented from complete pentration by intact inter-Sertoli cell tight junctional complexes (arrows)

tracers selected have been ferritin (Fawcett *et al.*, 1970), peroxidase (Vitale *et al.*, 1973) and lanthanum (Dym and Fawcett, 1970; Neaves, 1973; Dym and Cavicchia, 1977; Connell, 1978). Evaluation of the permeability of the blood–testis barrier is achieved by the simple method of addition of 2% lanthanum nitrate to a fixative solution of 5% glutaraldehyde buffered in 0.2 M collidine, pH 7.8. All post-fixation and dehydration procedures up to absolute alcohol contain 2% lanthanum. If a physiological saline solution is used to clear the testis of blood, it is recommended that the saline contains no phosphate since insoluble lanthanum phosphate will cause precipitation of particles large enough to inhibit successful perfusion.

The effects of agents on spermatogenesis are often evaluated by quantitative assessments of this process. Accurate evaluation of the germ cell population is only possible by the use of quantitative techniques. In animals such as the rat where an easily defined seminiferous cycle is present, quantitative evaluation can be obtained by selecting a specific stage of the cycle and counting the number of each germ cell type in 25 tubules cut in cross-section which are at the particular stage. However, in some experimental procedures, it is not possible to identify the specific stages and it then becomes necessary to count the germ cell population in 25 cross-sections of seminiferous tubules selected at random in each experimental animal.

Where changes in the Sertoli or Leydig cells are to be evaluated or where ultrastructural changes in germ cells are to be studied, it is necessary to use other techniques based on morphometry. The principles of morphometry and stereology have only recently been applied to the mammalian testis (Bergh and Damber, 1978; Bergh and Helander, 1978; Frankenhuis *et al.*, 1979; Hochereau-de Reviers *et al.*, 1979; Kerr *et al.*, 1979a; Christensen and Peacock, 1980; Mori and Christensen, 1980; Zirkin *et al.*, 1980) in an attempt to quantitate the alterations in number, size and relative volume occupancy of specific tissue types, cells or cellular organelles which may accompany changes in the activity of the testis. In summary, these procedures make use of tissue sections fixed by perfusion and the relative area of a given histological feature within the testis is measured by direct light microscopic observation using eyepiece grids containing a square lattice. The number of intersections on the particular feature is recorded and its density is calculated by dividing the sum of points falling on the structure by the total points lying on the tissue. This method provides information for the numerical density of a feature per unit area or volume of testis for seminiferous epithelium, intertubular tissue, or any structure within the intertubular tissue.

Stereological analysis of the number and volume occupancy of any cell type within the testis may be performed at the electron microscope level using similar methods of relative point counting or grids containing lines of known length whose intersections with relevant surface contours within the cell of interest are recorded. Details of these techniques applied to the testis are available in Christensen and Peacock (1980) and Mori and Christensen (1980).

2.2 Human

2.2.1 *Testicular Biopsy*

Whole testes are rarely available for study and consequently, small pieces of tissue obtained by biopsy are all that is usually available. Such tissue should be obtained by techniques that have been described previously (Rowley and Heller, 1966) in which a small incision in the tunica albuginea allows the testicular tissue to protrude and to be excised by a sharp scalpel blade used parallel to the surface of the testis. The tissue must be handled gently and placed in Bouin's or Cleland's fixative for processing into paraffin.

2.2.2 *Fixation and Quantitation Methods*

Fixation procedures for light or electron microscopy are similar to the methods described for laboratory species. If a testis becomes available for perfusion fixation, the spermatic cord should be retained for 3–5 cm to facilitate cannulation of the testicular artery, and perfusion of the testis requires similar procedures described for the laboratory species.

In the human testis, quantitative histological methods of counting the numbers of germ cells in cross-sectional views of sections of seminiferous tubules have demonstrated a rise in serum FSH levels to be correlated with disruption of spermatogenesis and infertility (de Krester *et al.*, 1972; Franchimont *et al.*, 1972; Leonard *et al.*, 1972). Measurement of serum FSH levels provides a simple index of spermatogenic activity; however, in man no specific germ cell type is linked to the control of FSH secretion (de Kretser *et al.*, 1974) suggesting that methods used for detection of abnormalities of spermatogenesis must examine the numbers and structure of the germ cells and the Sertoli cells.

3 METHODS FOR ASSESSMENT OF SERTOLI CELL FUNCTION

3.1 Secretory Capacity

Until recently, the Sertoli cells could only be evaluated by observation of their morphology using light and electron microscopic techniques. Developments in our understanding of Sertoli cell function have been recently reviewed (Ritzen *et al.*, 1980) and it is now recognized that Sertoli cells are responsible for the production of androgen binding protein (ABP), seminiferous tubule fluid and inhibin. These secretory properties associated with the Sertoli cell have allowed the development of simple tests of Sertoli cell function. ABP production by the Sertoli cell is impaired following spermatogenic damage induced by agents such as surgical cryptorchidism, fetal irradiation, vitamin A deficiency of drug treatments (Hagenas and Ritzen, 1976; Rich and de Kretser, 1977a; Jegou and

Table 1   Effect of treatment on levels of ABP in the testis and caput epididymis

	TESTIS ABP		APIDIDYMAL ABP	
	pmol/mg protein	pmol/testis	pmol/mg protein	pmol/caput
Normal adult male	0.41	17.41	6.03	28.08
Hydroxyurea treated	0.39	6.52*	4.02*	7.27*
Vitamin A-deficient	0.45	5.23*	ND	ND
Fetal X-irradiated	0.68	3.31*	1.33*	1.08*

Results are expressed as mean value of duplicate estimations of two cytosols, each prepared from tissues pooled from five animals.
*P < 0.01 (Dunnett's t-test); ND, not detectable.
(Reproduced with permission from Rich, K. A. and de Kretser, D. M. (1977). *Endocrinology* **101**, 959–968, © 1977, The Endocrine Society.)

de Kretser, 1979; Kerr *et al.*, 1979b). The measurement of ABP production is regarded as being a sensitive test for Sertoli cell function since brief exposure of the testis to 43 °C for 15 minutes results in marked impairement of ABP secretion (Rich and de Kretser, 1977b). It is emphasized that expression of the concentration of ABP (per mg protein) in testes exhibiting spermatogenic damage may not differ significantly from that measured in normal testes. However, calculation of the total amount of ABP per testis (Table 1) has to date demonstrated diminished secretory capacity of the Sertoli cell in all conditions of spermatogenic damage and emphasizes the need to consider that these cells are susceptible and sensitive to noxious agents. The decrease in ABP production by the damaged testis is proportional to the severity of spermatogenic disruption (Rich and de Kretser, 1977a) but whether noxious agents simultaneously alter the function of both the Sertoli and germ cells remains unknown.

Since the Sertoli cells are responsible for fluid secretion within the seminiferous tubules, measurement of the production of fluid by Sertoli cells suspected of being damaged is simply measured by ligation of the vasa efferentia; comparison of the weight of the ligated testis to the non-ligated contralateral testis following 16 hours' ligation provides an index of fluid production (Smith, 1962). Accumulation of the total volume of fluid secreted by damaged testes after ligation is markedly diminished in proportion to the severity of spermatogenic disruption, a result in agreement with the associated reduction in ABP production by Sertoli cells within the damaged testis (Figure 5; Rich and de Kretser, 1977a). ABP production rate may be obtained by comparing the ABP content of the ligated and non-ligated testis and provides a more dynamic test of Sertoli cell function.

Inhibin production by Sertoli cells provides a factor capable of selectively regulating the release of FSH from the pituitary. A disturbance of normal Sertoli cell function in conditions of spermatogenic damage is expected to alter the

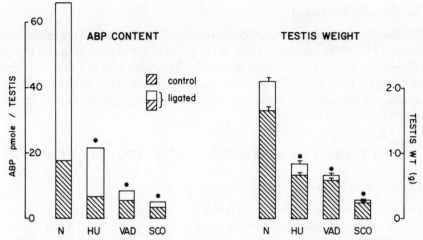

Figure 5 Production of ABP and seminiferous tubule fluid after efferent duct ligation (EDL). In normal animals, unilateral EDL results in an increase in weight of the ligated testis of 27% after 16 h. In damaged testes, a marked decrease in the total volume of fluid (weight decrease) secreted by the testis is seen after ligation, as well as a diminution in fluid secretion by the testis per unit weight of testis. The rise in testicular ABP content after EDL is markedly reduced in each damaged testis in proportion to the severity of the spermatogenic destruction. N, Normal; HU, hydroxyurea treatment; VAD, Vitamin A-deficient diet; SCO, fetal irradiation. Testicular weight is expressed as the mean $\pm$ s.e. of individual testes ($n = 10$). The ABP content per testis is expressed as the mean value of duplicate estimations of two cytosols, each prepared from tissues pooled from five animals. $*P < 0.01$. (Reproduced with permission from Rich, K. A. and de Kretser, D. M. (1977) *Endocrinology* **101**, 959–968, © 1977, The Endocrine Society.)

production of inhibin which in turn results in alterations of FSH secretion from the pituitary.

In rodents, damage to the seminiferous epithelium is accompanied by elevated serum FSH levels, as shown by disruption of spermatogenesis in cryptorchidism (Walsh and Swerdloff, 1973; Kerr *et al.*, 1979b). Similar results have been noted following spermatogenic damaged induced by drugs (Debeljuk *et al.*, 1973; Gomes *et al.*, 1973; Rich and de Kretser, 1977a) or irradiation of fetal (Rich and de Kretser, 1977a) or adult rats (Verjans and Eik-Nes, 1976).

In general, the severity of spermatogenic damage is correlated with the resultant elevation in FSH levels in serum, therefore allowing radioimmunoassay of serum FSH as a simple index of spermatogenic activity.

A more direct and precise assessment of inhibin production is obtained by a quantitative bioassay technique of inhibin production using cultures of anterior pituitary cells (Steinberger and Steinberger, 1976, 1977; Scott *et al.*, 1980). The extent of the selective inhibition of FSH release or cellular FSH content from dispersed anterior pituitary cell cultures provides an index of inhibin production.

3.2 Receptor Properties

The demonstration that Sertoli cells contain FSH receptors (Orth and Christensen, 1977, 1978) which are markedly reduced in states of damage to the testis (Hagenas *et al.*, 1978; Risbridger *et al.*, 1981a) provides a further test of the index of the state of Sertoli cells in testes suspected of being influenced by agents capable of disrupting spermatogenesis. The reason for the decline in FSH receptor numbers is unknown.

4 METHODS FOR ASSESSMENT OF LEYDIG CELL FUNCTION

4.1 Secretory Capacity

The functional status of the Leydig cells within the intertubular tissue of the testis may be evaluated from their secretory and receptor properties. The concept that a variety of conditions interfering with spermatogenesis had minimal effects upon Leydig cell function was based upon light microscopic observations of the Leydig cells which commonly appeared unchanged or more plentiful compared to normal. In summary the changes occuring to Leydig cells within the damaged testis include alterations in cell volume and content of organelles associated with steroidogenesis, changes in receptor numbers for luteinizing hormone (LH) or human chorionic gonadotrophin (hCG) and changes in the capacity of Leydig cells to secrete testosterone in response to trophic stimulation.

Measurement of serum testosterone and LH levels by radioimmunoassay provides a useful and rapid indication of Leydig cell function since states of testicular damage if severe are associated with Leydig cell dysfunction as reflected by low serum testosterone levels and elevated serum LH levels. A more accurate and sensitive assessment of the secretory capacity of the Leydig cell may be obtained from the assay of serum testosterone following hCG stimulation *in vivo*. Maximal stimulation of testosterone secretion by the testis is determined from dose–response studies of 10–50 iu of hCG in 0.5 ml saline injected intravenously. Control groups are given 0.5 ml saline alone. Blood samples are obtained under light anaesthesia from the jugular vein immediately prior to and 60 minutes after injection. All injections should be performed at the same time of day to reduce the effects of diurnal fluctuations in peripheral testosterone levels. Blood is allowed to clot at room temperature, serum is separated and stored at − 20°C until assayed. The ability of the Leydig cells to secrete testosterone is assessed from the incremental rise in stimulated minus basal testosterone production compared to normal animals.

Testicular damage may be associated with altered blood flow to the testis possibly due to lowered delivery of gonadotropic hormone to Leydig cells or decreased outflow of testosterone elaborated in response to *in vivo* stimulations (Damber *et al.*, 1978). Thus, hCG stimulation of whole testis suspensions or

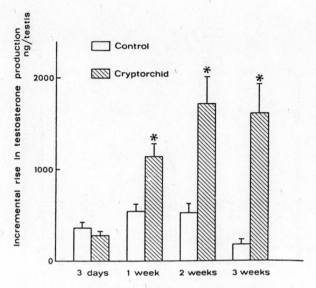

Figure 6 Response of testes to gonadotropin *in vitro* following testicular damage induced by experimental cryptorchidism. The incremental rise in testosterone production (stimulated minus basal) shows an enhanced response *in vitro* compared to normal testis. Mean ± s.e. ($n = 5$); *$P < 0.01$ compared to incremental rise in T production by control testes. (Reproduced with permission from de Kretser, D. M., Kerr, J. B., Rich, K. A., Risbridger, G. P. and Dobos, M. (1980). In Steinberger, A. and Steinberger, E. (Eds.) *Testicular Development, Structure and Function.* Raven Press, New York.)

isolated Leydig cells *in vitro* is also necessary to assess the secretory characteristics of the Ledig cell in damaged testes. If evaluation of testosterone production by whole testes in required, they are incubated for 4 hours in Krebs–Ringer bicarbonate buffer in the presence or absence of hCG and the testosterone content of the medium is measured (Figures 6, 7) (de Kretser *et al.*, 1979). Isolated Leydig cells may also be studied by identical techniques and the testosterone secretion per cell can be assessed (Schumacher *et al.*, 1978; Payne *et al.*, 1980).

4.2 Receptor Properties

Androgen production by the Leydig cell is regulated by the action of LH on the cell and in studies designed to assess the number of receptors for LH on the Leydig

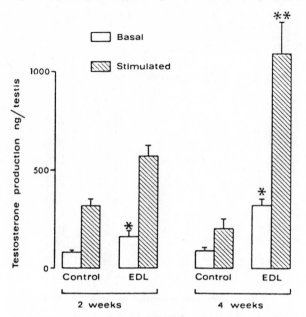

Figure 7 Response of testes to gonadotropin stimulation *in vitro* following testicular damage induced by efferent duct ligation. At both time intervals after ligation, the testosterone response to gonadotropin stimulation *in vitro* was elevated compared to controls, but a significant difference ($P < 0.01$) was only observed 4 weeks postoperatively. Mean $\pm$ s.e. ($n = 5$). *$P < 0.01$. compared to basal T production by control testes; **$P < 0.01$ compared to stimulated T production by control testes

cells, hCG is frequently used since its biological and immunological properties closely resemble those of LH. Several studies have demonstrated that damage to the seminiferous epithelium is accompanied by 50–60% loss of testicular LH/hCG receptors following surgical cryptorchidism (de Kretser *et al.*, 1979) fetal testicular irradiation (Rich and de Kretser, 1979) or efferent duct ligation (Risbridger *et al.*, 1981b). Although the cause of the reduction in the number of receptor sites for LH/hCG is not understood, the experimental induction of unilateral testicular damage by cryptorchidism or efferent duct ligation showed loss of these receptors whereas the contralateral intact testis showed no reduction in receptor number (Risbridger *et al.*, 1981a,b). These studies suggest that the function of Leydig cells in states of testicular damage is influenced by local factors elaborated from the damaged seminiferous epithelium, and emphasizes the interaction between the seminiferous tubules and the intertubular tissue.

Measurement of the binding of ^{125}I-hCG to testicular tissue *in vitro* thus provides a further indication of alterations to Leydig cell function.

The use of these methods in an evaluation of testicular function provides data on the integrity of the germ cells, the Sertoli cells and Leydig cells and assessment of the status of these cells is clearly important in understanding the sequence of events which may result in the disruption of the spermatogenic process. The techniques described in this report stress the importance of considering the structure and function of various cell types within the testis and requires that in assessing the effects of agents which disrupt testicular function, the testis should be considered as a whole and not simply as two or more functionally independent components.

5 REFERENCES

Bennett, H. S. and Luft, J. H. (1959). *s*-Collidine as a basis for buffering fixatives. *J. biophys. biochem. Cytol.* **6**, 113–114.

Bennett, H. S., Wyrick, A. D., Lee, S. W. and McNeil, J. H. (1976). Science and art in preparing tissues embedded in plastic for light microscopy, with special reference to glycol methacrylate, glass knives and simple stains. *Stain Technol.* **51**, 71–97.

Bergh, A. and Damber, J. E. (1978). Morphometric and functional investigation on the Leydig cells in experimental unilateral cryptorchidism in the rat. *Int. J. Androl.* **1**, 549–562.

Bergh, A. and Helander, H. F. (1978). Testicular development in the unilaterally cryptorchid rat. *Int. J. Androl.* **1**, 440–458.

Christensen, A. K. (1965). The fine structure of testicular interstitial cells in guinea pigs. *J. Cell Biol.* **26**, 911–935.

Christensen, A. K. and Peacock, K. C. (1980). Increase in Leydig cell number in testes of adult rats treated chronically with an excess of human chorionic gonadotropin. *Biol. Reprod.* **22**, 383–391.

Connell, C. J. (1978). A freeze-fracture and lanthanum tracer study of the complex junction between Sertoli cells of the canine testis. *J. Cell. Biol.* **76**, 57–75.

Damber, J. E., Bergh, A. and Janson, P. O. (1979). Testicular blood flow and testosterone concentrations in the spermatic venous blood in rats with experimental cryptorchidism. *Acta endocrinol.* **88**, 611–618.

Debeljuk, L., Arimura, A. and Schally, A. V. (1973). Pituitary and serum FSH and LH levels after massive and selective depletion of the germinal epithelium in the rat testis. *Endocrinology* **92**, 48–54.

de Kretser, D. M., Burger, H. G., Fortune, D., Hudson, B., Long, A. R., Paulsen, C. A. and Taft, H. P. (1972). Hormonal, histological and chromosomal studies in adult males with testicular disorders. *J. clin. Endocrinol. Metab.* **35**, 392–401.

de Kretser, D. M., Burger, H. G. and Hudson, B. (1974). The relationship between germinal cells and serum FSH levels in males with infertility. *J. clin. Endocrinol. Metab.* **38**, 787–793.

de Kretser, D. M., Sharpe, R. M. and Swanston, I. A. (1979). Alterations in steroidogenesis and human chorionic gonadotrophin binding in the crystorchid rat testis. *Endocrinology* **105**, 135–138.

Dym, M. (1973). The fine structure of the monkey (Macaca) Sertoli cell and its role in maintaining the blood-testis barrier. *Anat. Rec.* **175**, 639–656.

Dym, M. and Cavicchia, J. C. (1977). Further observations on the blood testis barrier in monkeys. *Biol. Reprod.* **17**, 390–403.

Dym, M. and Fawcett, D. W. (1970). The blood–testis barrier in the rat and the physiological compartmentation of the seminiferous epithelium. *Biol. Reprod.* **3**, 308–326.

Fawcett, D. W. (1975). Ultrastructure and function of the Sertoli cell. In Hamilton, D. W. and Greep, R. O. (Eds.) *Handbook of Physiology*, Vol. V Section 7: *Endocrinology*, pp. 21–55. Williams and Wilkins, Baltimore, Maryland.

Fawcett, D. W., Leak, L. V. and Heidger, P. M. (1970). Electron microscopic observations on the structural components of the blood–testis barrier. *J. Reprod. Fertil. Suppl.* **10**, 105–122.

Forssmann, W. G., Ito, S., Weine, E., Aoki, A., Dym, M. and Fawcett, D. W. (1977). An improved perfusion fixation method for the testis. *Anat. Rec.* **188**, 307–314.

Franchimont, P., Millet, D., Vendrely, E., Letane, J., Legros, J. J. and Netter, A. (1972). Relationship between spermatogenesis and serum gonadotrophin levels in azoospermia and oligospermia. *J. clin. Endocrinol. Metab.* **34**, 1003–1008.

Frankenhuis, M. T., Wiegeriuck, M. A. H. M., Schoorl, M., Kremer, J. and Wensing, C. J. G. (1979). The origin of orchiopexy-induced testicular lesions in the pig. *Fertl. Steril.* **32**, 583–587.

Gomes, W. R., Hall, R. W., Jain, S. K. and Boots, L. R. (1973). Serum gonadotrophin and testosterone levels during loss and recovery of spermatogenesis in rats. *Endocrinology* **93**, 800–809.

Hagenas, L. and Ritzen, E. M. (1976). Impaired Sertoli cell function in experimental cryptorchidism in the rat. *Mol. Cell Endocr.* **4**, 25–34.

Hagenas, L., Ritzen, E. M., Svensson, J., Hansson, V. and Purvis, K. (1978). Temperature dependence of Sertoli cell function. *Int. J. Androl. Suppl.* **2**, 449–456.

Hochereau-de Reviers, M-T., Blanc, M. R., Cahoreau, C., Courot, M., Dacheaux, J. L. and Pisselet, C. (1979). Histological testicular parameters in bilateral cryptorchid adult rams. *Ann. Biol. Anim. Biochim. Biophys.* **19**, 1141–1146.

Ito, S. and Karnovsky, M. J. (1968). Formaldehyde-glutaraldehyde fixatives containing trinitro compounds. *J. Cell Biol.* **39**, 168a–169a.

Jegou, B. and de Kretser, D. M. (1979). Early effects of experimental cryptorchidism on the rat testis and epididymis. *Proc. 11th Annual Conference, Australian Society for Reproductive Biology*, Perth. Abstract 39.

Karnovsky, M. J. (1965). A formaldehyde-glutaraldehyde fixative of high osmolarity for use in electron microscopy. *J. Cell Biol.* **27**, 137a.

Kerr, J. B. and de Kretser, D. M. (1975). Cyclic variations in Sertoli cell lipid content throughout the spermatogenic cycle in the rat. *J. Reprod. Fertil.* **43**, 1–8.

Kerr, J. B., Rich, K. A. and de Kretser, D. M. (1979a). Alterations of the fine structure and androgen secretion of the interstitial cells in the experimentally cryptorchid rat testis. *Biol. Reprod.* **20**, 409–422.

Kerr, J. B., Rich, K. A. and de Kretser, D. M. (1979b). The effects of experimental cryptorchidism on the ultrastructure and function of the Sertoli cell and peritubular tissue of the rat testis. *Biol. Reprod.* **21**, 823–838.

Leonard, J. M., Leach, R. B., Coutoure, M. and Paulsen, C. A. (1972). Plasma and urinary FSH levels in oligospermia. *J. clin. Endocrinol. Metab.* **34**, 209–214.

Mori, H. and Christensen, A. K. (1980). Morphometric analysis of Leydig cells in the normal rat testis. *J. Cell Biol.* **84**, 340–354.

Neaves, W. B. (1973). Permeability of Sertoli cell tight junctions to lanthanum after ligation of ductus deferens and ductuli efferentes. *J. Cell Biol.* **59**, 559–572.

Orth, J. and Christensen, A. K. (1977). Localisation of ^{125}I-labelled FSH in the testes of hypophysectomised rats by autoradiography at the light and electron microscope levels. *Endocrinology* **101**, 262–278.

Orth, J. and Christensen, A. K. (1978). Autoradiographic localisation of specifically bound ^{125}I-labelled follicle-stimulating hormone on spermatogenesis of the rat testis. *Endocrinology* **103**, 1944–1951.

Payne, A. H., Downing, J. R. and Wong, K-L. (1980). Luteinising hormone receptors and testosterone synthesis in two distinct populations of Leydig cells. *Endocrinology* **106**, 1424–1429.

Rich, K. A. and de Kretser, D. M. (1977a). Effects of differing degrees of destruction of the rat seminiferous epithelium on levels of serum FSH and androgen binding protein. *Endocrinology* **101**, 959–968.

Rich, K. A. and de Kretser, D. M. (1977b). Changes in the levels of FSH and LH in serum and androgen binding protein in the testis and epididymis of the rat following exposure of the testis to local heating. *Proc. Endocrine Soc. Aust.* **20**, p. 43 Abst.

Rich, K. A. and de Kretser, D. M. (1979). Effect of fetal irradiation on testicular receptors and testosterone response to gonadotrophin stimulation in adult rats. *Int. J. Androl.* **2**, 343–352.

Risbridger, G. P., Kerr, J. B. and de Kretser, D. M. (1981a). An evaluation of Leydig cell function and gonadotropin binding in unilateral and bilateral cryptorchidism: evidence for local control of Leydig cell function by the seminiferous tubules. *Biol. Reprod.* **24**, 534–540.

Risbridger, G. P., Kerr, J. B., Peake, R. A. and de Kretser, D. M. (1981b). An assessment of Leydig cell function after bilateral or unilateral efferent duct ligation: further evidence for local control of Leydig cell function. *Endocrinology* **109**, 1234–1241.

Ritzen, E. M., Hansson, V. and French, F. S. (1980). The Sertoli cell. In Burger, H. G. and de Kretser, D. M. (Eds.). *The Testis*, pp. 171–194. Raven Press, New York.

Rowley, M. J. and Heller, C. G. (1966). The testicular biopsy: surgical procedure, fixation and staining techniques. *Fertil. Steril.* **17**, 177–186.

Russell, L. D. (1978). The blood–testis barrier and its formation relative to spermatocyte maturation in the adult sat: a lanthanum tracer study. *Anat. Rec.* **190**, 99–112.

Russell, L. D. (1980). Sertoli-germ cell interrelations: a review, *Gamete Res.* **3**, 179–202.

Schumacher, M., Schafer, G., Holstein, A. F. and Hilz, H. (1978). Rapid isolation of mouse Leydig cells by centrifugation in Percoll density gradients with complete retention of morphological and biochemical integrity. *Fedr. Eur. Biochem. Soc. Lett.* **91**, 33–338.

Scott, R. S., Burger, H. G. and Quigg, H. (1980). A simple and rapid in vitro bioassay for inhibin. *Endocrinology* **107**, 1536–1542.

Smith, G. (1962). The effects of ligation of the vasa efferentia and vasectomy on testicular function in the adult rat. *J. Endocrinol.* **23**, 385–399.

Stefanini, M., De Martino, C. and Samboni, L. (1967). Fixation of ejaculated spermatozoa for electron microscopy. *Nature (London)* **216**, 173–174.

Steinberger, A. and Steinberger, E. (1976). Secretion of an FSH-inhibiting factor by cultured Sertoli cells. *Endocrinology* **99**, 918–921.

Steinberger, A. and Steinberger, E. (1977). Inhibition of FSH by a Sertoli cell factor *in vitro*. In Troen, P. and Nankin, H. R. (Eds.) *The Testis in Normal and Infertile Men*, pp. 271–279. Raven Press, New York.

Verjans, H. L. and Eik-Nes, K. B. (1976). Hypothalamic–pituitary–testicular system following testicular X-irradiation. *Acta Endocrinol.* **83**, 190–200.

Vitale, R. Fawcett, D. W. and Dym, (1973). The normal development of the blood–testis barrier and the effects of clomiphene and estrogen treatment. *Anat. Rec.* **176**, 333–344.

Walsh, P. C. and Swerdloff, R. S. (1973). Experimental cryptorchidism: effect on serum FSH and LH in the rat. *Urol. Res.* **1**, 22–26.

Zirkin, B. R., Ewing, L. L., Kromann, N. and Cochran, R. C. (1980). Testosterone secretion by rat, rabbit, guinea pig, dog and hamster testes perfused *in vitro*: correlation with Leydig cell ultrastructure. *Endocrinology* **107**, 1867–1874.

Methods for Assessing the Effects of Chemicals on Reproductive Functions
Edited by V. B. Vouk and P. J. Sheehan
© 1983 SCOPE

Morphological and Chemical Methods of Semen Analysis for Quantitating Damage to Male Reproductive Function in Man

RUNE ELIASSON

1 INTRODUCTION

This review will provide only a few references to publications dealing with adverse effects of chemicals or drugs. The main aim is to present techniques and principles for the analysis of human semen. However, recent publications are listed giving further important details of semen analysis and interested readers should consult these publications (Belsey *et al.*, 1980; Eliasson, 1981).

The analysis of human semen has been formerly carried out mainly when a couple had an infertility problem and the woman had been found more or less free from pathology that could explain the barren union. This and other forms of bias in the selection of men have given most clinicians and scientists a wrong view of the 'normal' values for various semen variables. Only analysis of semen specimens from men who are representative of the normal male population should be used to assess the 'normal limits'. Such limits are generally defined as equal to the 95% confidence limits which can be calculated in different ways (see Martin *et al.*, 1975). There is no reason to believe that the limits for 'normal' are the same for semen from young and older men. Nor should we expect the 'normal' limits to be the same in all countries or among all ethnic groups.

The limits for 'normal' should not be linked with 'fertility' since it is well documented that an 'abnormal' semen sample is not necessarily incompatible with fertility. For future work on the relation between semen qualities and environmental chemicals and drugs we urgently require access to relevant data from different well-characterized male populations. In addition, all semen samples must be collected, transported and analysed according to standards permitting comparative studies.

Disturbances in semen quality can be caused not only by such exogenous factors as chemicals, radiation, and heat but also by a number of more or less trivial or short illnesses, such as a throat infection, a virus infection with fever, or vaccinations. Control samples and control groups are therefore essential in most

263

studies related to the possible effects of various environmental factors on semen quality.

Although it is known that supervening diseases, drugs, and chemicals can influence semen qualities such as sperm count, motility and morphology, it should be emphasized that some methods discussed in this review have not as yet been proven to be useful in the study of environmental hazards. In this respect experience is still limited.

2 GENERAL EXAMINATION OF MAN

In studies aiming at an understanding of the possible effects of environmental factors on the male reproductive organs it is not sufficient to restrict the investigations to semen analysis. One must perform careful clinical examinations of the man to exclude malformations, 'silent' or subclinical infections and other diseases. Production by the testes of spermatozoa (but not of hormones) is well correlated with testicular size, and measurements of the testes are therefore important. Testicular size should be given in ml and the easiest and most accurate method is to assess it with a standard orchidometer like that of Prader (see Eliasson, 1978; Eliasson and Johannisson, 1978; Johannison and Eliasson, 1978).

3 COLLECTION OF SEMEN

In normal clinical research and clinical laboratory procedures it is suggested that all methods should be carefully standardized. If we know that fasting of a patient is likely to influence the variable we are measuring (e.g. cholesterol or blood sugar) the patient should be instructed to follow certain rules, e.g. fasting for 12 hours. Within-individual, interindividual, and interlaboratory comparison of data is possible only if the techniques for collection and analysis of semen have been previously standardized.

Since the *duration of abstinence* before collection of a semen sample can influence its properties (e.g. volume and count) this variable must be standardized. According to present recommendations from WHO the time interval should be 2–5 days (Belsey *et al.*, 1980; see also Schwartz *et al.*, 1979).

Semen should be *collected* by masturbation and not during coitus. Interrupted intercourse frequently results in the loss of the first (sperm-rich) portion of the ejaculate and also carries the risk of contamination with vaginal fluid which might cause a decrease in motility and viability of the spermatozoa. Plastic condoms can be used provided one has found that they do not interfere with any of the analyses. Rubber condoms contain spermicidal compounds which might affect chemical analyses.

4 VOLUME

The volume of semen is influenced by the admixture of the accessory genital glands which in turn depends on the secretory output of these glands, and the time interval between ejaculations. The volume should be assessed by weight or with a calibrated centrifuge tube but not with a pipette. Samples exhibiting excess viscosity can be accurately measured only by the weight method. Normal values for men between 20 and 50 years of age are 2–6 ml.

Low volumes can be due to a disturbed secretory function of the seminal vesicles, sometimes combined with a low secretory function of the prostate, and also, partially, to retrograde ejaculation; examination of a urine sample taken immediately after ejaculation can in most cases provide the correct explanation. The combination of a very low volume (< 0.5 ml) with azoospermia, low pH (6.4–6.7) and lack of fructose in the seminal plasma is typical for semen of a man with congenital absence of the seminal vesicles and the ampullae of the deferent ducts. Frequently such men also lack the vas deferentia and parts of the epididymides.

5 SPERM COUNT

Most techniques require a dilution of the semen before a sample is taken for the assessment of sperm count. For this purpose it is essential to use a completely liquefied and well-mixed specimen before the semen is diluted and the sperm concentration determined. The degree of dilution (e.g. 1 : 10, 1 : 50 or 1 : 100) depends upon the initial sperm concentration. The dilution must be precise and the subsequent mixing carefully carried out. A suitable diluent is composed of 50 g $NaHCO_3$, 10 ml of 35% formalin, 5 ml saturated aqueous gentian violet, and distilled water up to 1000 ml. When a phase-contrast microscope is used, it is unnecessary to use gentian violet. After a drop of the diluted semen has been transferred to the counting chamber it should be left in a moist chamber for at least 10–15 minutes to allow the cells to sediment. The commonly used white blood cell pipette does not give an accurate enough dilution or mixing (see Freund and Carol, 1964). At dilution higher than 1 : 100 there is a risk of adhesion of the spermatozoa to the glass surface which will introduce a significant error.

Since the volume of the seminal plasma is not regulated by a homoeostatic mechanism, one should express the final result of semen analysis by giving the sperm *count per ejaculate.* and not merely in terms of concentration per ml. A 2 ml semen sample with a total of 120 million spermatozoa will have 60 million/ ml, but a 6 ml sample with a total of 120 million spermatozoa would have only 20 million/ml. To report one of these samples as 'normal' and the other as 'oligozoospermic' is incorrect, particularly if one is interested in the output of spermatozoa in semen.

The normal limits (for the Swedish population) are from 25 to 400 million spermatozoa per ejaculate. However, sperm counts below 25 million per ejaculate are *not* incompatible with fertility. In studies aiming at the early detection of adverse effects—and thereby making it possible to prevent damages to the germinal epithelium—one should primarily look for *changes* in the sperm output (and sperm motility, morphology, etc.) and pay less attention to the results from single analysis.

6 MOTILITY OF SPERMATOZOA

There is a good correlation between sperm motility soon after ejaculation and male fertility and there is evidence that motility is a very sensitive indicator of sperm function. The motility of the spermatozoa must always be evaluated with regard to three variables:

(1) progressive (or qualitative) motility, usually expressed in terms of a mean progressive motility score like good, medium, poor, and none (in protocol often coded as 0 = none, 1 = poor, etc.);
(2) percentage of motile spermatozoa, usually presented with 5% intervals since the precision is not higher; and
(3) time after ejaculation, expressed in hours.

Human spermatozoa can show good motility and viability in the seminal plasma 24 hours after ejaculation but in some semen samples the motility declines much faster. A rapid decline in motility could be due to infections (e.g. *E. coli*), a prostatic dysfunction or a disturbed order of emission of fluids from the prostate and seminal vesicles, but in many instances one is unable to identify the cause. There is no known correlation between 'survival' in the seminal plasma and fertility. One reason could be that spermatozoa soon after ejaculation leave the seminal plasma and enter the cervical mucus.

Addition of human serum albumin to semen immediately after the ejaculation can lead in about 50% of samples characterized by a rapidly declining sperm motility to a significant prolongation of the motility. This indicates that the composition of the seminal plasma is of importance for normal sperm motility and viability (see Lindholmer, 1974).

Several methods for objective registration of sperm motility have recently been published (see Jouannet *et al.*, 1977; Makler, 1978; Dott, 1979), but despite this, most laboratories are using the subjective rating and with experienced technicians this shows a good reproducibility (see Jouannet, 1977).

Values compatible with fertility are > 40% motile spermatozoa with a mean progressive motility score of 'medium' or 'good' less than 1 hour after ejaculation. Low motility of ejaculated spermatozoa is probably a more sensitive indicator of disturbed testicular (and epididymal) function than sperm count, and there are several reports that motility declines before there is a decrease in sperm output when men or animals are exposed to toxic chemicals.

Sperm motility in either cervical mucus or some other suitable medium is of great value in the work-up of men with an infertility problem but the usefulness of such laboratory tests for studies on potentially harmful xenobiotic factors is unknown. It seems safe to assume that environmental factors will not primarily induce production of sperm immobilizing or agglutinating antibodies. The tests would therefore most likely only reflect the general motility of the spermatozoa.

7 SUPRAVITAL STAINING TECHNIQUES

It is important to distinguish between live and dead spermatozoa when there is < 40% motile spermatozoa. This can be done with a supravital stain like eosin Y.

(1) A 0.5% solution of eosin Y in 0.15 M phosphate buffer is mixed with an equal volume of semen and after 1 minute a thin smear is made on a clean microscope slide. The smear is dried in air and then examined with a microscope with *negative* (i.e. anopthral) phase-contrast equipment and an 100 × objective (oil immersion). The live cells are light bluish (or violet) and the dead ones are yellow. Some cells are 'half-stained' and this can cause confusion. If a part of the cell is bright yellow it should be classified as 'dead'.

(2) Many laboratories are not equipped with a negative phase-contrast microscope, and in this case the following technique can be used. One volume of semen (usually a drop) is mixed with two volumes of an eosin Y solution (1% in distilled water). After 30 seconds three volumes of a 10% nigrosin solution (in distilled water) are added and the sample is mixed. A thin smear is then made immediately and air dried. Such a smear can be examined under normal oil immersion microscopy (100 × objective). Live spermatozoa are unstained (white) and the dead ones are red. (For ref. see Eliasson and Treichl, 1971; Eliasson, 1977.)

8 MORPHOLOGY

To assess properly the sperm morphology one must employ a staining technique which visualizes not only the head (incl acrosome) but also the midpiece, protoplasmic droplet (if present) and tail. Acceptable staining techniques are for example the slight modification of the Papanicolaou, the Blom, and the Bryan–Leishman techniques. (For details see Belsey *et al.*, 1980; Eliasson, 1981.)

In the past, most studies have been restricted to the morphology of the sperm head. Furthermore, in some publications immature germ cells have been included in defining the frequency distribution of the spermatozoa. This is unfortunate as illustrated by the following example. If a semen sample contains 30% 'immature cells', 20% 'oval heads', etc., the observer has actually counted 70 sperm heads (= 70 spermatozoa) plus 30 'immature cells'. The true frequency of 'oval heads' per 100 *spermatozoa* is then 29% (20/70 = 0.29). It is therefore difficult to compare results from such studies with those in which 'immature cells' were not included in the frequency distribution of 'spermatozoa'.

In the present review the term 'normal' morphology does not refer to anything other than 'a configuration which presently is defined as normal for head, midpiece, *and* tail'. To make comparisons between different laboratories possible, a common technique for assessment is necessary. Preferably the WHO recommendations should be generally accepted, thereby allowing a better agreement

Table 1   Principles for morphological assessment of human spermatoza

Classification	Length (μm)	Width (μm)	Remarks
Normal spermatozoa			
Head	3.0–5.0	2.0–3.0	Regular oval shape. Borderline forms are assessed as normal
Midpiece	5.0–7.0	Approx. 1	
Tail	40–50		
Abnormal head			
Too large	> 5.0	> 3.0	As long as the shape approximates an oval, it is to be counted primarily according to its size (large, small, tapering)
Too small	< 3.0	< 2.0	
Tapering	> 5.0	< 3.0	Ratio length: width > 1.8
	< 5.0	< 2.0	
Amorphous			Various irregular forms including those with a combination of irregular and elongated shape
Duplicate			
Pear-shaped			Between oval and tapering, regular shape. Irregular forms are regarded as amorphous. Borderline as normal
Abnormal midpiece	> 8.0	> 2.0	Missing or broken midpieces are also abnormal.
Abnormal cytoplasmic droplet.			When larger than half of the sperm head
Abnormal tail			e.g. broken, coiled (not bent nor asymmetrical insertion), or short tails

From Eliasson, R. (1981). Analysis of semen. In Burger, H. and de Kretser, D. (Eds.) *The Testis.* Raven Press, New York.

on what is 'normal' for different populations (see Belsey *et al.*, 1980; Eliasson, 1981).

Guidelines for classification of human spermatozoa are presented in Table 9.1. It is, however, impossible to learn how to classify spermatozoa from this table in such a way that accurate comparisons can be made with other observers; to classify spermatozoa, training with the assistance and supervision by an experienced person is required. Training centres and established ways for interlaboratory controls are therefore extremely important.

It appears that human male fertility is significantly affected when semen samples contain more than 50% abnormal sperm heads and/or more than 25% defective midpieces and/or more than 25% defective tails.

There is no doubt that chemicals (and perhaps also smoking and alcohol) can induce changes in the morphology of the human spermatozoa. We don't know whether—or to what extent—such changes will affect subsequent generations, nor do we know to what degree different changes in morphology will affect fertility (for reference see Wyrobek and Bruce, 1978; Joffe, 1979). When semen samples from the same individual are analysed over a period of many years the sperm morphology is surprisingly constant (Hartman *et al.*, 1964; MacLeod, 1974; Eliasson and Samuelsson, to be published). A *change* in morphology is therefore an indicator of exposure to a mutagenic agent (provided one can exclude factors like infections, allergic reactions, etc.) and should always be given attention.

In summary, sperm morphology is probably a sensitive indicator of adverse effects. However, we do need many more well-planned and well-conducted studies to understand the significance of different abnormalities.

9 QUANTITATIVE ASSESSMENT OF CELLS OTHER THAN SPERMATOZOA IN THE SEMEN

As discussed earlier, spermatids and other immature cells resulting from spermatogenesis should not be reported as part of the differential count of the spermatozoa. Spermatids, spermatocytes, white blood cells (WBC), etc. should instead be recorded as number of cells of each type per ml of per ejaculate. One method to do this is to count the number of a given cell type (X-cells) found in the stained smear within the same fields as *100 spermatozoa* and then apply the formula:

$$\text{number of X-cells per ml} = \frac{\text{Spz} \times X}{100}$$

where Spz is the number of spermatozoa per ml in the ejaculate and Y is the number of X-cells counted in the same fields as those containing 100 spermatozoa. A normal semen sample should not contain any immature cells. Their occurrence is a sign of disturbance in the testis. The occurrence of immature cells in semen from men exposed to potentially toxic factors should always be regarded as an indication of an adverse effect.

Normal semen does not contain leucocytes. Their presence can indicate a genital infection, an allergic or immune reaction in the accessory glands, or be due to a long period of abstinence (> 10 days). The absence of leucocytes in semen is no proof that there is no infection or inflammation in the accessory genital glands. Haemospermia is frequently a sign of an inflammation in the seminal vesicles or in the prostate but may also occur without any demonstrable dysfunction or disease in these glands.

10 CHROMATIN DECONDENSATION

During their passage through the epididymis spermatozoa undergo a maturation process. One example of such a change is the increased stability and condensation of the chromatin. Epididymal spermatozoa undergo decondensation and swelling in the presence of sodium dodecyl sulphate (SDS). Ejaculated spermatozoa from all subhuman mammalian species studied are, on the other hand, resistant when exposed to SDS. Pretreatment of ejaculated spermatozoa with thiol reducing agents (e.g. dithiothreitol) induces immediate swelling in a SDS solution. The resistance to SDS alone is therefore most likely reflecting a degree of maturation of the spermatozoa (Bedford *et al.*, 1973b). When the spermatozoon has entered the egg, the chromatin must undergo a decondensation to form the male pronucleus which then fuses with the female equivalent. A disturbed ability to undergo decondensation at the right time can therefore be a serious abnormality.

Ejaculated human spermatozoa are less resistant than those from subhuman species. In semen from fertile men one usually finds 10–30% spermatozoa which have undergone swelling if exposed to a 1% solution of SDS (Bedford *et al.*, 1973a; Kvist and Eliasson, 1980). In semen samples from men with an infertility problem it is not uncommon to find > 40% of the spermatozoa to be affected by SDS indicating a relation between chromatin decondensation ability and fertility (Eliasson and Enquist, 1981). The SDS test is, however, not a specific measure of 'epididymal maturation' of human spermatozoa since the composition of the seminal plasma can influence the reactivity and this must therefore be controlled (Kvist *et al.*, 1980; Kvist and Eliasson, 1980).

To test the nuclear decondensation ability, one part of semen (or washed spermatozoa) is mixed with nine parts of 1% SDS in 0.05 M sodium borate buffer, pH 9.0. The reaction is stopped after 2 hours by adding an equal volume of 2.5% glutaraldehyde in 0.05 M sodium borate buffer, pH 9.0. The degree of nuclear swelling is semi-quantitatively assessed under phase-contrast microscopy (500 × magnification) and scored as indicated in Table 2.

Men taking the drug sulphasalazine usually have semen samples with a lower than normal percentage of stable spermatozoa (observations to be published). In

Table 2   Classification of the swelling of the heads of ejaculated human spermatozoa exposed to sodium dodecyl sulphate

Classification	Description
Stable	No visible change in sperm head configuration or light refraction
Moderately swollen	Nucleus has started to swell, darkened and the light refraction almost disappeared.
Grossly swollen	The 'size' of the head has increased > 5 times and the nucleus has almost the same light transmission as the background

another unpublished study we have noted that spermatozoa from men moderately exposed to lead had spermatozoa which were more resistant than those from a control group of unexposed men. If this could be confirmed it would indicate that lead may in some way interact with, an stabilize, the S–S bonds in the chromatin. Spermatozoa unable to undergo decondensation cannot fertilize an egg and the observation is thus of a general biological interest. It should be emphasized that the within-individual variations are small under normal conditions and changes should therefore be regarded as a sign of an adverse effect.

11 ETHIDIUM BROMIDE UPTAKE BY SPERMATOZOA

Ethidium bromide (EB) binds specifically to double-stranded polynucleotides and the amount can be assessed by microspectrofluorimetric analysis. The uptake of this fluorescent stain decreases with maturation of the spermatozoa; ejaculated normal human spermatozoa have about 50–60% of the fluorescence value found in spermatides of the Sab type (Johannisson *et al.*, 1982).

A thin smear of semen is made on a clean glass slide and immediately fixed for 30 min with methanol. The smear is stained with EB (7.5 μg/ml distilled water), air dried and examined under oil immersion (objective 54 $\times$) in a microfluorometer equipped for incident light. The excitation light is 546nm and the emission observed at 590 nm. The fluorescence emission is measured using a photomultiplier highly sensitive for red fluorescence light and expressed in arbitrary units with a standard population of lymphocytes as diploid reference cells.

The RNA interference can be eliminated (and quantitatively measured) by treatment of separate smears with RNAse for 30 min at 37 °C before staining with EB (see Johannisson *et al.*, 1982).

Spermatozoa from men taking sulphasalazine and from men with infertility problems frequently have higher fluorescence values than spermatozoa from men whose wives are pregnant in the first trimester (Johannisson and Eliasson, 1981). It is unlikely that the difference is due to different amounts of DNA and the assessment of EB uptake by the spermatozoa is therefore of value in the analysis of the post-testicular sperm 'maturation' (see also Gledhill, 1970).

12 RELEASE OF ENZYMES FROM SPERMATOZOA

Spermatozoa from many species contain an isoenzyme of lactic dehydrogenase (LDH-X or LDH-C4) which is sperm specific. The occurrence of this isoenzyme in the seminal plasma can be used for assessing damage to the sperm membranes (see Eliasson *et al.*, 1967). Most likely other sperm-specific isoenzymes could also be used for such an assessment.

Our present technique for separating and analysing the LDH-C4 activity in human seminal plasma is the same as previously published (Eliasson *et al.*, 1967) with minor modifications. The semen sample (> 0.8 ml) is allowed to liquefy and then placed in a water bath at 37 °C for 4 hours. The sample is centrifuged twice at 1000 × g and the seminal plasma removed for further analysis. The total LDH activity is assayed by the NADH method. The electrophoresis is performed on agarose gels at pH. The bands are identified with the nitro-blue tetrazolium staining method and the quantitative assessment is made with a densitometer. The activity is expressed in nanokatal per 10^8 spermatozoa.

Semen from fertile men have a mean releases of 10 nkat/10^8 spermatozoa (95% confidence limits 5–27). There is a significantly higher activity in many semen samples from men with a barren union (mean for the whole group 20 nkat/10^8 spermatozoa). In a separate group of men taking sulphasalazine the mean activity of LDH-C4 was about 40 nkat/10^8 spermatozoa and there are reasons to believe that this is due to the drug and not the underlying disease. The occurrence of testicular cells in the semen will give false high values. (Eliasson *et al.*, 1980, and to be published).

13 FORMATION OF LIPID PEROXIDES BY THE SPERMATOZOA

Disintegration of biological membranes is accompanied by the formation of lipid peroxides (LPO) and measurements of LPO formation by spermatozoa could therefore reflect stability of the membranes. The method has only been used in a few studies on human spermatozoa and its usefulness for detecting toxic factors is unknown. There are, however, significant differences in the LPO formation by spermatozoa from different men. The secretory function of the prostate and seminal vesicles, respectively, seems to be of importance for the LPO forming capacity by *washed* human spermatozoa.

14 DETERMINATION OF ZINC AND OTHER IONS IN SPERMATOZOA

Seminal plasma is very rich in zinc (and many other metal ions) and the spermatozoa must therefore be separated from the plasma before an analysis of their zinc content can be made. Ordinary washing procedures involve a great risk of zinc losses and for the isolation procedure one should therefore use centrifugation through an indifferent medium (e.g. Ficoll or sucrose) (For reference see Arver and Eliasson, 1980).

We know that zinc can influence several functional properties of the spermatozoa. We also know that spermatozoa from men with a disturbed prostate function have an abnormal uptake of zinc and that spermatozoa from 'fertile' men have lower zinc content than spermatozoa from 'infertile' men. The zinc content of spermatozoa can be of importance for their fertilizing ability and it should therefore be of interest to further clarify how the content of zinc and other metal ions is influenced by different endogenous and exogenous factors.

15 SECRETORY FUNCTION OF THE ACCESSORY GENITAL GLANDS

The secretory function of the accessory genital glands should be assessed in all studies related to the functional properties of the spermatozoa since the composition of the plasma can influence the functional properties of the spermatozoa. The secretory function of the prostate is evaluated by analysing e.g. acid phosphatase activity, citric acid, zinc, and/or magnesium. The secretory function of the seminal vesicles is usually assessed from the fructose concentration but prostaglandins are also specific products. Since the different glands are functionally 'multiglandular' it is recommended that more than one factor from each gland be studied. No factor has been proven suitable for evaluation of the secretory function of human epididymis or bulbourethral glands.

The volume of the seminal plasma is not regulated by homoeostatic mechanisms and one should therefore always give due attention to the volume when specific secretory products are analysed or give the total amounts (or activity) instead of concentrations or relative activities.

During ejaculation the different glands discharge their products in a specific sequence. In the healthy human male the first part of the ejaculate contains fluids from the prostate and the ampullae of the deferent ducts and thus also the bulk of the spermatozoa. The last part contains mainly fluid from the seminal vesicles.

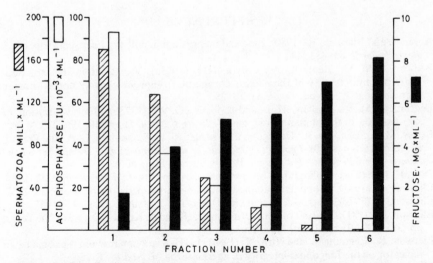

Figure 1   Distribution of spermatozoa, acid phosphatase activity, and fructose concentration in six fractions of split ejaculate. (From Eliasson, R. and Lindholmer, C. (1976). Functions of male accessory genital organs. In Hafez, E.S.E. (Ed.) *Human Semen and Fertility Regulation in Men*. The C. V. Mosby Co., St. Louis.)

The distribution patterns can be studied by collecting the semen as a 'split-ejaculate' in at least four portions; they are illustrated in Figure 9.1 (Lundquist, 1979; Eliasson and Lindholmer, 1976). Since each individual has a specific pattern and there is no guarantee that even the same man at different occasions will have the same amount of fluid in each fraction one cannot pool the data and calculate means and standard deviations.

The collection of an ejaculate with the split-ejaculate technique is very helpful in studies of the excretion of specific products into the semen and it also permits one to understand the nature and magnitude of ejaculatory dysfunctions. Even minor disturbances of the nerves regulating the emission could have a serious effect on the ejaculation process. If the spermatozoa are discharge together with the vesicular fluid instead of the prostatic fluid their motility and survival are adversely affected. (For reference see Eliasson and Lindholmer, 1976).

The possible importance of the accessory genital glands and their secretory products for the functional properties of the human spermatozoa and for male fertility has long been neglected and our knowledge in this field is therefore limited. However, extended biochemical analyses of the seminal plasma will in the future give information of importance for an early detection of disease and adverse effects of xenobiotic factors on the accessory genital glands and also increase our understanding of the role of these glands in human reproduction. The published evidence supporting these views should stimulate research in this field.

16 REFERENCES

Arver, S. and Eliasson, R. (1980). Zinc and magnesium in bull and boar spermatozoa. *J. Reprod. Fertil.* **60**, 481–484.

Bedford, J. M. M., Bent, J., and Calvin, H. I. (1973a). Variations in the structural character and stability of the nuclear chromatin in morphologically normal human spermatozoa. *J. Reprod. Fertil.* **33**, 19–29.

Bedford, J. M. M., Calvin, H. I. and Cooper, G. W. (1973b). The maturation of spermatozoa in the human epididymis. *J. Reprod. Fertil. Suppl.* **18**, 199–213.

Belsey, M. A., Eliasson, R., Gallegos, A. J., Moghissi, K. S., Paulsen, C. A. and Prasad, M. R. N. (Eds.) (1980). *Laboratory Manual for the Examination of Human Semen and Semen–Cervical Mucus Interaction.* Press Concern, Singapore.

Dott, H. M. (1979). Bibliography on spermatozoan motility. *Bibliogr. Reprod.* **32**, 1–84.

Eliasson, R. (1977). Supravital staining of human spermatozoa. *Fertil. Steril.* **28**, 1257.

Eliasson, R. (1978). Diagnosis in male infertility. *Int. J. Androl. Suppl.* **1**, 53–65.

Eliasson, R. (1981). Analysis of semen. In Burger, H. and de Kretser, D. (Eds.) *The Testis*, pp. 381–399. Raven Press, New York.

Eliasson, R., Eliasson, L. and Virji, N. (1980). LDH-X in human seminal plasma as an indicator of the functional integrity of spermatozoa. *J. Androl.* **1**, 76.

Eliasson, R. and Enqvist, A. M. (1981). Chromatin stability of the human spermatozoa in relation to male fertility. *Int. J. Androl. Suppl.* **3**, 73–74.

Eliasson, R., Häggman, K. and Wiklund, B. (1967). Lactate dehydrogenase in human seminal plasma. *Scand. J. clin. Lab. Invest.* **20**, 353–359.

Eliasson, R. and Johannisson, E. (1978). Cytological studies of prostatic fluids from men with and without abnormal palpatory findings of the prostate—II. Clinical application. *Int. J. Androl.* **1**, 582–588.

Eliasson, R. and Lindholmer, C. (1976). Functions of male accessory genital organs. In Hafez, E. (Ed.) *Human Semen and Fertility Regulation*, pp. 321–331. Mosby Co., St. Louis.

Eliasson, R. and Treichl, L. (1971). Supravital staining of human spermatozoa. *Fertil. Steril.* **22**, 134–137.

Freund, M. and Carol, B. (1964). Factors affecting haemocytometer counts of sperm concentration in human semen. *J. Reprod. Fertil.* **8**, 149–155.

Gledhill, B. L. (1970). Changes in nuclear stainability associated with spermateliosis, spermatozoal maturation, and male infertility. In Wied, G. L. and Bahr, G. F. (Eds.) *Introduction to Quantitative Cytochemistry—II*, pp. 125–151. Academic Press, New York, San Francisco, London.

Hartman, C. G., Schoenfeld, C. and Coperland, E. (1964). Individualism in the semen picture of infertile men. *Fertil. Steril.* **15**, 231–253.

Joffe, J. M. (1979). Influence of drug exposure of the father on perinatal outcome. *Clin. Perinatol.* **6**, 21–36.

Johannisson, E. and Eliasson, R. (1978). Cytological studies of prostatic fluids from men with and without abnormal palpatory findings of the prostate. *Int. J. Androl.* **1**, 201–212.

Johannisson, E. and Eliasson, R. (1981). Ethidium bromide uptake by spermatozoa from fertile and infertile men. *Int. J. Androl. Suppl.* **3**, 72–73.

Johannisson, E., Norén, S., Riotton, G. and Eliasson, R. (1982). Microfluorometrical assessment of the sperm maturation in testicular biopsies from men with histological normal or reduced spermatogenesis. *Int. J. Androl.* **5**, 11–12.

Jouannet, P., Volochine, B., Deguert, P., Serres, C., and David, G. (1977). Light scattering determination of various characteristic parameters of spermatozoa motility in a series of human sperm. *Andrologia*, **9**, 36–49.

Kvist, U., Afzelius, B. and Nilsson, L. (1980). The intrinsic mechanism of chromatin decondensation and its activation in human spermatozoa. *Develop. Growth Differ.* **22**, 543–554.

Kvist, U. and Eliasson, R. (1980). Influence of seminal plasma on the chromatin stability of ejaculated human spermatozoa. *Int. J. Androl.* **3**, 130–142.

Lindholmer, C. (1974). The importance of seminal plasma for human sperm motility. *Biol Reprod.* **10**, 533–542.

Lundqvist, F. (1949). Aspects of the biochemistry of human semen. *Acta physiol. scand.* **19**, Suppl. **66**.

MacLeod, J. (1974). Effects of environmental factors and of antispermatogenic compounds on the human testis as reflected in seminal cytology. In Mancini, R. E. and Martini, L. (Eds.) *Male Fertility and Sterility*, pp. 123–148. Academic Press, New York, San Francisco, London.

Makler, A. (1978). A New multiple exposure photography method for objective human spermatozoal motility determination. *Fertil. Steril.* **30**, 192–199.

Martin, H. F., Gudzinowicz, B. J. and Fanger, H. (1975). *Normal Values in Clinical Chemistry*. Marcel Decker, Inc., New York.

Schwartz, A., Laplanche, P., Jouannet, P. and David, G. (1979). Within-Subject variability of human semen in regard to sperm count, volume, total number of spermatozoa and length of abstinence. *J. Reprod. Fertil.* **57**, 391–395.

Wyrobek, A. J. and Bruce, W. R. (1978). The induction of sperm-shape abnormalities in mice and humans. In Hollaender, A. and de Serres, F. J. (Eds.) *Chemical Mutagens: Principles and Methods for Their Detection*, Vol. 5, pp. 257–285. Plenum Press, New York.

Methods for Assessing the Effects of Chemicals on Reproductive Functions
Edited by V. B. Vouk and P. J. Sheehan
© 1983 SCOPE

The Mammalian Embryo and Fetus in vitro

D. A. T. NEW

1 CULTURE SYSTEMS

Culture systems have a number of advantages for the study of mammalian embryos. They allow close and continuous observation at all stages of embryonic development, and of embryos too small to be observed in the uterus. They also allow precise control of experimental conditions, and enable a clear distinction to be made between direct effects of a treatment on the embryo and those resulting from interaction between the treatment and the maternal metabolism.

For a culture system to be of value in assessing the effects of chemicals, it is essential that it be capable of supporting normal growth of 'control' embryos. Although all stages of embryo/fetal development can be maintained in culture, there are at present only two periods of development that can be supported with a high level of reliability. They are:

(1) egg to blastocyst (preimplantation stages)—particularly of mouse and rabbit;
(2) early fetus (organogenesis)—of mouse and rat.

Methods for culturing eggs and blastocysts have been available for many years and are well known. They provide a simple method for testing the effects of chemicals on the earliest stages of development. However, these preimplantation embryos have considerable capacity for recovery after injury, and it is the later stages of development, particularly during early organogenesis, which are the most susceptible to permanent damage. Culture methods that will maintain embryos during organogenesis (New, 1978a) seem therefore likely to be of particular value for assessing embryotoxic effects of chemicals, and most of the following account will be concerned with them.

1.1 Types of Embryo Culture Systems

The main types of culture systems in use in our laboratory are shown in Figure 1.

(a) petri dish cultures. The nutrient medium is placed either as drops under a layer of mineral oil, or is contained in a watchglass. Such cultures with static

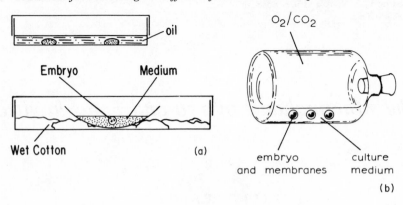

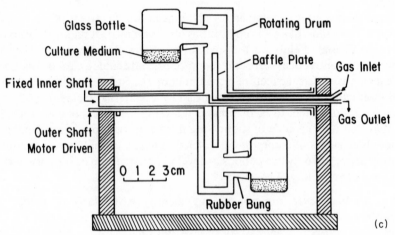

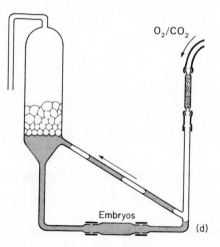

Figure 1 Embryo culture systems. (a) Petri dish cultures; (b) roller bottle; (c) rotator; (d) circulator

(non-flowing) medium support the growth of eggs and blastocysts, and of postimplantation embryos up to early limb-bud stages (25–30 somites).

(b) Roller bottles. The culture vessels are small cylindrical bottles in which part of the available volume is filled with nutrient medium (usually rat serum) and the remainder with the required $O_2/N_2/CO_2$ mixture. The bottles are laid horizontally on rollers and rotated at 30–60 rev/min during incubation. This method supports better development of postimplantation embryos, and to more advanced stages, than can be obtained in static medium. It is also particularly useful in experiments to test the effect of an agent on embryonic development; the continuous movement ensures maximum and even exposure of the embryo to the agent.

(c) Rotator. In this system, small culture bottles are attached to a hollow rotating drum. The oxygenating gas is passed continuously through the drum during the culture period. The method provides a constant O_2 and CO_2 level and minimum variation of pH in the culture medium.

(d) Circulator. The embryos are anchored in a small chamber through which a continuous flow of medium is maintained. The medium is oxygenated and caused to flow by a stream of bubbles passing up a sloping tube. Because the

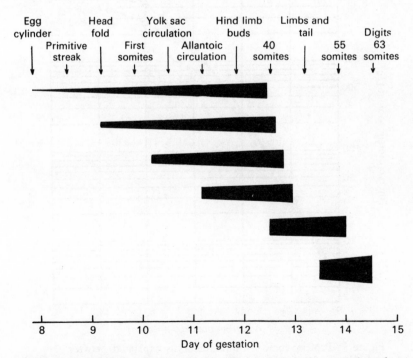

Figure 2 Periods of development in culture of rat embryos explanted at different stages of organogenesis

embryos are fixed in position, the method allows them to be observed continuously throughout the culture period.

1.2 Duration and Rate of Growth

Figure 2 shows the periods of development of postimplantation rat embryos that can be maintained in culture. Embryos placed in culture at egg-cylinder (8 day) stage can be maintained for 4–5 days and grow to 30–40 somite stages. Embryos placed in culture at later stages develop for progressively shorter periods.

Figure 3 compares rates of protein synthesis by rat embryos *in vivo* and *in vitro*. Up to the $11\frac{1}{2}$-day stage, the rate of protein synthesis *in vitro* is indistinguishable from that *in vivo*; after this, the embryos *in vitro* grow more slowly (although rates of organ differentiation remain nearly normal). The

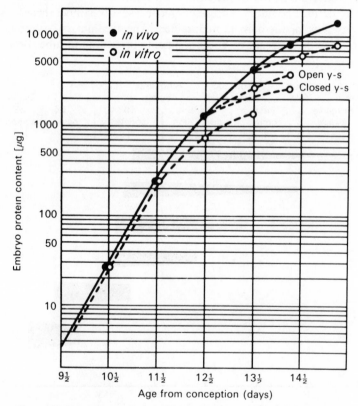

Figure 3   Protein content of rat embryos explanted between 9 and 14 days of gestation and grown *in vitro* (open circles), compared with growth *in vivo* (solid circles)

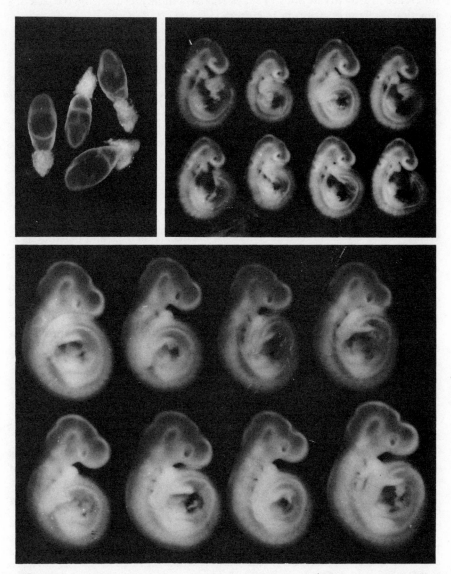

Figure 4 Top left: head-fold embryos as explanted at $9\frac{1}{2}$ days' gestation. Top right: Embryos grown for 32 hours *in vivo* (upper row) and *in vitro* (lower row). All eight embryos are from the same rat. Bottom: Embryos grown for 48 hours *in vivo* (upper row) and *in vitro* (lower row). All eight embryos are from the same rat. (All the photographs are at the same magnification ($\times 11$)) (New *et al.*, 1976b)

difference in growth rate after $11\frac{1}{2}$ days almost certainly results from the lack of a functional allantoic placenta in culture.

1.3 Reliability

The culture systems are extremely reliable for rat embryos during the 48 hour period between head-fold and early limb-bud stages ($9\frac{1}{2}$–$11\frac{1}{2}$ days). Over 95% of the embryos form a blood circulation and develop normally during this period, with rates of protein synthesis and differentiation indistinguishable from those *in vivo* (New *et al.*, 1976b). This can be particularly well shown by comparing the development in culture of the embryos from one uterine horn of a rat with that of the embryos left to grow *in situ* in the other uterine horn (Figure 4).

1.4 Sensitivity

Observations on the immediate effects of chemicals on eggs and blastocysts in culture can often be augmented by study of long-term effects after the egg/blastocysts have been returned to the uterus.

Postimplantation embryos cannot be returned to the uterus for continued development. However, extensive organogenesis occurs within a 2–3 day culture period, and by combining morphological and histological observations with determinations of heart rate, protein and DNA content etc., the system provides a sensitive test of the action of toxic agents. If increased sensitivity and/or discrimination is needed, it may be obtained by:

(1) Increasing the numbers of embryos cultured. Because the culture systems are both simple and reliable, it is feasible to use 50–100 embryos for each dosage of a test agent, and to detect abnormalities appearing in only a few per cent of exposed embryos.
(2) Making detailed measurements of selected parts of the embryos. This method was used in a study by Cockroft and New (1978) of the effects of

Table 1   Mean protein, crown–rump length and somite numbers of rat embryos cultured at different temperatures

Temperature	No. of embryos	Turned embryos	Protein (μg $\pm$ s.e.)	Crown–rump (mm $\pm$ s.e.)	Somites ($\pm$ s.e.)
38.0°C	18	17	185 $\pm$ 10	3.38 $\pm$ 0.08	25.9 $\pm$ 0.2
40.0°C	18	18	186 $\pm$ 8	3.35 $\pm$ 0.08	26.4 $\pm$ 0.3
40.5°C	18	7	122 $\pm$ 10	2.63 $\pm$ 0.09	23.8 $\pm$ 0.7[1]
41.0°C	18	1	92 $\pm$ 6	2.14 $\pm$ 0.06	–[2]

[1] $n = 11$, others uncountable.
[2] No somite counts possible.
From Cockroft and New, 1978.

Table 2 Frequency of certain abnormalities found in a embryos cultured at different temperatures

				Type of abnormality		
Temperature	No. of embryos	Abnormal embryos	Micro-cephaly	Pericardial oedema	Neural folds fused ant–post	Open neural tube
38.0°C	18	0	0	0	0	0
40.0°C	18	1	1	0	0	0
40.5°C	18	10	10	1	0	0
41.0°C	18	18	16	16	3	1

From Cockroft and New, 1978.

hyperthermia. Embryos were incubated at 38 °C, 40 °C, 40.5 °C and 41 °C. The embryos at 40.5°C and 41°C were obviously abnormal. Those at 40°C showed no clear malformations and the protein content was similar to that of the controls at 38°C (Tables 1 and 2). However, it was suspected that they might be microcephalic, and this was confirmed by detailed comparison of head measurements with those of controls, and by determination of head/embryo protein ratios (Figure 5 and Tables 3 and 4)

(3) Injection methods. New and Brent (1972) examined the effect of yolk-sac antibody (sheep anti-rat-yolk-sac gammaglobulin) on rat embryos in culture. At concentrations of 0.1 mg/ml, the antibody caused gross retardation of growth and differentiation. It was suspected that the primary

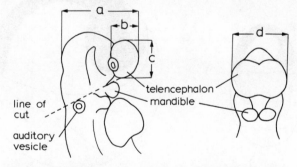

Figure 5 Diagrams showing side view (left) and front view (right) of head region of rat embryo explanted at $9\frac{1}{2}$ days of gestation and grown in culture for 48 hours. The diagrams show the four head dimensions that were measured and the position of the cut made for separate head and body protein determinations. a, head length; b, length of telencephalon; c, height of telencephalon; d, width across telencephalon (Cockroft and New, 1978)

Table 3   Comparison of head/embryo protein content ratios of groups of rat embryos matched for total protein content after culture at 38 and 40 °C

Temperature	No. of embryos	Total embryo protein (μg $\pm$ s.e.)	Head/embryo protein ratio ($\pm$ s.e.)
38°C	18	167 ± 9	0.295 ± 0.003
40°C	18	167 ± 9	0.278 ± 0.005
			$P < 0.02$

From Cockroft and New, 1978.

    effect was on the yolk-sac endoderm. Supporting evidence was provided by injection of the antibody into selected regions of the conceptus, particularly into the amniotic cavity and extra-embryonic coelom (Figure 10.6). In neither of these sites was the antibody in contact with yolk-sac endoderm (although in contact with most other tissues of the conceptus) and the embryo developed normally.

(4) Prolonged development of parts of the embryo. In a study of the action of 5-bromodeoxyuridine (BudR), an analogue of the nucleoside thymidine, Agnish and Kochhar (1976) used a two-stage culture procedure. Whole 11 day mouse embryos (24–34 somites) were cultured for 12–24 hours in a medium containing 50–150 μg/ml Bud R, and the forelimbs were then excised

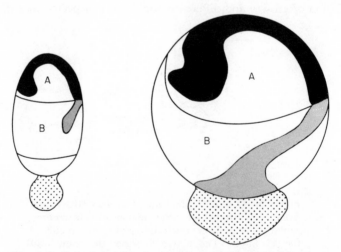

Figure 6   Injection sites in explants at $9\frac{1}{2}$ and $10\frac{1}{2}$ days' gestation. A, Amniotic cavity. B, Space between amnion and yolk sac (extra-embryonic coelom). Heavy stipple, embryo. Medium stipple, allantois. Light stipple, ectoplacental cone (New and Brent, 1972)

Table 4 Comparison of head dimensions of groups of rat embryos matched for crown–rump length after culture at 38 and 40°C

Temperature	No. of embryos	Crown–rump (mm ± s.e)	(a) Length of head (mm ± s.e.)	(b) Length of telencephalon (mm ± s.e.)	(c) Height of telencephalon (mm ± s.e.)	(d) Width of telencephalon (mm ± s.e.)
38 °C	22	3.19 ± 0.04	1.52 ± 0.04	0.63 ± 0.02	0.73 ± 0.02	1.03 ± 0.03
40 °C	22	3.19 ± 0.04	1.42 ± 0.02	0.57 ± 0.01	0.66 ± 0.01	1.03 ± 0.02
			$P < 0.01$	$P < 0.02$	$P < 0.02$	

For details of measurements see Figure 4.
From Cockroft and New, 1978.

and cultured separately for a further 9 days in drug-free medium. The results showed significant and dose-related inhibition of limb chondrogenesis by the drug, particularly in limbs taken from embryos that had been exposed to the drug at the 26–29 somite stage.

Further illustration of the possibilities of embryo culture methods for assessing the effects of chemicals will be given by indicating some of the studies made with these methods in different laboratories. The following selection is intended only to illustrate the range of applications possible; it is not a comprehensive review. Further discussion of both the advantages and limitations of embryo culture can be found in New, 1978a,b; Wilson, 1978.

2 BLASTOCYSTS

2.1 Action of Various Agents on Rabbit Blastocysts (Lutwak-Mann *et al.*, 1969).

Blastocysts were taken from the uterine horns of rabbits at 6 days of gestation. The blastocysts were transferred to small watchglasses of culture medium in petri dishes, and incubated in a gas chamber containing 95% O_2/5% CO_2. Each watchglass contained 4–5 blastocysts in 1 ml of medium TC 199 with 0.02 mg bovine plasma albumin.

Substances tested in this system, at various dosages and for various durations, included the following:

Antimetabolites: 2-deoxyglucose, 2-deoxyglucose-6-phosphate 2-deoxygalactose, 6-mercaptopurine riboside, DL-ethionine, isoniazid, vitamin B_{12} analogues;
Enzyme inhibitors: DL-glyceraldehyde, sodium salicylate, bromoacetyl-DL-carnitine, *p*-chloromercuribenzoate, sodium fluoride;
Antimitotic agents: colcemid, aminopterin;
Cytostatic agents: actinomycin D, cytochalasin B;
Hormones: polyoestriol phosphate, growth hormone.

Results were assessed by noting any effects of the test substance on:

(1) expansion of the blastocoelic cavity;
(2) the embryonic disc: size and shape, frequency of dividing cells, abnormal mitotic figures, metaphase arrest, cellular degeneration.
(3) the trophoblast: frequency of dividing cells, abnormal mitotic figures, metaphase arrest, cellular degeneration.

Many of the substances, at concentrations of 0.1–1.0 mg/ml, showed effects on the blastocysts after 6–8 hours incubation. But the pattern of effects varied from one substance to another. For example, 6-mercaptopurine riboside caused degeneration in the embryonic disc but had little effect on the trophoblast, DL-glyceraldehyde was more harmful to trophoblast than to disc, and aminopterin damaged both disc and trophoblast. A few of the agents were damaging at exceptionally low concentrations; e.g. *p*-chloromercuribenzoate suppressed all growth at 1 μg/ml.

Effects of the substances *in vitro* sometimes differed from those *in vivo*. For example 2-deoxyglucose was less harmful at equivalent concentrations *in vitro* than *in vivo*, perhaps indicating that *in vivo* a metabolic modification may increase its action on embryos. Conversely, aminopterin was without effect *in vivo* but at 0.2 mg/ml resulted in inhibition of cell division and degeneration of the blastocysts *in vitro*.

When agents were administered *in vivo* and the blastocysts then explanted (on day 6) and cultured in agent-free medium, many of the blastocysts showed partial or total recovery.

Overall, these experiments showed that blastocysts in culture provide a simple method for evaluating toxic effects of chemicals on this stage of development. However, the effects may not always be the same as *in vivo*, and if the blastocysts are not too severely damaged they may recover when the agent is removed.

3 RAT AND MOUSE EMBRYOS DURING ORGANOGENESIS

3.1 Tribromoethanol; Cadmium, Lead, Arsenic

Kaufman and Steele (1976) examined the development of head-fold stage rat embryos exposed in culture to the anaesthetic Avertin (tribromoethanol). In a 'standard dose' of Avertin (0.02 ml of a 1.2% solution of Avertin per ml of serum) growth of the embryos, as assessed by synthesis of new protein, was significantly less than that of controls. Embryos exposed to twice the standard dose showed further retardation of growth and various other abnormalities including poorly developed somites and heart, and a failure of the embryo to rotate to the fetal position. The results demonstrated a teratogenic action of this anaesthetic and emphasized the clinical importance of determining whether any of the anaesthetic agents commonly used in human practice have similar embryotoxic action when administered during early pregnancy.

A study of the effects of cadmium has been made by Klein *et al.* (1980). In one series of experiments serum was prepared from rats at intervals of 1, 4, 8, 16 and 24 hours after injection of a high but sublethal dose (2.13 mg/kg Cd) of cadmium chloride. Head-fold stage rat embryos were then incubated in the sera for 48 hours. The 1 hour and 4 hour sera were rapidly lethal to the embryos. Sera taken after 8 hours allowed survival for 48 hours but the embryos showed various abnormalities, including failure of closure of the fore- and midbrain, and retarded growth (Table 5). In 16 and 24 hours sera, embryos appeared morphologically normal but smaller than controls.

Table 5   Protein and DNA contents of embryos cultured for 48 hours in serum from rats injected with 2.13 mg cadmium/kg

Hours after injection	No. rats serum donors	No. embryos analysed	Protein/embryo (μg $\pm$ s.e.)	DNA/embryo (μg $\pm$ s.e.)
1	4	9	13.8 $\pm$ 0.7	0.9 $\pm$ 0.1
4	3	6	12.2 $\pm$ 1.5	1.5 $\pm$ 0.3
8	2	6	68.0 $\pm$ 6.6	6.9 $\pm$ 0.2
16	2	6	84.7 $\pm$ 7.2	6.4 $\pm$ 0.6
24	2	6	86.2 $\pm$ 3.7	7.0 $\pm$ 0.8
Control	4	8	96.7 $\pm$ 6.9	8.7 $\pm$ 0.6

Adapted from Klein *et al.*, 1980.

These results are interesting in showing how the culture system can be used to determine the changes in toxicity of an agent over a period of time as it interacts with the maternal metabolism. Klein *et al.* (1980) also examined the effects on rat embryos in culture of 1.6–2.0 μM cadmium added to serum from untreated rats. The response was quite variable and embryos in the same culture vessel included those that were normal, abnormal or failed to survive the culture period. The abnormal embryos showed extensive haemorrhages but the neural tubes closed normally. Altogether, the pattern of response of the embryos in serum with direct addition of cadmium was very different from that in sera from injected animals.

Beaudoin and Fisher (1981) have combined maternal treatment with *in vitro* culture in evaluating a number of teratogens, including cadmium, lead and arsenic. Embryos were explanted at 10 days of gestation (5–9 somites) from rats which had been treated with the agent 4–24 hours previously. The embryos were then grown for 24–42 hours in culture medium without teratogen. In culture many of these embryos showed failure or slowing of axial rotation and neural tube closure, as well as retarded somite and limb-bud formation, compared with cultured control embryos from untreated rats. An advantage of the procedure is that it allows study of effects of embryonic development following exposure of the intact mother–placenta–embryo unit to an agent for a brief and precisely defined period of gestation.

3.2 Depletion of Glucose, Amino Acids, Vitamins

Cockroft (1979) used the culture system to study some of the nutrient requirements of rat embryos during organogenesis. The culture serum was first dialysed against a balanced salt solution and then supplemented with various combinations of glucose, pyruvate, vitamins and amino acids. The results are shown in Tables 6 and 7.

Growth was minimal when there was no energy source, but the addition of glucose restored both growth and differentiation to control levels. The inclusion

Table 6 Mean ± s.e.m. protein contents, somite numbers and crown–rump lengths of presomite rat embryos cultured for 48 h in whole rat serum, or dialysed serum supplemented with various combinations of glucose, pyruvate, vitamins and amino acids

	No. of embryos	Protein (µg)	No. of somites	Crown–rump length (mm)
(A) Whole serum	12	158 ± 13	26.5 ± 0.3	3.36 ± 0.11
Dialysed serum†	12	11 ± 1*	—	0.68 ± 0.03*
Dialysed serum† + glucose	12	153 ± 10	26.9 ± 0.3	3.28 ± 0.08
Dialysed serum† + glucose + pyruvate	12	108 ± 6*	23.1 ± 0.7*	2.67 ± 0.07*
Dialysed serum† + pyruvate	12	28 ± 5*	—	0.62 ± 0.02*
(B) Whole serum	18	177 ± 8	26.4 ± 0.2	3.23 ± 0.07
Dialysed serum ‡	18	44 ± 6*	—	1.51 ± 0.17*
Dialysed serum ‡ + vitamins	18	172 ± 9	26.1 ± 0.5	3.15 ± 0.08
Dialysed serum ‡ + vitamins + amino acids	18	185 ± 6	27.1 ± 0.2	3.38 ± 0.04
Dialysed serum ‡ + amino acids	18	53 ± 5*	—	1.79 ± 0.15*

* Significantly different from value with whole serum, P ≤ 0.001.
† Including amino acids and vitamins.
‡ Containing 1·5 mg glucose/ml.
From Cockroft, 1979, by permission of *Journals of Reproduction and Fertility Ltd.*

Table 7   Mean ± s.e.m. protein contents, somite numbers, crown–rump lengths and abnormalities in presomite rat embryos cultured for 48 h in dialysed rat serum supplemented with glucose, amino acids and various combinations of vitamins

Pantothenic acid (1.0 mg/l)	Choline chloride (1.0 mg/l)	Folic acid (1.0 mg/l)	i-Inositol (2.0 mg/l)	Nicotinamide (1.0 mg/l)	Pyridoxal HCl (0.1 mg/l)	Riboflavin (0.1 mg/l)	Thiamine HCl (0.0 mg/l)	No. of embryos	Protein (μg)	No. of somites	Crown–rump length (mm)	Abnormal embryos
(A) +	+	+	+	+	+	+	+	8	162 ± 10	27.0 ± 0.3	3.43 ± 0.13	—
−	−	−	−	−	−	−	+	8	59 ± 13	—	2.10 ± 0.23	7
−	+	+	+	+	+	+	+	8	83 ± 19	—	2.30 ± 0.34	5
+	−	+	+	+	+	+	+	8	173 ± 15	26.5 ± 0.3	3.31 ± 0.07	—
+	+	−	+	+	+	+	+	8	142 ± 12	25.8 ± 0.5	3.25 ± 0.11	3
+	+	+	−	+	+	+	+	8	161 ± 11	26.6 ± 0.3	3.29 ± 0.11	—
+	+	+	+	−	+	+	+	8	156 ± 8	26.9 ± 0.3	3.36 ± 0.08	—
+	+	+	+	+	−	+	+	8	170 ± 11	27.1 ± 0.4	3.51 ± 0.13	—
+	+	+	+	+	+	−	+	8	27 ± 16	26.4 ± 0.8	2.98 ± 0.30	3
+	+	+	+	+	+	+	−	8	178 ± 9	26.8 ± 0.3	3.44 ± 0.06	—
(B) +	+	+	+	+	+	+	+	12	180 ± 11	26.8 ± 0.3	3.48 ± 0.07	—
+	−	−	−	−	−	−	−	12	145 ± 11	25.0 ± 0.3	3.28 ± 0.09	3
+	−	−	−	−	−	+	+	12	157 ± 11	25.8 ± 0.2	3.29 ± 0.08	3
+	+	+	+	−	−	+	+	12	162 ± 13	25.8 ± 0.3	3.36 ± 0.08	—
+	+	+	−	−	−	+	+	12	198 ± 10	27.0 ± 0.3	3.58 ± 0.05	1

From Cockroft, 1979, by permission of *Journals of Reproduction and Fertility, Ltd.*

of pyruvate with glucose had an adverse effect on development and pyruvate alone supported very little development.

The presence of free amino acids appeared to be relatively unimportant, but vitamins were essential. The vitamin whose absence produced the most marked effect was pantothenic acid: protein content and crown–rump lengths were significantly reduced, and most of the embryos were abnormal. Absence of riboflavin or folic acid also affected growth and differentiation but to a lesser extent. Absence of *i*-inositol caused developmental abnormalities (open neural tubes) but did not reduce protein synthesis.

Cockroft's work has provided an excellent example of the possibilities provided by the culture system for detailed and precise analysis of the nutrient requirements of embryos. It could be relevant to any toxicological studies involving changes in the balance of serum constitutents.

3.3 Excess Glucose; Excess and Deficient Insulin

Cockroft and Coppola (1977, and personal communication) found that extra D-glucose added to the culture medium in excess of 6 mg/ml resulted in severe malformations of rat embryos, including abnormal fusion of the neural folds, microcephaly and eye defects. The glucose levels of such cultures were similar to those occurring in the blood of severely diabetic patients. The effects seemed specific to D-glucose, because L-glucose produced no abnormalities of development in culture and only a general retarding of growth.

Addition of extra insulin to the cultures stimulated embryo growth (20–25% increase in protein synthesis) without causing malformations.

Sadler (1980) has found that 5 mg/ml extra glucose added to cultures of mouse embryos caused neural tube defects. He also obtained similar defects in mouse embryos cultured in serum taken from rats rendered diabetic with streptozotocin (The serum was taken only after all trace of the drug had disappeared). The glucose level in this serum was 4 mg/ml but the insulin level ($9 \mu U/ml$) did not differ significantly from that of control serum. In serum from more severely diabetic rats (glucose 6 mg/ml, insulin $1 \mu U/ml$) the mouse embryos showed both neural tube defects and reduced protein synthesis.

Diabetes in human mothers is known to result in increased incidence of congenital malformations, stillbirths and abortions. Until recently, a major obstacle in the study of the mechanisms involved has been the lack of an experimental model. The culture system makes possible study of the separate effects of hyperglycaemia, hypoinsulinaemia, etc. on embryos, and avoids any confusing effects resulting from drugs (e.g. streptozotocin).

Studies by Shepard and his colleagues at the University of Washington (Shepard *et al.*, 1970) demonstrated some of the pathways of energy metabolism in the rat embryo in culture. They added ^{14}C-glucose to the culture medium and traced the fate of this glucose in terms of the amount of lactate

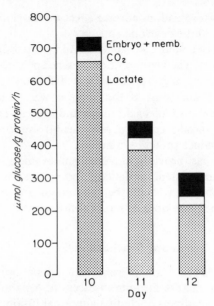

Figure 7   Utilization of glucose by rat embryos in culture. (Reproduced from Shepard *et al.*, 1970, by permission of Academic Press, Inc.)

released into the medium, amount of respiratory carbon dioxide give off, and the amount that finished up in the embryo and membranes. The embryos were of three different ages, 10,11 and 12 days, which approximately spans the period of major organogenesis. The results (Figure 7) showed that during this period, rates of glucose uptake and lactate production are declining rapidly which, together with other evidence, strongly suggests that the energy pathways are changing over from anaerobic glycolysis to the Krebs cycle and electron transport system.

In a study by Robkin and Cockroft (1978), embryos were cultured for 18 hours in a gas mixture containing 1-10% carbon monoxide. Although differentiation (somite formation) was unaffected, the growth rate (protein synthesis) was reduced, while glucose consumption, lactate production and the lactate/glucose ratio were all increased. Similar but more pronounced effects were obtained in cultures where the CO was omitted and the O_2 of the gas phase reduced below the optimum level. The two sets of results indicated that under anoxia, resulting from either CO poisoning or from reduced environmental O_2, the midterm embryo can adjust its metabolism to obtain more energy from anaerobic glycolysis to compensate for the reduced activity of the Kreb's cycle and electron transport system. The compensation is only partial and is insufficient to support normal rates of protein synthesis, but may sometimes be adequate to support differentiation of organs similar to that in control embryos.

3.4 Excess Oxygen

At the earlier stages of organogenesis, rat embryos develop normally in culture in a gas phase containing 5–10% oxygen. This is equivalent to oxygen pressures between about 40 mmHg and 80 mmHg, which are close to the values usually found in the uterine vein and artery, respectively. When the oxygen is raised to 20% many of the embryos show a failure of closure of the cephalic neural folds, as in the early stages of exencephaly (New *et al.*, 1976a). This suggests that exposure to little more than twice the normal amount of oxygen is sufficient to cause major abnormalities of development. The effects on the neural folds are associated with loss of apical microfilament bundles from the lateral cells, and reduction of neural crest migration and programmed cell death (Morriss and New, 1979).

3.5 Effects of Temperature and Drugs on the Heart Rate

Detailed records of the heart beat of the early embryo were obtained by Robkin *et al.* (1972). Rat embryos explanted at $11\frac{1}{2}$ days of gestation were cultured in a circulation system and transilluminated with a low-power laser beam. A lens focused the image of the embryo into a photomultiplying tube and the flicker produced by the beating heart could then be detected by an oscilloscope and recorded on a strip chart recorder (Figure 8). Heart rates (i.e. the frequencies of heart beat) in embryos of this age at 38 °C were about 160 per min but with some variation from one embryo to another; lowering the temperature gave a reduction in heart rate of about 7% for each degree drop in temperature.

Robkin *et al.* (1974, 1976) also studied the response of the embryonic heart to drugs which are known to affect the heart rate of the adult. The drugs were added to the circulating medium of cultures of $10\frac{1}{2}$–11 day rat embryos (Figure 8). The addition of isoproterenol, a drug which stimulates the adrenergic beta-receptors, resulted in an immediate increase of heart rate in $10\frac{1}{2}$ day embryos (10–15 somites). The effect could be quickly terminated by the administration of propranolol, which competitively blocks the adrenergic beta-receptors, but which did not prevent a further increase obtained by administering theophylline. Methoxamine had no effect. Trials with atropine, carbamylcholine, curare (*d*-tubocurarine chloride) and nicotine demonstrated the development of cholinergic receptors in the heart about half a day later (11 days, 21–26 somites) than the formation of the adrenergic receptors.

These studies by Robkin have indicated the feasibility of using the culture system to detect effects of toxic chemicals on cardiac physiology from the earliest stages of heart formation in the embryo.

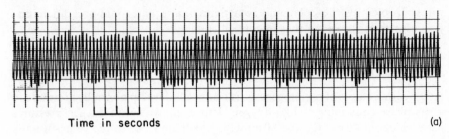

Time in seconds   (a)

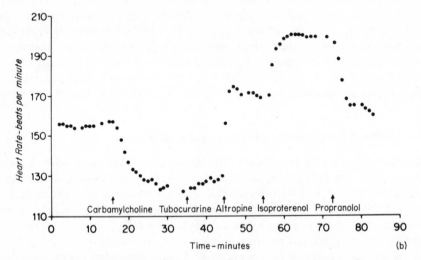

Figure 8   (a) Strip chart recording of heart-beats of 11-day rat embryo in culture. (b) Heart rate response to different drugs. (Reproduced from Robkin *et al.*, 1972, 1976, by permission of Alan R. Liss, Inc. and the *Society for Experimental Biology and Medicine*)

3.6 Cyclophosphamide

It is well established that administration of cyclophosphamide to pregnant laboratory rodents causes embryo malformations, but there has been controversy as to whether the cyclophosphamide affects the embryos directly or only after activation by the maternal metabolism.

Fantel *et al.* (1979) have used rat embryos in culture to resolve this. Embryos were explanted at head-fold stage and grown in human serum in a roller-bottle system. To the cultures were added various combinations of cyclophosphamide (CP), liver microscome fraction (S-9 fraction), and cofactors for a monooxygenase system (NADPH and glucose-6-phosphate).

Table 8 summarizes the results. No malformations or significant differences in growth rate were found in embryos in serum only, serum with S-9 + cofactors, serum with cyclophosphamide alone, or serum with

Table 8 Effects of various combinations of cyclophosphamide, S-9 liver fraction, and cofactors on embryo growth in culture

Cyclophosphamide	−	−	+	+	+
S-9	−	+	−	+	+
Cofactors	−	+	+	−	+
Embryo protein (μg)	172	218	207	206	128
Malformations (%)	0/12	0/15	0/12	0/18	12/16

Adapted from Fantel *et al.*, 1979.

CP + S-9. Only when CP,S-9 and cofactors were all present, were the embryos affected. The number of malformations and amount of growth retardation increased with increasing concentrations of the CP.

The experiment demonstrated that cyclophosphamide requires activation before it becomes teratogenic, probably by a cytochrome P-450 dependent monooxygenase system present in the liver.

3.7 Detection of Toxic Chemicals in Human Serum

Human serum has generally been found to be a poor medium for culturing rat embryos at the earliest stages of organogenesis. However, Chatot *et al.* (1980) have found that the embryos develop satisfactorily if the serum is supplemented with additional glucose (2–3 mg/ml).

This has enabled these workers to use the culture system for detecting teratogens or other embryotoxic agents in human serum. They have shown that

Table 9 Growth of rat embryos in serum from patients receiving cancer chemotherapy or anticonvulsants

	Subject	No. embryos	No. abnormal	Protein (μg/embryo)
Controls	1–19	118	20	76
Cancer chemotherapy				
Vincristine, etc.	21	3	lethal	9
(post-treatment)	21	3	0	82
(no treatment)	22	3	0	87
Methotrexate, etc.	24	3	3	54
Tamoxifen	25	3	3	88
Anticonvulsants				
Tegretol	26	3	3	63
Peganone etc.	27	3	3	61
Primidone etc.	28	3	3	14
Tegretol etc.	29	3	3	83
Tegretol etc.	30	3	3	79

Adapted from Chatot *et al.*, 1980.

sera from patients undergoing cancer chemotherapy, and patients receiving anticonvulsants are often lethal or teratogenic to embryos (Table 9). The work has provided a valuable method for studying the embryotoxicity of the products of interaction between a chemical substance and the human metabolism. But one problem to be overcome is the greater variability of embryo growth in 'control' human serum (particularly between sera from different individuals) than in rat serum.

4 REFERENCES

Agnish, N. D. and Kochhar, D. M. (1976). Direct exposure of postimplantation mouse embryos to 5-bromodeoxyuridine *in vitro* and its effect on subsequent chondrogenesis in the limbs. *J. Embryol. exp. Morphol.* **36**, 623–638.

Beaudoin, A. R. and Fisher, D. L. (1981). An *in vivo/in vitro* evaluation of teratogenic action. *Teratology* **23**, 57–61.

Chatot, C. L., Klein, N. W., Piatek, J. and Pierro, L. J. (1980). Successful culture of rat embryos on human serum: Use in the detection of teratogens. *Science (Washington, DC)* 207, 1471–1473.

Cockroft, D. L. (1979). Nutrient requirements of rat embryos undergoing organogenesis *in vitro*. *J. Reprod. Fertil.* **57**, 505–510.

Cockroft, D. L. and Coppola, P. T. (1977). Teratogenic effects of excess glucose on headfold rat embryos in culture. *Teratology* **16**, 141–146.

Cockroft, D. L. and New, D. A. T. (1978). Abnormalities induced in cultured rat embryos by hyperthermia. *Teratology* **17**, 277–284.

Fantel, A. G., Greenaway, J. C., Juchau, M. R. and Shepard, T. H. (1979). Teratogenic bioactivation of cyclophosphamide *in vitro*. *Life Sci.* **25**, 67–72.

Kaufman, M. H. and Steele, C. E. (1976). Deleterious effect of an anaesthetic on cultured mammalian embryos. *Nature (London)* **260**, 782–784.

Klein, N. W., Vogler, M. A., Chatot, C. L. and Pierro, L. J. (1980). The use of cultured rat embryos to evaluate the teratogenic activity of serum: cadmium and cyclophosphamide. *Teratology* **21**, 199–208.

Lutwak-Mann, C., Hay, M. F. and New, D. A. T. (1969). Action of various agents on rabbit blastocysts *in vivo* and *in vitro* *J. Reprod. Fertil.* **18**, 235–237.

Morriss, G. M. and New, D. A. T. (1969). Effect of oxygen concentration on morphogenesis of cranial neural folds and neural crest in cultured rat embryos. *J. Embryol exp. Morphol.* **54**, 17–35.

New, D. A. T. (1978a). Whole-embryo culture and the study of mammalian embryos during organogenesis. *Biol. Rev. Cambridge Phil. Soc.* **53**, 81–122.

New, D. T. A. (1978b). Whole embryo explants and transplants. In Wilson, J. G. and Fraser, F. C. (Eds.) *Handbook of Teratology*, Vol. 4, Chapter 4. Plenum Press, New York.

New, D. A. T. and Brent, R. L. (1972). Effect of yolk-sac antibody on rat embryos grown in culture. *J. Embryol. exp. Morphol.* **27**, 543–553.

New, D. A. T., Coppola, P. T. and Cockroft, D. L. (1976a). Improved development of headfold rat embryos in culture resulting from low oxygen and modifications of the culture serum. *J. Reprod. Fertil.* **48**, 219–222.

New, D. A. T., Coppola, P. T. and Cockroft, D. L. (1976b). Comparison of growth *in vitro* and *in vivo* of post-implantation rat embryos. *J. Embryol. exp. Morphol.* **36**, 133–144.

Robkin, M. A. and Cockroft, D. L. (1978). The effect of carbon monoxide on glucose metabolism and growth of rat embryos. *Teratology* **18**, 337–342.

Robkin, M. A. Shepard, T. H. and Baum, D. (1974). Autonomic drug effects on the heart rate of early rat embryos. *Teratology* **9**, 35–44.

Robkin, M. A., Shepard, T. H. and Dyer, D. C. (1976). Autonomic receptors of the early rat embryo heart: growth and development. *Proc. Soc. exp. Biol. Med.* **151**, 799–803.

Robkin, M. A., Shepard, T. H. and Tanimura, T. (1972). A new *in vitro* culture technique for rat embryos. *Teratology* **5**, 367–376.

Sadler, T. W. (1980). Effects of maternal diabetes on early embryogenesis: I. The teratogenic potential of diabetic serum. II Hyperglycemia-induced exencephaly. *Teratology* **21**, 339–347 and 349–356.

Shepard, T. H., Tanimura, T. and Robkin, M. A. (1970). Energy metabolism in early mammalian embryos. *Devel. Biol Suppl.* **4**, 42–58.

Wilson, J. G. (1978). Survey of *in vitro* systems: their potential use in teratogenicity screening. In Wilson, J. G. and Frases, F. C. (Eds.) *Handbook of Teratology*, Vol. 4, Chapter 5. Plenum Press, New York.

Methods for Assessing the Effects of Chemicals on Reproducting Functions
Edited by V. B. Vouk and P. J. Sheehan
© 1983 SCOPE

Methods for Evaluating and Predicting Human Fetal Development

J. E. JIRÁSEK

1. INTRODUCTION

Whenever a pregnant woman is exposed to infectious agents, ionizing radiation or chemicals, including drugs, there is always a possibility that such exposures may have adverse effects on the development of the fetus. A therapy that may be of great benefit to the sick mother, may be at the same time hazardous to the fetus.

A teratogen may be defined as a physical, chemical or biological agent producing structural or functional abnormalities in an organism exposed to it before birth. The sensitivity of the conceptus to an exogenously induced damage varies widely depending on the stage of development (Wilson, 1972). At the early stage of ontogenesis, before blastogenesis is completed (in humans during the first three weeks after conception) the conceptus, if exposed to a noxious agent such as ionizing radiation, tends to have an "all-or-none" response (Russel and Russel, 1954). The embryo survives without any anatomical damage, or dies and is aborted. During organogenesis, approximately 4–12 weeks after conception, the sensitivity of embryo to morphologic malformations is high, the peak of sensitivity being during the fifth and sixth week after conception. The period of peak sensitivity to teratogens includes the constitution of embryochorionic circulation and early differentiation of many organs. There are "critical periods" in morphogenesis of all structures (Schwalbe, 1906; Saxén and Rapola, 1969). Adverse influences at critical periods may involve not only morphologic malformations, but may result in adverse changes of postnatal functions as well.

Possible teratogens are tested using several species of animals. In spite of similarities in the developmental pattern, the peculiarities of some species make the comparisons extremely difficult. For instance, inversion of the germ-layers in mice and rats and the resulting temporary yolk sac placenta does not occur in other mammals. Also the metabolism of chemicals in the maternal organism may differ significantly between species.

299

Table 1 Comparative classification of prenatal development of quadruped vertebrates

Comparative stages	Stage	Human		Monkey		Rat		Mouse	
		Length in mm	Age in days	Length in mm	Age in days	Length in mm	Age in days	Length in mm	Age in days
Unicellular	1	0.2	0–2	0.15	1		1		1
Blastomeric (16–20 blastomers)	2	0.2	2–4	0.15	2–4		2–3		2–3
Blastodermic	3	0.4	4–6	0.2–0.3	7–9		4–5		4–4½
Bilaminar embryo stage:									
bilaminar plate	4–1	0.1	6–14	0.3	10–13		6–7		5
primary yolk sac	4–2								
secondary yolk sac	4–3	0.2–0.4							6½
Trilaminar embryo stage:									
with primitive streak	5–1	0.4–1.0	15–17	0.5	17–19		8–9		7
with a notochordal process	5–2	1.0–2.0	17–20	1.5					
Early somite stage:									
completely open neural groove	6–1	1.5–2.0	20–21	1,9	21–24		9½		8
neural tube closing, both ends open	6–2	1.5–4.0	21–26	4.0	24	1.3–3.0	10–10-3/4		

6-3	one or both neuropores closed	3-5	26-30	4.0-6.0	24-26	3-4.1	11	1.8-3	9½
7-1	Stage of limb development: bud of proximal extremity	4-6	28-32	6.0	26	4-4.5	11	2-3.3	9½-10
7-2	buds of proximal and distal extremities	5-8	31-35	8.0	27	4-6	11.5	7.9	10½
7-3	proximal extremity two segments	7-10	35-38			5.8-8	13		11
7-4	proximal and distal extremity two segments	8-12	37-42	7-9		8-9.5	13½		
7-5	digital rays, foot plates	10-14	42-44	10	34	10	14	11.5	13
7-6	digital tubercles	13-21	44-51	9-11	36	12.5	15½	13	14
7-7	digits, toe tubercles	19-24	51-53	19	41	16	17	14	
8-1	Late embryonal stage: differentiated extremities	22-23	52-56	22	44	19	17½	14-17	18
8-2	using eyelids	27-35	56-60	39-44	52	22	19½	22	16-18
9	Fetal period	31-200	60-182+	40-260	53-170	25	19-21	22-25	18-10
10	Perinatal period	201-450	180-266+	Post-natal	Post-natal	Post-natal			

The goal of teratogenicity tests is to determine the dose which is embryotoxic in animals causing intrauterine death or growth retardation, or which is teratogenic, producing anatomical malformations. The mechanism of damage is not often investigated. General mechanisms of interference with prenatal growth and differentiation include inhibition of cell proliferation related to altered synthesis of proteins, carbohydrates and lipids, or to limited energy supply; inhibition of placental transfer and protein synthesis; interference with fetal and fetoplacental circulation; and altered or inhibited formation of secretory products.

The type of malformation is related to the stage at which embryo is exposed to a teratogen. For instance, a human conceptus aborted during third gestational month after exposure to aminopterin (a folic acid antagonist) showed trophoblastic necrosis, thrombosis of the intervillous space and damaged fetal hematopoiesis within the liver (Shaw, 1972). If the fetus survived, a typical aminopterin syndrome was characterized by malformations in the central nervous system, craniofacial dysplasia, clubhands and clubfeet, and mental retardation (Thiersch, 1952; Howard and Rudd, 1977).

The effects of the chemicals which have been tested may be classified as expected and unexpected. The expected effects are gross malformations, abortion and clefts resulting from inhibition of growth observed after administration of aminopterin, busulfan, chlorambucil, cyclophosphamide and tolbutamid in the first trimester of pregnancy (Schiff et al., 1970). Growth retardation may result from the treatment with cortisone (Warrel and Taylor, 1968). Masculinization of female fetuses is an expected consequence of administration of androgenic substances such as testosterone and its derivatives (Grumbach and Ducharme, 1960). The interference of diethylstilbestrol (Herbst et al., 1971) with normal regression of paramesonephric epithelium within the vaginal plate leading to vaginal adenosis should be considered as a predictable effect since vagina is a known target of estrogens. Tetracyclin is known to form chelates with calcium, and after application to pregant women it is deposited in the fetal bone mineral and deciduous teeth (Toaff and Ravid, 1968). A less expected effect is the deposition of tetracycline into the lenses leading to cataracts (Harley et al., 1964). Understandable is the eighth nerve damage related to neomycin, streptomycin and quinine and the formation of fetal goiter after administration of anti-thyroid drugs during pregnancy.

Unexpected teratogenic effects are the effects which are difficult to predict even if the metabolism of the chemical is known. For instance, the phenocopy of the stippled epiphyses syndrome (or chondrodysplasia punctata) which develops after administration of dicumarol anticoagulants (such as warfarin) during the first three months is difficult to predict (Shaul and Hall, 1977). Similarly, the properties of thalidomide do not forewarn the character of the now well-known syndrome. Unexpected effects may be sometimes detected in animal experiments. However, it should always be understood that extrapolation of animal experiments to man is valid only to a limited degree.

Teratologists and experimental embryologists have provided much information on the developmental mechanisms and their disturbances in different vertebrates. To make the interpretation of results easier, we have proposed a comparative classification of prenatal development of quandrupeds in which corresponding stages are marked by the same system of numbers. The prenatal development of man, macaccus, rat and mouse is compared in Table 1.

2 MOTHER-FETUS AND FETUS-MOTHER TRANSFER; THE PLACENTAL BARRIER

The transfer of substances from the maternal into the fetal compartment takes place either across the placenta or across fetal membranes. Only under therapeutical or experimental conditions substances are administered directly into the amnion, or into the peritoneal cavity of the fetus (intrauterine fetal transfusion). Transport mechanisms are related to the anatomy of the biological barrier, to the uterochorionic and uteroplacental (maternal) circulation and to the embryo-chorionic or feto-placental (fetal) circulation.

The total maternal uterine blood flow is considered to be 94–127 ml/minute/kg at 10–28 gestational weeks and approximately 150 ml/minute/kg at the term (Assali et al., 1960). The blood flow entering intervillous space is intermittent, and the blood pressure in the terminal uterine arteries is 70–80 mmHg (Alvarez and Caldeiro-Barcia, 1950). The blood pressure in the intervillous space is approximately 10 mmHg, and increases during uterine contractions up to 30–50 mmHg. The pressure in the maternal veins leaving the intervillous space is about 8 mmHg. The blood pressure within the intervillous space is lower than that within the chorionic (fetal) vessels. The blood pressure in the umbilical arteries is approximately 48–50 mmHg and in the vein 24 mmHg (Margolis and Orcutt, 1960). These conditions favor feto-maternal transport.

The paraplacental transfer is effected by a transport from decidual cells across the chorion into the amnion. For instance, prolactine released from decidual cells crosses the chorion and amnion and diffuses into the amnionic fluid (Riddick and Masler, 1981). The transport of decidual prolactine requires active protein synthesis and an intact microtubular system. The permeability of amniochorion can be easily studied in vitro (Seeds *et al.*, 1980).

The placental transfer takes place by diffusion, by facilitated diffusion, by active transport (against the gradient), by endocytosis, or by other poorly understood mechanisms, and depends on the physicochemical properties of chemicals, such as molecular weight, ionization, lipid solubility and protein binding (Mirkin, 1976)

Compounds with low molecular weight diffuse more rapidly. If the molecular weight exceeds 1000u, the passage across the placenta is usually slow. Molecules in non-ionized state cross the placental barrier more rapidly than in ionized state. Lipid solubility facilities the transport. There is a substantial difference between protein binding in the maternal and fetal blood plasma. This difference may exert a significant influence on the transfer of chemicals, especially if the free substance crosses the placental barrier slowly. There are some specific placental transfer systems involving specific conjugation of the substance crossing the placenta to a complex which is cleaved before the substance is released after the transport across the trophoblast.

The placenta, especially the trophoblast, contains enzymes metabolizing endogenous as well as xenobiotic substrates (Hagerman, 1969). Some of them are of fundamental physiological importance, for example, the monoamine oxidase (De Maria, 1963) which deaminates a number of substrates such as epinephrine, norepinephrine, dopamine, serotonine and some amphetamines; diamine oxidase (histaminase) (Weingold and Southern, 1968); catechol-O-methyltransferase which inactivates epinephrine and norepinephrine; several peptidases, such as cystine aminopeptidase (oxytocinase) (Mathur and Walker, 1968; choline acetytransferase (Bull *et al.*, 1961); 3β-hydroxysteroid dehydrogenase, 17β-hydroxysteroid dehydrogenase, a very potent steroid arylating system, and others.

The effects of chemicals on the placental vasculature can be studied in vitro in perfusion experiment (Mancini and Gautier, 1964). Serotonin, norepinephrine, LSD and some other hallucinogens, morphine and codeine are potent constrictors of placental vessels, at least in vitro (Gant and Dyer, 1971). Prostaglandin $F_{2\alpha}$ enhances the effect of oxytocin (Jungmannová *et al.*, 1975).

It is evident that placental enzymatic systems can metabolize a large number of endogenous as well as exogenous substances. Hydrolyzable substrates are usually hydrolyzed, and vasoactive substances and hormonal peptides are metabolized to inactive substances. Placental conjugations, with a possible exception of acetylation, seem not to occur.

3 PRENATAL DETECTION OF FETAL MALFORMATIONS AND CHROMOSOMAL AND GENETIC DISEASES

Techniques used for prenatal detection of fetal disorders can be classified as invasive and non-invasive. Invasive techniques, such as amniocenthesis and fetoscopy, include penetration into the amniotic cavity. Non-invasive techniques are based on X-ray or ultrasound procedures, or on different kinds of fetal monitoring.

3.1. Procedures Based on Amniocenthesis

Amniocenthesis is usually performed at 16–18 weeks of gestation. The volume of amniotic fluid at this stage is approximately 120–300 ml, from which 5–20 ml are withdrawn and used for analysis. The risk of complications related to amniocenthesis is less that 0, 5% (Simpson and Martin, 1976). Potential maternal complications include intra-abdominal bleeding, puncture of the bladder or intestine and Rh-immunization. Possible fetal complications are injuries to the fetus by the needle, bleeding from placental vessels, intraovular infection and abortion. Leakage of amniotic fluid has also been reported.

The amniotic fluid sample is centrifuged, and the cells are used for cytologic examination, cultivation and subsequent chromosomal and metabolic analysis. The fluid can be examined by biochemical methods.

3.1.1 Cytology of Amniotic Cells

Centrifuged cells from amniotic fluid are spread on a microscopic slide, fixed in formalin in vapor and, if an open neural tube defect is suspected, the smear is checked for the presence of glial elements (Brock, 1978). The glial elements are bipolar, elongated and detectable by a glial protein S-100 exhibiting a specific immunofluorescence (Sarkar *et al.*, 1980). Analysis for X-chromatin and Y-chromatin in uncultivated amniotic cells can be easily performed; however, the results are far less informative than karyotyping.

3.1.2 Amniotic Cells Tissue Cultures

Centrifuged cells from amniotic fluid are cultivated for approximately 2–4 weeks in a nutrient medium containing calf serum and antibiotics. The cultivation is successful in 70–99% of cases. If karyotyping is required, colchicine is added to the growing culture (mitoses are arrested at metaphase), the medium of the culture is hypotonized and acetic acid-methanol fixative added; cells are spread on microscopic slides and stained by different banding techniques. Using this method all numerical chromosomal abnormalities can be detected. The most common is the monosomy for the X-chromosome (45,X). The other quite frequently occurring pathologic karyotypes are 47,XXY; 47,XXX; 47, + 21; 47, + 18; 47, + 13.

The detection of structural chromosomal anomalies depends on the extent of chromosomal lesions. Minor abnormalities may remain undetected. Structural chromosomal abnormalities involve deletions, translocations and rearrangements resulting in the formation of isochromosomes, incomplete chromosomes, fragments, ring-chromosomes, etc. Chromosomal breaks are observed after X-ray irradiation.

The most important indication for prenatal karyotyping of the fetus are chromosomal abnormalities (such as balanced translocation or inversion) in either parent, advanced maternal age or existence of individuals affected by chromosomal aneuploidy, or another chromosomal abnormality in the family.

Cultures from amniotic fluid of fetuses with open neural tube defects contain glial cells which are elongated, bi-polar and exceptionally adhesive (rapid adherent or RA cells), and contain a specific glial protein (Sarkar *et al.*, 1980).

Cultures of amniotic cells can also be used to detect many metabolic diseases with known biochemical basis. The biochemical defect is usually identified by enzyme assays in cultured cells. About 75 different metabolic disorders (such as mucopolysacharidoses, glycogenoses, lipidoses, aminoacidopathies, etc.) can now be diagnosed prenatally (Golbus *et al.*, 1976; Rhine, 1976).

3.1.3 Biochemical Analysis of Amniotic Fluid

(a) *Alpha-fetoprotein (AFP)*. AFP is synthesized in fetal endodermal structures such as the yolk sac, liver and gut. AFP in amniotic fluid originates probably from fetal urine, and its amniotic concentration decreases with advancing gestational age (Brock and Sutchiffe, 1972). Elevated concentrations of AFP are encountered in open neural tube defects (anencephaly, open spina bifida) and have also been reported in sacrococcygeal teratoma, omphalocele and congenital nephrosis and in pregnancies with fetal deaths; elevated AFP is sometimes present also in fetuses with atresias of digestive tube, polycystic kidneys, annular pancreas, hydrocephalus, Fallot's tetralogy and congenital skin defects. Normal concentrations of amniotic AFP during gestational weeks 16–18 are between 20 and 7 ng/ml. In fetuses with open neural tube defects, the AFP values exceed 25 ng, reaching in some cases 400–500 ng/ml (Brock, 1978). Contamination of the amniotic fluid with fetal blood is the most common source of false positive results.

(b) *Hormones in amniotic fluid*. Fetal sex can be predicted from the amniotic concentration of testosterone, FSH and LH. In male fetuses, testosterone concentration is much higher, and FSH and LH concentration lower than in female.

The differences in amniotic concentrations of testosterone, FSH and LH during gestational weeks 16–18 are shown in Table 2.

Estimation of amniotic concentration of FSH and 3, 3′, 5′-triodothyronine (RT$_3$) could be useful for prenatal diagnosis of fetal hypotheyroidism, either congenital or induced by exposure of pregnant women to strumigens (Chopra and Crandall, 1975). Elevated amniotic 17-hydroxyprogesterone was observed in fetuses affected by adrenal cortical hyperplasia due to C-21 steroid hydroxylase deficiency (Pang et al., 1980).

Table 2   Differences in hormone levels in the fetal amniotic fluid of males and females*

Amniotic concentration during 16–18 gestational weeks	Males	Females
T	140–190 pg/ml	20–30 pg/ml
FSH	0.05–0.12 ng/ml	0.5–0.7 ng/ml
LH	3–4 ng/ml	9–12 ng/ml

* Data from Clements *et al.*, 1976; Dawood and Saxena, 1977; Jírasek *et al.*, 1980.

3.2 Fetoscopy

Direct visual observation of the fetus is performed by a fetoscope, a special fiberoptic endoscope. Although simultaneous visualization of the entire fetus is not possible, isolated portions of the fetus such as scalp, eyes, lips, fingers, toes, external genitalia and the anterior body wall, including the insertion of umbilical cord, may be directly examined. In some cases the visualization of a structure, whose anatomy is to be examined may be very difficult because of the contamination of amniotic fluid either by meconium or by blood. In our hospital, fetoscopy is performed under general anesthesia. The Wolf fetoscope (3, 2 mm diameter) is inserted into the uterus under visual control after a small laparotomy has been performed; a suture is inserted around the fetoscope insertion. The localization of the placenta is always determined ultrasonically and the transplacental route of fetoscope insertion is strictly avoided. The risk of fetal death and abortion after fetoscopy is approximately 20%. Abortions are related to leakage of amniotic fluid and subsequent amniochorionitis, rarely to intra-amniotic bleeding. Chronic leakage of amniotic fluid during the third trimester requires a long-term hospitalization in approximately 30% of patients. Fetoscopy allows prenatal diagnosis of all major external morphological malformations such as facial clefts, deformed external ears, defects of CNS, gross malformations of limbs (phocomelia, arthrogryposis), oligodactylies, polydactylies, syndactylies, defects of anterior body wall and some malformations of external genitalia.

Fetoscopy is indicated in syndromes which do not exhibit chromosomal or biochemical abnormalities inherited according to Mendelian laws, and which are characterized by constant anatomical malformations.

Diagnostic fetoscopy has been performed in our hospital by Zwinger in 47 cases; 20 of them were therapeutically aborted. Malformations were found in 18 cases. In two cases in which the fetuses were diagnosed fetoscopically as malformed, the diagnosis was not confirmed after abortion. Unwanted abortion occurred in four patients with healthy fetuses. Pre-term deliveries occurred in three cases, two pre-term newborns died. Twenty patients delivered healthy children at full-term. Leakage of amniotic fluid occurred in six of them. Using fetoscope we detected following defects: familial cleft-lip and palate (6 cases), Treacher Collins' syndrome (2 cases), anencephaly (previously diagnosed ultrasonically, 2 cases), ectrodactyly (1 case), Saldino-Noonan syndrome (1 case), Majewski syndrome (1 case), syndactyly type V (1 case), Roberts syndrome (1 case), arthrogryposis (1 case), Apert syndrome (1 case). Lip pit-cleft lip syndrome (1 case).

Sampling of fetal tissue under fetoscopic control. The needlescope, which has a rather limited visual field for a general fetoscopy is a good tool for visualization of chorionic veins in the placental plate. After a suitable vein is visualized, a heparinized needle is directed into the lumen of the vessel. By this method pure fetal blood can be obtained and used for prenatal diagnosis of hemoglobin disorders (MacKenzie and Maclean, 1980).

Fetoscopy controlled intrauterine skin and muscle biopsies are possible and promising for diagnoses of disorders which are not detectable from amniotic fibroblasts. Fetoscope can be also used for the control of intrauterine transfusion.

3.3 Non-Invasive Methods in Prenatal Diagnosis

3.3.1 Ultrasonography

Using real-time ultrasonic instruments, the conceptus can be visualized during 5th or 6th gestational weeks, and its growth, position and localization of the placenta can be monitored (Joupilla and Piiroinen, 1975). The increase in the biparietal diameter is normally used for general growth evaluation (Queehan *et al.*, 1976). Estimations of fetal body and head volumes are performed to diagnose intrauterine growth retardation (Jordan and Clark, 1980).

The fetal heart rate and the beat of umbilical arteries can be also visualized ultrasonically. The following malformations can be diagnosed prenatally by ultrasound procedures: anencephaly at the beginning of the second trimester; myelomeningoceles, but diagnosis may be difficult (Campbell, 1977); hydrocephalus and microcephaly in the third trimester; iniencephaly; sacrococcygeal teratomas; multicystic or polycystic kidneys or hydronephrosis and omphaloceles visualized as masses in a characteristic location (Bartley et al., 1977). In some cases, the shape of external geintalia allows the diagnosis of sex. In the last trimester, the heart valves and cavities can be visualized and the diagnosis of gross congenital heart anomalies is possible (Patel and Goldberg, 1976).

3.3.2 Radiography

The use of direct radiography for diagnosis of skeletal defects is limited to the third trimester. During second trimester even gross anomalies such as achondroplasia are undetectable (Golbus and Hall, 1974). Prenatal radiographic diagnosis (after 30th gestational week) of anencephaly, hydrocephaly, microcephaly and of most of the gross skeletal anomalies has been reported. Contrast radiography with a water-soluble radio-contrast dyes has been used in the third trimester for visualization of absent fetal swallowing in cases of gastrointestinal atresia.

4 CONCLUSIONS

The elucidation of genetic, biochemical and physiological mechanisms involved in prenatal morphogenesis and embryonic function is a necessary prerequisite for attempting the prediction of adverse effects of chemical agents on the exposed mother and fetus. To predict the effects of xenobiotic substances on prenatal development, the stage of pregnancy at which the fetus was exposed and the exposure concentration need to be known. Predictions based on animal embryotoxicity and teratogenicity are, however, of limited value.

For detection of inadequate fetal growth, chromosomal and metabolic diseases and external anatomical malformations, the following methods can be used: cytology of cells exfoliated into the amniotic fluid, direct biochemical tests of amniotic fluid, karyotyping of amniotic cells grown in tissue cultures, biochemical analysis of amniotic cells grown in tissue cultures, fetoscopy, analysis of fetal blood withdrawn under fetoscopical control, ultrasonography and radiography of the fetus.

5 REFERENCES

Alvarez, H., and Caldeiro-Barcia, R. (1950). Contractility of the human uterus recorded by new methods. *Surg. Gynecol. Obstet.*, **91**, 1–13.

Assali, N. S., Rauramo, L., and Peltonen, T. (1960). *Measurement of uterine blood flow and uterine metabolism. Amer. J. Obstet. Gynecol.*, **79**, 86–98.

Bartley, J. A., Golbus, M. S., Filly, R. A., and Hall, B. D. (1977). Prenatal diagnosis of dysplastic kidney disease. *Clin. Genet.*, **11**, 375–378.

Brock, D. J. H. (1978). Alpha-fetoprotein in the prenatal diagnosis of neural tube defects. In Littlefield J. W., de Grouchy, J., and Ebling I. J. B. (Eds.). *Birth Defects*, Proc. 5th International Conference, Excerpta Med. Found., Amsterdam and Oxford.

Brock, D., and Sutchiffe, R. (1972). Alpha-fetoprotein in the antenatal diagnosis of anencephaly and spina bifida. *Lancet*, **2**, 197–199.

Bull, H., Hebb, C., and Ratkovic, C. (1961). Choline acetylase in the human placenta at different stages of development. *Nature (London)*, **190**, 1202.

Campbell, S. (1977). Early prenatal diagnosis of neural tube defects by ultrasound. *Clin. Obstet. Gynecol.*, **20**, 351–359.

Chopra, I. J., and Crandall, B. F. (1975). Thyroid hormones and thyrotropin in amniotic fluid. *New Engl. J. Med.*, **293**, 740–743.

Clemenes, J. A., Reyes, F. I., Winter, J. S., and Faiman, C. (1976). Studies of human sexual development. III. Fetal pituitary, serum and amniotic fluid concentration of LH, CG and FSH. *J. Clin. Endocrinol. Metab.*, **42**, 9–19.

Dawood, M. Y., and Saxena, B. B. (1977). Testosterone and dihydrotestosterone in maternal and cord blood and in amniotic fluid. *Amer. J. Obstet. Gynecol.*, **129**, 37–42.

De Maria, J. F. (1963). The histochemical demonstration in the human placenta of monoamine oxidase activity by tetrazolium salts. *Amer. J. Obstet. Gynecol.*, **87**, 27–32.

Gant, D. W., and Dyer, D. C. (1971). d-Lysergic acid diethylamine (LSD-25) a constrictor of human umbilical vein. *Life Sci.*, **10**, 235–240.

Golbus, M. S., Kan, Y. W., and Naglich-Craig, M. (1976). Fetal blood sampling in midtrimester pregnancies. *Amer. J. Obstet. Gynecol.*, **124**, 653–655.

Golbus, M. S., and Hall, B. D. (1974). Failure to diagnose achondroplasia in utero. *Lancet*, **1**, 629.

Grumbach, M. M., and Ducharme, J. R. (1960). The effects of androgens on fetal sexual development. *Fertil. Steril.*, **11**, 157–180.

Hagerman, D. D. (1969). Enzymology of the placenta. In Klopper, A., and Diczfalusy, E. (Eds.). *Fetus and Placenta*, pp. 413–469, Blackwell, Oxford.

Harley, J. D., Farrar, J. F., Gray, J. B., and Dunlop, I. C. (1964). Aromatic drugs and congenital cataracts. *Lancet*, **1**, 472.

Herbst, A. L., Ulfelder, H., and Poskanzer, D. C. (1971). Adenocarcinoma of the vagina. Association of maternal stibestrol therapy with tumor appearance in young women. *New Engl. J. Med.*, **284**, 878–881.

Howard, J., and Rudd, N. L. (1977). The natural history of aminopterin-induced embryopathy. In Bergsma, D., and Lowry, R. B. (Eds.). *Birth Defects Orig. Art. Ser.*, Vol. XIII, No. 3C, pp. 85–90, March of Dimes.

Jirások, J. E., Štroufová, A., Zwinger, A., Židovský, J. (1980). Prenatal determination of fetal sex and testosterone amniotic concentration. (in Czech), *Česk. Gynekol.*, **101**, 104–106.

Jordan, H. V. F., and Clark, W. B. (1980). Prenatal determination of fetal brain and somatic weight by ultrasound. *Amer. J. Obstet. Gynec.*, **136**, 54–59.

Jouppilla, P. and Piiroinen, O. (1975). Ultrasonic diagnosis of fetal life in early pregnancy. *Obstet. Gynecol.* **46**, 616–620.

Jungamannová, C., Havránek, F., Hodr, J., and Zidovský, J. (1975). In vitro interaction of prostaglandin $F_{2\alpha}$ and oxytocin in placental vessels. *J. reprod. Med.*, **14**, 52–54.

MacKenzie, Z., and Maclean, D. A. (1980). Pure fetal blood from the umbilical cord obtained at fetoscopy: Experience with 125 consecutive cases. *Amer. J. Obstet. Gynecol.*, **138**, 1214–1218.

Mancini, R., and Gautier, R. F. (1964). Effect of certain drugs on perfused human placenta: IV Detection of specific receptor sites. *J. pharm. Sci.*, **53**, 1476.

Mathur, V. S., and Walker, J. M. (1968). Oxytocinase in plasma and placenta in normal and prolonged labor. *Brit. med. J.*, **3**, 96–97.

Margolis, A. J., and Orcutt, R. E. (1960). Pressures in human umbilical vessels in utero. *Amer. J. Obstet. Gynecol.*, **80**, 573–576.

Mirkin, B. L. (1976). *Perinatal Pharmacology and Terapeutics*. Academic Press, New York, San Francisco, and London.

Pang, S., Levina, L. S., Cederqvist, L. L. *et al.* (1980). Amniotic fluid concentrations of Δ^5 and Δ^4 steroids in fetuses with congenital adrenal hyperplasia due to 21-hydroxylase deficiency and in anencephalic fetuses. *J. clin. Endocrinol. Metab.*, **51**, 223–229.

Patel, J., and Goldberg, B. B. (1976). Prental genetic diagnosis and ultrasougrophy. *Clin. Obstet. Gynecol.*, **19**, 893–907.

Queehan, J. T., Kubarych, S. F., Cook, M. N. *et al.* (1976). Diagnostic ultrasound for detection of intrauterine growth retardation. *Amer. J. Obstet. Gynecol.*, **124**, 865–873.

Rhine, S. (1976). Prenatal genetic diagnosis and metabolic disorders. *Clin. Obstet. Gynecol.*, **19**, 855.

Riddick, D. H., and Masler, I. A. (1981). The transport of prolactin by human fetal membranes. *J. Clin. Endocrinol. Metab.*, **52**, 220–224.

Russel, L. B., and Russel, W. L. (1954). An analysis of the changing radiation response of the developing mouse embryo. *J. cell. comp. Physiol.*, *Suppl. I*, **39**, 103–147.

Sarkar, S., Chang, H. C., Porreco, R. P., and Jones, O. W. (1980). Neural origin of cells in amniotic fluid. *AMER. J. Obstet. Gynecol.*, **136**, 67–72.

Saxén, L., and Rapola, J. (1969). Congenital Defects. Holt, Rinehart Winston, New York.

Schiff, D., Aranda, J. V., and Stern, L. (1970). Neonatal thrombocytopenia and congenital malformations associated with the administration of tolbutamide to the mother. *J. Pediat.*, **77**, 457–458.

Schwalbe, E. (1906). *Missbildungslehre (Teratologie)*, Fischer, Jena.

Seeds, A. E., Leung, L. S., Stys, S. J. *et al.* (1980). Comparison of human and sheep chrion laeve, permeability of glucose, β-hydroxybutyrate and glycerol. *Amer. J. Obstet. Gynecol.*, **138**, 604–614.

Shaw, E. B. (1972). Fetal damage due to maternal aminopterin ingestion. *Amer. J. Dis. Child.*, **124**, 93–96.

Shaul, W. L., and Hall, J. G. (1977). Multiple cogenital anomalies associated with oral anticoagulants. *Amer. J. Obstet. Gynecol.*, **127**, 191–198.

Simpson, J. L., and Martin, A. C. (1976). Prenatal diagnosis of cytogenetic disorders. *Clin. Obstet. Gynecol.*, **19**, 841–853.

Thiersch, J. B. (1952). Therapeutic abortions which a folic acid antagonist, 4-aminopteroylglutamic acid administered by the oral route. *Amer. J. Obstet. Gynecol.*, **63**, 1298–1304.

Toaff, R., and Ravid, R. (1968). In Meyer, L., and Peci, H. M. (Eds.). *Drug Induced Diseases*, Excerpta Med. Found., Amsterdam.

Warrel, D. W., and Taylor, R. (1968). Outcome for the fetus of mothers receiving prednisolone during pregnancy. *Lancet*, **1**, 117–119.

Weingold, A. B., and Southern, A. L. (1968). Diamine oxidase as an index of the fetoplacental unit. *Obstet. Gynecol.*, **32**, 593–600.

Wilson, J. G. (1972). Environmental effects on development teratology. In Assali, N. S. (Ed.). *Pathophysiology of Gestation*, Vol. II, pp. 270–320, Academic Press, New York.

Methods for Assessing the Effects of Chemicals on Reproductive Functions
Edited by V. B. Vouk and P. J. Sheehan
© 1983 SCOPE

Experimental Methods in Embryotoxicity Risk Assessment

RICHARD JELÍNEK AND OTAKAR MARHAN

1 SUMMARY*

Embryotoxicity is a hazard to the fetus arising from environmental, infectious, genetic and other agents. The manifestations of embryotoxicity include prenatal death, structural and functional defects and, in their mildest form, growth retardation of the conceptus. The embryotoxic outcomes have a 'normal' or 'spontaneous' occurrence in human populations upon which are superimposed any additional cases possibly arising from exposures to drugs, food additives, cosmetics and other chemicals from environmental sources.

Although it would be most desirable to have integrated screening systems capable of predicting a broad range of effects from mutagenesis to behavioural defects and, perhaps, carcinogenesis, such comprehensive test systems are not yet available. The development of such systems is dependent upon future research, and must be based on an understanding of the basic biological relationships between mutagenesis, teratogenesis and carcinogenesis.

Direct evidence for the embryotoxic potential of a substance can usually be secured only from animal experiments. However, animal tests are considered by some experts to be of low predictive value for man; only a few chemicals have been proven as teratogens in man compared to the hundreds exhibiting the embryotoxic potential in laboratory animals.

Screening for reproductive toxicity became a matter of legislation as long as 15 years ago in many countries. The currently used official procedures, especially those that are believed to mimic features of human teratogenesis, are considered by many to afford satisfactory safeguards. Alternative methods adapted from basic teratological research employ simple experimental systems ranging from individual cells and more or less isolated parts of mammalian fetoplacental units to embryos of non-mammalian species. According to a widespread opinion, these techniques represent an important complement to teratological research, but generally cannot replace the official procedures for regulatory purposes.

* Only the summary is included here because of space limitations. The full report can be requested from the authors.

313

More fundamentally, however, it must be recognized that a reliable test system should not only examine various features of embryotoxicity but must also be capable of screening for human embryotoxic metabolites if the *in vitro* techniques (including the avian embryo) are to be valid.

Probably the specificity of embryotoxic action of chemicals in humans resides neither in the basic morphogenetic processes nor in the unusual properties of placental transfer of xenobiotics alone, but also often in metabolic transformation within the maternal organism which frequently differs between species. Thus, any procedure using a non-human pregnant animal suffers from the possible introduction of an additional unknown variable. For this reason it is desirable to test not only the parent substance but also metabolites occurring in man. Blood sera of the exposed human individuals can in some cases be employed as their source.

In basic teratological research it is recommended to cease the search for an animal similar to man and turn to the more useful activity of investigating the possibility of using *in vitro* techniques for more exact estimation of the embryotoxicity dose range for a pregnant mammal. The major task of basic research, however, remains the investigation of the functional properties of embryonic, fetal, perinatal and postnatal morphogenetic systems and the factors underlying the sensitivity of their constituent cell populations to toxic agents coming from the environment. As to testing needs, an approach involving multilevel screening procedures starting with *in vitro* techniques is suggested as a priority selection system.

In the area of applied research, practical tests need to be devised starting from the most promising developments in basic teratological research. Such tests would then be eligible for trial and for standardization.

The regulatory agencies will need to collect and evaluate critically the information necessary for proposing new guidelines for embryotoxicity testing that will cover the range of chemicals to which man may be exposed in the present society. Meanwhile, basic research must aim towards a better understanding of the biological inter-relationships of the various possible effects on the fetus such as mutagenesis, teratogenesis and carcinogenesis arising from exposure to toxic chemicals.

More detailed discussion of methods and procedures for teratogenicity testing developed in Czechoslovak laboratories may be found in the papers published by the authors and their collaborators listed below.

2 REFERENCES

Dostál, M. and Jelínek, R. (1973). Sensitivity of embryos and intraspecies differences in mice in response to prenatal administration of corticoids. *Teratology* **8**, 245–252.

Jelínek, R. (1977). The chick embryotoxicity screening test (CHEST). In Neubert, D., Merker, H. J. and Kwasigroch, T. E. (Eds.). *Methods in Prenatal Toxicology*, pp. 381–386. G. Thieme, Stuttgart.

Jelínek, R. (1979). Embryotoxicity assay on morphogenetic systems. In Benešová, O., Rychter, Z. and Jelinek, R. (Eds.). *Evaluation of Embryotoxicity, Mutagenicity and Carcinogenicity Risks in New Drugs*, pp. 195–205. Univerzita Karlova, Praha.

Jelínek, R., Benešová, O., Peterka, M., Souček, K. and Žatecká, I. (1978). Embryotoxicity of maprotiline (Ludiomil, Ciba-Geigy) in a semiclinical experiment. *Act. Nerv. Super.* (*Prabha*) **20**, 300.

Jelínek, R., Benešová, O. and Souček, K. (1980). The use of chick embryotoxicity screening test (CHEST) in evaluating blood sera of patients treated with antidepressants. *Pol. J. Pharmacol. Pharm.* **32**, 205–209.

Jelínek, R. and Dostál, M. (1973). Species specificity in teratology in the light of analyzing the intraspecies differences in mice. *Folia Morphol.* (*Prague*) **21**, 94–96.

Jelínek, R. and Rychter, Z. (1979). Morphogenetic systems and the central phenomena of teratology. In Persaud, T. V. N. (Ed.). *New Trends in Experimental Teratology*, pp. 41–67. M. T. P. Press, Lancaster.

Jelínek, R. and Rychter, Z. (1980). Morphogenetic systems and screening for embryotoxicity. *Archs Toxicol. Suppl.* **4**, 267–273.

Jelínek, R., Volhová, I. and Loštický, C. (1975). Interference of heterologous vertebrate sera with chick embryo development. *Folia Morphol.* (*Prague*) **23**, 136–144.

Marhan, O. and Jelínek, R. (1979a). Efficiency of the embryotoxicity testing procedures. I. A compromise approach. *Toxicol. Lett.* (*Amsterdam*) **4**, 385–388.

Marhan, O., and Jelínek, R. (1979b). Efficiency of the embryotoxicity testing procedures. II. Comparison between the official, MEST and CHEST methods. *Toxicol. Lett.* (*Amsterdam*) **4**, 389–392.

Marhan, O., Jelínek, R., Rychter, Z. and Řežábek, K. (1979). Seventeen drugs compared in embryotoxicity tests using pregnant animals and a morphogenetic system. In Benešová, O., Rychter, Z. and Jelínek, R. (Eds.). *Evaluation of Embryotoxicity, Mutagenicity and Carcinogenicity Risks in New Drugs*, pp. 219–227. Univerzita Karlova, Praha.

Methods for Assessing the Effects of Chemicals on Reproductive Functions
Edited by V. B. Vouk and P. J. Sheehan
© 1983 SCOPE

Perinatal Exposure and Teratological Endpoints: Some Principles and Possibilities

RICHARD DOHERTY

1 INTRODUCTION

Prenatal exposure to toxic environmental chemicals could affect male or female germ cells, or the various somatic organs. Goals for reproductive screening of potentially toxic chemicals are to determine the magnitude of possible germ cell or somatic damage and to estimate resultant impact on reproductive capacity or somatic functional capacity throughout the life cycle. Prenatal exposure to toxic chemicals could result in sterility or spontaneous abortion, reducing overall fertility. Even more worrisome, however, are lesser somatic effects which allow survival of individuals with varying degrees of mental and physical handicap or reductions in physiological adaptive capacities, who are, or will become, significantly handicapped during their lifetimes.

Concepts of normal and abnormal early mammalian development that may contribute to prenatal and postnatal reproductive screening strategies are briefly reviewed. Possible teratological and toxic effects of chemical agents on the developing organism must be evaluated within the context of rather extensive embryofetal, perinatal wastage and postnatal developmental and reproductive morbidity due to other environmental and genetic causes. Multiplication and differentiation of functional units during early development and effects on functional reserve adaptive capacity in the developmentally mature organism provide a conceptual framework for evaluating adverse effects of chemical agents.

The importance of valid dose–effect, dose–response relationships as an essential basis for hazard evaluation is stressed and is illustrated with the few available human examples.

Finally, lactation as a route of exposure is discussed because it represents a unique early postnatal nutritional stage during which the rapidly developing suckling infant is completely dependent on mother's milk, which, if contaminated with toxic pollutant chemicals; could pose a significant threat to early postnatal growth and development.

317

2 BIOLOGICAL ASPECTS OF HUMAN DEVELOPMENT RELATING TO EVALUATION OF ADVERSE REPRODUCTIVE EFFECTS OF CHEMICALS

During the course of normal prenatal human development the human conceptus increases from one cell, the fertilized egg, to $\sim$ 1000 billions of cells in the newborn infant. From this quantitative dimension alone, to say nothing of the qualitative complexities of differentiation and interaction of at least 100 histologically distinguishable types of cells, it is not surprising to find that abnormalities of development are frequent. There is great opportunity for interference with early developmental processes due to abnormal intrinsic (genetic) capacity, as well as from adverse environmental influences (e.g. chemical pollutants) which may impact the developmental sequence. We have very little knowledge of details of developmental processes or the mechanisms by which they are impeded.

With this developmental perspective, it is not so surprising to learn that a large fraction of embryos and fetuses fail to develop with sufficient capacity to survive to birth. Recent clarification of the major contribution of chromosomal causes of early embryofetal wastage has provided insight that fetal incapacity due to chromosomal abnormalities and malformations of unknown cause contribute a large fraction of embryofetal wastage due to inability of abnormal embryos and fetuses to survive. In addition to the 15–20% of pregnancies which end in perceived spontaneous abortions, it is currently estimated that 40–50% of total conceptions do not survive to live birth, a phenomenon that is also observed widely in other mammalian species (Carr, 1977; see Warburton, this publication). Yet this extensive prenatal biological filtering by spontaneous abortion is not complete. Approximately 1 in 200 newborns has a detectable chromosomal abnormality, and it is conservatively estimated that 3–5% of human infants are born with medically significant birth defects or mental retardation. Yet, there are few proven human teratogens and it has been predicted that drugs and environmental chemicals cause less than 1% of congenital malformations (Wilson, 1973; Brent and Harris, 1976). A measure of the primitiveness of current knowledge is the admission that we are unable to assign specific causes for 60–70% of malformations observed in human infants at birth (Wilson, 1973). Since most birth defects are of unknown aetiology it is possible that some additional portion could be due to prenatal exposure to toxic chemicals.

Approximately 3% of the US population is considered mentally retarded (IQ < 70). About 10% of these individuals are severely retarded (IQ < 50). It is currently thought that the majority of severe mental retardation represents discontinuous phenotypes due to chromosomal, environmental, Mendelian and multifactorial causes (Opitz, 1980). The numbers of mild to moderately retarded persons who may have been adversely affected by prenatal or perinatal exposure to toxic environmental chemical agents cannot currently be estimated. Recently, the first strong evidence has been presented that childhood (non-occupational) exposure to unidentified ambient sources of lead can cause neuropsychological deficits that may interfere with classroom performance (Needleman *et al.*, 1979, 1982). The frequency of non-adaptive classroom behaviour increased in a dose-related fashion relative to dentine (tooth) lead levels, at doses below those producing signs or symptoms severe enough to be diagnosed clinically.

To evaluate possible adverse effects of prenatal chemical exposure, toxic effects of chemicals must be distinguished from the rather high background frequencies of prenatal growth retardation, birth defects, mental retardation and learning or other behavioural disorders of unknown cause. The formidable task of determining valid dose–response relationships in prenatally and perinatally exposed populations has infrequently been accomplished to date. Exceptions are the dentine lead–school performance study of Needleman *et al.* described briefly above, and the Iraqi methylmercury outbreak described in more detail below.

Animal models provide powerful tools for investigating mechanisms of teratological effects but currently applied teratogenicity tests seems very limited in terms of their capacity to predict human teratogens (Brent, 1972). Lack of fundamental knowledge of mammalian developmental biology is the most serious handicap we face in designing rational and reliable non-human reproductive screening tests. Thus present approaches to teratogenicity and developmental toxicity testing must be empirically derived. This situation could be improved by informative comparative pharmacokinetic studies among mammalian species as promoted by Rall and others (Freireich *et al.*, 1966) coupled with further development of more sensitive structure – function assessment of postnatal end-points such as as those described by Rodier (see below). However, as commented by Wilson (1977): 'The absence of embryotoxicity in a well-conducted animal study, at doses representing reasonable multiples above estimated environmental levels, does not assure the safety of any chemical.'

Ultimately, direct observational studies in human populations must provide the most reliable test of whether or not exposure is associated with adverse health effects in humans. Possible end-points include a spectrum of effects from sterility, reduced fertility or spontaneous abortion or stillbirth, through intrauterine growth retardation, to survival with non-lethal congenital malformations or with aberrant or reduced functional capacities of various organs, especially the reproductive system or the central nervous system.

Stein and coworkers argue persuasively the importance of constructing pre-experiment design and evaluating post-experiment interpretation of environmental health studies of chemical agents in terms of statistical power analysis (Strobino *et al.*, 1978; see Warburton, this publication). Power is a measure of the capacity of a study to detect an effect. Most observers would support extension of well-designed epidemiological surveillance studies to monitor possible effects of environmental chemical agents potentially injurious to exposed subsets or in some instances possibly to the population at large (see PCBs below). However, it must be emphasized that none of the major human teratogens has been identified by epidemiological methods (Miller, 1970), or by screening for teratogenicity using animals tests. Rather they have been discovered by alert, observant medical practitioners often aided by patients or related lay observers.

3 TOXIC OR TERATOLOGICAL EFFECTS ON FUNCTIONAL UNITS AND RESERVE ADAPTIVE CAPACITY

Concepts of development and regulation which have been originated or promoted by Goss (1964, 1966, 1978a, b) have potentially significant implications for understanding and evaluating teratological and toxicological effects of environmental chemicals on developing mammals. Goss' classification of tissues in terms of their mitotic or regenerative growth capacities provides a relevant general developmental framework.

Renewing tissues such as the epidermis, mucosal epithelium of the gut, seminiferous epithelium of testis, and blood cells, are in a continual state of multiplication, i.e. cellular losses are kinetically balanced by replacements (Figures 1, 2). For example, approximately one million new erythrocytes are constructed every second to replace an equivalent number which are destroyed during the same time interval. The germinative zones of these tissues, spatially distinct from the resultant differentiated cells, are populated with

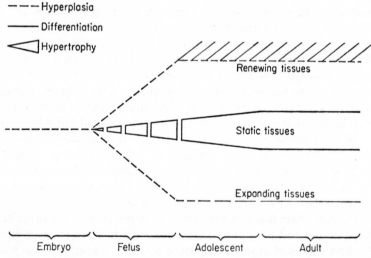

Figure 1 Alternate pathways of growth and differentiation in tissues and organs. *Renewing tissues* continue to proliferate throughout life, generating decendants that differentiate into non-mitotic cells. *Static tissues* permanently lose the capacity to divide as they differentiate early in life; thereafter they grow by hypertrophy. *Expanding tissues* do not stop dividing until body growth ceases, despite their fully differentiated condition. (Reproduced with permission from Goss, 1967)

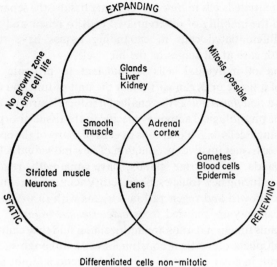

Figure 2 Relationship between static, renewing, and expanding tissues. *Static tissues* differ from the others in their lack of mitotic potential. *Renewing tissues* have growth zones spatially distinct from the differentiated compartment, and the life spans of their cells are relatively short. *Expanding tissues* are capable of cell division in the fully differentiated state; their specific products are secreted from the cells and the functions are, in general, chemical in nature. As indicated, some tissues and organs of the body share attributes in common with more than one of these categories. (Reproduced with permission from Goss, 1967)

relatively undifferentiated progenitor ('stem') cells in a state of constant proliferation.

In *expanding tissues* such as most endocrine glands there is no spatial incompatibility between proliferation and differentiation. Dividing cells are diffusely distributed. There is no need for a germinative compartment separate from differentiated cells since all cells apparently are capable of division.

Mitotically *static tissues*, e.g. the nervous system and striated muscle, do not proliferate beyond early stages of development when neuroblasts and myoblasts begin to differentiate into neurons and muscle fibres. Cells of these static tissues, like those in expanding organs, are capable of living as long as the organism as a whole survives. Differentiated cells of both static and renewing tissues cannot divide. In static tissues the germinative cell population compartment is separated from the differentiated cells in *time*; in renewing tissues, the separation is *spatial*. In contrast to the inability of differentiated cells to renew and static tissues to proliferate, differentiated cells in expanding tissues have the capacity to proliferate with ease at all stages of the life cycle.

Proliferation of individual cells is sufficient to promote full functional competence of a tissue or organ *only* when the unit of function is the cell. Goss (1964) defines a *functional unit* as the smallest irreducible structure still capable of performing the physiological activities specific to the tissue or organ. Functional units may be single cells, e.g. blood cells or cells of many of the endocrine glands. Growth in these tissues involves production of new individual cells. Organs such as thyroid glands, or exocrine glands, have apparently retained unlimited capacity for producing new follicles, or secretory acini, and are therefore capable of remarkable growth and regeneration. Organs with this type of growth and regenerative capacity are referred to as *indeterminate organs.*

In some organs functional units are multicellular and they cannot be increased simply by multiplication of their constituent cells, although such cell multiplication can result in enlargement of individual functional units and in a limited increase in functional capacity. It would seem to have been to the advantage of the organism if such organs were capable of proliferating (or regenerating) at the organizational level of their functional units, yet the evolutionary sequence has eliminated regenerative capacity. Some organs such as the mammalian kidney are unable to increase their numbers of multicellular functional units. The number of nephrons in the kidney is fixed early in life and cannot be increased after developmental maturation (Figure 3). Compensatory growth of a kidney after removal of the other kidney of a pair is achieved by cellular hyperplasia and hypertrophy, resulting in larger nephrons with some increase in functional capacity, but mature kidneys are unable to regenerate nephrons. Organs incapable of regenerating functional units after maturity include lung (alveoli), small intestine (villi) and testes (seminiferous tubules) (Figure 3). Growth is possible in these *determinate organs* only by increasing size but not number of functional units.

It is apparent that toxic chemical agents (or other adverse genetic or environmental factors) could reduce total *reserve adaptive capacity* of *determinate organs* (1) by interfering with formation of the absolute number or anatomic distribution of functional units generated during early development, or (2) by destroying functional units after maturity when they can no longer be replaced. Both effects permanently reduce reserve capacity and render the organism liable to debilitating or even life-threatening effects if the numbers of functional units are further depleted by other physical, chemical or biological injurious influences, or by aging.

Thus, if an organ (*indeterminate*) can multiply its functional units it is capable of unlimited growth (hyperplasia) and regeneration to maintain functional efficiency. Conversely, *determinate* organs can compensate for developmental

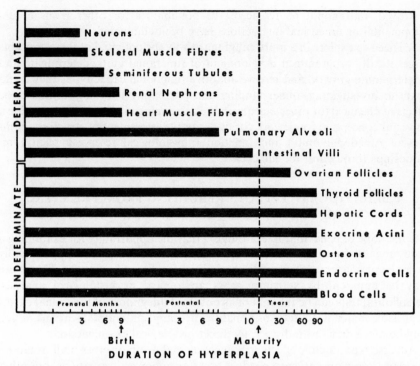

Figure 3 Duration of hyperplasia in various histological structures in man. Organs in which substructures cease to multiply before maturity have *determinate* numbers of structural units and restricted capacities for growth beyond normal adult dimensions. Those which retain their hyperplastic abilities throughout life can grow potentially without limit, and therefore have *indeterminate* numbers of structural units. (Reproduced with permission from Goss, 1966)

reductions or mature losses of functional units only to a limited extent by enlarging the remaining functional units (hypertrophy). It is not yet apparent why certain organs are endowed with unlimited powers of growth while some of the most vitally essential organs of the body, the brain, the heart, the lungs and the kidneys, cannot augment their specified populations of functional units (Goss, 1967). Therefore, it is not surprising that these determinate organs, indispensable for survival, are susceptible to effects of adverse environmental effects which sooner or later may contribute to debilitation or lethality.

I do not mean to imply that there are not other important mechanisms for causing permanent injury to organs of developing mammals. Damage to the genome or interference with cell–cell interactions both during development and in the mature central nervous system are important possible mechanisms of teratological and structural toxic effects at the cellular or organ level. Nevertheless, if cells or functional units are not initially generated or are destroyed and cannot be replaced, the possibilities for other levels of developmental or functional interactions have been eliminated.

We need to explore in a more enlightened way the potential of these concepts of genetically programmed development of functional units, determinate and indeterminate growth, and reserve adaptive functional capacity, as they could relate to investigating, understanding and preventing teratological and toxic effects of chemical (or other) agents on the developing mammal. They provide a powerful conceptual framework for quantitative assessment of structure (numbers of functional units) and function (physiological reserve capacity) relationships throughout the life cycle.

4 BEHAVIOURAL EFFECTS RESULTING FROM PRENATAL EXPOSURE TO TERATOGENIC AND TOXIC CHEMICALS

It is the hope of behavioural teratologists that the opportunity for examining a wide range of functional activities and responses after exposure to potentially toxic chemical agents will provide possibilities for discerning subtler effects than may be apparent by standard gross anatomical or histological analysis. Behavioural tests can be thought of as potential integrators of functional effects of possible minor structural abnormalities in many anatomical locations, which may be more difficult to discern by direct histological examination.

Adverse reproductive effects may include fetal death or gross malformation. Postnatal survivors can have residual gross or minor malformations, but other individuals may have subtler physical defects, or functional brain deficits expressed as reduced intelligence or aberrant behavioural responses, which would not be discerned by prenatal evaluation. Postnatal evaluation of effects of potential teratogens in animals is an important screening objective, since it is mainly this class of adverse effects, resulting in handicapped human survivors, which is of major concern to society.

Significantly abnormal function of most critical organ systems is usually expressed in mortality data. Physiological deviations compatible with survival require more demanding efforts to discern. Failure or impaired function of reproductive organs and impaired higher functions of the central nervous system are better tolerated than deficits in most other organ systems, since they have less drastic direct impact on survival of the individual. Therefore, these organ systems, especially the central nervous system, provide sensitive useful indicators of adverse effects of chemical agents.

The developing mammalian central nervous system is especially vulnerable because of its long developmental sequence continuing throughout much of embryofetal development and extending well beyond birth into infancy. While neurogenesis is only one of many complex events in the development of the nervous system, it is critical, for a nervous system lacking a full complement of neurons would not be expected to develop and function normally.

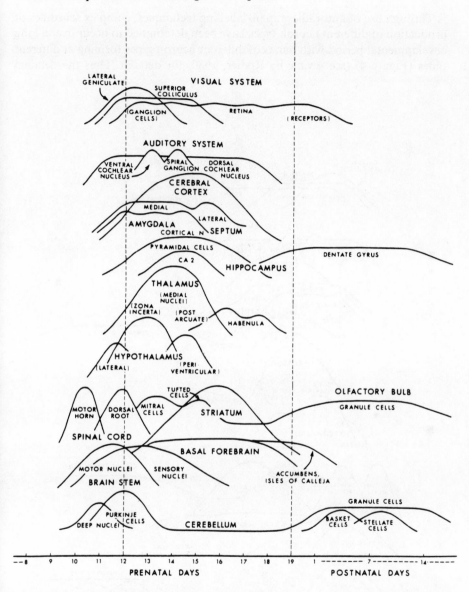

Figure 4 Chronology of proliferative bursts of neuron production in mouse CNS. Vertical line on E12 (prenatal day 12) represents last day of gestation when gross external malformations can be induced by interference with cell proliferation. Vertical line on day 19 represents time of birth. Parentheses enclose structures or cell type included as examples: for example, many thalamic nuclei are forming on E14—the medial nuclei are representative of a larger group. (Reproduced with permission from Rodier, P. M., 1980)

Through use of autoradiographic labelling techniques, complex schedules of production of different neuron types have been determined to occur over a long developmental period with bursts of different neuron types forming at different times (Figure 4) (see review by Rodier, 1980, for details). Thus the detailed

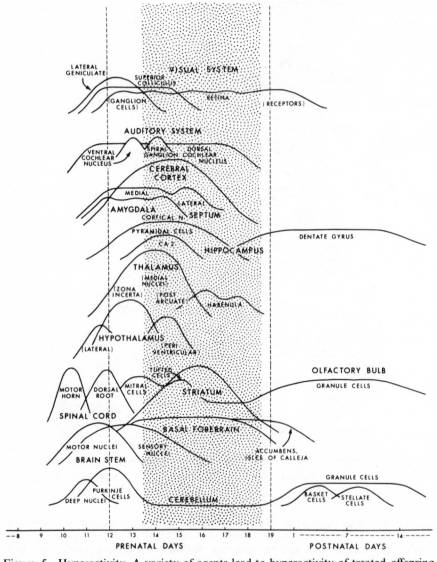

Figure 5   Hyperactivity. A variety of agents lead to hyperactivity of treated offspring when delivered during the period marked by stippling. (Reproduced with permission from Rodier, P. M., 1980)

chronology of production of different geographic populations of neurons becomes important for understanding the clinical relevance of timing of brain injury during development. Though absolute time schedules of the generation of neuron populations differ among mammals, relative temporal sequences of production of different types of neurons are similar.

Brain damage resulting from interference with neuron proliferation may have

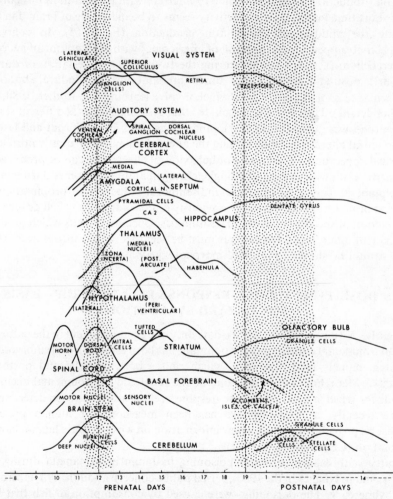

Figure 6 Hypoactivity, reflex delays, locomotor abnormalities. Critical period for syndromes combining hypoactivity with various reflex delays and motor abnormalities is biphasic. Both early and late insults seem to lead to these behaviours, while insults in between these periods have other effects. (Reproduced with permission from Rodier, P.M., 1980)

a variety of behavioural effects, since the systems that are damaged will differ from one developmental stage to another. Studies of specific temporal insults (exposures to X-irradiation or azacytidine) to cell proliferation have documented that the behavioural effects are as time dependent as the corresponding neuroanatomical effects (Hicks and D'Amato, 1961; Rodier and Gramann, 1979). Cell loss at different times produces different behavioural effects. Rodier (1980) has related critical periods for behavioural effects to critical periods for neuron production using azacytidine to interfere with proliferation of neurons over short time intervals. Hyperactivity seems to be indicative of brain damage during the middle part of neuron production (Figure 5). In contrast, hypoactivity appears to be the result of interference with proliferation of neurons of cerebellum (Figure 6) either during the twelfth day of gestation or during the first postnatal week. Other timed prenatal insults produce abnormal performance on a variety of tests which involve learning (see Rodier, 1980, for further details). Thus it can be concluded that systemic insults at different stages of neurogenesis during brain development may result in significant and lasting behavioural alterations while leaving the affected animals apparently normal in physical appearance. The variety of behavioural effects that can be produced is extensive, even with the use of a single teratogen at different times during brain development. Timing of exposure and temporal sequences of proliferation of specific brain cell populations are obviously critical variables which govern the production of specific behavioural teratologies. Chemical agents which produce permanent alterations of behaviour must be regarded as hazardous even when they cannot be shown to produce morphological changes.

5 DOSE–EFFECT, DOSE–RESPONSE RELATIONSHIP—BASIS FOR HAZARD EVALUATION

Recently, Wilson (1977) wrote: 'To date only one chemical agent in the nature of an environmental contaminant or pollutant has been established as embryotoxic in man, namely methylmercury, which causes both prenatal and postnatal toxicity.' Methylmercury is also one of the few toxic environmental chemical agents for which a valid adult dose–response relationship has been determined. More recently, a dose–response has been measured for human prenatal exposure, providing important new information on which to base human hazard evaluation (Clarkson *et al.*, 1981).

Large outbreaks of mercury poisoning in Japan in Minamata during the 1950s, and in Niigata in the 1960s, raised public concern about health hazards of methylmercury. The poisonings were caused by consumption of fish that had been contaminated by industrial discharge of methylmercury compounds (Tsubaki and Irukayama, 1977). When Swedish investigators discovered that inorganic mercury could be methylated by microorganisms in the environment to form methylmercury it was realized that the ecotoxicological threat was more widespread (WHO, 1976; NAS, 1978). Standards for maximum safe levels of methylmercury in edible fish were proposed by several nations, and WHO advised a tolerable weekly intake of methylmercury (WHO, 1972, 1978). These estimates were derived from best available data but there was an important need for quantitative human dose–effect, dose–response relationships and for identification of the most sensitive stage of the human life cycle. In Japan, it had been observed that asymptomatic mothers exposed to methylmercury during pregnancy could produce neurologically damaged offspring.

An unusual opportunity to obtain data for determining dose–response relationships was provided when a large outbreak of methylmercury poisoning occurred in Iraq during the winter of 1971–2 (Bakir *et al.*, 1973). Within approximately a 3-month period large numbers of rural families consumed homemade bread prepared from seed wheat which had been treated with a methylmercury fungicide. More than 6000 persons were hospitalized and approximately 450 hospital deaths were attributed to methylmercury poisoning. Many other individuals are known to have been seriously poisoned. The importance of this large outbreak as a unique opportunity to obtain detailed information on effects of prenatal exposure was appreciated and long-term studies were initiated to document both adult and prenatal fetal exposures and to observe toxic effects in resulting offspring.

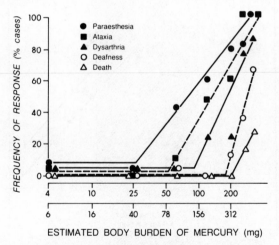

Figure 7 The relationship between frequency of signs and symptoms and the estimated body burden of methylmercury. Both scales of the abscissa refer to body burdens of methylmercury (mg) at the cessation of exposure. The two scales represented different methods of calculating the body burden as discussed in the text. (Adapted from Bakir *et al.*, 1973)

Dose–response relationships imply cause–effect relationships. Their importance as a basic input for human hazard evaluation is well recognized. The relationship between frequency of signs or symptoms and estimated body burden of non-pregnant adults in Iraq are shown in Figure 7 (Bakir *et al.*, 1973).

It was discovered that the concentration of mercury in hair at the time of its formation is directly proportional to simultaneous concentration in blood. Sequential, segmental analysis of hair mercury content provided a reliable, quantitative means of recapitulation of exposure for 2 years or longer prior to the time of hair sampling, since hair grows approximately 1 cm each month. Maternal hair mercury levels were determined through pregnancy intervals, providing an integrative index of fetal exposure, and enabling dose–response relationships to be developed for postnatally observed effects of fetal exposure (Figure 8). Maternal hair mercury levels were related to frequencies of motor retardation and other central nervous system signs in 82 mother–infant pairs (Figure 9) (Clarkson *et al.*, 1981).

These observations provide the first example of a dose–response relationship of human prenatal exposure to a toxic environmental chemical pollutant. The

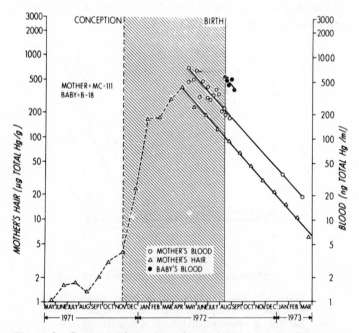

Figure 8   Concentration of total mercury in 1 cm segments of sample of mother's hair, whole blood, and baby's blood (prenatal exposure). (Reproduced with permission from Amin-Zaki *et al.* (1976) *Am. J. Dis. Child.* **130**, 1070–1076, Copyright 1976, American Medical Association)

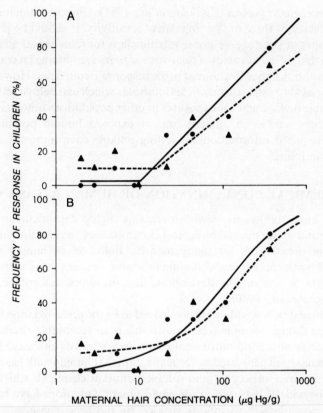

Figure 9 Frequency of abnormalities in prenatally exposed children versus the estimated maximum body burden in the mother during pregnancy. In Figure 13.9A, the estimated frequencies were obtained by the Hockey Stick method and in Figure 13.9B by logit analysis. 0———— Motor retardation is defined as failure to walk by the age of 18 months; Δ-------- CNS signs, moderate to severe central nervous system (CNS) signs were defined according to a scoring system ranging from mild (unity) to most severe (ten). Children with a score greater than three were defined as having CNS signs. The scoring was based on the results of examination by two independent neurologists. (Reproduced with permission from Clarkson *et al.*, 1981)

adult and prenatal dose–response relationships enable quantitative comparison of differential sensitivity at different life cycle stages, providing a more sound basis for human hazard evaluation.

From these dose–response relationships EC50 values have been calculated which indicate that the human fetus is more sensitive to methylmercury than the adult, non-pregnant person (Clarkson *et al.*, 1981). Current estimates indicate roughly a factor of three or four in relative sensitivity. It should be pointed out that the slopes of the dose–response relationships for fetus versus adult are not parallel, so that different values of relative sensitivity are obtained if comparisons are based on body concentrations at other response frequencies. However, these data can be used to estimate practical thresholds which can help in setting limits for acceptable methylmercury exposures in other populations potentially at risk. Thus mercury studies in animals and in exposed human populations are providing required information for setting reliable environmental and nutritional intake limits.

6 CHEMICAL CONTAMINATION OF HUMAN BREAST MILK

Following birth the human newborn remains highly dependent on maternal sustenance and under normal biological circumstances receives total nutritional intake from breast milk for many months. Pollution of human milk with widespread synthetic chemical contaminants raises concern for potential adverse health effects on the rapidly developing, and presumed susceptible, suckling infant (Rogan *et al.*, 1980).

Human breast milk is widely acknowledged to be the preferred food for human infants, even though formula-feeding by bottle is an acceptable alternative with apparent safety and good nutritional results in a majority of cases. Therefore, some alarm has been generated by the realization that human milk has often been found to contain a variety of lipid-soluble pollutant chemicals which are now known to be widely dispersed in the environment. Questions have been raised about the possible risk to infants suckled by mothers whose milk contains measurable quantities of a variety of synthetic organohalides such as the polychlorinated biphenyls (PCBs) and dichlorodiphenyl trichloroethane (DDT) (Barr, 1981).

Long-term low-level exposure to the organohalides results in gradual accumulation of residues in body fat, including the fat of breast milk (Rall, 1979). Lactation is the only route by which large amounts of such residues are known to be excreted. The fat content of breast milk varies widely among women, with some differences even in the same lactating mother from day to day, as well as significant increases in concentration even during a single feeding. Since these chemicals are nearly all partitioned in fat it is not surprising that there is considerable variation in reported milk levels. Concentrations of chemical residues in milk should be expressed on a fat content basis to aid in comparing results from different studies and over time.

A systematic survey of pesticides in mother's milk was sponsored by the Environmental Protection Agency (Savage, 1977). Of 1038 milk samples, 30% had levels above 0.05 parts per million (p.p.m.) on a whole milk basis, and 6.7% had levels above 0.1 p.p.m. More recently, breast milk samples from more than a thousand nursing mothers in Michigan were analysed for PCB residues (Wickizer *et al.*, 1981). All of the samples collected from 68 of the state's 83 counties contained measurable PCB residues, ranging from trace quantities to 5.1 p.p.m. (fat basis). The mean level was 1.496 p.p.m.; 17.4% had 2–3 p.p.m.; 6.14%, more than 3 p.p.m. It was estimated that an infant breast fed for 8 months by a woman with this average PCB milk level (1.496 p.p.m.) would have a cumulated body burden of approximately 0.89 mg/kg (p.p.m.) of PCBs. Nearly one-half of these sampled women had breast milk PCB concentrations equal to or above the present FDA tolerance limit (1.5 p.p.m./fat basis) for cow's milk. Blood PCB levels in infants ingesting PCB-contaminated breast milk may exceed those of their non-occupationally exposed mothers by as much as six-fold (Kuwabara *et al.*, 1979). The possible effects of this chemical contamination on the growth and development of infants are at present unknown.

Because of their chemical stability and resistance to biological decomposition, polychlorinated biphenyls have become ubiquitous environmental contaminants. It is estimated that more than 1.4 billion pounds have been manufactured and introduced into the marketplace since 1929, and that 750 million pounds are still in service and available to impact the environment (Sheffy, 1979). The high lipid solubility of PCBs facilitates their entry and progressive accumulation in the food chain leading to man, with the suckling human infant at the apex. Unfortunately, little toxicological information is available on which to base hazard evaluation. Of particular concern relating to possible prenatal exposure is Barr's recent report that PCBs enter the fetal brain compartment, though they do not seem to cross the adult blood–brain barrier (Barr, 1981).

Though these observations are reason for serious concern, the recommendation by the Wisconsin State Department of Health, in a letter to all Wisconsin physicians, stating that certain subsets of women should have their milk analysed for PCBs and insecticides, and that the Department of Health cannot recommend continuation of breast feeding if milk PCB levels in a mother are above the FDA tolerance limit, would seem premature and imprudent according to Kendrick (1980). A retrospective EPA study of the 1975–6 human milk survey and two prospective studies in progress in Wisconsin and in North Carolina may provide data which will aid in evaluating whether adverse health effects can be ascertained in human infants whose mother's milk has higher than average levels of PCBs.

7 METHYLMERCURY POISONING IN BREAST-FED INFANTS

That human infants can be severely damaged by ingestion of a mercury fungicide solely through dietary intake of exposed mothers has been demonstrated during the recent large outbreak of methylmercury poisoning in Iraq (Amin-Zaki *et al.*, 1976, 1980). The Iraqi outbreak of acute methylmercury poisoning from ingestion of bread made from seed wheat treated with a methylmercury fungicide

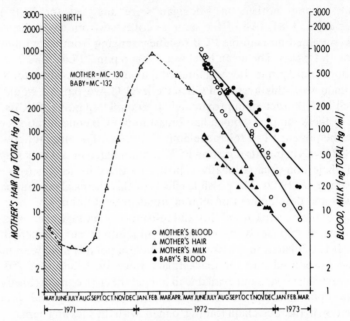

Figure 10   Concentration of total mercury in 1 cm segments of sample of mother's hair, whole blood, and milk, and baby's blood (postnatal exposure). Cencentrations in milk and blood are plotted according to dates of collection. (Reproduced with permission from Amin-Zaki *et al.* (1976) *Am. J. Dis. Child.* **130**, 1070–1076, Copyright 1976, American Medical Association)

provided an opportunity to measure methylmercury intake via suckling in infants born just prior to the time when their mothers began eating contaminated bread. As shown by the example in Figure 10, suckled infants' blood mercury concentrations were frequently raised to levels greater than those of their mothers by transfer of methylmercury in milk. A number of these infants were later observed to have suffered significant adverse neurological effects. (Amin-Zaki *et al.*, 1980).

Potentially large acute doses of chemical agents can also be transmitted from mother to suckled offspring. As much as 27% of a tracer dose of radioactive iodine administered to a lactating woman has been observed to cross the plasma–milk barrier (Nurnberger and Lipscomb, 1952). Recently, studies of mice in our laboratory have also shown that approximately 25% of an intravenous maternal dose of lead is transferred to the litter by suckling within four days, accounting for a significant fraction of the total lead excreted by the lactating mothers (Figure 11) (Keller and Doherty, 1980).

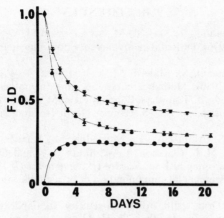

Figure 11   Whole-body retention (FID, Fraction of Initial Dose) of lead in lactating (Δ) and non-lactating (∇) female mice following i.v. lead administration and transfer of meternal lead to suckling pups (0). Vertical bars represent $\pm$ 1 s.e. Bars not shown when smaller than symbol dimensions. (Reproduced with permission from Keller and Doherty (1980) Lead and calcium distributions in blood, plasma and milk of the lactating mouse. *J. lab. clin. Med.* **95**, 81–89)

8 CONCLUSIONS

Potential teratological and toxic effects of chemical agents on the developing mammal can best be evaluated within the context of the rather extensive background of observed embryofetal and perinatal wastage, and postnatal developmental morbidity. Unfortunately, at present, our very limited knowledge of genetic and environmental factors affecting mammalian development precludes other than an empirical approach for evaluating adverse effects of environmental agents. Some general principles of development relating to embryological generation of functional units, regenerative capacities of determinate and indeterminate organ systems, and the concept of changes in reserve adaptive capacity throughout the life cycle are proposed as useful parameters for a conceptual framework with which to evaluate teratological and toxic effects of environmental agents on the developing mammal. The importance of examining dose–effect, dose–response relationships in terms of establishing quantitative estimates of prenatal or perinatal dose and evaluating quantitatively effects (response) and all subsequent postnatal stages in terms of adverse effects on reserve adaptive capacities of organ systems is emphasized.

9 REFERENCES

Amin-Zaki, L., Elhassani, S., Majeed, M. A., Clarkson, T. W., Doherty, R. A. and Greenwood, M. (1976). Perinatal methylmercury poisoning in Iraq. *Am. J. Dis. Child.* **130**, 1070–1076.

Amin-Zaki, L., Elhassani, S., Majeed, M. A., Clarkson, T. W., Doherty, R. A. and Greenwood, M. (1980). Methylmercury poisoning in mothers and their suckling infants. In Holmstedt, B., Lauwerys, R. and Mercer, M. (Eds.) *Mechanisms of Toxicity and Hazard Evaluation*, pp. 75–78. Elsevier/North Holland Biomedical Press, New York.

Bakir, F., Damluji, S., Amin-Zaki, L., Murtadha, M., Khalidi, A., Al-Rawi, N. Y., Tikriti, S., Dhahir, H. I., Clarkson, T. W., Smith, J. C. and Doherty, R. A. (1973). Methylmercury poisoning in Iraq. *Science (Washington, DC)* **181**, 230.

Barr, M. (1981). Environmental contamination of breast milk. *Am. J. Public Health* **71**, 124–126.

Brent, R. L. (1972). Drug testing for teratogenicity: its implications, limitations and applications to man. *Adv. exp. Biol.* **27**, 31–43.

Brent, R. L. and Harris, M. I. (1976). Environmental factors: miscellaneous. In *Prevention of Embryonic, Fetal and Perinatal Disease*, pp. 211–218. N. I. H., Bethesda, Maryland.

Carr, D. H. (1977). Detection and evaluation of pregnancy wastage. In Wilson, J. G. and Fraser, F. Clarke (Eds.) *Handbook of Teratology* 3, pp. 189–213. Plenum Press, New York.

Clarkson, T. W., Cox, C. Marsh, D. O., Myers, G. J. Al-Tikriti, S. K., Amin-Zaki, L., and Dabbagh, A. R. (1981). Dose-response relationship for adult and prenatal exposure to methylmercury. In Berg, G., Miller, M., and Maillie, D. (Eds.) *Measurement of Risk*, pp. 111–130, Plenum Press, New York.

Freireich, E. J., Gehan, E. A., Rall, D. P., Schmidt, L. H. and Skipper, H. E. (1966). Quantitative comparison of toxicity of anti-cancer agents in mouse, rat, hamster, dog, monkey and man. *Cancer Chemother. Rep.* **50**(4), 219–244.

Goss, R. J. (1964). *Adaptive Growth*. Academic Press, New York.

Goss, R. J. (1966). Hypertrophy versus hyperplasia. *Science (Washington, DC)* **153**, 1615–1620.

Goss, R. J. (1967). The strategy of growth. In Teir, H. and Ryfömaa, T. (Eds.) *Control of Cellular Growth in Adult Organisms*, pp. 3–27. Academic Press, New York.

Goss, R. J. (1978a). *The Physiology of Growth*. Academic Press, New York.

Goss, R. J. (1978b). Adaptive mechanisms of growth control. In Falkner, F. and Tanner, J. M. (Eds.) *Human Growth I. Principles and Prenatal Growth*, pp. 3–21. Plenum Press, New York.

Hicks S. P. and D'Amato, C. J. (1961). How to design and build abnormal brains using radiation during development. In Fields, W. S. and Desmond, M. M. (Eds.) *Disorders of the Developing Nervous System*, pp. 60–97. C. C. Thomas, Springfield, Illinois.

Keller, C. A. and Doherty, R. A. (1980). Lead and calcium distributions in blood, plasma and milk of the lactating mouse. *J. lab. clin. Med.* **95**, 81–89.

Kendrick, E. (1980). Testing for environmental contaminants in human milk. *Pediatrics* **66** (3), 470–472.

Kuwabara, K., Yakushiji, T. and Watanabe, S. (1979). Levels of polychlorinated biphenyls in blood of breast-fed children whose mothers are non-occupationally exposed to PCB's*Bull. Environ. Contam. Toxicol.* **21**, 458–462.

Miller, R. W. (1970). Teratology in 1970: the national scene. President's report to the Teratology Society. *Teratology* 3, 223–227.

NAS (National Academy of Sciences) (1978). *An Assessment of Mercury in the Environment*. National Academy of Sciences, Washington, DC.

Needleman, H. L., Gunnoe, C., Leviton, A., Reed, R., Peresie, H., Maher, C., and Barrett, P. (1979). Deficits in psychologic and classroom performance of children with elevated dentin lead levels. *New Engl. J. Med.* **300**, 689–695.

Needleman, H. L., Leviton, A., and Bellinger, D. (1982). Lead-associated intellectual deficit. *New Engl. J. Med.*, **306**, 367.

Nurnberger, C. E., and Lipscomb, A. (1952). Transmission of radioiodine (^{131}I) to infants through human maternal milk. *J. Amer. Med. Assoc.* **150**, 1398–1400.

Opitz, J. M. (1980). Mental retardation: biological aspects of concern to pediatricians. *Pediatrics in Review* **2(2)**, 41–50.

Rall, D. P. (1979). Secretion of foreign substances in breast milk. In *Breastfeeding and Food Policy in a Hungry World*, pp. 233–240. Academic Press, New York.

Rodier, P. M. (1980). Chronology of neuron development: animal studies and their clinical implications. *Devel. Med. Child Neurol.* **22**, 525–545.

Rodier, P. M., and Gramann, W. J. (1979). Morphologic effects of interference with cell proliferation in the early fetal period. *Neurobehav. Toxicol.* **1**, 129–135.

Rogan, W. J., Bangniewska, A. and Damstra, T. (1980). Pollutants in breast milk. *New Engl. J. Med.* **302**, 1450–1453.

Savage, E. P. (1977). *National Study to Determine Levels of Chlorinated Hydrocarbon Insecticides in Human Milk: 1975–76; Supplementary Report to the National Milk Study: 1975–1976*. National Technical Information Service, Springfield, Virginia.

Sheffy, T. B. (1979). Don't monkey with PCB's. *Wisconsin Natural Resources* **3**, 13.

Strobino, B. R., Kline, J. and Stein, Z. (1978). Chemical and physical exposure of parents: effects on human reproduction and offspring. *Early Hum. Dev.* **1(4)**, 371–399.

Tsubaki, T. and Irukayama, K. (1977). *Minamata Disease. Methylmercury poisoning in Minamata and Niigata, Japan*. Elsevier, Amsterdam.

WHO (1972). Evaluation of mercury, lead, cadmium and food additives, amaranth, diethylpyrocarbonate and octyl gallate. *Food Additive Series No. 4*. World Health Organization, Geneva.

WHO (1976). *Environmental and Health Criteria 1. Mercury*. World Health Organization, Geneva.

Wickizer, T. M., Brilliant, L. B., Copeland, R. and Tilden, R. (1981). Polychlorinated biphenyl contamination of nursing mothers' milk in Michigan. *Am. J. Public Health* **71**, 132–137.

Wilson, J. G. (1973). *Environment and Birth Defects*. Academic Press, New York.

Wilson, J. G. (1977). Environmental chemicals. In Wilson, J. G. and Fraser, F. C. (Eds.) *Handbook of Teratology* **1**, pp. 357–368. Plenum Press, New York.

Methods for Assessing the Effects of Chemicals on Reproductive Functions
Edited by V. B. Vouk and P. J. Sheehan
© 1983 SCOPE

Appraisal of Reproductive Failure in Wildlife

J. E. KIHLSTRÖM

1 FIELD OBSERVATIONS

A number of reports indicate that the seal populations (*Halichoerus grypus, Pusa hispida* and *Phoca vitulina*) in the Baltic area has decreased seriously during the last decades (Bergman, 1956; Hook and Johnels, 1972; Söderberg, 1975). Other observations also suggest decreasing population sizes of some terrestrial species, e.g., pheasants (Göransson, 1980). Simultaneously there has been increasing pollution of our environment, resulting in higher residue levels of DDT, PCBs, heavy metals and other toxic contaminants in the biotic and abiotic components of the ecosystem. Often the reproductive processes of mammals and birds are very sensitive to these toxic chemicals. Therefore, one possible explanation of the decreasing wildlife populations could be the increased incidence of reproductive failure caused by some of these substances.

2 FINDINGS IN INDIVIDUALS FROM DECREASING POPULATIONS

Helle *et al.* (1976a), found that only 27% of the adult female ringed seals (*Pusa hispida*) in the Baltic area are pregnant compared to 80–90% in other areas. Moreover, the non-pregnant individuals demonstrate higher concentrations of DDT and PCBs than the pregnant ones (Helle *et al.*, 1976a, b). About 40% of the studied animals show unilateral or bilateral occlusions of the uterine horns, preventing any passage between the oviduct and the body of the uterus (Helle *et al.*, 1976b). Animals with these pathological changes show even higher levels of DDT and PCBs than the non-pregnant females with normal uteri (Helle *et al.*, 1976b). Therefore, it is tempting to assume the high concentrations of PCBs and/or DDT interfere with fertilization, implantation of ova, fetal growth and/or the maintenance of pregnancy.

Because of some physiological and ecological similarities to the seals (a fish-eating species with delayed implantation), the mink (*Mustela vison*) has been used as animal 'model' in order to verify or falsify the above hypothesis experimentally. PCBs (a mixture of Clophen A 50 and Clophen A 60, prepared in order to obtain a PCB mixture similar to that extracted from Baltic herrings) and/or DDT/DDE (1/1) was given via the food daily for 666 days, including the mating season and the gestation period. The doses varied from 0.02 to 33 mg/kg food corresponding to 6–9900 μg/day per individual.

The reproduction of the mink was not influenced by DDT, even at the highest doses used, in spite of increased liver weights ($+12\%$), indicating a stimulation of the activity of the liver (Jensen *et al.*, 1977). On the other hand, there was a close dose–response relationship between the PCB residues in the tissues of the mothers and the number of whelps born. At a mean PCB residue of 48 mg/kg body fat, corresponding to a dose of 330 μg/day per individual (1.1 mg/kg food), the number of whelps significantly decreased; and at 280 mg PCB/kg fat (corresponding to 11 mg/kg food), no whelps were born. The fertilization rate and the duration of the gestation were not influenced by PCBs. Post-mortem examinations revealed normal numbers of implantations, even at the highest doses of PCBs used, but also showed a high frequency of dead and macerated fetuses (Jensen *et al.*, 1977). Later it was demonstrated that limiting the administration of PCBs (2700 μg/day per individual) to 10 days during the later part of the gestation period also resulted in fetal death (Kihlström *et al.*, 1983). Moreover, controls and experimental animals showed the same concentrations of progesterone throughout the pregnancy (Kihlström *et al.*, 1983).

It is generally believed that the persistent chemicals in the environment influence the reproduction via an increased catabolic activity of the liver, thus reducing the blood levels of the steroid hormones regulating the sexual processes. One important conclusion of the studies reviewed above is that this explanation cannot be the entire explanation. Alternative explanations may be an accumulation of the toxicants in the fetuses or a decreased transport of nutrients or excretion products across the placenta.

3 EXPERIMENTAL ANALYSIS

3.1 Placental Perfusion

Fetal death after administration of PCB substances to pregnant animals has been observed in the mink (Jensen *et al.*, 1977, technical PCBs), the rat (Örberg, 1978, 2, 2′, 4, 4′, 5, 5′-hexachlorobiphenyl), the mouse (Merson and Kirkpatrick, 1976, technical PCBs; Török, 1978, 2, 2′-dichlorobiphenyl), and the guinea pig (Brunström *et al.*, 1982, technical PCBs). In order to evaluate the reproductive disturbances caused by environmental pollutants, we have developed a technique for perfusion of the fetal part of the guinea pig placenta *in situ* (Kihlström and Kihlström, 1981). This technique provides viable conditions for the placenta as demonstrated by an active stereoselective transfer of alanine from the mother and by placental impermeability to trypan blue.

Using this method the transfer of [^{14}C] 2, 2′, 4, 4′, 5, 5′-hexachlorobiphenyl from the maternal circulation to the fetal part of the placenta was shown to proceed rapidly when blood or an albumin solution was used as perfusion medium (Kihlström, 1982). Identical concentrations of the chlorobiphenyl in the maternal and fetal compartments are obtained in 20 minutes. At that time, concentration of the chlorobiphenyl in the perfusion medium exceeds that of the maternal plasma and continues to rise throughout the perfusion (Kihlström, 1982). This placental transfer of hexachlorobiphenyl is highly dependent on the albumin concentration in the medium and fails to occur when albumin is excluded (Kihlström, 1982). In addition, there is an exponential relationship between the accumulation of PCBs in the perfusion medium and albumin concentrations (Kihlström, 1982). This fast penetration of hexachlorobiphenyl through the placenta may be one of the serious hazards to the fetuses.

The same method has been used to study the placental transfer of amino acids in mothers treated with environmental toxicants. Experiments with pregnant guinea pigs given triethyllead chloride (used as an antiknock agent in gasoline) indicate a decreased placental transfer of alanine (Kihlström and Odenbro, 1980). Similar experiments with PCB treated animals using a non-metabolizable amino acid are in progress. This method may become a useful tool for rapid screening of potentially fetotoxic substances.

3.2 Embryotoxic studies of embryonated hens' eggs

Injection of substances into embryonated hens' eggs is an inexpensive and simple method of studying embryotoxicity. However, a major problem is to find a proper vehicle for injection of lipophilic substances into the eggs. In order to find an appropriate vehicle, several different solvents containing a fat-soluble dye were injected on day 4 of incubation and the distribution of the dye studied. On the basis of these studies, an emulsion of lecithin, peanut oil and water has been chosen as the most suitable vehicle. Using this vehicle, a labelled lipophilic substance ($[^{14}C]$ 2, 2′, 4, 5′-tetrachlorobiphenyl) was injected on day 4 of incubation. By means of autoradiography the chlorobiphenyl was detected in the embryos one day later. Five and 25, but not 1, mg Aroclor 1248/kg egg injected into hens' eggs significantly decreased their hatchability. Eggs injected with 25 mg Aroclor 1248/kg exhibited anomalies (clearly visible at candling on day 7) localized in areas around the vessels of the yolk-sac (Brunström and Örberg, 1982). No teratogenic effects have been observed thus far.

Preliminary experiments using the same technique demonstrate that 2, 2′, 4, 5′-tetrachlorobiphenyl is, in this test, at least 100 times more toxic than 3, 3′, 4, 4′-tetrachlorobiphenyl (Brunström and Örberg, 1982), while toxaphenes and chlorinated paraffins seem to demonstrate low embryotoxicity (Brunström and Örberg, 1981). Therefore, this method may be a useful tool for an inexpensive and rapid screening of potentially embryotoxic contaminants.

4 CONCLUSIONS AND RECOMMENDATIONS

The PCB story (Jensen, 1972) and similar toxic chemical releases into the environment point out the necessity of assessing the potential impact of new chemicals before they become widespread in the environment. The reproductive functioning of wildlife is very sensitive to many pesticides, e.g., PCBs; DDT and organic mercurials. Consequently, there may be a reduction of the reproductive rate long before more easily detected effects become manifest. Therefore, there is a need for rapid and inexpensive methods for evaluating the reproductive hazards of the increasing number of potentially toxic chemicals. The two techniques, placental perfusion and the modified embryotoxic studies of embryonated hens' eggs described above, fulfil these demands and may thus become useful tools for a rapid and inexpensive appraisal of potential reproductive failures in wildlife.

5 REFERENCES

Bergman, G. (1956). Rarrikoittemme hyljekannasta. *Luonnon Tutkija* **60**, 81–91 (in Swedish).

Brunström, B. and Örberg, J. (1981). Unpublished observations.

Brunström, B. and Örberg, J. (1982). A method for studying embryotoxicity of lipophilic substances experimentally introduced into hens' eggs. *Ambio*, **11**, 209–211.

Brunström, B., Kihlström, I. and Lundkvist, U. (1982). Studies of foetal death and foetal weight in guinea pigs fed polychlorinated biphenyls (PCB). *Acta pharmac. tox.* **50**, 100–103.

Göransson, G. (1980). *Dynamics, Reproduction and Social Organization in Pheasant Phasianus Colchicus Populations in South Scandinavia*, pp. 1–112. Thesis, University of Lund.

Helle, E., Olsson, M. and Jensen, S. (1976a). DDT and PCB levels and reproduction in ringed seal from the Bothnian Bay. *Ambio* **5**, 188–189.

Helle, E., Olsson, M. and Jensen, S. (1976b). PCB levels correlated with pathological changes in seal uteri. *Ambio* **5**, 261–263.

Hook, O. and Johnels, A. G. (1972). The breeding and distribution of the grey seal (*Halichoerus grypus*, Fabr.) in the Baltic Sea, with observations of other seals of the area. *Proc. R. Soc. (London) B, Biol. Sci.* **8, 182**, 37–58.

Jensen, S. (1972). The PCB story. *Ambio* **1**, 123–131.

Jensen, S., Kihlström, J. E., Olsson, M., Lundberg, C. and Örberg, J. (1977). Effects of PCB and DDT on mink (*Mustela vison*) during the reproductive season. *Ambio* **6**, 239.

Kihlström, I. (1982). Influence of albumin concentration in the foetal circulation on the placental transfer of 2, 2′, 4, 4′, 5, 5′-hexachlorobiphenyl in the guinea pig. *Acta pharmac. tox.* **50**, 300–304.

Kihlström, I. and Odenbro, A. (1980). Report at the International Symposium on Primate and Non-Primate Placental Transfer, Rotterdam.

Kihlström, I. and Kihlström, J. E. (1981). An improved technique for perfusion of the guinea pig placenta *in situ* giving viable conditions demonstrated by placental transport of amino acids (L- and D-alanine). *Biol. Neonate* **39**, 150–159.

Kihlström, J. E., Olsson, M., Jensen, S., and Örberg, J. (1983). Effects of sublethal doses of DDT and PCB on mink (*Mustela vison*) and its reproduction. *Ambio* (in press).

Merson, M. H., and Kirkpatrick, R. L. (1976). Reproductive performance of captive white-footed mice fed a PCB. *Bull. environ. Contam. Toxicol.* **16**, 392–397.

Örberg, J. (1978). A comparison between two structurally defined chlorobiphenyls —2, 4′ 5-trichlorobiphenyl and 2, 2′, 4, 4′, 5, 5′-hexachlorobiphenyl—with regard to biological effects and behaviour in the animal body. *National Swedish Environment Protection Board, SNV PM* **932**, 1–72.

Söderberg, S. (1975). Sealhunting in Sweden. In Proceedings from the *Symposium on the Seal in the Baltic*, pp. 104–116. National Swedish Environment Protection Board, Solna.

Török, P. (1978). Verzögerte Implantation und Frühembryonale Keimachäden bei der Maus nach Applikation des PCB: 2, 2′-dichlorobiphenyl. *Archs. Toxicol* (Berlin) **40**, 249–254.

Methods for Assessing the Effects of Chemicals on Reproductive Functions
Edited by V. B. Vouk and P. J. Sheehan
© 1983 SCOPE

Methods for Assessment of the Effects of Pollutants on Avian Reproduction

DAVID B. PEAKALL

Tests of the effects of chemicals on avian reproduction can be divided into two broad categories: screening tests to provide an initial assessment of the chemical, and definitive studies to assess the actual hazard in a specific case.

1 SCREENING TESTS

1.1 Readily Available Species

For screening tests it is necessary to work with species that are readily available in large numbers. Additionally, there is merit in using a few well-studied species in order to facilitate comparison between chemicals. A list of these species with some of their basic characteristics is given in Table 1.

The first four species are indeterminate layers and have precocial young. This enables large numbers of eggs to be collected from each female (30–40 would be typical for the mallard, for example) so that eggs can be used for residue analysis, determination of eggshell thickness, nutritional studies, etc., without serious

Table 1 Species commonly used for screening tests

Name*	Minimum age of breeding (months)	Typical cage size (m)	Protocols
Mallard	10	1 × 1**	ASTM[†]/OECD
Bobwhite quail	2	1 × 2	ASTM/OECD
Japanese quail	2	0.5 × 0.3 × 0.3	—
Ring-necked pheasant	10	1.5 × 0.5 × 0.3	—
Ring dove	6	0.8 × 0.4 × 0.2	OECD

* Scientific names are given in Appendix.
[†] American Society for Testing and Materials.
** Game farm mallards only; wild-strain mallards require much larger cages.

disturbance of the study. Precocial young are essential if artificial incubation is to be used, otherwise it is virtually impossible to raise the young.

The ring dove is a determinate layer (clutch size of 2) and the young are dependent on the parent's crop secretions until the age of 14 days. Nevertheless, they can be bred readily in small cages throughout the year and are the easiest species for testing if it is desired to make the study with parental incubation and care of young.

There is interest in international harmonization of testing protocols and in the fact that the species should be representative of the fauna of the individual country. On these considerations the mallard is the clear choice. It is a common breading species in a broad belt across North America, Europe and Asia. Even outside this area replacement species such as the Australian black duck could be used with reasonable confidence. The bobwhite quail is confined to North America, the Japanese quail to central Europe and Asia, and the ring-necked pheasant and ring dove are largely domesticated species with rather obscure natural origins. The possibility of interchanging one species of quail for another is not considered valid (Heinz *et al.*, 1979).

There is a major movement towards international harmonization of testing protocols so that information produced in one country is accepted in other countries. The widest attempt to obtain international harmonization has been by the Organization for Economic and Cooperative Development (OECD). The agreement within the OECD that a specific set of information, the minimum premarket data (MPD), shall be produced for every new chemical and that the way that these data are generated shall conform to an agreed good laboratory practice is a major step in this direction. Similar, but rather more rigid guidelines are used by the European Economic Community. An MPD for birds is not prescribed but avian toxicology is part of the OECD step system approach to the testing of chemicals. An international approach to the safety of environmental chemicals is essential since no single country could afford to generate the necessary data, even MPD, let alone further testing.

1.2 Species Variation in Response to Toxic Chemicals

The problem of species variation is one that has bedevilled ecotoxicology from its inception. Even a first approximation of complete testing is obviously impossible when one considers that the total number of species in the world has been estimated at about three million. The total number of classes is more than 50 and little consideration has so far been given to such well-known classes as Amphibia or Reptilia, let alone more obscure ones such as Holothuroidea and Scyphozoa. Thus, while the problem of the variable response of individual species within a class is a serious one, it should be kept in perspective with the other difficulties of ecotoxicology.

A classical example of species variation in response to an environmental contaminant is DDE-induced eggshell thinning. Eggshell thinning was a major cause of the decline of several species of raptors, most notably the peregrine falcon, over wide stretches of its range in Europe and North America (Hickey, 1969; Newton, 1979). Experimental studies revealed that there is a wide variation of response of individual species; Peakall (1975) divided species into three categories: highly sensitive, moderately sensitive and insensitive. As specific examples, 10 p.p.m. in the diet† of the American kestrel causes 22% thinning, 40 p.p.m. causes 12% in the mallard and 300 p.p.m. does not affect the shell thickness of the chicken egg. The resistance of the Galliformes to eggshell thinning has given this order the reputation of being a tough group of species when the testing of chemicals is considered. This is not true in all cases: 20 p.p.m. of Aroclor 1254 (a polychlorinated biphenyl with 54% chlorine) causes almost complete reproductive failure in the chicken (Lillie *et al.*, 1974), whereas 25 p.p.m. has no effect on the mallard (Custer and Heinz, 1980).

Another example of variation of species response is the effect of ingested crude oil on seabirds. When nestling herring gulls were given a single small dose of crude oil they showed a marked reduction in the rate of weight gain (Miller *et al.*, 1978), whereas dosing the nesting adult had no discernible effect on reproduction (Butler, unpublished). In contrast, Leach's petrel chicks were not affected by an equivalent dosage of crude oil, whereas when adults were dosed, their chicks failed to gain weight normally and survival of chicks was severely affected (Miller *et al.*, 1980). Mallard ducklings required a dietary level of 5% South Louisiana crude oil in their diet (2.5% did not produce statistically significant differences) to retard the rate of growth (Szaro *et al.*, 1978), whereas only a single dose of 0.2 ml was needed to inhibit growth in the herring gull.

Ideally, the criteria for testing should be:

(1) that the tests should be carried out on the target species ;
(2) that the conditions of the test simulate those that occur in nature;
(3) that the collection of the data does not affect the test itself.

In practice, all of these criteria cannot be fully met.

1.3 Injection of Toxicants into Eggs

The fact that the avian embryo develops externally to its parent makes the study of this class of organisms much easier than is the case with mammals. Use of the technique of injecting chemicals into eggs to observe their effect dates back to the end of the last century (Féré, 1893). The technique of injecting chemicals into the yolk-sac of eggs for routine toxicological assessment has been described by McLaughlin *et al.* (1963). Dunachie and Fletcher (1969) tested the toxicity of 25

---

† Dietary levels, in parts per million, are usually expressed merely on a weight-added basis. With doves, quail and ducks, this is essentially on a dry weight basis, whereas with flesh-eaters it is on a wet weight basis. The reader is referred to the original references for exact details.

insecticides to chicken embryos and, although their results are difficult to interpret, the general trends (the cyclodienes being the most toxic of the organochlorines; the organophosphates being more toxic than the organochlorines) are in agreement with the results obtained from other methods of assessing the effects of chemicals on reproduction. Since the egg injection technique is inexpensive and simple, a rigorous examination of its value in predicting the effects of chemicals on avian reproduction would be worthwhile.

2 DEFINITIVE STUDIES

2.1 Breeding Target Species in Captivity

One approach to the problem of using target species has been to breed more species in captivity. The US Fish and Wildlife Service has been particularly active in this regard. The current state-of-the-art in this challenging and time-consuming aspect of avian testing is given in Table 2.

These breeding programmes have increased our capacity to carry out experiments on raptorial species which are at the top of food-webs. The requirements for these species are given in more detail below.

The American kestrel has been used for a number of studies of the effects of pollutants on reproduction of birds of prey. As a member of the genus *Falco* it is closely related to the peregrine, a species which has come to be a symbol for conservationists. Willoughby and Cade (1964) demonstrated that the American kestrel could be bred fairly readily in captivity and made observations on its breeding biology. The species has been bred successfully in large numbers at Patuxent Wildlife Research Center and their protocol has been described by Porter and Wiemeyer (1970).

Kestrels require good sanitary conditions and health care to breed well in captivity. Given this, it is a good model for raptorial birds. The kestrel breeds in its first year, has a large clutch size (4–5 eggs), is sexually dimorphic and will eat any animal material.

Screech owls and barn owls have been maintained in outside wire mesh cages (7 × 16 × 2 m) with a nest box and a three-sided shelter. Owls have been fed a diet of ground hamsters, mice, rats and chicken, with vitamin and calcium supplements.

Certainly the use of kestrels for testing DDT would have revealed the potential for eggshell thinning that was the major cause of the decline of the peregrine. But, despite the dedicated work of researchers, the number of species that it is feasible to breed in captivity in sufficient numbers at reasonable cost and with sufficient reliability to be used for toxicological experiments is small. The effort that would be involved in breeding a pelagic seabird for toxicological purposes would be enormous. There is a further point to be considered. Some effects on behaviour (such as decreased nest attentiveness leading to increased predation, Fox *et al.*, 1978) and on physiology (increased metabolic rate leading to an inability to

Table 2 Status of 'target' species bred in captivity for toxicological experiments

Species	Ecology	Research station(s)	Status*
Black-crowned night heron	Colonically nesting fish-eating heron	Patuxent Wildlife Research Center (PWRC)	Breeding success considered to be somewhat erratic. Has not yet been used for toxicological studies.
Black duck	Dabbling duck, mainly feeding on vegetation	PWRC	Bred successfully, Longcore and Stendell (1977).
Hooded merganser	Fish-eating diving duck	PWRC	Difficulties with feeding small young, not yet used for studies.
Kittiwake	Small pelagic gull	Netherlands Institute for Sea Research (NISR)**	Bred successfully in small numbers, no studies carried out.
Common murre/guillemot	Pelagic, fish-eating seabird	NISR	Difficulties with supplying food for small young
American kestrel	Small, flesh-eating hawk	PWRC, Cornell University; MacDonald Raptor Research Center	Bred successfully, Porter and Wiemeyer (1969).
Barn owl	Medium-sized, rodent-eating owl	PWRC	Breeds well in captivity.
Screech owl	Small, flesh-eating owl	PWRC	Bred successfully, McLane and Hall (1972).
Starling	Medium-sized passerine, omnivorous	PWRC Institute for Terrestrial Ecology, UK (ITE)	Bred successfully although fledging stage is difficult. Toxicological studies underway.
Bengalese finch	Small, seed-eating passerine	ITE	Readily bred in captivity (Jefferies 1967).

* A single reference to a toxicological study is given as an example.
** Details of the set-up for breeding seabirds is given in Sweenen (1977).

obtain enough food, Miller *et al.*, 1980) would not be discovered even if the target species or some near congener was available in captivity.

2.2 Multigeneration Studies

Another feature of environmental contaminants that is rarely investigated is whether or not their effects are intensified in subsequent generations. In the case of highly stable contaminants such as the organochlorines, PCBs and DDT, and the heavy metals, multigeneration exposure can be expected to occur.

Peakall *et al.* (1972) found that while the first generation of ring doves was unaffected by 10 p.p.m. of the PCB Aroclor 1254, the second generation hatched only 20% of eggs laid compared to 91% of the controls and the fledging success of the few eggs laid was 50% compared to 100% in the controls.

Carnio and McQueen (1973) exposed Japanese quail to a diet containing 15 p.p.m. of DDT for three generations. They found a marked decline in percentage of fertile eggs: 79% fertile in the first generation, 37% in the second and 20% in the third. A significant percentage of eggs without shell or with only a parchment-like shell were noted in the second and third generation (11.4% and 23.3% respectively), whereas none was recorded in the first generation or in the controls. Shellenberger (1978), using the same species at a dietary level of 50 p.p.m. *p, p'*-DDT, was unable to show any marked effect in a four-generation study. The reason for the difference between this study and that of Carnio and McQueen is unknown.

Dahlgren and Linder (1974) gave pheasants dieldrin weekly (4 or 6 mg) for two generations and cross-bred exposed and unexposed males and females. Egg production, fertility, hatchability and viability of chicks was erratic among the groups (including controls) and no clearcut relationship to dosage could be established.

The most detailed multigeneration study that has been undertaken was that of exposing the Mallard to 0.5 p.p.m. methylmercury dicyandiamide for three generations (Heinz, 1979). Methylmercury at this dose level had no significant effects on reproduction during the first generation. In each successive generation hens fed the mercury compound laid a greater percentage of their eggs outside the nesting box, although this was statistically significant only for the second generation and for all generations combined. The number of sound eggs was significantly reduced by the mercury compound in the third generation and for the experiment as a whole.

2.3 Effects of Pollutants on Reproductive Behaviour

The hypothesis that pollutants could have an effect on behaviour such that reproductive success is reduced has existed for a long time. Ratcliffe (1958) alluded to the possibility in a note in a local ornithological journal when referring to broken peregrine eggs, he stated: 'Having considered the evidence and the alternative explanations, it is difficult to avoid the conclusion that the majority of these broken eggs were eaten by one or the other of the owners. Should this be the correct explanation, the reason for this particular behaviour is even more obscure'.

Stickel (1975) in his excellent review of the effects of pollutants in terrestrial ecosystems comments: 'In general, behavioural changes in birds and mammals are exceedingly difficult to prove in the field for multiple factors are present, individual variability is high, and alternative explanations seldom can be ruled out' and, 'too much behavioural work is done with lethal or nearly lethal dosages; the reader often feels that he is simply learning how sick animals act'. Both these comments are borne in mind in the selection of papers for discussion here.

The most detailed laboratory studies have been made by Heinz and co-workers on the mallard and by a number of workers, including the author of this review, on the ring dove. The work on the mallard is summarized in Table 3.

The behaviour of the ring dove has been studied in great detail by Lehrman and co-workers (for summaries see Lehrman, 1964, and Silver, 1978) which forms a good basis against which to measure the changes caused by pollutants. The effects of the two organochlorines studied, DDE and PCBs, are similar and the results are consistent from study to study (Table 4).

An important question is how well these studies relate to the real world. The changes in the distribution pattern of the egg temperatures observed when ring doves were exposed to PCBs (Peakall and Peakall, 1973) are quite similar to those observed in herring gulls in the wild in an area of high contamination (Fox *et al.*, 1978). Increased time to lay was also noted when ring doves were exposed to organochlorines, a finding also noted by Jefferies (1967) in his study on the effect of DDT on Bengalese finches. Jefferies considered it probable that organochlorine pesticides were responsible for the late breeding of several species of

Table 3   Effect of low levels of pollutants on the behaviour of mallard duckling

	Pollutant	
Response	Methylmercury (0.5 p.p.m.)	DDE (3 p.p.m.)
Approach response to maternal call	Decreased	Increased
Avoidance response to frightening stimulus	Increased	Decreased
Locomotor activity	No significant effect	Not studied

After Heinz (1976, 1979)

Table 4 Effects of PCBs and *p,p'*-DDE on parental behaviour in ring doves

Chemical	Dose (p.p.m.)	Courtship behaviour	Time to lay	Nest attentiveness	Reproductive success	Reference
p,p'-DDE	40	—	Increased	—	Decreased	Haegele and Hudson (1973)
	10	Decreased	—	—	—	Haegele and Hudson (1977)
	50	Decreased	—	—	—	
	100	Decreased	Increased	Decreased	Decreased	Keith (1978)
	10	—	Increased	—	—	Richie and Peterle (1979)
	40	—	Increased	—	—	
PCBs	10	—	Increased	Decreased	Decreased	Peakall and Peakall (1973)
	25	Decreased	Increased	Decreased	Decreased	Farve (1978)
PCBs	8	Same	Increased	Decreased	Decreased	McArthur *et al.* (in press)
p,p'-DDE	2					
Mirex	0–3					
Photomirex	0.1					
PCBs	8	Decreased	Increased	—	Decreased	McArthur *et al.* (in press)
p,p'-DDE	5					
Mirex	0.9					
Photomirex	0.3					

birds reported in the early 1960s, although evidence is lacking. Herring gulls forced to renest as part of the egg-exchange experiment took longer to do so in the highly contaminated Lake Ontario colonies than they did on the much cleaner colonies on the Atlantic coast.

3 FIELD EXPERIMENTS

Another approach to the problem of target species and realistic conditions is to carry out experiments on free-living populations. There are a number of difficulties with this approach. First, there is the difficulty of getting the toxicant to the bird, especially if a chronic dose is to be tested or material is highly toxic, such as the chlorodioxins. Second, there is the lack of control over the experiment (weather, predation, vandalism) which are difficult to compensate for by increased sample size and third, there is the problem of the influence that the observer has on the reproduction of the birds that are being studied.

Some field toxicological experiments that have been carried out are listed in Table 5. This listing is confined to studies where experimental manipulation was carried out and thus excludes the numerous studies in which pollutant residue levels are correlated with reproductive effects. A good review of those studies on birds of prey has been given by Newton (1979).

Field experiments enable the observer to assess the impact of the pollutant on such critical nesting behaviour as nest defence and attentiveness. One of the most detailed studies was made with the herring gull colonies on the Great Lakes by the Canadian Wildlife Service. In the early and mid-1970s the overall reproductive success of this species on Lake Ontario was very low. Visually, these colonies were quite different form normal, with the adults leaving while the observer is several hundred metres away and only a few wheeling overhead.

Experiments were carried out using telemetered eggs which provided a record of the core and surface temperature and intensity of light falling on a receiver in the apex of the egg (Fox *et al.*, 1978). It was found that the nest attentiveness was lower in the Lake Ontario colonies compared to successful colonies in New Brunswick and that the unsuccessful nests were characterized by greater temperature variation and much longer absences of adults from the nest. The high rate of egg loss, together with decreased nest defence and nest attentiveness, indicates that behavioural changes were involved.

Embryonic mortality could be caused by toxicants within the egg or by inadequate care, or by a combination of these two factors. In order to separate these two factors, the intrinsic and extrinsic, an egg-exchange experiment was devised. In theory this is a simple experiment. There are two colonies, one 'clean' and one 'dirty'. Eggs are moved from the clean colony and placed in the dirty colony and vice versa. There are four sets of conditions: clean adults incubating clean eggs, clean adults incubating dirty eggs, dirty adults incubating clean eggs

Table 5　Species on which field toxicological experiments have been carried out

	General description	Food	Advantages
Leach's petrel	Small pelagic seabird, colonial nesting in individual burrows	Microorganisms on surface of ocean	Nests readily located; adults and young can be handled readily using trapdoor over nesting cavity
Prairie falcon	Medium-sized falcon, solitary nesting	Small birds and mammals	
Osprey	Large bird of prey, small colonies or solitary	Fish	
Herring gull	Large coastal or inland aquatic species, nests colonially on open ground	Opportunistic with fish usually predominant	Colonies readily located; species common
Puffin	Medium-sized pelagic seabird nesting colonially in individual burrows or rock crevices	Fish	Nests readily located
Black guillemot	Medium-sized pelagic seabird nesting in crevices, more or less solitary	Fish	Young readily handled without apparent effect
Starling	Medium-sized, hole-nesting passerine	Omnivorous	Will use nesting boxes, large clutch size
House wren	Small passerine, nests in cavities	Insectivore	Will nest in nesting box; large clutch size, high breeding success
White-throated sparrow	Small woodland passerine, ground or near ground nesting	Largely seed eaters	Relatively common

Species	Disadvantages	Reference	
Leach's petrel	Colonies remote; single egg clutch; noctural habits make behavioural observing virtually impossible	General:	Lockley (1961)
		Specific:	Miller et al. (1980)
Prairie falcon	Species relatively scarce; readily disturbed by observer; nests relatively inaccessible	Specific:	Enderson and Berger (1970)
Osprey	Nests hard to climb to; species relatively scarce	Specific:	Wiemeyer et al. (1975)
Herring gull	Adults hard to retrap without major disturbance; biologist effect is serious	General:	Tinbergen (1953)
		Specific:	Gilman et al. (1978) Fox et al. (1978) Peakall et al. (1980a) Butler and Lukasiewicz (1979)
Puffin	Colonies remote; hard to extract adults and young from same burrows	General:	Lockley (1962)
		Specific:	Osborn and Harris (1979)
Black guillemot	Nests hard to locate; adults difficult to capture	Specific:	Peakall et al. (1980b)
Starling	Nesting box approach requires considerable lead time	Specific:	Powell and Gray (1980)
House wren	Otherwise nests hard to locate	General:	Armstrong (1955)
		Specific:	Bart (1976)
White-throated sparrow	High predation rate of observed nests	Specific:	Pearce and Busby (1980)

Table 6   Results from the 1968/69 osprey and 1975 harring gull egg exchange experiments

			Osprey*		Herring gull**	
Adult	Egg	Information obtained	n	% hatch-ed	n	% hatch-ed
Clean	Clean	Normal reproduction	47	36	85	86
Clean	Dirty	Intrinsic factors only	24	12	41	10
Dirty	Clean	Extrinsic factors only	45	42	41	7
Dirty	Dirty	Both intrinsic and extrinsic factors	18	11	49	2
Artification	Incubation					
—	Clean	Normal reproduction	—	—	109	60
—	Dirty	Instrinsic factors only	—	—	86	37

* Summarized from Wiemeyer *et al.* (1975).
** Peakall *et al.* (1980a).

and dirty adults incubating dirty eggs. The experimental design and expected resultant information is shown in Table 6.

In practice all sorts of complications occur. There are, obviously, the effects of transportation on the viability of the eggs. Thus, it is necessary to transport control eggs and return them to the colony from which they were removed so that they correspond to the eggs that were moved from colony to colony. Also, nesting occurs at different times in different areas.

Experiments involving egg exchange have been carried out on the osprey (Wiemeyer *et al.*, 1975) and herring gull (Peakall *et al.*, 1980a). An overview of the results is tabulated in Table 6.

The experiments with the osprey eggs show that, for this species, the behavioural component is not important since the 'clean' eggs hatch equally well under 'clean' or 'dirty' adults. In the case of the herring gull, both intrinsic and extrinsic factors are working. Attempts were made to mimic the intrinsic factor by injection of contaminants extracted from Lake Ontario herring gull eggs into 'clean' eggs on the Atlantic seaboard. Despite the fact that the embryonic uptake of pollutants was similar to that occurring in naturally contaminated eggs, no increase of embryonic or chick mortality was observed (Gilman *et al.*, 1978). It is possible that the critical pollutant was not injected or that the pollutants need to be ingested before the egg is laid in order to exert their toxic effect. The injection technique only tests the toxic effects of the material contained within the egg on the developing embryo. Effects on genetic material and on the formation of the egg itself would be missed by this approach. Marked effects that have been found in the second generation of multigeneration studies of birds exposed to PCBs (Peakall *et al.*, 1972) and DDE (Carnio and McQueen, 1973) indicate that these effects can be important.

There are considerable difficulties in dosing adult birds in the wild to simulate environmental pollution. Direct dosing of the adult after capture can be carried out for some species such as Leach's petrel which is readily captured in its burrow and does not desert its nest but for many species this procedure cannot be carried out without excessive disturbance to the breeding cycle.

Enderson and Berger (1970) exposed nesting prairie falcons to dieldrin by tethering contaminated starlings near to their nesting sites. The dieldrin levels achieved were measured in subcutaneous fat (taken by biopsy from the captured adult) and by collection of one egg from each clutch. The results of this study are difficult to interpret because of the high levels of DDE also found in these birds, an example of the difficulties encountered with field studies. The technique of Enderson and Berger is limited to birds living on live prey or to carrion eaters. It could not be readily used on birds feeding on fish, seeds or insects. A technique capable of much wider application has been devised by Osborn and Harris (1979). These workers implanted PCBs contained in an open polydimethyl-siloxane tube below the skin of puffins. The birds were mist-netted, the implantation carried out using a local anaesthetic (ethyl chloride), the incision closed with one or two sutures, and the birds held in captivity for 6–10 hours before release. Observations on the colony indicated that the procedure caused no more stress than is involved in ringing the birds. It is likely that this approach will play an important role in future field studies. Nevertheless, the problems of simulating chronic, natural exposure and proving that one has done so make field experimentation difficult.

The effect of the biologist on the species being studied can be a serious one, especially in some colonial species such as gulls and open-nesting passerines. In studies under the surveillance programme on the Great Lakes, an assessment based on three visits has been used (Weseloh *et al.*, 1979). The first visit is made late in incubation to determine the total number of nests. The second visit is when most young in the colony are about 3 weeks old and the chicks are marked, and the third visit is made on the following day and total chick population calculated by the mark–recapture index. From these data and the number of active nests established from the first visit, the number of young produced per pair can be calculated.

4 EXPERIMENTAL DESIGN

Sample size is a critical factor in experiments involving non-standard species carried out over a considerable period of time. The number of individuals available is generally limited and the cost per individual of running the experiment is considerable. The sample size needed is related to the dosage level used. If a high dosage level is used, then the sample size can be small, but the results, even though statistically significant, may have little relevance to environmental conditions. One solution is to have two or more dosage levels. This has considerable scientific merit as effects that can be related to dose are much more convincing, but again this approach increases the number of animals that must be used. The best compromise may be a three-group experiment: control, environmentally relevant level and a dosage level several-fold higher than the environmental level.

For some variables, individuals can serve as their own controls. Some of the variation of reproductive success can be removed by using experienced breeders, but this involves the cost of taking all the birds through an entire breeding cycle before starting the main experiment. For some physiological characteristics such as blood chemistry, it is feasible to use individuals as their own controls. For others, such as hepatic enzyme induction, it is not possible to make the measurement without killing the bird, or at least performing a major surgery.

The sample size needed is also related to the type of measurement being made. Some physiological factors, such as levels of plasma electrolytes, should show little individual variation, whereas others, such as hepatic enzyme levels are highly variable. Intestinal transport of amino acids and sugars in gulls shows a good deal of variation from run to run; the nutritional history of the bird may well be important here. In contrast, the effects on osmoregulation, either via plasma sodium levels or $Na^+ K^+$ ATPase activity in the nasal gland, are relatively easy to demonstrate as the control values are highly consistent.

Field experiments are liable to additional hazards, although experience varies greatly from species to species. The reproductive success of gulls is quite variable and both experimentals and controls should be in the same subcolonies. Other species, such as the burrow-nesting petrels and hole-nesting passerines, have high and reasonably consistent breeding success.

5 INTEGRATED LABORATORY/FIELD STUDIES

A careful examination of specific environmental problems requires a combination of detailed laboratory work with the extension of this information into the field. Initially, studies can be carried out under strictly controlled conditions in the laboratory and then the results applied in the field to confirm that the results are consistent and, more importantly, to assess their practical importance. Otherwise one can go no further than the pious statement so often made at the end of a paper, 'these effects can be expected to reduce survival of the species', but the question is 'does it really have an effect'? As an example of the integrated approach, initial studies on ingested oil were carried out on nestling herring gulls in captivity (Miller *et al.*, 1978) which showed that the rate of weight gain was significantly reduced; also a number of physiological measurements (transient drop in plasma sodium, increased nasal gland size, decreased intestinal transport of amino acids) were made. Subsequently, a field experiment was carried out (Butler and Lukasiewicz, 1979) which demonstrated the retardation of weight gain and also decreased survival of the treated nestlings. In the field experiment the physiological studies were less detailed as no individuals were sacrificed since one wished to follow the survival of the birds.

It is now possible to make many chemical studies with modest blood samples collected without serious damage to the individual. Using this approach, we have been able to document pollutant-induced changes in plasma sodium levels in the black guillemot (Peakall *et al.*, 1980b) and alterations of circulating hormone levels in several species of seabirds (Peakall *et al.*, 1981). The technique of radioimmunoassay permits the determination of hormones to be carried out rapidly and accurately on small (20–100 μl) samples of blood and has revolutionized the field of endocrinology. Nevertheless, very little work has been done on the alterations of hormone levels by pollutants, and their meaning in terms of behavioural change, but the technique of assaying hormone levels from small samples of blood provides the possibility of quantitative measurements both in the laboratory and in the field.

Another potentially valuable technique for assessing the impact of pollutants on free-living birds is the heavy water method of measuring metabolic rate. Animals can be injected with doubly labelled water (either $^3H_2^{18}O$ or $D_2^{18}O$) and the rates of change in the ratios of $^3H:H$ and $^{18}O:^{16}O$ in blood (50 μl samples) enable the average metabolic rate to be calculated (Lifson and McClintock, 1966). The method has been used for a number of energy budget calculations in free-living birds (Weathers and Nagy, 1980). No pollutant work with this technique has been reported, but the alteration of corticosterone and thyroxine levels in Leach's petrels exposed to oil, and the inability of these birds to provide enough food for their young (Peakall *et al.*, 1981; Trivelpiece, in press), suggests that metabolic changes are occurring.

6 CONCLUSIONS AND RECOMMENDATIONS

(1) International harmonization of screening tests is essential so that data produced in different countries are mutually understood and accepted.

(2) Tests with additional species are necessary to study the variation of the response of different avian species to chemical pollutants that exist in the environment in appreciable concentrations or that display problems at the screening test stage. The use of egg-injection technique as a screening tool should be critically evaluated.

(3) Some target species can be bred in captivity; good representatives of the Anseriformes, Falconiformes, Galliformes, Columbiformes, Strigiformes and Passeriformes are available, but expansion of this list would be costly.

(4) Some behavioural effects can be studied in captivity, but the impact of behavioural changes on survival is difficult to assess.

(5) Field experiments take into account some of the problems outlined above, but have severe problems of their own. These include lack of control over the

experimental conditions, difficulties in chronic dosing of the birds and the effect of the observer on the performance being measured.

(6) Integrated laboratory/field studies is a good approach if the scale of the problem is large enough to warrant the cost. Biochemical determinations are particularly useful as these often have less variability than behavioural measurements.

ACKNOWLEDGEMENTS

I am most grateful for the constructive comments of W. H. Stickel, G. M. Heinz and S. Haseltine of the US Fish and Wildlife Service and G. A. Fox and J. A. Keith of the Canadian Wildlife Service.

APPENDIX

Scientific Names of Species Listed in Text

Leach's petrel *(Oceanodroma leucorhoa)*
Black-crowned night heron *(Nycticorax nycticorax)*
Mallard *(Anas platyrhynchos)*
Black duck *(Anas rubripes)*
Australian black duck *(Anas superciliosa)*
Hooded merganser *(Lophodytes cucullatus)*
Osprey *(Pandion haliaetus)*
Prairie falcon *(Falco mexicanus)*
Peregrine falcon *(Falco peregrinus)*
American kestrel *(Falco sparverius)*
Bobwhite *(Colinus virginianus)*
Japanese quail *(Coturnix coturnix)*
Ring-necked pheasant *(Phasianus colchicus)*
Herring gull *(Larus argentatus)*
Kittiwake *(Rissa tridactyla)*
Common murre *(Uria aalge)*
Puffin *(Fratercula arctica)*
Black guillemot *(Cepphus grylle)*
Ring dove *(Streptopelia risoria)*
Barn owl *(Tyto alba)*
Screech owl *(Otus asio)*
House wren *(Troglodytes aedon)*
Starling *(Sturnus vulgaris)*
Bengalese finch *(Lonchura striata)*
White-throated sparrow *(Zonotrichia albicollis)*

7 REFERENCES

Armstrong, E. A. (1955) *The Wren*. Collins, London.

Bart, J. (1976). *The Effects of Orthene, Serin and Dimilin on Birds*. M.Sc. Thesis, Cornell Univ.

Butler, R. G. and Lukasiewicz, P. (1979). A field study of the effect of crude oil on Herring Gull (*Larus argentatus*) chick growth. *Auk* **96**, 809–812.

Carnio, J. S. and McQueen, D. J. (1973). Adverse effects of 15 ppm of *p, p'*-DDT on three generations of Japanese Quail. *Can. J. Zool.* **51**, 1307–1312.

Custer, T. W. and Heinz, G. H. (1980). Reproductive success and nest attentiveness of Mallard ducks fed Aroclor 1254. *Environ. Pollut. Ser. A. Ecol. Biol.* **21**, 313–318.

Dahlgren, R. B. and Linder, R. L. (1974). Effects of dieldrin in penned pheasants through the third generation. *J. Wildl. Manage.* **38**, 320–330.

Dunachie, J. F. and Fletcher, W. W. (1969). An investigation of the toxicity of insecticides to birds eggs using the egg-injection technique. *Ann. appl. Biol.* **64**, 409–423.

Enderson, J. H. and Berger, D. D. (1970). Pesticides: Eggshell thinning and lowered production of young in Prairie Falcons. *BioScience* **20**, 355–356.

Farve, M. A. (1978). *Effects of PCB's on Ring-dove Courtship Behaviour*. M.Sc. Thesis, Ohio State Univ.

Féré, C. (1893). Note sur l'influence sur l'incubation de l'oeuf de poule d'injections préalables dans l'albumen de solutions de sel, de glucose, de glycérine. *C. R. Soc. Biol. Paris* **45**, 831–834.

Fox, G. A., Gilman, A. P., Peakall, D. B. and Anderka, F. W. (1978). Behavioural abnormalities in nesting Lake Ontario Herring Gulls. *J. Wildl. Manage.* **42**, 477–483.

Gilman, A. P., Hallett, D. J., Fox, G. A., Allan, L. J., Learning, D. J. and Peakall, D. B. (1978). Effects of injected organochlorines on naturally incubated Herring Gull eggs. *J. Wildl. Manage.* **42**, 484–493.

Haegele, M. A. and Hudson, R. H. (1973). DDE effects on reproduction of Ring-doves. *Environ. Pollut.* **4**, 53–57.

Haegele, M. A. and Hudson, R. H. (1977). Reduction of courtship behaviour induced by DDE in male ringed turtle doves. *Wilson Bull.* **89**, 593–601.

Heinz, G. H. (1976). Behaviour of Mallard ducklings from parents fed 3 ppm DDE. *Bull. Environ. Contamin. Toxicol.* **16**, 640–645.

Heinz, G. H. (1979). Methylmercury: reproductive and behavioural effects on three generations of Mallard ducks. *J. Wildl. Manage.* **43**, 394–401.

Heinz, G. H., Hill, E. F., Stickel, W. H. and Stickel, L. F. (1979). Environmental contaminant studies by the Patuxent Wildlife Research Center. In Kenaga, E. E. (Ed.) *Avian and Mammalian Wildlife Toxicology*, pp. 9–35. ASTM STP 693.

Hickey, J. J. (Ed.), (1969). *Peregrine Falcon Populations, Their Biology and Decline*. Univ. of Wisconsin Press, Madison, Wisconsin.

Jefferies, D. J. (1967). The delay in ovulation produced by *p,p'*-DDT and its possible significance in the field. *Ibis* **109**, 266–272.

Keith, J. O. (1978). *Synergistic Effects of DDE and Food Stress in Reproduction in Brown Pelicans and Ring-doves*. Ph.D. dissertation, Ohio State Univ.

Lehrman, D. S. (1964). The reproductive behaviour of Ring-doves. *Sci. Am.* **211**, 48–54.

Lifson, N. and McClintock, R. (1966). Theory and use of the turnover rates of body water for measuring energy and material balance. *J. Theor. Biol.* **12**, 46–74.

Lillie, R. J., Cecil, H. C., Bitman, J. and Fries, G. F. (1974). Differences in response of caged White Leghorn layers to various polychlorinated biphenyls (PCB's) in the diet. *Poult. Sci.* **53**, 726–732.

Lockley, R. M. (1961). *Shearwaters*. Doubleday and Co. Inc., New York.

Lockley, R. M. (1962). *Puffins.* Doubleday and Co. Inc., New York.

Longcore, J. R. and Stendell, R. C. (1977). Shell thinning and reproductive impairment in Black Ducks after cessation of DDE dosage. *Arch. environ. Contam. Toxicol.* **6**, 293–304.

McArthur, M. L. B., Fox, G. A., Peakall, D. B. and Philogene, B. A. R. (in press) Ecological significance of behavioral and humoral anomolies in breeding Ring-dove fed organo-chlorine mixture. Arch. environ. Contam. Toxicol.

McLane, M. A. R. and Hall, L. C. (1972). DDE thins Screech Owl eggshells. *Bull. Environ. Contam. Toxicol.* **8**, 65–68.

McLaughlin, J., Jr., Marliac, J.-P., Vernett, M. J., Mutchler, M. K. and Fitzhugh, O. G. (1963). The injection of chemicals into the yolks of fertile eggs prior to incubation as a toxicity test. *Toxic. appl. Pharmac.* **5**, 760–771.

Miller, D. S., Peakall, D. B. and Kinter, W. B. (1978). Ingestion of crude oil: Sublethal effects in Herring Gull chicks. *Science, (Washington, D.C.)* **199**, 315–317.

Miller, D. S., Butler, R. G., Trivelpiece, W. Jans-Butler, S., Green, S., Peakall, B., and Peakall, D. B. (1980). Crude oil ingestion by seabirds: possible metabolic and reproductive effects. *Bull. Mt. Desert Island Biological Lab.* **20**, 137–138.

Newton, I. (1979). *Population Ecology of Raptors.* Buteo Books. Vermillion, S. Dakota.

Osborn, D. and Harris, M. P. (1979). A procedure for implanting a slow release formulation of an environmental pollutant into a free-living animal. *Environ. Pollut.* **19**, 139–144.

Peakall, D. B. (1975). Physiological effects of chlorinated hydrocarbons on avian species. In Haque, R. and Freed, V. H. (Eds.) *Environmental Dynamics of Pesticides*, pp. 343–360. Plenum Press, New York.

Peakall, D. B., Fox, G. A., Gilman, A. P., Hallett, D. J. and Norstrom, R. J. (1980a). Reproductive success of Herring Gulls an indicator of Great Lakes water quality. In Afghan, B. K. and Mackay, D. (Eds.) *Hydrocarbons and Halogenated Hydrocarbons in the Aquatic Environment* pp. 337–344. Plenum Press, New York.

Peakall, D. B., Hallett, D. J., Miller, D. S., Butler, R. G. and Kinter, W. B. (1980b). Effects of crude oil on Black Guillemots: a combined field and laboratory study. *Ambio* **9**, 28–30.

Peakall, D. B., Lincer, J. L. and Bloom, S. E. (1972). Embryonic mortality and chromosomal alterations caused by Aroclor 1254 in Ring-doves. *Environ. Health Perspect.* **1**, 103–104.

Peakall, D. B. and Peakall, M. L. (1973). Effect of a polychlorinated biphenyl on the reproduction of artificially and naturally incubated dove eggs. *J. appl. Ecol.* **10**, 363–868.

Peakall, D. B., Tremblay, J., Kinter, W. B. and Miller, D. S. (1981). Endocrine dysfunction in seabirds caused by ingested oil. *Environ. Res.* **24**, 6–14.

Pearce, P. A. and Busby, D. G. (1980). Research on the effects of Fenitrothion on the White-throated Sparrow. *Seventh Annual Forest Pest Control Forum, Ottawa.* Appendix 23.

Porter, R. D. and Wiemeyer, S. N. (1969). Dieldrin and DDT: effects on Sparrow Hawk eggshells and reproduction. *Science (Washington, DC)* **165**, 199–200.

Porter, R. D. and Wiemeyer, S. N. (1970). Propagation of captive American Kestrels. *J. Wildl. Manage.* **34**, 594–604.

Powell, G. V. N. and Gray, D. C. (1980). Dosing free-living nestling Starlings with an organophosphate pesticide, Famphin. *J. Wildl. Manage.* **44**, 918–921.

Ratcliffe, D. A. (1958). Broken eggs in Peregrine eyries. *Br. Birds* **51**, 23–26.

Richie, P. J. and Peterle, T. J. (1979). Effect of DDE on circulating luteinizing hormone levels in Ring-doves during courtship and nesting. *Bull. environ. Contam. Toxicol.* **23**, 220–226.

Shellenberger, T. E. (1978). A multigeneration toxicity evaluation of *p, p'*-DDT and dieldrin with Japanese Quail. I. Effects on growth and reproduction. *Drug Chem. Toxicol.* **1**, 137–146.

Silver, R. (1978). The parental behaviour of Ring-doves. *Sci. Am.* **66**, 207–215.

Stickel, W. H. (1975). Some effects of pollutants in terrestrial ecosystems. In McIntyre, A. D. and Mills, C. F. (Eds.). *Ecological Toxicology Research*, pp. 25–74. Plenum Press, New York.

Sweenen, C. (1977). *Practical Investigation into the Possibility of Keeping Seabirds for Research Purposes*. Report, Netherlands Institute for Sea Research.

Szaro, R. C., Dieter, M. P., Heinz, G. H. and Ferrell, J. F. (1978). Effects of chronic ingestion of South Louisiana crude oil on Mallard ducklings. *Environ. Res.* **17**, 426–436.

Tinbergen, N. (1953). *The Herring Gull's World*. Collins, London.

Trivelpiece, W., Butler, R. G., Miller, D. S. and Peakall, D. B. (1983). Crude oil ingestion of adult Leach's Petrels reduces survival and growth of their chicks. *Science (Washington, DC)* (in press).

Weathers, W. W. and Nagy, K. A. (1980). Simultaneous doubly labeled water ($^3HH^{18}O$) and time budget estimates of daily energy expenditure in *Phainopepla nitens*. *Auk* **97**, 861–867.

Weseloh, D. V., Mineau, P. and Hallett, D. J. (1979). Organochlorine contaminants and trends in reproduction in Great Lakes Herring Gulls, 1974–1978. *Trans. 44th N. Amer. Wildl. Resources Conf.*, pp. 543–557.

Wiemeyer, S. N., Spitzer, P. R., Krant, W. C., Lamont, T. G. and Cromartie, E. (1975). Effects of environmental pollutants on Connecticut and Maryland Ospreys. *J. Wildl. Manage.* **39**, 124–139.

Willoughby, E. J. and Cade, T. J. (1964). Breeding behaviour of the American Kestrel (sparrow hawk). *Living Bird* **3**, 75–96.

Methods for Assessing the Effects of Chemicals on Reproductive Functions
Edited by V. B. Vouk and P. J. Sheehan
© 1983 SCOPE

Methods to Test and Assess Effects of Chemicals on Reproduction in Fish

EDWARD M. DONALDSON and EBERHARD SCHERER

1 INTRODUCTION

Attempts to evaluate environmental risk of man-made chemicals often focus on fish. Beyond their immediate economic value to man, fish represent the upper trophic, bioaccumulatory levels of aquatic ecosystems whose primary element, water, acts globally as a most effective transport medium or sink for environmental toxicants.

'Acute bioassays', i.e. acute lethal tests that determine the concentration of a chemical killing 50% of test fish in 96 hours, were the main and often the only means of hazard assessment till the 1970s. Ecotoxicologists became increasingly aware, however, that acute death or survival in a short-term test would not provide adequate information on the effects of chemicals. More insidious (if less conspicuous) sublethal and chronic effects, and tests capable of detecting and quantifying them, have been receiving more and more attention over recent years. A multitude of effects on reproductive function in fish, from gonad differentiation over larval development to spawning has become known (see reviews by Waldichuck, 1973; EIFAC, 1975, 1978; Donaldson, 1976; FAO, 1977; Sprague, 1976; Brungs et al., 1978; ICES, 1978; Birge et al. 1979a, b; Cole, 1979; Spehar et al., 1980; McIntyre and Pearce, 1980).

Some previous reviews specifically emphasized the importance of reproductive impairment criteria for toxicity assessment (Rosenthal and Alderdice, 1976; Macek and Sleight, 1977; McKim, 1977). So far, however, very little of this knowledge on effects has been utilized for or transformed to standardized toxicity test methods.

Our paper will look at:

(1) effects of chemical pollutants on reproducing fish and early life stages;
(2) test methods, procedures and approaches available to determine such effects;
(3) research needs regarding our present knowledge of effects or mechanisms, and gaps between effects described and tests proposed.

2. EFFECTS OF CHEMICALS ON REPRODUCTION

The effects of chemicals on reproduction in fish can be segregated according to ontogenetic stage. In some cases the effect of a xenobiotic on reproduction is observed directly in the life history stage which is exposed, while in other situations the effect is observed in a later ontogenetic stage or in the offspring produced by the exposed parents. In this section reproductive effects will be considered from gametes to gonadal maturation in adults, and finally effects transmitted to offspring and full life cycle testing will be considered.

2.1 Gametes and Fertilization

External fertilization is the reproductive mode of the majority of teleosts. The release of gametes into and direct exposure to the aquatic medium is a critical stage during which the presence of a chemical pollutant can either have a direct lethal effect on spermatozoa or ova, cause gene damage, interfere with the motility of the spermatozoon, or impair its ability to enter the micropyle and successfully fertilize the ovum. Many economically important species of fish such as herring, salmonids and eels migrate to specific spawning locations and the spawning event is characterized by marked seasonality. The investigation of the effect of chemicals on gametes in these species would not be relevant outside the above space–time relationship. On the other hand, the presence of a xenobiotic in the water at the spawning location at the time when spawning occurs could have a devastating effect. In this context it has been noted (Johnston, 1978) that the Ekofisk oil well blow-out had only a minor impact as it occurred in a mackerel spawning area but one month before the time of spawning.

The motility of trout sperm and subsequent egg fertilization rate were reduced by detergents at 5–10 p.p.m. (Mann and Schmid, 1961). Continuous exposure of plaice (*Pleuronectes platessa*) eggs from before fertilization to vinyl chloride byproducts at 50 and 100 p.p.m. had no effect on fertilization rate but resulted in cessation of embryonic development in the late stages of gastrulation (Braaten *et al.*, 1972). Exposure of steelhead trout (*Salmo gairdneri*) spermatozoa at 1.0 p.p.m. methylmercuric chloride for 30 minutes markedly reduced their fertilizing capacity (McIntyre, 1973). Cadmium exposure up to 10 p.p.m. did not affect the fertilization of Pacific herring eggs but resulted in dose and exposure-time related poor survival at hatching (Rosenthal and Alderdice, unpublished, in Rosenthal and Alderdice, 1976).

Billard and co-workers have developed methodologies for the examination of the effect of pollutants on spermatozoa and ova separately prior to fertilization. To obtain test periods of up to 60 minutes spermatozoa were exposed to pollutants in the presence of 2g/1KCl, which inhibits sperm motility (Billard and Jalabert, 1974). After dilution of the potassium ion the fertilizing ability was tested at 1/10,000 and 1/1000 sperm dilutions. To prevent closure of the micropyle, ova were immersed in a physiological solution containing TRIS–glycol buffer 250 mosmol, pH 9.0 (Billard, 1977). Using these techniques a polychlorobiphenyl was shown to inhibit fertilization by effects on both sperm and eggs over a dose range of 4–400 p.p.b. (Billard *et al.*, 1978). Hexadecanol and octadecanol exposure for 20 or 40 minutes reduced the fertilizing ability of a 10^{-4} dilution of trout sperm over a dose range 1–1000 mg/l while octadecanol exposure for 60 minutes over a dose range of 100–1000 mg/l significantly reduced the fertility of trout ova (Billard, 1978a). In further tests using this technique the organochlorine pesticide lindane was shown to lower the fertilization rate at 25 p.p.m., and Hg, Fe, Cu and Cr were shown to be the most toxic metals for gametes (Billard, 1978b).

2.2 Cytological and Cytogenetic Effects on Eggs

The examination of egg chromosomes, rate of chromosome division (mitotic index) in the yolk-sac membrane and general cell state has recently been used to evaluate the possible effect of pollutants in the oceanic microlayer on Atlantic mackerel eggs (*Scomber scombrus*) in the surface waters of the New York Bight (Longwell and Hughes, 1980). Cytogenetic abnormalities observed included chromosome bridging, chromosome breakage and translocation, and chromosomes outside the mitotic spindle at telophase. In the early stage of the investigation mortality–moribundity estimates were calculated for the cleavage, morula, blastula, gastrula–early embryo and tail bud–tail-free stages and estimates were made for the number of telophases per embryo and percentage of embryos with < 15 telophases at the gastrula–early embryo and tail bud–tail-free stages. In later stages of the investigation yolk-sac viability was estimated on the basis of cell state, mitotic index and mitotic irregularity. Computer comparison of these indices with chemical analysis at sample locations indicated associations between the cytological and cytogenetic parameters, microlayer levels of heavy metals and toxic hydrocarbons. To obtain more meaningful correlations future intensive studies may involve a greater amount of chemical sampling and analysis at fewer locations. Concentration on specific mutagenic events in the yolk-sac membrane may reduce the problem of separating the natural and unnatural components of zygote mortality (Longwell and Hughes, 1980). Important factors in the methodology include adequate sample size, control sampling from pollutant-free areas and simultaneous physical and chemical studies in the sample areas (Sinderman *et al.*, 1980).

2.3 Early-life-history Stages

The term 'early-life-history stages' encompasses embryonic development, hatching, yolk-sac larvae and the stages of larval development after first feeding. An overwhelming amount of effort has been devoted to the investigation of the effect of chemical pollutants on all stages of early development in fish. The subject has been thoroughly reviewed on a number of occasions (Rosenthal and Alderdice, 1976; McKim, 1977; Macek and Sleight, 1977) and a number of specific test methodologies have been developed (e.g. Birge *et al.*, 1979a; Macdonald, 1979; Anon, 1981a, b). The specific effects of pollutants on the various early-life-history stages have been reviewed by Rosenthal and Alderdice (1976) and are summarized in Table 1. It has been suggested (Birge *et al.*, 1979a) that early-life-history tests are unlikely to produce 'false negative' results providing that exposure is maintained from fertilization through 4–7 days post-hatching; the

Table 1   Effects induced by chemical pollutants which affect gametes or early-life-history stages

GAMETES
Spermatozoa
   reduced mortality
   abnormal appearance in electron microscope
   reduced fertilization of normal eggs
   gene damage
Ova
   reduced fertilization by normal spermatozoa
   gene damage
   delayed effect on hatching

FERTILIZATION
Reduced fertilization rate

EGG CHARACTERISTICS POST-FERTILIZATION
Altered rate of water hardening
Increased fragility
Reduced adhesiveness in normally adhesive eggs
Reduced egg volume
Reduced bursting pressure
Reduced osmolality of perivitelline fluid
Altered buoyancy

EMBRYONIC DEVELOPMENT
Prehatch embryonic mortality
Embryonic malformation
Cytogenetic abnormalities
   chromosome bridging, breakage, translocation
   chromosome(s) outside spindle during telophase
   number of telophases per embryo
Arrested differentiation or dedifferentiation
Altered embryonic movement—behavioural change
Decreased enzyme activity
Change in respiratory rate
Histopathological changes, e.g. in integument
Altered rate of yolk utilization
Altered heat rate

Table 1 *(Contd.)*

HATCHING
Alteration in percentage hatch
Failure to hatch
Changed time of hatching, earlier or later than normal
Decreased weight and/or length at hatch
Altered body size to yolk-sac size relationship

YOLK-SAC LARVAE (ALEVINS)
Mortality
Deformity
Reduced or uneven yolk utilization
Reduced growth
Changed buoyancy
Retarded morphological development
Retarded behavioural development
Inability to swim
Poor equilibrium
Change in respiratory rate
Histopathological changes, e.g. in branchial epithelium

LARVAE (FRY)
Mortality
Deformity
Failure to feed
Retarded growth rate
Reduced swimming ability
Disturbed equilibrium
Behavioural changes
Lowered disease resistance
Abnormal gonad differentiation
Change in respiratory rate
Change in osmoregulatory ability

EMBRYONIC DEVELOPMENT IN VIVIPAROUS FISH
Embryo mortality
Deformity
Reduced brood size
Reduced body length at birth
Change in interval between broods

reason being that a wide range of biochemically and physiologically mediated toxic effects on early developmental stages are possible including effects on cell differentiation and growth, cellular differentiation, metabolism, systemic functions, hatching and initial accommodation to a free-living existence (Birge *et al.*, 1979a). To permit an evaluation of the effect of xenobiotics on the critical period of transition from the endogenous food source, yolk, to an exogenous source of natural or formulated feed would require extension of the test period beyond the 4–7 days post-hatch proposed by Birge *et al.* (1979b).

2.3.1 *Effects of Organic Compounds on Early-life-history Stages*

Organochlorine compounds   Attempts to relate egg hatchability in hatchery salmonids to levels of PCBs and other organochlorine compounds accumulated in the eggs in the natural environment have so far failed to show a clear relationship (Zitko and Saunders, 1979; Stauffer, 1979; Broyles and Noveck, 1979). An earlier study had shown that the PCB Aroclor 1242 caused 75% mortality at 30 days in rainbow trout eggs which contained 2.7 $\mu g/g$ PCBs (Hogan and Brauhn, 1975). Continuous exposure of brook trout eggs to the organochlorine pesticide toxaphene from 21 days before hatching did not affect hatching, but caused complete mortality 30 or 60 days after hatching at 502 and 288 ng/l respectively (Mehrle and Mayer, 1975). The effect of halogenated organic compounds produced by chlorination of sewage effluent and cooling water has been tested by exposing carp embryos from fertilization to hatching to synthetic mixtures. The percentage survival of eggs at hatching was used to estimate the LC_{50} (Trabalka and Burch, 1978). It has been pointed out that in the case of 5-chlorouracil, hatched embryos with malformations which prevent them from entering the reproductive pool should be added to the direct mortalities (Eyman *et al.*, 1975). The effect of 2, 4-D on oxygen consumption during early embryonic development in the loach has been examined using Cartesian divers. Fertilization of eggs in a 15 mM solution of 2, 4-D reduced oxygen consumption at 7 hours, while fertilization in water followed by transfer to herbicide solution had a lesser effect on oxygen consumption and addition of 2, 4-D four hours after fertilization had no effect (Klekowski *et al.*, 1977). These differences in response to different exposure timing relate to changes in egg permeability after fertilization. The effect of 2, 4-D has been tested on fertilized eggs and freshly hatched larvae of bleak (*Alburnus alburnus*). 2, 4-D stopped development of embryos, caused behavioural changes and morphological alterations, and the LC_{50} values ranged from 12.9 to 159.4 mg/l for embryos and from 51.6 to 111.2 mg/l for larvae depending on time of exposure (Biro, 1979). The information was used to obtain a maximum acceptable toxicant concentration (MATC).

Organophosphates   Cholinesterase-inhibiting organophosphate insecticides, such as fenitrothion, have been shown to be less toxic to salmonid embryos and alevins than to later-life-history stages (Klaverkamp *et al.*, 1977). As a consequence, early-life-history tests may not be appropriate for organophosphates.

Oil and oil dispersants   A number of recent studies have been conducted on the effects of oil pollution on early-life-history stages. In the killifish (*Fundulus heteroclitus*), exposure to oil decreased the interval between fertilization and hatching (Linden *et al.*, 1979) and the early embryonic stages were more sensitive than the later embryonic and larval stages, perhaps as a result of the decreasing permeability of the vitelline membrane to naphthalene. The water-soluble fraction depressed developmental rate, hatching success and larval survival, and increased developmental abnormalities (Sharp *et al.*, 1979). In pink salmon *Oncorhynchus gorbuscha*, on the other hand, alevins and fry were more sensitive than embryos to crude oil (Rice *et al.*, 1975). In the Pacific herring *Clupea pallasi*, exposure of embryos to the water-soluble fraction of crude oil resulted in reduced size at hatching. It also resulted in body flexure which caused failure to swim and in nature would prevent filling of the swimbladder at the surface and failure to maintain position in the water column and feeding. The scanning electron microscope revealed deformed mouths which would also affect feeding (Smith and Cameron, 1979). The egg of the medaka (*Oryzias latipes*) has been suggested as a promising candidate for toxicant testing. The adult female spawns daily for 3–4 months in the laboratory and the chorion is transparent, permitting observation of prehatch developmental stages. Exposure to crude oil reduced hatching time by up to 33% and produced smaller larvae with larger than normal yolk-sacs. The premature hatching was thought to be the result of increased respiratory rate or irritation which had caused increased opercular movement and ruptured the hatching glands (Leung and Bulkley, 1979). Some earlier publications reviewed in the above paper showed crude oil or its components to delay hatching. The difference is thought to be related to differences in the ratio of individual toxicants. Oil dispersants also have significant effects on embryonic development in fish. In the cod (*Gadus morhua*) there was high sensitivity in early embryos, a decrease after gastrulation and an increase again after hatching (Lonning and Falk-Petersen, 1979).

2.3.2 *Effects of Inorganic Compounds on Early-life-history Stages*

Acid precipitation Acid precipitation resulting from industrial sulphur dioxide emission into the atmosphere has lowered the pH in a number of freshwater systems and had a severe impact on the reproductive capacity and consequent survival of many fish species in the affected areas (Beamish, 1976). The impact on reproduction has been at both the early-life-history stages and at the adult stages. Exposure of brook trout embryos to pH 4.65 resulted in a significantly lower survival to hatching (Trojnar, 1977). In Atlantic salmon (*Salmo salar*) and brown trout (*Salmo trutta*) exposure of eggs to pH 4.5 and above did not affect hatching rate, while pH 3.5 was lethal to all eggs in 10 days (Carrick, 1979). Embryonic mortality and morbidity were found in lake trout (*Salvelinus namaycush*) inhabiting a lake experimentally acidified over a 3 year period to a mean summer epilimnion pH of 5.84 and hypolimnion pH of 6.2 (Kennedy, 1980). A recent detailed study of the effects of acidic pH on embryos and alevins in Atlantic salmon has shown sublethal alterations in the integument, gill and blood vascular structures of all live alevins at pH 5.0 and lower. Below pH 4.5 injuries also occurred in brain, optic retina, kidney, spleen and erythrocytes. In prehatch and post-hatch embryos, injury to the integument and branchial epithelium respectively were believed to be the primary cause of death as a result of impairment of respiration and ion homoeostasis (Daye and Garside, 1980). In field tests in an acid lake, survival of rainbow trout eggs and fry was improved by incubation over a limestone substrate (Gunn and Keller, 1980).

Metals   The effects of cadmium on the fertilized egg of the Pacific herring *Clupea pallasi* have been investigated in detail by Alderdice, Rosenthal and collaborators. Incubation of herring eggs in seawater containing 1 p.p.m. cadmium delayed attainment of the primary maximum bursting pressure and reduced both the primary and secondary bursting pressure maxima. The decrease in strength of the egg envelope appeared to be caused by cadmium binding to the jelly coat and resulted in increased susceptibility of the eggs to mechanical damage (Alderdice *et al.*, 1979a, b, c). Exposure of Pacific herring eggs to cadmium between 0.5 and 30 hours after fertilization reduced total egg volume.

It was proposed that cadmium interfered with the water-hardening process by competing with calcium for binding sites. In pelagic eggs a change in egg volume could affect egg buoyancy (Alderdice *et al.*, 1979b). Exposure to cadmium also reduced the osmolality of the perivitelline fluid especially at high salinities (Alderdice *et al.*, 1979c). To explain the above effects Alderdice *et al.* (1979c) proposed that binding of cadmium to the jelly coat of the egg caused it to harden more slowly. At higher concentrations cadmium penetrates the egg, altering the capsule structure and forming complex ions and molecules in the perivitelline fluid. This reduces the osmotic pressure of the perivitelline fluid and causes less water to be imbibed, thus decreasing egg volume. In the bluegill (*Lepomis macrochirus*) as in other species the embryo and larval stages are much more sensitive to cadmium than adult fish. The difference between the safe chronic and acute mortality values was 200-fold (Eaton, 1974). In rainbow trout exposure of alevins to cadmium caused erratic swimming and blood clotting. Alevins from cadmium-exposed eggs survived longer during cadmium exposure than alevins from unexposed eggs (Beattie and Pascoe, 1978). In the Atlantic silverside *Menidia menidia*, an estuarine teleost, cadmium-induced larval mortality was highest at low salinity (10 per thousand) and lowest at high salinity (30 per thousand) (Voyer *et al.*, 1979). These workers devised a fluctuating salinity test system for estuarine which simulates the cyclic changes which occur in estuarine salinity. In an investigation of the combined effects of cadmium, copper and lead on herring (*Clupea harengus*) eggs and larvae, 'viable hatch' was found to be a much more sensitive indicator than embryonic survival up to the time of hatching. The effects of cadmium and copper were additive (Westernhagen *et al.*, 1979).

The zebrafish *Brachydanio rerio* has been extensively used for toxicity testing on the basis of its transparent eggs, the fact that the adults breed year round and the sensitivity of its early-life-history stages. Exposure of prolarvae and larvae to lead ions induced epithelioma, poor absorption of yolk and tail erosions while copper induced spirality of the nervous system. Lead appeared to antagonize the effect of copper (Ozoh, 1979). Removal of the shell membrane from the developing egg (dechorionation) increased embryonic sensitivity to copper (Ozoh, 1980). This is opposite to the effect of dechorionation during zinc exposure.

A detailed method has been described for the investigation of the effect of copper on Pacific herring eggs and larvae. Embryo mortality occurred at 35 μg/l while larval mortality occurred at 300 μg/l (Rice and Harrison, 1977). In freshwater species the larval stage is the more sensitive early-life-history stage to copper. Investigation of the effect of copper on two other marine species has shown that the Atlantic silverside, an estuarine spawner, is more sensitive to copper than the spot (*Leiostomus xanthurus*), an oceanic spawner. Copper was most toxic to the eggs of the silverside at hatching. The percentage mortality at hatching was compared with number of eggs alive 24 hours after fertilization (Engel and Sunda, 1979). In the zebra ciclid *Cichlasoma nigrofasciatum*, exposure of prolarvae and larvae to copper caused malformation of the nervous system while zinc caused mortality without obvious malformation. The combination of 32 p.p.b. zinc and 16 p.p.b. copper had a synergistic effect on mortality expressed as percentage hatch. The lesser sensitivity in this ciclid to copper malformation compared to the zebra fish was related to the lower amount of yolk present in the egg of the latter species (Ozoh and Jacobson, 1979).

Exposure of carp (*Cyprinus carpio*) eggs and larvae to nickel has shown that eggs are more sensitive than larvae for the same exposure time; however, the larval stage lasts longer than the embryonic stage and is thus more sensitive to extended exposure (Blaycock and Frank, 1979). Silver caused premature hatching of eggs and retarded alevin development in rainbow trout at concentrations of 0.17–0.69 μg/l. Mortality prior to swim-up was 52% at 0.69 μg/l. The 'no effect' concentration between 0.09 and 0.17 μg/l indicates that silver is one of the most toxic metals to fish (Davies *et al.*, 1978). In the USSR the effects of the organometallic compound ethylmercuric chloride have been tested on the early-life-history stages of the loach. Eggs were most sensitive at gastrulation and at hatching. After hatching, larvae were reared in freshwater for 2 weeks to determine mortality. The maximum tolerable concentration was 0.005 mg/l (Bykova, 1979).

Arsenic   Early-life-history tests in the muskellunge (*Esox masquinongy*) have shown that larvae undergoing swim-up are more sensitive by far than either earlier or later developmental stages (Spotila and Paladino, 1979). In addition to causing mortality arsenic has been shown to lower the critical thermal maximum for muskellunge fry (Paladino and Spotila, 1978).

Chlorine   Chlorine is used as a biocide in power generating facilities and sewage treatment plants. Eggs from stripped bass (*Morone saxatilis*), white perch (*Morone americana*) and blueback herring (*Alosa aestivalis*) were exposed to chlorine until hatching. Hatching was reduced, larvae were shorter at hatching, larval development was inhibited and in the herring abnormal larvae were produced (Morgan and Prince, 1978). A test system for simulating the effect of the simultaneous rise in temperature and total residual chlorine exposure that occurs in power plant condenser systems has been devised. Using this system the effect of chlorine on striped bass eggs and prolarvae was investigated. Eggs were more resistant to the combined effects of chlorine and temperature than prolarvae. For prolarvae there was a second order linear interaction between chlorine and temperature (Burton *et al.*, 1979). In the zebra fish chlorine was more toxic to newly hatched larvae than to eggs (Yosha and Cohen, 1979).

Nitrate, ammonia and hydrogen sulphide   Fish can be exposed to nitrate from agricultural fertilizers or from hatchery water re-use. Exposure of salmonids to nitrate from water hardening of eggs through to first feeding showed that rainbow and steelhead trout were the most sensitive. In the latter species, 5 mg/1 caused significant egg mortality. Mortality was lower in surviving fry (Kincheloe *et al.*, 1979).

Exposure of rainbow trout eggs and alevins to un-ionized ammonia caused mortality at or after hatching, retarded larval growth, inhibited yolk-sac absorption and in some cases resulted in hypertrophy of the gill epithelium. The lethal threshold concentration (LC_{50}) for alevins was 0.25 mg/1 NH_3-N (Burkhalter and Kaya, 1977).

Hydrogen sulphide is generated by decomposition of organic material or is present in effluents. Concentrations exceeding 0.025 mg/1 retard growth, extend the incubation period and result in deformed fry. The effects are accentuated at low oxygen concentrations (Smith and Oseid, 1972). In northern pike *Esox lucius* hydrogen sulphide had similar effects; anatomical malformations included lordosis, congestion, gelatinous lesions, malformed bodies and uneven resorption of yolk (Adelman and Smith, 1970).

2.4 Sexually Maturing Adult Fish

The effects of chemicals on reproductive development in fish manifest themselves in a number of different ways, ranging from histopathological effects to changes in the production and metabolism of gonadotropin and the sex steroids. A number of recorded and potential effects, some of which may be suitable as tests, are listed in Table 2. In the following sections some recently described effects on reproduction in adult fish will be presented according to the nature of the pollutant chemical.

Table 2 Reproductive effects of pollutants during sexual maturation and spawning

SEXUALLY MATURING ADULT
Changes in gonad development
  sterilization
  delay in appearance of secondary sexual characteristics
  delayed maturation
  abnormal gross appearance of gonads
  change in gonadosomatic index
  histopathological changes in gonads
  change in ratio of somatic to spermatogenic tissue in testis
  inhibition of spermatogenesis, blockage of spermatogonial mitosis
  regression of testis
  inhibition of vitellogenesis (yolk deposition)
  reduction in plasma calcium in female
  regression of ovary
Changes in endocrine control mechanisms
  reduction in hypothalamic content of gonadotropin-releasing factor
  altered gonadotropin levels in pituitary and plasma
  change in number of receptors for gonadotropin, androgens and oestrogens*
  altered ovarian ^{32}P uptake
  decreased gonadal 3β-hydroxysteroid dehydrogenase activity
  increase in ovarian cholesterol concentration
  altered gonadal steroidogenesis *in vitro*
  change in plasma concentrations of adrogens, oestrogens and progestogens*
  change in timing of gonadal hormone cycles
  altered turnover time, metabolic clearance rate and secretion rates of gonadal steroids*
Changes in activity of ovarian and testicular enzymes involved in intermediary metabolism
  altered rate of hepatic metabolism of sex hormones *in vitro*
  stimulation of hepatic microsomal enzyme activity, e.g. cytochrome P-450

SEXUALLY MATURE ADULT
Failure to spermiate
Reduced number of mature ova in ovary
Delay or failure of oocyte final maturation
Failure to ovulate
Increased number of atretic ova
Inhibition of sensitivity to sexual aggregating pheromone

SPAWNING
Change in intervals between spawnings
Change in time of spawning
Impairment of spawning behaviour
Behavioural displacement from spawning location
Failure or inhibition of spawning
Reduced eggs released per spawning or per day
Reduction in number of spawnings per female

* Potential effects

2.4.1 *Effects of Organic Compounds on Sexual Maturation*

Organochlorine compounds   A study at the West Vancouver laboratory at the beginning of the last decade (Harvey, 1972) revealed that the feeding of DDT at low levels in the diet to coho salmon (*Oncorhynchus kisutch*) significantly increased the rate of *in vitro* 17β-oestradiol metabolism by liver slices. There was no significant change in oestradiol metabolic clearance rate *in vivo* suggesting that oestradiol was already being metabolized at a maximal rate (Harvey, 1972). The effect on *in vivo* oestradiol clearance rate may have been significant if maturing rather than immature salmon had been used as the former fish have higher plasma oestrogen concentrations.

Exposure of brook trout to a subethal level of polychlorinated biphenyls (PCBs) in the water for 21 days increased the concentration of polar steroid metabolites produced during *in vitro* incubation of the testis. Furthermore, the hatching rate was reduced in eggs produced by treated females (Freeman and Idler 1975). Reproductive effects were also obtained when Atlantic cod (*Gadus morhua*) were fed PCBs (Aroclor 1254) at 1 to 50 mg/kg diet for several months. *In vitro* incubation of testicular tissue from treated fish with ^{14}C-progesterone indicated a marked stimulation of testosterone and 11-ketotestosterone biosynthesis at 5 mg/kg PCBs and an inhibition of 11-ketotestosterone biosynthesis at 10 and 50 mg/kg PCBs. During the experiment plasma androgen levels increased in control fish as sexual maturation proceeded. On the other hand, plasma androgen levels remained low in PCB-treated cod. These marked endocrine changes in PCB-exposed cod were not accompanied by any changes in the gross appearance of the fish (Freeman and Sangalang, 1977a; Freeman *et al.*, 1978).

Examination of enzyme activity in the testes of cod exposed for $5\frac{1}{2}$ months to PCBs in the above experiment indicated increases in supernatant malic dehydrogenase and supernatant aspartic aminotransferase at the higher PCB concentrations and depression of mitochondrial alanine aminotransferase. A number of other enzymes involved in intermediary metabolism were unaffected (Mounib and Eison, 1978). To determine whether there is a correlation between PCB-stimulated hepatic microsomal enzyme activities and plasma sex hormone concentrations trout and carp were administered PCBs intraperitoneally at a dose of 25 mg/kg body weight per week for 4 weeks. The plasma androgen level decreased significantly in trout after 3 weeks and in male carp after 4 weeks. The plasma oestrogen concentration decreased significantly in trout and carp after 4 weeks. These decreases in androgen and oestrogen concentrations were correlated with a significant increase in hepatic cytochrome P-450 activity in both trout and carp (Sivarajah *et al.*, 1978a). Exposure of female catfish *Heteropneustes fossilis* to the organochlorine insecticide endrin for 96 hours resulted in reduced ovarian ^{32}P uptake *in vivo* and reduced pituitary and serum gonadotropin concentrations as measured by stimulation of ^{32}P uptake *in vivo*. Endrin treatment either enhanced at a safe concentration or did not interfere, at a higher concentration, with the stimulation of ovarian ^{32}P uptake by luteinizing hormone or catfish pituitary extract. Thus the effect of endrin on reproduction in the catfish is at the hypothalamic or pituitary level (Singh and Singh, 1980a). The effect of endrin on reproduction in catfish was confirmed during a 4 week exposure at safe and sublethel concentrations. Ovarian ^{32}P uptake was reduced at all phases of the reproductive cycle. The effect on pituitary and serum gonadotropin concentrations was particularly significant during the prespawning and spawning phases (Singh and Singh, 1980b). In addition to its effect on gonadotropin, endrin induced a significant increase in ovarian cholesterol concentration during the prespawning and spawning phases. This increase may reflect a decreased rate of steroid hormone biosynthesis (Singh and Singh, 1980c). Similar changes have been reported in the female catfish after aldrin treatment (Singh and Singh, 1981a). Recently male catfish have been shown to respond to endrin in a similar manner to the females (Singh and Singh, 1980d).

Gonadal histopathological changes have been identified as a result of PCB treatment. In the cod testis these ranged from thickening of the lobule wall to disintegration of spermatogenic elements (Freeman *et al.*, 1980). Electron microscopic investigation of trout and carp gonads exposed to PCBs revealed enlargement and proliferation of the endoplasmic reticulum in the developing oocytes and damage to spermatozoa in the testis. The effect of PCBs on the spermatozoa may have been direct or may have been caused by an alteration in circulating androgen concentrations (Sivarajah *et al.*, 1978b).

It has been recently shown that the effects of the organochlorine insecticides aldrin and endrin have two mechanisms of action which interfere with reproduction in the female catfish. They reduce the hypothalmic content of gonadotropin-releasing factor and also decrease ovarian sensitivity to gonadotropin measured by suppression of ovarian ^{32}P uptake in hypophysectomized fish (Singh and Singh, 1981b).

Organophosphate and other non-chlorinated pesticides The effects of the organophosphate insecticides malathion and parathion on ovarian ^{32}P uptake, pituitary and serum gonadotropin and ovarian and testicular cholesterol in the catfish were generally similar to those reported above for endrin (Singh and Singh, 1980a,b,c,d, 1981a). Malathion and parathion appear to have a single mode of action in the female catfish by reducing the hypothalamic secretion of gonadotropin-releasing hormone. They do not suppress ovarian sensitivity to gonadotropin (Singh and Singh, 1981b). Exposure of carp to safe and sublethal doses of fenitrothion for 6 months significantly reduced testicular and ovarian 3β-hydroxysteroid dehydrogenase (HSD) activity. The effect may be secondary to the inhibition of gonadotropin secretion (Kapur *et al.*, 1978). Exposure of *Channa punctatus* to the 180 day LC_{50} concentrations of fenitrothion (1.5 p.p.m.) and carbaryl (2 p.p.m.) reduced or inhibited respectively, the production of mature oocytes and increased the proportion of atretic oocytes and decreased ovarian weight over 150 days (Saxena and Garg, 1978). Carbaryl exposure of fathead minnows (*Pimephales promelas*) for 9 months at 0.68 mg/l reduced the number of eggs per female and number of eggs per spawning and prevented hatching. The ovaries of treated fish contained flaccid ova which appeared to be atretic (Carlson, 1971). Treatment of male guppies in sublethal concentrations of parathion for 40 days caused a dose-related inhibition of spermatogenesis resembling the effect of hypophysectomy and suggesting an effect on gonadotropin (Billard and Kinkelin, 1970). Recently the insecticide Lebaycid® (Fenthion) has been shown to cause total atresia of the ovaries of *Tilapia leucosticta* (Kling, 1981).

Oil   Exposure of a marine fish, the cunner (*Tautogolabrus adspersus*) to a surface slick of crude oil for 6 months resulted in a significant reduction in the testicular somatic index (Payne *et al.*, 1978). Oil exposure of this same species for a period of only 14 days resulted in no obvious reproductive effect (Kiceniuk *et al.*, 1980). A test of the effect of petroleum on trout reproduction by administration of a diet containing 1% crude petroleum also failed to show any effect (Hodgins *et al.*, 1977). On the other hand, examples of apparent environmental oil-induced hepatic mixed-function oxygenase (MFO) activity in fish have been reviewed by Stegeman (1980). Changes in MFO could have effects on the turnover rate of gonadal steroids.

2.4.2 *Effects of Inorganic Compounds on Sexual Maturation*

Acid precipitation   In addition to having effects on the survival of early-life-history stages, acidification of fresh waters has been shown to have significant reproductive effects on adult fish. In George Lake in Ontario progressive acidification resulted in failure to reproduce and consequent disappearance of small mouth bass, walleye and burbot at pH 6.0 to 5.5, lake trout and trout perch at pH 5.5 to 5.2, white sucker, brown bullhead and rock bass at pH 5.2 to 4.7 and lake herring, yellow perch and lake chub at pH 4.7 to 4.5. Examination of fish after the normal spawning period revealed that they had failed to release their ova (Beamish *et al.*, 1975; Beamish, 1976). Sexual maturation in female teleosts is characterized by an oestrogen-stimulated increase in serum calcium concentration (for review see Holmes and Donaldson, 1969). Female white suckers in George Lake did not show the characteristic rise in serum calcium characteristic of normal maturing fish. The rise in calcium was, however, seen in George Lake suckers transferred to water of normal pH and in females of other species which were still reproducing successfully in the acidified water of George Lake (Beamish *et al.*, 1975; Lockhart and Lutz, 1977). Recent investigation of the effect of low pH on oogenesis in the flagfish *Jordanella floridae* has shown that exposure to pH 6.0, 5.5, 5.0 and 4.5 interfered with the formation of mature eggs, in particular the deposition of secondary yolk was inhibited. At pH 4.5 primary yolk deposition was also affected (Ruby *et al.*, 1977). In a parallel test on male flagfish over the same pH range, production of mature sperm was reduced, the ratio of reproductive to somatic tissue in the testis was decreased and at pH 4.5 there was an increase in the number of tubules devoid of spermatozoa. Comparison with ovarian data suggested that testicular development was less sensitive than ovarian development to low pH (Ruby *et al.*, 1978).

Metals Sangalang and O'Halloran (1972, 1973) reported cadmium-induced testicular injury in maturing brook trout. Exposure to 25 p.p.b. cadmium for 24 hours followed by fresh water for 6 days or 10 p.p.b. until death (LT_{50} 21 days) induced gross changes in testicular colour and abnormal vascularization. Histology revealed haemorrhagic necrosis and a reduction in the lipid content (Sudan Black B stain) and disintegration of the lobule boundary cells. *In vitro* incubation of testicular tissue from 25 p.p.b. cadmium-treated brook trout with ^{14}C-pregnenolone indicated a reduction in 11β-hydroxytestosterone and testosterone biosynthesis and a failure in 11-ketotestosterone biosynthesis. *In vitro* incubation of normal brook trout testis with ^{14}C-pregnenolone in the presence of $10-1000$ μg cadmium/g tissue resulted in inhibition of 11-ketotestosterone biosynthesis and an alteration in the pattern of radioactive metabolites produced (Sangalang and O'Halloran, 1973). Long-term exposure of maturing brook trout to 1 p.p.b. cadmium did not influence spermatogenesis, affect the onset of secondary sexual characteristics or alter the time of functional maturity. However, measurement of plasma androgen concentrations indicated that 11-ketotestosterone levels were higher than those in control fish and continued to increase after maturity when concentrations were decreasing in control fish. In cadmium-treated trout testosterone concentrations rose later during maturation than in controls and continued to increase during testicular regression which occurred 2 weeks earlier in treated fish (Sangalang and Freeman, 1974). As treatment was initiated only a month before functional maturity, it is not clear what effect earlier treatment would have had on the timing of sexual maturity. The utility of changes in steroid hormone metabolism as a test method has been reviewed by Freeman and Sangalang (1977b) and Freeman *et al.* (1980).

Mercuric chloride has been shown to influence enzymic activity in the ovary of the freshwater teleost (*Channa punctatus* (Sastry and Agrawal, 1979a). Exposure of fish to the 96-hour LC_{50} concentration (1.8 mg/l) for 96 hours reduced ovarian alkaline phosphatase, glucose-6-phosphatase and lipase activity while exposure to a sublethal concentration (0.3 mg/l) for 30 days significantly reduced ovarian glucose-6-phosphatase and lipase activity. Sastry and Agrawal (1979b) have also investigated the effect of lead nitrate on ovarian enzymes in *Channa punctatus*. Exposure to the 96-hour LC_{50} concentration (13.2 mg/l) for 96 hours or to a sublethal concentration (3.8 mg/l) for 30 days significantly reduced ovarian acid phosphatase, alkaline phosphatase, glucose-6-phosphatase and lipase activity. The effect was greatest after 30 days, indicating a cumulative action of lead.

A T-maze system has been developed for examining the sensitivity of zebra fish to a sexual aggregating pheromone produced by conspecifics (Bloom and Perlmutter, 1977). Using this system it has been shown that exposure of female zebra fish to 5 p.p.m. zinc for 9 days eliminated their preference for female, pheromone-containing, donor water. The zinc may have had a direct effect on the ability of the nasal or gustatory epithelium to detect the sexual aggregating pheromone (Bloom *et al.*, 1978).

Cyanide   Exposure of fathead minnows to 0.019 mg/l cyanide for 256 days resulted in a decrease in egg production (Lind *et al.*, 1977). In brook trout the number of eggs spawned per female was reduced by treatment with 0.012 mg/l cyanide for 144 days (Koenst *et al.*, 1977) while short-term exposure of rainbow trout to 0.01 mg/l cyanide inhibited yolk deposition (Lesniak, 1977). In the juvenile male rainbow trout, exposure to 0.01 or 0.03 mg/l HCN for 18 days reduced the numbers of dividing spermatogonia by 13% and 50% respectively (Ruby *et al.*, 1979). Cyanide affected mitotic spindle formation giving rise to multipolar spindles and multinucleate interphase cells. Blockage of mitosis resulted in an increase in the number of spermatogonia in prophase. Spermatogonial necrosis at the higher concentration suggested that cyanide may cause permanent damage to the final number of spermatogonia present in the testis and thus lower reproductive capacity.

2.5   Behavioural Displacement from Spawning Location

For successful spawning of migrating fishes, 'homing' to suitable spawning sites is essential. Hasler and his co-workers (Walker and Hasler, 1949; Hasler and Wisby, 1951, 1958; Hasler, 1960) investigated the homing mechanisms of salmon, concluding that the response to an imprinted or conditioned odour of the home creek is essential for guiding the fish to their spawning locations. Pollutants may interfere with this mechanism, either by impairing chemosensory capabilities, or by the repellent action of certain toxicants. Of course, visual navigation and swimming stamina may also be affected. Saunders and Sprague (1967) observed that pollution from a base metal mine on a tributary of the Miramichi River in New Brunswick 'caused adult Atlantic salmon, which were on their normal up-stream spawning migration, to return prematurely downstream... Downstream returns of salmon rose from between 1 and 3 percent during 6 years before pollution to between 10 and 22 percent during 4 years of pollution' (Saunders and Sprague, 1967, p. 419). This effect was attributed to increased levels of Cu^{2+} and Zn^{2+}. An avoidance response to these and other pollutants was also demonstrated in laboratory experiments under controlled conditions

(Sprague and Drury, 1969). A number of laboratory techniques have been developed to detect such avoidance reactions (Shelford, 1917; Jones, 1948; Höglund, 1953; Sprague, 1964; Hansen, 1969; Scherer and Nowak, 1973; Scherer, 1979). This literature shows that not only anadromous and catadromous fishes are affected, but any species using chemoreception for selecting and maintaining suitable spawning habitats within their range of distribution.

2.6 Effects of Partial and Full-life-cycle Exposure on Reproduction and Transmission of Effects to Offspring

Up to this point the effects which have been described are those which have a direct impact on reproduction at some point during the life cycle of the individual fish. In a number of studies the effects of long-term exposure of maturing fish on the viability of the succeeding generation have been investigated. In these experiments parameters such as number of eggs ovulated may be reported in addition to such indices as egg mortality and failure to hatch in the succeeding generation (Table 3). In some cases the offspring were incubated and reared in water which contains the pollutant to which the adults were exposed, while in others the progeny were reared in unpolluted water. As before, these long-term studies or tests have been subdivided according to the nature of the pollutant and

Table 3   Reproductive effects of xenobiotics which may be quantified during partial- or complete-life-cycle tests

---

EFFECT OF CHRONIC EXPOSURE DURING SEXUAL MATURATION ON ADULTS
Delay in maturation
Inhibition of spawning
Reduction in eggs produced per female

EFFECT OF EXPOSURE DURING MATURATION OR DURING MATURATION AND SUBSEQUENT EARLY-LIFE-HISTORY STAGES ON EARLY-LIFE-HISTORY STAGES
Egg weight
Egg fertility
Prehatch mortality
Hatching rate
Larval survival
Egg to smolt survival in salmonids
Correlation of xenobiotic levels in adult gonads or eggs with egg and fry mortality

IN VIVIPAROUS FISH, IMPACT OF ADULT EXPOSURE ON
Embryo mortality
Total number of embryos
Time to birth of first brood

---

in most cases, only recent work is cited as these papers contain adequate references to the earlier literature.

2.6.1 *Effects of long-term exposure to organic compounds*

Chlorinated hydrocarbons   A number of studies have attempted to relate the concentration of chlorinated hydrocarbons in the ovaries of different salmonid populations with subsequent egg and fry mortality. Comparing rainbow trout from five lakes in New Zealand, Hopkins *et al.* (1969) found that the population with the highest ovarian DDT level produced eggs with the highest prehatch mortality. There was no effect on fry survival which made it difficult to conclude that egg mortality was definitely related to ovarian DDT in the parents (Burdick *et al.*, 1964). A recent report on hatchery-produced lake trout (*Salvelinus namaycush*) indicates that ovarian p,p'-DDT levels have decreased since the prohibition of DDT use in 1966 and that mortality of fry has also decreased (Dean *et al.*, 1979).

In brook trout, treatment of adults with 0.2 p.p.m. PCBs (Aroclor 1254) resulted in a decrease in hatching rate from 92% to 72% for eggs reared in fresh water. Rearing of eggs from PCB-treated adults in water containing the same concentration of PCBs resulted in zero hatch while less than 1% of eggs from control adults survived to hatch in water containing PCBs (Freeman and Idler, 1975). Chronic exposure of fathead minnows to PCBs at concentrations similar to the 30 day LC_{50} did not interfere with either egg production or hatching and it was concluded that larvae were the most sensitive stage for the chronic biassay of PCBs (Defoe *et al.*, 1978). The sheepshead minnow fry were more sensitive to PCBs than were embryos, juveniles or adults (Schimmel *et al.*, 1974).

Organophosphates   Complete inhibition of reproduction occurred when flag-fish were exposed to diazinon for 21 days with a peak concentration of 130 μg/l (Allison, 1977). Using much lower concentrations of diazinon, Goodman *et al.* (1979) have shown that the number of eggs produced per female in sheepshead minnows is a very sensitive test for organophosphate insecticides. Diazinon over the dose range 0.47–6.5 μg/l significantly reduced the egg production/female per day from 32.8 in controls to from 22.6 to 14.9 in treated fish. In this study number of eggs/female was a more sensitive indicator than either adult survival or egg fertility and survival and growth of progeny.

Linear alkylbenzene sulphonates   The toxicity of the detergent component linear alkylbenzene sulphonates (LAS) increases according to alkyl chain length. Complete-life-cycle tests on fathead minnows conducted according to USEPA (1972) procedures indicated that $C_{11.7}$ LAS had no effect on reproduction up to 1.09 mg/l. On the other hand, $C_{13.3}$ LAS at 0.25 mg/l reduced egg production or inhibited spawning. This same concentration significantly reduced the survival of first generation larvae. The survival of second generation larvae was also low, but the difference in this case was not significant owing to variability between replicates (Holman and Macek, 1980).

Mutagens A model test system has been developed using the viviparous teleost *Poecilia reticulata* to examine the effect of mutagens on fish reproduction. Mature males were either injected with (0.1, 0.2 and 0.4 mg/kg) or immersed in the same concentration of the mutagen triethylenemelamine. The males were then mated 24 hours after initiation of treatment and 10 days following mating the number of live and dead embryos was determined by dissection. There was a dose-related increase in embryo mortality and decrease in the total number of embryos. The guppies were more sensitive to injection than immersion, however, the latter treatment more closely simulated environmental exposure (Mathews *et al.*, 1978).

2.6.2 *Effects of Long-term Exposure to Inorganic Compounds*

Metals Chronic exposure of blugill to cadmium up to 2140 μg/l did not appear to affect the number of spawnings. Embryo survival for the first 6 days was reduced at 239 μg/l and above. At 30 days survival was low at 80 μg/l and there was no survival above this concentration. Chronic exposure at 31 μg/l in 200 mg/l hardness of water had no significant effect on reproduction (Eaton, 1974). The effect of life cycle exposure of flagfish to cadmium-zinc mixtures on reproduction was determined by assessing spawnings per female, total embryos produced, embryos per female and hatchability (Spehar *et al.*, 1978). Sexual maturity was not delayed; however, spawning behaviour was decreased. The number of spawnings per female and embryo production was lower in all Cd (4.3–8.5μg/l)-Zn (73.4–127.0 μg/l) mixtures tested. Larvae previously exposed as embryos were less sensitive than larvae not previously exposed. Exposure of male and female zebrafish to a threshhold concentration of 5 p.p.m. zinc for 9 days prior to spawning delayed spawning. Treated adults produced lower numbers of eggs (165 compared to 434). These eggs were less viable (21% compared to 90%) than control eggs. Survival to hatching in normal water was 0.9% in eggs from Zn exposed adults and 63.3% in controls (Speranza *et al.*, 1977). Possible effects of zinc on sockeye salmon *Oncorhynchus nerka* during freshwater residency were investigated by exposing adults for 3 months prior to spawning and embryonic to smolt stages for 18 months from fertilization (Chapman, 1978). Parameters measured were maturation time, fecundity, egg weight, fertility and egg to smolt survival. Zinc concentrations up to 112 μg/l in the adult stage and 242 μg/l in the embryo to smolt period did not have any deleterious affect. Life cycle exposure of fathead minnows to zinc revealed that egg adhesiveness and fragility were sensitive indicators at 145 μg/l and above. These were direct effects of zinc during water hardening and were not related to parental exposure. Hatchability and larval survival were reduced at 295 μg/l and above (Benoit and Holcombe, 1978). Life cycle and partial chronic testing of the effect of zinc on reproduction in brook trout indicated no harmful effects up to 534 μg/l. At 1360 μg/l zinc reduced egg chorion strength and reduced embryo and 12-week larval survival (Holcombe *et al.*, 1979). The guppy has been used as a test species for zinc to determine the effect on development without direct contact with water. There was no effect on interval between broods but brood size was significantly reduced at 0.88 and 1.70 μg/l and the standard length of young at birth was also significantly reduced (Uviovo and Beatty, 1979). In a recent long-term study on the effect of zinc on reproduction in the guppy, the most sensitive indicator was delay in female maturation. Fewer females were mature after 70-day exposure at 0.173 mg/l. At 0.607 mg/l fewer females gave birth and the time until birth of the first brood was increased. Transfer of zinc from adult to embryo occurs during pregnancy and second generation guppies were less sensitive to zinc exposure (Pierson, 1981). White suckers (*Catostomus commersonii*) have been shown in a field study to respond to decreased spawning success, egg size, egg and larval survival and life span induced by Zn, Cu and Cd by compensatory increases in growth rate and fecundity and earlier maturation (McFarlane and Franzin, 1978).

To establish a no effect concentration of copper, yearling brook trout were exposed to 4.5–9.4 μg Cu/l through spawning to 3-month juveniles. Measurement of Cu levels in ova indicated that no Cu was passed from parent to egg at 9.4 μg/l or below and no significant adverse effects of reproduction were observed (number of mature males and females, number of females spawning, mean spawnings per female, mean viable eggs spawned per female). Hatchability was significantly reduced in one replicate at 9.4 μg/l but not in the other (McKim and Benoit, 1974). In bluegills spawning was inhibited after 22 months exposure to 162 μl/l Cu but not below this concentration. On the other hand, survival of larvae from non-exposed parents was reduced at 40–162 μg/l Cu (Benoit, 1975). Chronic exposure of fathead minnows to copper for 0.3 and 6 months prior to spawning reduced the number of eggs produced per female. Egg production was correlated with concentration and was significant at 37 μg/l and above but was not correlated with time of exposure (Pickering *et al.*, 1977).

To determine the effect of chronic lead exposure on reproduction, 3-year-old rainbow trout were exposed to 6–30 μg/l Pb for 9 months in soft water prior to spawning. Natural spawning (recommended by Brungs, 1969, for determination of MATC) was not achieved and the fish were spawned artifically. Successful hatching and viable fry were obtained from at least one out of each pair of trout at each concentration. The early-life-history stages were more sensitive than adults especially when exposure was initiated at the egg stage (Davies *et al.*, 1976). Exposure of zebrafish to mercury in the form of phenylmercuric acetate (used in the pulp and paper industry) at 1 μg/l or above reduced the number of eggs spawned, possibly by influencing muscular contraction during the spawning process. Eggs from exposed females incubated in pure water showed a lower percentage hatch down to 0.2 μg/l, the lowest concentration tested by Kihlström *et al.*, (1971). In a three-generation study on brook trout the MATC for methylmercury was shown to fall to between 0.93 and 0.29 μg Hg/l (McKim *et al.*, 1976).

High pH The chronic effect of an alkaline environment has been examined by exposure of the guppy to sodium hydroxide. Fecundity was decreased and maturity was either late or premature. At 25 mg/l NaOH, only 66.6% of females produced progeny while at 75 mg/l and above no fish reached sexual maturity (Rustamova, 1979).

Cyanide Life cycle testing of hydrogen cyanide in bluegills has indicated that spawning inhibition is the most sensitive reproductive indicator. Spawning was completely inhibited after chronic exposure to 5.2 μg/l and above. On the other hand, fry survival was reduced at 15.6–19.4 μg/l and juveniles were not affected below 53.1 μg/l (Kimball *et al.*, 1978).

In the fathead minnow the number of eggs per female was significantly reduced at 19.6 μg/l HCN and egg hatchability was significantly reduced at 44.2 μg/l and above. Computer simulation indicated that a population would be driven to extinction by an 80% reduction in recruitment to the spawning stock. This would occur between 44.2 and 63.6 μg/l based on reduced fecundity alone (Lind *et al.*, 1977). Studies on brook trout which involved exposure 144 days prior to spawning and 90 days into the next generation indicated that the MATC was between 5.7 and 11.2 μg/l HCN based on reproduction data, especially eggs spawned per female (Koenst *et al.*, 1977).

3 ACTUAL OR POTENTIAL TESTS BASED ON EFFECTS ON REPRODUCTION

In this section potential tests will be discussed in the context of specific ontogenetic stages. In considering the suitability of a potential test method it is important to consider its feasibility and practicality, its chances of wide acceptance, its sensitivity to xenobiotics and its cost effectiveness. With respect to the latter criterion rapid or short-term tests would normally be expected to have a cost advantage over life cycle tests; however, some potential rapid tests involve the use of relatively sophisticated equipment in an appropriate laboratory environment. Another significant aspect of the suitability of a test is its applicability. To be relevant it must be applicable to species of fish which are important from a commercial, recreational or aesthetic point of view. Preferably it must also be applicable to a range of chemicals or particularly suited to a specific group of chemicals. In the case of migratory species the test must be applicable during the life-history stage that the fish are exposed. In this section some potential or partially developed tests will be briefly reviewed.

3.1 Gametes and Fertilization

In the majority of teleosts the gametes are released directly into the aquatic environment and fertilization is external. The testing for direct effects of chemicals on gametes by measuring percentage fertilization after exposure has merit for its rapidity and its relevance to situations where fish are exposed to pollutants on the spawning grounds. The procedure developed by Billard permits extension of the normally very brief period between gamete release and fertilization with a consequent increase in sensitivity (Billard, 1978a, b; Billard *et al.*, 1978). This is accomplished by exposing spermatozoa in a medium containing potassium, and by hatching eggs during exposure in a buffer solution which maintains their capacity to be fertilized. Percentage fertilization can be determined by examining intact or cleared eggs using a low power microscope hours or days after fertilization, depending on species and temperature of incubation.

3.2 Mortality Tests During Early-life-history Stages

For early-life-history mortality tests in fish there has been considerable discussion in the literature concerning the time to initiate exposure, and the time to terminate exposure and assess the total mortality. It is generally accepted that the egg is permeable up to the time of water hardening after which the chorion becomes relatively impermeable. Thus more pollutant is liable to enter the egg if it is exposed immediately after fertilization. On the other hand, in some species where egg fertility is normally relatively low, exposure is not initiated until the number of unfertilized eggs has been assessed or they have been removed. In this respect, salmonid eggs have the advantage of high fertility (98–99% for *Oncorhynchus* species at the West Vancouver Laboratory). With regard to the duration of exposure prehatch embryonic mortality can be assessed but it is usually advantageous to wait at least until hatching, as successful hatching is a very sensitive and also clear-cut parameter. The next milestone is the survival and successful utilization of the yolk reserve during the yolk-sac larva or alevin stage culminating in the successful initiation of feeding. To achieve the greatest sensitivity and allow for the fact that some chemicals are more toxic at one early-life-history stage rather than another, e.g. sensitivity of muskellunge to arsenic at swim-up (Spotila and Paladino, 1979) it is necessary to expose from fertilization through to first feeding. For the reasons mentioned above, some tests start after assessment of egg fertility and many are terminated prior to first feeding. Others have been continued through to a later stage e.g. smolting (preparation for seawater entry) in salmonids.

McKim (1977) reviewed 56 partial- and complete-life-cycle tests involving 34 organic and inorganic chemicals to determine the most sensitive life history stage for testing purposes. The reviewed tests were conducted according to methods recommended by the US Environmental Protection Agency Committee on Aquatic Bioassays (USEPA, 1972) on fathead minnows, bluegills, brook trout, and flagfish. In all but 10 of these tests the embryo–larval or early juvenile stages were the most sensitive and the MATC estimate using these early-life-history stages was similar to the actual MATC values determined by partial-life-cycle tests (juvenile through adult spawning to 3 months after hatching of offspring) or complete-life-cycle tests (embryos or newly hatched larvae through adult spawning to 3 months after hatching of offspring). In 10 of the tests the early-life-history stages were not the most sensitive, adult spawning, growth or mortality being approximately twice as sensitive. These 10 tests involved effects of cadmium, lead and zinc in the flagfish, methylmercury, chloramine, Guthion®, lindane and trifluralin in the fathead minnow and atrazine in the brook trout. In the case of cadmium, repeat tests in the foregoing species indicated that the early-life-history stages were the most sensitive. In the case of lead, zinc and methylmercury, the early-life-history stages were the most sensitive when other test species were used (McKim, 1977).

Macek and Sleight (1977) have also compared early-life-history tests with life cycle tests. They have identified three criteria that must be met to permit the use of early-life-history tests to determine application factors. First, the chemical must not exhibit significant cumulative toxicity; second, there must be a single mode of action which manifests its effect in a relatively short time and third, the effect must be most deleterious in the early life stages. Chemicals reported by Macek and Sleight (1977) which do not meet these criteria include zinc, lead, chromium, malathion, toxaphene, diazinon and phosphorus. Of these, lead, chromium and diazinon are cumulative and zinc and elemental phosphorus are known to have more than one mode of action.

3.3 Proposed Medaka Embryo Test

Further savings in time and resources over those achieved with the embryo–larval test may be possible with a proposed test based on the use of the transparent eggs of the medaka (*Oryzias latipes*) (Stoss and Haines, 1979). Ten eggs were placed soon after fertilization in 20 ml test solution in 23 ml screw top vials. Mortalities and developmental abnormalities were noted up until and including hatching. Using toluene as a test toxicant, the embryos were more sensitive than larvae. Stoss and Haines (1979) consider that the method may provide a simple and rapid tool for estimating MATC. The use of medaka eggs for tests has also been advocated by Leung and Bulkley (1979).

3.4 Proposed Guppy Embryo Test

A model test system for the evaluation of water-borne mutagens has been proposed which involves injection of male guppies, followed by determination of embryo mortality and total number of embryos in females fertilized by the treated males (Mathews *et al.*, 1978). Embryonic development in the guppy has also been used as a test for zinc. In this case, the criterion was the size of young at birth (Uviovo and Beatty, 1979).

3.5 Cytogenetic Tests for Embryos

Recently the potential for using cytogenetic abnormalities in Atlantic mackerel (*Scomber scombrus*) eggs as a field test for xenobiotics in the natural environment has been investigated (Longwell and Hughes, 1980; Sinderman *et al.*, 1980). After further research on the quantification of specific mutagenic events and comparison with appropriate controls the test may be validated for the monitoring of planktonic marine eggs in the field in areas contaminated by heavy metals and toxic hydrocarbons.

3.6 Tests Based on Hormonal Control Mechanisms

Reproductive development and spawning depends in fish as in other vertebrates on the precise orchestration and seqencing of number of inter-related events. These events are largely coordinated by the endocrine system through changes in the production and/or release of hormones from the hypothalamus, pituitary and gonads (Figure 1). It is to be expected therefore, that the deleterious effects of chemicals on reproductive development will appear first as changes in one or more facets of the control mechanism and later as impairments of gonadal development and/or spawning. Although only a limited amount of research effort has been devoted to date to the investigation of the effects of pollutant chemicals on reproductive control mechanisms, it is already apparent that there are several approaches which may lead to test methodologies. One technique explored by Freeman and co-workers involves *in vitro* incubation of gonadal tissue from exposed fish with radiolabelled steroid precursor molecules to determine changes in steroidogenic pathways leading to the production of sex steroids (Freeman *et al.*, 1980). A second technique involves the direct quantification of reproductive hormone concentrations in the endocrine glands or tissues or in the blood plasma of exposed fish. Changes in androgen or oestrogen concentrations have been monitored by Sangalang and Freeman (1974) and Sivarajah *et al.* (1978a) and changes in gonadotropin and gonadotropin-releasing hormone have been monitored by Singh and Singh (1980a, b, 1981b). There is much scope for further research in this area using radioimmunoassay and radioreceptor assay techniques to monitor changes in the above hormones and other hormones which are involved in reproduction such as the prostaglandins, corticosteroids and thyroid hormones. Cortisoteroid measurement has already been used to quantify the classical stress response in fish to pollutants (Donaldson, 1981). A third test methodology which relates to hormonal control

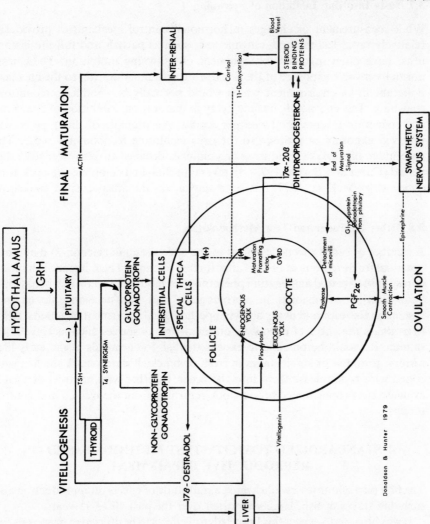

Figure 1 Endocrine control of vitellogenesis, final maturation and ovulation in teleosts. Hormonal pathways which may respond to xenobiotics are indicated, dashed lines indicate possible pathways. ACTH, corticotropin; TSH, thyrotropin; T_4, thyroxine; $PGF_{2\alpha}$, prostaglandin $F_{2\alpha}$; GVBD, germinal vesicle breakdown; GRH, gonadotropin-releasing hormone. (E. M. Donaldson and G. A. Hunter, unpublished, 1979)

mechanisms is the measurement of changes in the hepatic mixed-function oxidase system (MFO) and its influence on gonadal steroid metabolism. These effects can be monitored by measuring levels of MFO activity in the field or in the laboratory (Lee *et al.*, 1980) or by measuring changes in the rate of gonadal steroid metabolism in exposed fish *in vitro* (Harvey, 1972) or *in vivo* using techniques similar to those which have been developed for the quantification of corticosteroid half-lives, metabolic clearance rates and secretion rates in fish (Donaldson and Fagerlund, 1970, 1972; Fagerlund and Donaldson, 1970).

3.7 Tests Involving Inhibition of Spawning

While measurement of changes in hormonal control mechanisms provides a relatively rapid test method, chronic tests such as partial- and full-life-history tests, have often involved measurement of spawning inhibition. These tests normally involve exposure of the fish during sexual maturation to the chemical pollutant in an environment which would normally be conducive to natural spawning. Test end-points include delay in maturation, inhibition of spawning and reduction in eggs produced per female. An example of this type of test involved exposure of medaka to the organochlorine Kepone at 1 p.p.b. The percentage of medaka producing egg clutches declined to zero over a 25 day period (Curtis and Beyers, 1978). In several partial- and complete-life-cycle tests reviewed by McKim (1977) failure to spawn was the most sensitive indicator.

3.8 Other Reproduction Test Methodologies

A number of other effects described in the effects section (section 2) may have potential for development of tests after further research. These include inhibition of response to sexual aggregating pheromone, inhibition of spawning behaviour, quantification of changes in steroidogenic and non-steroidogenic enzyme systems in the testis and ovary and histopathological assessment of gonads. Also, to evaluate the effect of chemicals on anadromous species such as the Pacific salmon, it should be possible to expose the fish to chemicals in the early-life-history, presmolt or smolt stages in fresh or brackish water, mark the fish with coded wire tags, release them into the ocean together with controls and later evaluate the proportion of brook stock returning from the treated and control groups.

4 STANDARDIZED TOXICITY TEST METHODS BASED ON REPRODUCTIVE IMPAIRMENT

The first part of our review illustrated a multitude of effects on reproduction and early life stages of fish, largely reported over the past 10 or 15 years.

It was obvious to expect this knowledge of effects to be utilized in proposals for more advanced testing ('hazard assessment') procedures. This development has taken place indeed, although a lag of several years between presentation of data in the primary literature and their application and verification in standardized and generally accepted test methods and procedures is inevitable.

4.1 APHA, AWWA and WPCF Tests

The 14th edition of *Standard Methods for the Examination of Water and Waste Water* published jointly by the American Public Health Association, the American Water Works Association and the Water Pollution Control Federation in 1976, was the first to include partial- and complete-life-cycle tests which could reveal effects on reproduction. A partial-life-cycle test usually determines effects on one to two life stages of the fish, e.g. egg and alevin, fry, juvenile, adult. Complete-life-cycle testing covers and exceeds one generation, e.g. from F_1 adult to eggs by F_2. The latest (15th) edition of *Standard Methods* (Anon, 1981a) describes test protocols for two freshwater fish (*Salvelinus fontinalis, Pimephales promelas*) and two marine or estuarine species (*Cyprinodon variegatus, Menidia menidia*). These procedures are presented as 'tentative', i.e. future modifications are expected. The four species chosen are intended to serve as examples or models for working with other fish. A list of 58 more species 'that have been used' (in various kinds of tests) is given. 'However, only about 15 species have been used extensively and of these, only a few freshwater species have been used in life-cycle tests. Until recently, few marine fish were cultured, reared in the laboratory, or used for testing' (Anon, 1981a, p. 723).

The recommended partial-life-cycle test description using the brook trout (*Salvelinus fontinalis*) presents technical and apparative requirements in some detail, e.g. shape and size of growth chambers and spawning tanks, boxes and screen egg retainers, following largely Benoit (1974). Also given are guidelines for flow rates, temperature and light regimens, feeding density, toxicant delivery, diluent water quality etc. If the test is begun with juveniles, they are to be collected no later than March 1 for acclimation to test temperature and water quality over at least 1 month. Exposure should start no later than April 1, to allow an exposure of about 4 months before secondary or rapid growth of gonads. Recorded are: number, weights and lengths of immature males and females at the beginning of the test, after 3 months, and when terminating the test; individual weights and total lengths of normal, deformed and injured fish; number maturing; mortality during the test; number of spawnings and eggs; hatchability and fry survival; growth and deformities; mean incubation time. Results are compiled for each test concentration and analysed statistically for significant differences from controls.

Mainly because of its short life span and ease of handling, the fathead minnow (*Pimephales promelas*) became a popular 'bioassay' species (Mount and Stephan, 1969; Brungs, 1969; Pickering and Thatcher, 1970; Eaton, 1974), and was included in *Standard Methods* as the recommended freshwater fish for whole-life-cycle testing.

The apparatus, equipment and requirements for flow rate, aeration, cleaning etc., are in general similar to those described for the brook trout. Since fathead minnows deposit their eggs on the undersides of submerged objects, inverted halves of tile, each end readily accessible to the fish, are placed in the spawning tanks. Regardless of the actual date the test is started, photoperiods are adjusted so that the estimated or mean spawning date of the fish used to start the experiment corresponds to the Evansville, Indiana day length of December 1. This is meant to provide consistent, comparable prespawning exposure.

The test is begun with fifty 1–5-day-old larvae in duplicate spawning tanks for each test concentration. At day 60 ($\pm$ 1 or 2) of the test, injured or crippled individuals are removed and the number of fish in each tank is reduced to 15. When fish appear mature and ready to spawn, 'spawning tiles' are introduced into each tank. Eggs are removed daily at a fixed time. Fifty unbroken, randomly selected eggs from a single spawning are placed in egg incubators to determine viability and hatchability. Each day live and dead eggs in incubator cups are counted. After 4–6 days, larvae begin to hatch. If enough larvae are found alive, 40 are selected at random and transferred to a larval growth chamber to determine survival and growth of the second generation. From eggs in duplicate tanks, larvae are used for 30- and 60-day growth and survival exposures. Procedures for the F_1 generation are repeated to determine effects on eggs, larvae and juveniles of the F_2 generation. Recorded are: 'total number and length of normal and deformed individuals in each tank at the end of 30 and 60 days for each generation; total length, weight, and number of each sex, both normal and deformed, at the end of tests; mortality during the tests; number of spawnings and eggs produced in each and total egg production by each generation; percentage of the eggs hatching; number and percentage of larvae surviving and growth of fry as well as deformities produced (Anon, 1981a, pp. 736–737).

Comparatively few marine and estuarine fishes have been cultured in the laboratory; difficulties in rearing them past yolk-sac absorption seem to persist. One of the more manageable species is the euryhaline and eurytherm sheepshead minnow, *Cyprinodon variegatus*. Eggs can be obtained by natural spawning or by inducing egg production artificially through injecting females intraperitoneally with 50 IU of human chorionic gonadotropic hormone. Average production is about 8 eggs per pair per day; hatching occurs after 5 days at 30 °C and a salinity between 15 and 20%. After placing the eggs in hatching chambers for each toxicant concentration and controls, hatching is monitored. Survival and growth of embryos and fry, providing the parental stock F_1, is recorded daily. During the first 2 weeks, newly hatched brine shrimp nauplii are fed, supplemented over the following 2 weeks with dry trout pellets or dry mollie flakes. Growth, weight, survival and deformities for each test concentration and controls are documented at 4 weeks after start of test. The fish are then placed in growth chambers, subjected to a prescribed feeding regimen (each batch of food checked for possible chemical contamination) and measured again at 8 weeks. When fish mature, separate pairs are put in spawning chambers, 10 pairs for each test concentration and controls. When fertilized eggs are produced, they are placed in hatching chambers, continuing the exposure and monitoring procedures as for F_1, with records of time required to hatch, hatching success and survival of embryos. After enough eggs for exposure of the F_2 generation and for statistical comparisons of fecundity, fertility and survival of embryos and fry have been obtained, the spawning pairs are measured, weighted and terminated. Eggs are then exposed and monitored for each toxicant concentration, and held as controls in the same manner as for the F_1 generation. At the end of another 4 weeks the test is stopped.

The fourth and last test suggested in *Standard Methods* uses the Atlantic silverside, *Menidia menidia*, a species occurring in estuarine areas of the North American east coast, ecologically important as food for predacious fishes. Although its life history and biological requirements seem to be well known, it is difficult to maintain for extended periods in the laboratory; this fish, particularly in its larval stage, is very susceptible to damage by physical handling. Therefore, only partial-life-cycle testing is proposed, beginning with ripening adults or fertilized eggs. Spawning occurs from March to August, with about 500 eggs per female. Mature adults collected in the field are held in water of 2.4–2.6% salinity at 22 °C, with control of light intensity and periodicity. They are fed with dry fish food, brine shrimp, copepods and minced clams or mussels. Ripe females and males are stripped, milt and eggs are fertilized by stirring. The gelatinous egg masses adhere readily to nylon or polyethylene strings; these are then suspended in flow-through exposure and control tanks. Normally hatching will be completed before day 12 after fertilization. At this stage of the test, the egg clumps are examined, and if there are no indications of further hatching, the test is terminated. The end-points compared are the numbers of live active larvae, deformed larvae, unhatched eggs, and their developmental stage.

4.2 ASTM Draft Guideline for Toxicity Tests with Early Life Stages of Fishes

As mentioned above, the tests described or outlined in *Standard Methods* are novel, tentative and subject to revision and upgrading through experience and on-going research. The American Society for Testing and Materials (ASTM) is currently providing a vehicle for arriving at further methodological developments by use of its panels of experts, e.g. Subcommittee E-35.23 on Safety to Aquatic Organisms, Subcommittee E-47.01 on Toxic Effects on Aquatic Organisms, with a special Task Group on Early Life Stage Tests with Fishes.

A revised draft of a proposed 'standard practice for conducting toxicity tests with the early life stages of fishes' was produced in 1981. No complete-life-cycle testing is attempted, rendering the test procedures shorter and easier. Still, according to this expert group, estimations of chemical hazards derived from these tests have been shown to be similar to those based on whole-life-cycle tests (see McKim, 1977; Macek and Sleight, 1977). The following list of recommended test species is provided:

Freshwater	Saltwater
Coho salmon, *Oncorhynchus kisutch*	Sheepshead minnow, *Cyprinodon variegatus*
Chinok salmon, *O. tshawytscha*	
Rainbow trout, *Salmo gairdneri*	Silversides, *Menidia* spp.
Brown trout, *S. trutta*	
Brook trout, *Salvelinus fontinalis*	
Lake trout, *S. namaycush*	
Northern pike, *Esox lucius*	
Carp, *Cyprinus carpio*	
Fathead minnow, *Pimephales promelas*	
Channel catfish, *Ictalurus punctatus*	
White sucker, *Catostomus commersoni*	
Bluegill, *Lepomis macrochirus*	
Channel catfish, *Ictalurus punctatus*	

The equipment prescribed (holding and acclimation tanks, test chambers, embryo cups) is generally similar to that in *Standard Methods*, and to descriptions in the primary literature. Added are numerous very specific stipulations, e.g.: 'To minimize leaching, dissolution, and sorption, either glass, # 316 stainless steel, polyamides (nylon) or fluoroplastics must be used' (Anon, 1981b, p. 7); 'test chambers can be made by welding, not soldering # 316 stainless steel or by gluing doublestrength or stronger window glass with clear silicone adhesive' (Anon, 1981b, p. 9); 'test chambers or toxicant delivery system must be constructed so that the organisms are not stressed by turbulence' (Anon, 1981b, p. 9).

General guidelines are provided for obtaining, holding and handling of brood fish, ova and sperm, supplemented by species-specific data. A minimum of five exposure concentrations of the test chemical and at least one control is recommended. The highest concentration should not exceed the 96-hour LC_{50} for the larval or juvenile stage of the species used. The test is begun with embryos, either (most commonly) by placing the eggs in exposure chambers after fertilization in dilution water, or (if the test chemical is suspected to be teratogenic or to impair gametes) by fertilizing them in the treatment water. Duration of the test depends on the species, ranging from 28 to 120 days' exposure.

Parameters used to determine differences between controls and experimentals are: percentage survival of embryos to hatching; time required for hatching; survival of hatched fish to termination of tests; overall survival from beginning to termination of test; growth of young fish. It is also recommended to consider biochemical, histological and physiological effects on embryos, larvae and juveniles, as well as abnormal post-hatch behaviour such as hyperventilation, uncoordinated swimming etc.

5 CONCLUSIONS, GAPS AND RESEARCH NEEDS

Our review shows that criteria of reproductive impairment in fish have been recognized as being important, if not essential, for hazard assessment, and that these criteria are being incorporated into standard testing procedures. A good deal of effort is currently expended in the area of test development internationally. Essential elements of the ASTM guideline for early-life-stage testing are being considered for inclusion in a test package of the OECD Chemicals Testing Programme (Hueck, pers. comm.), and certainly we can expect proposals with alternate species and/or modified procedures to originate from various countries.

A number of questions have remained unresolved so far:

(1) Selection of test species. Viewpoints used for selection include: availability, commercial value, suitability/hardiness for holding and culturing, sensitivity, ecological significance. Certainly, not all test species proposed satisfy all these viewpoints equally well; in fact, some of them may be mutually exclusive.

(2) Criteria for reproductive impairment from effects on gametes over egg and larval development to maturation of adults: no agreement appears to exist as to which of these criteria are more significant or sensitive than others, and whether or not all of them should be included in standard tests.

(3) Sensitivity: none of the species and criteria proposed has been systematically applied to all major kinds or groups of organic and inorganic pollutants. Consequently, no generalized statements about the sensitivity of these various species and criteria appear possible at present.

(4) Details of test methods in terms of apparatus, quality of dilution water, quality and acclimation of test fish, and statistical analysis are still widely lacking (the ASTM guidelines seem to be most advanced in these aspects).

(5) Laboratory versus field techniques: all of the more standardized methods are designed for laboratory use; field techniques (on-site testing in cages etc.) are conceivable and desirable, but at present, insufficiently developed.

(6) Multispecies tests determining interspecific ecological consequences (predator/prey relations, competition for ecological niches etc.) are not available.

(7) Single and multispecies tests to determine either possible build-up of resistance or cumulative detrimental effects in repeated and multigeneration exposures are insufficiently developed.

ACKNOWLEDGEMENTS

We wish to thank Dr. M. Waldichuk, Mr. G. Miller, Mrs. K. Day and Mr. E. Marshall for assistance in the location of reference material, Drs. J. F.

Klaverkamp and M. Waldichuk for their constructive comments on the manuscript and M. Young for typing the manuscript.

6 REFERENCES

Adelman, J. R. and Smith, L. C. (1970). Effect of hydrogen sulphide on Northern pike eggs and sac fry. *Trans. Am. Fish. Soc.* **9**, 501–509.

Alderdice, D. F., Rosenthal, H. and Velsen, F. P. J. (1979a). Influence of salinity and cadmium on capsule strength in Pacific herring eggs. *Helgol. wiss. Meeresunters.* **32**, 149–162.

Alderdice, D. F., Rosenthal, H. and Velsen, F. P. J. (1979b). Influence of salinity and cadmium on the volume of Pacific herring eggs. *Helgol. wiss. Meeresunters.* **32**, 163–178.

Alderdice, D. F., Rao, T. R. and Rosenthal, H. (1979c). Osmotic responses of eggs and larvae of the Pacific herring to salinity and cadmium. *Helgol. wiss. Meeresunters.* **32**, 508–538.

Allison, D. T. (1977). *Use of Exposure Units for Estimating Aquatic Toxicity of Organophosphate Pesticides.* U. S. Environmental Protection Agency, National Environmental Research Center, Ecological Research Series EPA-600/3-77-077.

Anon (1981a). *Standard Methods for the Examination of Water and Waste Water*, 15th edn, xlvii + 1134 pages. American Public Health Association, Washington, DC.

Anon (1981b). *Standard Practice for Conducting Toxicity Tests with the Early Life Stages of Fishes (draft)*, 53 pages. American Society for Testing and Materials, Philadelphia.

Beamish, R. J. (1976). Acidification of lakes in Canada by acid precipitation and the resulting effects on fishes. *Water Air Soil Pollut.* **6**, 501–514.

Beamish, R. J., Lockhart, W. L., Van Loon, J. C. and Harvey, H. H. (1975). Long term acidification of a lake and resulting effects on fishes. *Ambio* **4**, 98–102.

Beattie, J. H. and Pascoe, D. (1978). Cadmium uptake by rainbow trout, *Salmo gairdneri*, eggs and alevins. *J. Fish Biol.* **13**, 631–637.

Benoit, D. A. (1974). Artificial laboratory spawning substrate for brook trout (*Salvelinus fontinalis* Mitchell). *Trans. Am. Fish Soc.* **103**, 144–145.

Benoit, D. A. (1975). Chronic effects of copper on survival, growth and reproduction of the bluegill (*Lepomis marcochirus*). *Trans. Am. Fish. Soc.* **104**, 353–358.

Benoit, D. A. and Holcombe, G. W. (1978). Toxic effects of zinc on fathead minnows *Pimephales promelas* in soft water. *J. Fish Biol.* **13**, 701–708.

Billard, R. (1977). Utilisation d'un système tris-glycocolle pour tamponner le dileur d'insemination pour truite. *Bull. Fr. Piscic.* **264**, 103–112.

Billard, R. (1978a). Effets des alcools gras sur la fécondation et les gametes de la truite arc-en-ciel. *Bull. Fr. Piscic.* **271**, 3–8 (in French)

Billard, R. (1978b). Effects of heat pollution and organo-chlorinated pesticides on fish reproduction. In *Final Reports on Research Sponsored under the First Environmental Research Programme (indirect action)*, pp. 265–267. Commission of the European Communities, ISBN 92-825-0185-X, Published by CEC, Brussels.

Billard, R., Cazin, J. C., Dequidt, J., Erb, F. and Colein, P. (1978). Toxicité du prayaléne 3010 sur les ovules et les spermatozoides la truites arc-en-ciel avant et pendant l'insemination. *Bull. Fr. Piscic.* **270**, 238–249.

Billard, R., and Jalabert, B. (1974). L'insemination artificielle de la truite (Richardson) II. Comparaison des effects diluers sur la conservation de la fertilité des gametes avant et après insemination. *Ann. Biol. anim. Biochim. Biophys.* **14**, 601–610.

Billard, R. and Kinkelin, P. (1970). Sterilization of the testicles of guppies by means of non-lethal doses of parathion. *Ann. Hydrobiol.* **1**, 91–99.

Birge, W. J., Black, J. A., Hudson, J. E. and Bruser, D. M. (1979a). Embryo-larval toxicity tests with organic compounds. In Marking, L. L. and Kimerle, R. A. (Eds.) *Aquatic Toxicology ASTM STP 667*, pp. 131–147. American Society for Testing and Materials, Philadelphia.

Birge, W. J., Black, J. A. and Westerman, A. G. (1979b). Evaluation of aquatic pollutants using fish and amphibian eggs as bioassay organisms. In *Animals as Monitors of Environmental Pollutants*, pp. 108–118. National Academy of Sciences, Washington, DC.

Biro, P. (1979). Acute effects of the sodium salt of 2, 4-D on the early developmental stages of bleak, *Alburnus alburnus*. *J. Fish Biol.* **14**, 101–109.

Blaycock, B. G. and Frank, M. L. (1979). A comparison of the toxicity of nickel to the developing eggs and larvae of carp (*Cyprinus carpio*). *Bull. environ. Contam. Toxicol.* **21**, 604–611.

Bloom, H. D. and Perlmutter, A. (1977). A sexual aggregating pheromone system in the zebrafish *Brachydanio rerio* (Hamilton-Buchanan). *J. exp. Zool.* **199**, 215–226.

Bloom, H. D., Perlmutter, A., and Seeley, R. J. (1978). Effect of a sublethal concentration of zinc on an aggregating pheromone system in the zebrafish *Brachydanio rerio* (Hamilton-Buchanan). *Environ. Pollut.* **17**, 127–132.

Braaten, B., Mollerud, E. E. and Solemdal, P. (1972). The influence of some by-products from vinylchloride production on fertilization, development and larval survival on plaice, cod and herring eggs. *Aquaculture* **1**, 81–90.

Broyles, R. H. and Noveck, M. I. (1979). Uptake and distribution of 2,4,5,2′,4′,5′-hexachlorobiphenyl in fry of lake trout and chinook salmon and its effects on viability. *Toxic. appl. Pharmac.* **50**, 299–308.

Brungs, W. A. (1969). Chronic toxicity of zinc to the fathead minnow, *Pimephales promelas* Rafinesque. *Trans. Am. Fish. Soc.* **98**, 272–279.

Brungs, W. A., Carlson, R. W., Horning, W. B., McCormick, J. H., Spehar, R. L. and Yount, J. D. (1978). Effects of pollution on freshwater fish. *J. Water Pollut. Control Fedn.* **1978**, 1582–1637.

Burdick, G. E., Harris, E. J., Dean, H. J., Walker, T. M., Shea, J. and Colby, D. (1964). The accumulation of DDT in lake trout and the effect on reproduction. *Trans. Am. Fish. Soc.* **93**, 127–136.

Burkhalter, D. E. and Kaya, C. M. (1977). Effects of prolonged exposure to ammonia on fertilized eggs and sac fry of rainbow trout (*Salmo gairdneri*). *Trans. Am. Fish. Soc.* **106**, 470–475.

Burton, D. T., Hall, L. W., Margrey, S. L. and Small, R. D. (1979). Interactions of chlorine, temperature change (ΔT), and exposure time on survival of striped bass (*Morone saxatilis*) eggs and prolarvae. *J. Fish Res. Board Can.* **36**, 1108–1113.

Bykova, A. V. (1979). The toxicity of granosan for loach eggs. *Veterinariya* (*Mosc*) **(1)**, 74–75.

Carlson, A. R. (1971). Effects of long term exposure to carbaryl (Sevin) on survival growth and reproduction of the fathead minnow (*Pimephales promelas*). *J. Fish. Res. Board Can.* **29**, 583–587.

Carrick, T. R. (1979). The effect of acid water on the hatching of salmonid eggs. *J. Fish Biol.* **14**, 165–172.

Champman, G. L. (1978). Effects of continuous zinc exposure on sockeye salmon during adult to smolt freshwater residency. *Trans. Am. Fish. Soc.* **107**, 828–836.

Cole, H. A. (Ed.) (1979). The assessment of sublethal effects of pollutants in the sea. *Phil. Trans. R. Soc. Lond. B Biol. Sci.*, **286**, 1–235. (Also available in book form, title as above. The Royal Society, London, 235 pages.)

Curtis, L. R. and Beyers, R. J. (1978). Inhibition of oviposition in the teleost *Oryzias latipes*, induced by subacute Kepone exposure. *Comp. Biochem. Physiol.* **66**C, 15–16.

Davies, P. H., Goeltl, J. P. and Sinley, J. R. (1978). Toxicity of silver rainbow trout (*Salmo gairdneri*). *Water Res.* **12**, 113–117.

Davies, P. H., Goeltl, J. P., Sinley, J. R. and Smith, N. F. (1976). Acute and chronic toxicity of lead to rainbow trout *Salmo gairdneri* in hard and soft water. *Water Res.* **10**, 199–206.

Daye, P. G. and Garside, E. T. (1980). Structural alterations in embryos and alevins of the Atlantic salmon *Salmo salar* L., induced by continuous or short-term exposure to acidic levels of pH. *Can. J. Zool.* **58**, 27–43.

Dean, H. D., Skea, J. C., Colquhoun, J. R. and Simonin, H. A. (1979). Reproduction of lake trout in Lake George. *N. Y. Fish Game J.* **26**, 188–191.

DeFoe, D. L., Veith, G. D. and Carlson, R. W. (1978). Effects of Arochlor 1248 and 1260 on the fathead minnow (*Pimephales promelas*). *J. Fish. Res. Board Can.* **35**, 997–1002.

Donaldson, E. M. (1976). Physiological and physiochemical factors associated with maturation and spawning. In *Workshop on Controlled Reproduction of Cultivated Fishes*. EIFAC Tech. Paper No. 25, 53–71.

Donaldson, E. M. (1981). The pituitary-interrenal axis as an indicator of stress in fish. In Pickering, A. D. (Ed.) *Stress and Fish*, Chapter 2, pp. 11–47. Academic Press, London.

Donaldson, E. M., and Fagerlund, U. H. M. (1970). Effect of sexual maturation and gonadectomy at sexual maturity on cortisol secretion rate in sockeye salmon (*Oncorhynchus nerka*). *J. Fish. Res. Board Can.* **27**, 2287–2296.

Donaldson, E. M., and Fagerlund, U. H. M. (1972). Corticosteroid dynamics in Pacific salmon. *Gen. comp. Endocrinol., Suppl.* **3**, 254–265.

Eaton, J. G. (1974). Chronic cadmium toxicity to the bluegill (*Lepomis macrochirus* Rafinesque). *Trans. Am. Fish. Soc.* **103**, 729–735.

EIFAC (1975). Report on fish toxicity testing procedures. *European Inland Fisheries Advisory Commission Technical Paper No 24, EIFAC/T 24*, 25 pp.

EIFAC (1978). The value and limitations of various approaches to the monitoring of water quality for freshwater fish. *European Inland Fisheries Advisory Commission Technical paper No 32 EIFAC/T32*, 27 pp.

Engel, D. W. and Sunda, W. G. (1979). Toxicity of cupric ion to eggs of the spot *Leiostomus xanthrus* and the Atlantic silverside *Menidia menidia*. *Mar. Biol. (Berlin)* **50**, 121–126.

Eyman, L. D., Gehrs, C. W. and Beauchamp, J. J. (1975). Sublethal effect of 5-chlorouracil on carp (*Cyprinus carpio*) larvae. *J. Fish. Res. Board Can.* **32**, 2227–2229.

Fagerlund, U. H. M. and Donaldson, E. M. (1970). Dynamics of cortisone secretion in sockeye salmon (*Oncorhynchus nerka*) during sexual maturation and after gonadectomy. *J. Fish. Res. Board Can.* **27**, 2323–2331.

FAO (1977). Manual of methods in aquatic environment research. Part 4: Basis for selecting biological tests to evaluate marine pollution. *FAO Fisheries Technical Paper. No. 164* (FIRI/TI64), Food and Agriculture Organization of the United Nations, Rome.

Freeman, H. C. and Idler, D. R. (1975). The effect of polychlorinated biphenyl on steroidogenesis and reproduction in the brook trout (*Salvelinus fontinalis*). *Can. J. Biochem.* **53**, 666–670.

Freeman, H. C. and Sangalang, G. (1977a). The effects of polychlorinated biphenyl (Arochlor 1254) contaminated diet on steroidogenesis and reproduction in the Atlantic cod (*Gadus morhua*). ICES CM 1977/E:67, 7 pages (mimeo).

Freeman, H. C. and Sangalang, G. (1977b). Changes in steroid hormone metabolism as a sensitive method of monitoring pollutants and contaminants. *Environment Canada, Environmental Protection Service Surveillance Report*, E. P. S.-5-AR-77-1, 123–132.

Freeman, H. C., Sangalang, G. and Flemming, B. (1978). The effects of a polychlorinated biphenyl (PCB) diet on Atlantic cod (*Gadus morhua*). ICES CM 1978/E: 18, 7 pages (mimeo).

Freeman, H. C., Uthe, J. F. and Sangalang, G. (1980). The use of steroid hormone metabolism studies in assessing the sublethal effects of marine pollution. *Rapp. P.-V. Réun. Cons. int. Explor. Mer.* **179**, 16–22.

Goodman, L. R., Hansen, D. J., Coppage, D. L., Moor, J. C. and Mathews, E. (1979). Diazinon: chronic toxicity to, and brain acetyl cholinesterase inhibition in the sheepshead minnow, *Cyprinodon variegatus. Trans. Am. Fish. Soc.* **108**, 479–488.

Gunn, J. M. and Keller, W. (1980). Enhancement of the survival of rainbow trout (*Salmo gairdneri*) eggs and fry in an acid lake through incubation in limestone. *Can. J. Fish. Aquat. Sci.* **37**, 1522–1530.

Hansen, D. J. (1969). Avoidance of pesticides by untrained sheepshead minnows. *Trans. Am. Fish. Soc.* **98**, 426–429.

Harvey, B. J. (1972). *The Effect of DDT upon the Metabolism of Estradiol in Coho Salmon* (*Oncorhynchus kisutch*). M. Sc. Thesis, Dept. of Zoology, University of British Columbia.

Hasler, A. D. (1960). Guideposts of migrating fishes. *Science (Washington, DC)* **132**, 785–792.

Hasler, A. D. and Wisby, W. J. (1951). Discrimination of stream odors by fishes and its relation to parent stream behavior. *Am. Nat.* **85**, 223–238.

Hasler, A. D. and Wisby, W. J. (1958). The return of displaced largemouth bass and green sunfish to a 'home' area. *Ecology* **39**, 289–293.

Hodgins, H. O., Gronlund, W. D., Mighell, J. L., Hawkes, J. W. and Robisch, P. A. (1977). Effect of crude oil on trout reproduction. In Wolfe, D. A. (Ed.) *Fate and Effects of Petroleum Hydrocarbons in Marine Organisms and Ecosystems*, pp. 143–144. Pergamon Press, New York.

Hogan, J. W. and Brauhn, J. L. (1975). Abnormal rainbow trout fry from eggs containing high residues of PCB (Arochlor 1242). *Prog. Fish-Cult.* **37**, 229–230.

Höglund, L. B. (1953). A new method of studying the reactions of fishes in gradients of chemical and other agents. *Oikos* **3**, 247–267.

Holcombe, G. W., Benoit, D. A. and Leonard, E. N. (1979). Long term effects of zinc exposures on brook trout (*Salvelinus fontinalis*). *Trans. Am. Fish. Soc.* **108**, 76–87.

Holman, W. F. and Macek. K. J. (1980). An aquatic safety assessment of linear alkyl-benzene sulfonates (LAS): chronic effect on fathead minnows. *Trans. Am. Fish. Soc.* **109**, 122–131.

Holmes, W. N. and Donaldson, E. M. (1969). Body compartments and distribution of electrolytes. In Hoar, W. S. and Randall, D. J. (Eds.) *Fish Physiology*, Vol. 1, pp. 1–89. Academic Press, New York.

Hopkins, C. L., Solly, S. R. B. and Ritchie, A. R. (1969). DDT in trout and its possible effect on reproductive potential. *N. Z. J. Mar. Freshwater Res.* **3**, 220–229.

Hueck, H. J. (1981). Personal communication.

ICES (1978). On the feasibility of effects of monitoring. *ICES Cooperative Res. Rep. No. 75*, 42 pages.

Johnston, R. (1978). Ekofisk blowout and after. *Scott. Fish. Bull.* **44**, 44–47.

Jones, J. R. E. (1948). A further study of the reactions of fish to toxic solutions. *J. exp. Biol.* **25**, 22–34.

Kapur, K., Kamaldeep, K. and Toor, H. S. (1978). The effect of fenitrothion on reproduction of a teleost fish *Cyprinus carpio communis* Linn: a biochemical study. *Bull. environ. Contam. Toxicol.* **20**, 438–442.

Kennedy, L. A. (1980). Teratogenesis in lake trout (*Salvelinus namaycush*) in an experimentally acidified lake. *Can. J. Fish. aquat. Sci.* **37**, 2355–2358.

Kiceniuk, J. W., Fletcher, G. L. and Misra, R. (1980). Physiological and morphological changes in a cold torpid marine fish upon acute exposure to petroleum. *Bull. environ. Contam. Toxicol.* **24**, 313–319.

Kihlström, J. E., Laudberg, C. and Halth, L. (1971). Number of eggs and young produced by zebrafishes (*Brachydanio rerio*, Hamilton-Buchanan) spawning in water containing small amounts of phenylmercuric acetate. *Environ. Res.* **4**, 355–359.

Kimball, G. L., Smith, L. L. and Broderius, S. J. (1978). Chronic toxicity of hydrogen cyanide to the bluegill. *Trans. Am. Fish. Soc.* **107**, 341–345.

Kincheloe, J. W. Wedemeyer, G. A. and Koch, D. L. (1979). Tolerance of developing salmonid eggs and fry to nitrate exposure. *Bull. environ. Contam. Toxicol.* **23**, 575–578.

Klaverkamp, J. F., Duangsawasdi, M., MacDonald, W. A. and Majewski, H. S. (1977). An evaluation of fenitrothion toxicity at four life stages of rainbow trout *Salmo gairdneri*. In Mayer, F. L. and Hamelink, J. L. (Eds.) *Aquatic Toxicology and Hazard Evaluation ASTM STP 634*, pp. 231–240. American Society for Testing and Materials, Philadelphia.

Klekowski, R. Z., Korde, B. and Kaniewska-Prus, M. (1977). The effect of sodium salt of 2, 4-D on oxygen consumption of *Misgurnus fossilis* L. during embryonal development. *Pol. Arch. Hydrobiol.* **24**, 413–421.

Kling, D. (1981). Total atresia of the ovaries of *Tilapia leucosticta* (Cichlidae) after intoxication with the insecticide Lebaycid. *Experientia* **37**, 73–74.

Koenst, W. M., Smith, L. L. and Broderius, S. J. (1977). Effect of chronic exposure of brook trout to sublethal concentrations of hydrogen cyanide. *Environ. Sci. Tech.* **11**, 883–887.

Lee, R., Davies, J. M., Freeman, H. C., Ivanovici, A., Moore, M. N., Stegeman, J. and Uthe, J. F. (1980). Biochemical techniques for monitoring biological effects of pollution in the sea. *Rapp. P.-V. Réun. cons. int. Explor. Mer.* **179**, 48–55.

Lesniak, J. A. (1977). *A Histological Approach to the Study of Sublethal Cyanide Effects on Rainbow Trout Ovaries*. M. Sci. Thesis, Concordia University, Montreal.

Leung, S. T. and Bulkley, R. V. (1979). Effects of petroleum hydrocarbons on length of incubation and hatching success in the Japanese medaka. *Bull. environ. Contam. Toxicol.* **23**, 236–243.

Lind, D. T., Smith, L. L. and Broderius, S. J. (1977). Chronic effects of hydrogen cyanide on the fathead minnow. *J. Water Pollut. Control Fedn* **49**, 262–268.

Linden, O., Sharp, J. R., Laughlin, R. and Neff, J. M. (1979). Interactive effects of salinity, temperature and chronic exposure to oil on the survival and developmental rate of embryos of the estuarine killifish *Fundulus heteroclitus*. *Mar. Biol.* (*Berlin*) **51**, 101–109.

Lockhart, W. L. and Lutz, A. (1977) Preliminary biochemical observations of fishes inhabiting an acidified lake in Ontario, Canada. *Water Air Soil Pollut.* **7**, 317–332.

Longwell, A. C. and Hughes, J. B. (1980). Cytologic, cytogenetic, and developmental state of Atlantic mackeral eggs from sea surface water of the New York bight, and prospects for biological effects monitoring with ichthyo plankton. *Rapp. P.-V. Réun. cons. int. Explor. Mer.* **179**, 275–291.

Lonning, S. and Falk-Petersen, I. B. (1979). The effects of oil dispersants on marine eggs and larvae. *Astarte* **11**, 135–138.

MacDonald, W. A. (1979). Testing embryonic and larval life history stages of fish. In Scherer, E. (Ed.) *Toxicity Tests for Freshwater Organisms*, pp. 131–138. Can. Spec. Publ. Fish. Aquat. Sci. No. 44.

Macek, K. J. and Sleight, B. H., III (1977). Utility of toxicity tests with embryos and fry of fish in evaluating hazards associated with the chronic toxicity of chemicals to fishes. In Mayer, F. L. and Hamelink, J. L. (Eds.) *Aquatic Toxicology and Hazard Evaluation, ASTM STP 634*, pp. 137–146. American Society for Testing and Materials, Philadelphia.

Mann, H. and Schmid, O. J. (1961). Der Einfluss von Detergentien auf Sperma,

Befruchtung und Entwicklung bei der Forelle. *Int. Rev. ges. Hydrobiol. Hydrogr.* **46**, 419–426 (in German).

Mathews, J. G., Favor, J. B. and Crenshaw, J. W. (1978). Dominant lethal effects of triethylenemelamine in the guppy *Poecilia reticulata. Mutat. Res.* **54**, 149–157.

McFarlane, G. A., and Franzin, W. G. (1978). Elevated heavy metals: a stress on a population of white suckers *Catostomus commersoni* in Hamell Lake, Saskatchewan. *J. Fish. Res. Board Can.* **35**, 963–970.

McIntyre, J. D. (1973). Toxicity of methylmercury for steelhead trout sperm. *Bull. environ. Contam. Toxicol.* **9**, 98–99.

McIntyre, A. D. and Pearce, J. B. (Eds.) (1980). Biological effects of marine pollution and the problems of monitoring. *Rapp. P.-V. Réun. cons. int. Explor. Mer.* **179**, 1–346.

McKim, J. M. (1977). Evaluation of tests with early life stages of fish for predicting long-term toxicity. *J. Fish. Res. Board Can.* **34**, 1148–1154.

McKim, J. M. and Benoit, D. A. (1974). Duration of toxicity tests for establishing 'no effect' concentrations for copper with brook trout (*Salvelinus fontinalis*). *J. Fish. Res. Board Can.* **31**, 449–452.

McKim, J. M., Olson, G. F., Holcombe, G. W. and Hunt, E. P. (1976). Long-term effects of methylmercuric chloride on three generations of brook trout (*Salvelinus fontinalis*): toxicity, accumulation, distribution, and elimination. *J. Fish Res. Board Can.* **33**, 2726–2739.

Mehrle, P. M. and Mayer, F. L. Jr. (1975). Toxaphene effects on growth and development of brook trout (*Salvelinus fontinalist*). *J. Fish. Res. Board Can.* **32**, 609–613.

Morgan, R. P. and Prince, R. D. (1978). Chlorine effects on larval development of striped bass (*Morone saxatilis*), white perch (*M. americana*) and blueback herring (*Alosa aestivalis*). *Trans. Am. Fish. Soc.* **107**, 636–641.

Mounib, M. S. and Eison, J. S. (1978). Effects of polychlorinated biphenyl (Arochlor 1254) on some dehydrogenases and amino transferases in the testes of Atlantic cod (*Gadus morhua*). ICES CM 1978/E:17, 9 pages (mimeo).

Mount, D. J. and Stephan, C. E. (1969). Chronic toxicity of copper to the fathead minnow (*Pimephales promelas*) in soft water. *J. Fish. Res. Board Can.* **26**, 2449–2457.

Ozoh, P. T. E. (1979). Malformations and inhibitory tendencies induced to *Brachydanio rerio* (Hamilton-Buchanan) eggs and larvae due to exposures in low concentrations of lead and copper ions. *Bull. environ. Contam. Toxicol.* **21**, 668–675.

Ozoh, P. T. E. (1980). Effects of reversible incubations of zebrafish eggs in copper and lead ions with or without shell membranes. *Bull. environ. Contam. Toxicol.* **24**, 270–275.

Ozoh, P. T. E. and Jacobson, C. O. (1979). Embryotoxicity and hatchability in *Cichlasoma nigrofasciatum* (Guenther) eggs and larvae briefly exposed to low concentrations of zinc and copper ions. *Bull. environ. Contam. Toxicol.* **21**, 782–786.

Paladino, F. V. and Spotila, J. R. (1978). The effect of arsenic on the thermal tolerance of newly hatched muskellunge fry (*Esox masquinongy*). *J. therm. Biol.* **3**, 223–227.

Payne, J. F., Kiceniuk, J. W., Squires, W. R. and Fletcher, G. L. (1978). Pathological changes in a marine fish after a 6-month exposure to petroleum. *J. Fish. Res. Board Can.* **35**, 665–667.

Pickering, Q. H., Brungs, W. and Gast, M. (1977). Effects of exposure time and copper concentration on reproduction of the fathead minnow (*Pimephales promelas*). *Water Res.* **11**, 1079–1083.

Pickering, Q. H. and Thatcher, T. O. (1970). The chronic toxicity of linear alkylate sulfonate (LAS) to *Pimephales promelas* Rafinesque. *J. Water Pollut. Control Fedn* **42**, 243–254.

Pierson, K. B. (1981). Effects of chronic zinc exposure on the growth, sexual maturity, reproduction and bioaccumulation of the guppy, *Poecilia reticulata. Can. J. Fish. Aquat. Sci.* **38**, 23–31.

Rice, D. W. and Harrison, F. L. (1977). Copper sensitivity of Pacific herring *Clupea harengus pallasi* during its early life history. *Nat. mar. Fish. Bull.* **76**, 347–356.

Rice, S. D., Moles, D. A. and Short, J. W. (1975). The effect of Prudhoe Bay crude oil on survival and growth of eggs, alevins and fry of pink salmon *Oncorhynchus gorbuscha. Proc. 1975 Conf. on Prevention and Control of Oil Pollution.* American Petroleum Institute, Washington, DC.

Rosenthal, H. and Alderdice, D. F. (1976). Sublethal effects of environmental stressors, natural and pollutional on marine fish eggs and larvae. *J. Fish. Res. Board Can.* **33**, 2047–2065.

Ruby, S. M. Aczel, J. and Craig, G. R. (1977). The effects of depressed pH on oogenesis in flagfish *Jordanella floridae. Water Res.* **11**, 757–762.

Ruby, S. M., Aczel, J. and Craig, G. R. (1978). The effects of depressed pH on spermatogenesis in flagfish *Jordanella floridae. Water Res.* **12**, 621–626.

Ruby, S. M., Dixon, D. G. and Leduc, G. (1979). Inhibition of spermatogenesis in rainbow trout during chronic cyanide poisoning. *Archs environ. Contam. Toxicol.* **8**, 533–544.

Rustamova, Sh. A. (1979). The chronic effect of alkali on the growth development and fecundity of the guppy. *Hydrobiol. J.* **13**, 83–85.

Sangalang, G. B. and Freeman, H. C. (1974). Effects of sublethal cadmium on maturation and testosterone and 11-ketotestosterone production *in vivo* in brook trout. *Biol. Reprod.* **11**, 429–435.

Sangalang, G. B. and O'Halloran, M. J. (1972). Cadmium induced testicular injury and alterations of androgen synthesis in brook trout. *Nature* **240**, 470–471.

Sangalang, G. B. and O'Halloran, M. J. (1973). Adverse effects of cadmium on brook trout testis and on *in vitro* testicular androgen synthesis. *Biol. Reprod.* **9**, 394–403.

Sastry, K. V. and Agrawal, M. K. (1979a). Mercuric chloride induced enzymological changes in kidney and ovary of a teleost fish, *Channa punctatus. Bull. environ. Contam. Toxicol.* **22**, 38–43.

Sastry, K. V. and Agrawal, M. K. (1979b). Effects of lead nitrate on the activities of a few enzymes in the kidney and ovary of *Heteropneustes follilis* (actually *Channa punctatus*). *Bull. environ. Contam. Toxicol.* **22**, 55–59.

Saunders, R. L. and Sprague, J. B. (1967). Effects of copper–zinc mining pollution on a spawning migration of Altantic salmon. *Water Res.* **1**, 419–432.

Saxena, P. K. and Garg, M. (1978). Effect of insecticidal pollution on ovarian recrudescence in the freshwater teleost *Channa punctatus* (Bl.). *Indian J. exp. Biol.* **16**, 689–691.

Scherer, E. (1979). Avoidance testing for fish and invertebrates. In Scherer, E. (Ed.) *Toxicity Tests for Freshwater Organisms*, pp. 160–170. Can. Spec. Publ. Fish. Aquat. Sci. No. 44.

Scherer, E. and Nowak, S. (1973). Apparatus for recording avoidance movements of fish. *J. Fish. Res. Board Can.* **30**, 1594–1596.

Schimmel, S. C., Hansen, D. J. and Forester, J. (1974). Effects of Aroclor 1254 on laboratory-reared embryos and fry of sheepshead minnows (*Cyprinodon variegatus*). *Trans. Am. Fish. Soc.* **103**, 582–586.

Sharp, J. R., Fucik, K. W. and Neff, J. M. (1979). Physiological basis of differential sensitivity of fish embryonic stages to oil pollution. In Vernberg, W. B. Thurberg, F. P., Calabrese, A. and Vernberg, F. J. (Eds.) *Marine Pollution: Functional Responses*, pp. 85–108. Academic Press, New York.

Shelford, V. E. (1917). An experimental study of the effects of gas waste upon fishes, with special reference to stream pollution. *Ill. State Lab. Nat. Hist. Bull.* **11**, 380–412.

Sindermann, C. J., Bong, F. B., Christensen, N. O., Dethlefsen, V., Harshberger, J. C., Mitchell, J. R. and Mulcahy, M. F. (1980). The role and value of pathobiology in pollution effects monitoring programs. *Rapp. P.-V. Réun. cons. int. Explor. Mer.* **179**, 135–151.

Singh, H. and Singh, T. P. (1980a). Short-term effect of two pesticides on the survival, ovarian ^{32}P uptake and gonadotrophic potency in a freshwater catfish, *Heteropneustes fossilis* (Bloch). *J. Endocrinol.* **85**, 193–199.

Singh, H. and Singh, T. P. (1980b). Effect of two pesticides on ovarian ^{32}P uptake and gonadotropin concentration during different phases of annual reproductive cycle in the freshwater catfish, *Heteropneustes fossilis* (Bloch). *Environ. Res.* **22**, 190–200.

Singh, H. and Singh, T. P. (1980c). Effect of two pesticides on total lipid and cholesterol contents of ovary, liver and blood serum during different phases of the annual reproductive cycle in the freshwater teleost *Heteropneustes fossilis* (Bloch). *Environ. Pollut. Ser. A. Ecol. Biol.* **23**, 9–17.

Singh, H. and Singh, T. P. (1980d). Effects of two pesticides on testicular ^{32}P uptake gonadotrophic potency, lipid and cholesterol content of testis, liver, and blood serum during spawning phase in *Heteropneustes fossilis* (Bloch). *Endokrinologie.* **76**, 288–296.

Singh, H. and Singh, T. P. (1981a). Effect of parathion and aldrin on survival, ovarian ^{32}P uptake and gonadotrophic potency in a fresh-water catfish *Heteropneustes fossilis* (Bloch). *Endokrinologie* **77**, 173–178.

Singh, H. and Singh, T. P. (1981b). Effect of pesticides on hypothalamo-hypophyseal-ovarian axis in the freshwater catfish *Heteropneustes fossilis* (Bloch). *Environ. Pollut. Ser. A. Ecol. Biol.* **27**, 283–288.

Sivarajah, K., Franklin, C. S. and Williams, W. P. (1978a). The effects of polychlorinated biphenyls on plasma steroid levels and hepatic microsomal enzymes in fish. *J. Fish Biol.* **13**, 401–409.

Sivarajah, K., Franklin, C. S. and Williams, W. P. (1978b). Some histopathological effects of Arochlor 1254 on the liver and gonads of rainbow trout, *Salmo gairdneri* and carp, *Cyprinus carpio*. *J. Fish Biol.* **13**, 411–414.

Smith, L. L. and Oseid, D. M. (1972). Effects of hydrogen sulphide on fish eggs and fry. *Water Res.* **6**, 711–720.

Smith, R. L. and Cameron, J. A. (1979). Effect of water soluble fraction of Prudhoe Bay crude oil on embryonic development of Pacific herring. *Trans. Am. Fish. Soc.* **108**, 70–75.

Spehar, R. L., Carlson, R. W., Lemke, A. E., Mount, D. I., Pickering, Q. H. and Snarski, V. M. (1980). Effects of pollution on freshwater fish. *J. Water Pollut. Control Fedn*, **52**, 1703–1768.

Spehar, R. L., Leonard, E. N. and DeFoe, D. L. (1978). Chronic effects of cadmium and zinc mixtures on flagfish (*Jordanella floridae*). *Trans. Am. Fish. Soc.* **107**, 354–360.

Speranza, A. W., Seeley, R. J., Seeley, V. A. and Perlmutter, A. (1977). The effect of sublethal concentrations of zinc on reproduction in the zebrafish *Brachydanio rerio* Hamilton-Buchanan. *Environ. Pollut.* **12**, 217–222.

Spotila, J. R. and Paladino, F. V. (1979). Toxicity of arsenic to developing muskellunge fry (*Esox masquinongy*). *Comp. Biochem. Physiol.* **62C**, 67–69.

Sprague, J. B. (1964). Avoidance of copper-zinc solutions by young salmon in the laboratory. *J. Water Pollut. Control Fedn*, **36**, 990–1004.

Sprague, J. B. (1976). Current status of sublethal tests of pollutants on aquatic organisms. *J. Fish. Res. Board Can.* **33**, 1988–1992.

Sprague, J. B. and Drury, D. E. (1969). Avoidance reactions of salmonid fish to representative pollutants. In Jenkins, S. H. (Ed.) *Advances in Water Pollution Research, Proc. of the Fourth International Conference held in Prague*, pp. 169–179. Pergamon Press, Oxford.

Stauffer, T. M. (1979). Effects of DDT and PCB's on survival of lake trout eggs and fry in a hatchery and in Lake Michigan 1973–1976. *Trans. Am. Fish. Soc.* **108**, 176–186.

Stegeman, J. J. (1980). Mixed function oxygenase studies in monitoring for effects of organic pollution. *Rapp. P.-V. Réun. cons. int. Explor. Mer.* **197**, 33–38.

Stoss, F. W. and Haines, T. A. (1979). The effects of toluene on embryos and fry of the Japanese medaka *Oryzias latipes* with a proposal for rapid determination of maximum acceptable toxicant concentration. *Environ. Pollut.* **20**, 39–148.

Trabalka, J. A. and Burch, M. B. (1978). Investigation of the effects of halogenated organic compounds produced in cooling systems and process effluents on aquatic organisms. In Jolley, R. L., Gorchev, H. and Hamilton, D. H. (Eds.) *Water Chlorination. Environmental Impact and Health Effects*, Vol. 2, pp. 163–173. Ann Arbor Science Publishers, Inc., Ann Arbor, Michigan.

Trojnar, J. R. (1977). Egg hatchability and tolerance of brook trout (*Salvelinus fontinalis*) fry at low pH. *J. Fish. Res. Board Can.* **34**, 574–579.

USEPA (1972). Committee on Aquatic Bioassays. *Recommended Bioassay Procedures for Brook Trout* (Salvelinus fontinalis), *Bluegill* (Lepomis macrochirus), *Fathead Minnow* (Pimephales promelas), and *Flagfish* (Jordanella floridae) *chronic tests.* EPA Environ. Res. Lab., Duluth, Minnesota.

Uviovo, E. J. and Beatty, D. D. (1979). Effects of chronic exposure to zinc on reproduction in the guppy (*Poecilia reticulata*). *Bull. environ. Contam. Toxicol.* **23**, 650–657.

Voyer, R. A., Heltsche, J. F. and Kraus, R. A. (1979). Hatching success and larvae mortality in an estuarine teleost *Menidia menidia* (Linnaeus), exposed to cadmium in constant and fluctuating salinity regimes. *Bull. environ. Contam. Toxicol.* **23**, 475–481.

Waldichuk, M. (1973). Trends in methodology for evaluation of effects of pollutants on marine organisms and ecosystems. *CRC Crit. Rev. environ. Cont.*, Feb. 1973, pp. 167–211.

Walker, T. J. and Hasler, A. D. (1949). Detection and discrimination of odors of aquatic plants by the bluntnose minnow *Hyborhynchus notatus. Physiol. Zool.* **22**, 45–63.

Westernhagen, H. V., Dethlefsen, V. and Rosenthal, H. (1979). Combined effects of cadmium, copper and lead on developing herring eggs and larvae. *Helgol. wiss. Meeresunters.* **32**, 257–278.

Yosha, S. F. and Cohen, G. M. (1979). Effect of intermittent chlorination on developing zebrafish embryos (*Brachydanio rerio*). *Bull. environ. Contam. Toxicol.* **21**, 703–710.

Zitko, V. and Saunders, R. L. (1979). Effect of PCB's and other organochlorine compounds on the hatchability of Atlantic salmon (*Salmo salar*) eggs. *Bull. environ. Contam. Toxicol.* **21**, 125–130.

Methods for Assessing the Effects on Chemicals on Reproductive Functions
Edited by V. B. Vouk and P. J. Sheehan
© 1983 SCOPE

Assessment of the Effects of Chemicals on the Reproductive Functions of Reptiles and Amphibians

AnnLouise Martin

1 INTRODUCTION

Amphibians and reptiles are regarded as rather primitive vertebrates. They are poikilothermic, in which they differ from birds and mammals; on the other hand, reptiles, like birds, produce eggs, while amphibians mostly produce spawn, like fish.

The risk in not maintaining a uniform body temperature lies in vulnerability to extreme temperatures. There are advantages: food intake is proportional to the actual body temperature; this is not only economic, but it is a survival mechanism when the environment is hostile.

Reptiles and amphibians are most abundant in the tropics but are, as well, spread far in the temperate zones. They are very prolific with a high degree of environmental adaptation. The economic benefit of these groups is limited except for crocodiles, alligators, green turtles and frogs.

Reproduction differs in amphibia and reptiles. Most reptiles produce eggs; but there are differences, e.g. tortoises and geckoes have hard-shelled eggs, laid in dry places, while in other species the eggs may have soft, flexible shells laid in moist sand or earth or dead vegetation. In a few species the eggs are retained within the body of the mother. In all cases the newly hatched young are minor copies of the parents, and all are independent. Amphibians produce eggs, with a gelatinous coating, usually laid in water. They hatch into tadpoles, which eat and grow before metamorphosing into young, parent-like animals. Only a few genera give birth to larvae or fully formed infants, or lay eggs which hatch into metamorphosed young. The larvae, or tadpoles, normally live in water.

This discussion of reproductive injury is primarily concerned with the effects of chemicals on the formation of eggs and sperm, embryogenesis, larval development, and growth and metamorphosis.

There is little information available on the toxic effects of environmental contamination on amphibians and reptiles compared, for example, to birds.

405

Specific information on the effects of external factors on reproduction is even more poorly documented.

In addition to the threat of pesticides to these groups, injury can occur from heavy metals, such as copper and cadmium, oil spills in water, as well as a low pH of water. Genetic damage may occur from a number of chemicals. Environmental contamination seems to affect amphibians and reptiles to about the same degree as other animals.

Physiological differences will, however, contribute to differences in response. For example, the water-vapour conductance in eggs is highly variable in turtles and reptiles. A snapping turtle egg (*Chelydra serpentia*) has a conductance to water 55 times higher than the avian egg, whereas the soft-shell turtle egg (*Trionyx spiniferus*) has a conductance only 5–6 times higher than the avian egg and that of the American alligator (*Alligator mississippiensis*). This implies possible differences in the intake of water-soluble agents by the egg, in this case the difference is about 10 times (Packard *et al.*, 1979). It has been shown that insecticides (DDT and dieldrin) do enter the eggs of the cottonmouth snake (*Agkistrodon mokeson*) (Fleet, *et al.*, 1972).

In anurans, the skin is the important organ for water uptake, lessening the need for actual drinking. Thus, a water-soluble agent may be absorbed into the body from the aqueous environment whereas a water-living snake can drink from uncontaminated water.

2 EFFECTS ON OOGENESIS AND SPERMATOGENESIS

In the African clawed toad (*Xenopus laevis*), the early cleavage stages of the eggs are sensitive to a halogenated analogue of the normal thymidine, incorporated during DNA synthesis. This pyrimidine, 5-bromodeoxyuridine, will be mistaken for thymidine during mitosis and block development at the blastula stage, leading to point mutations in the newly formed DNA strands. The effect is greater with echinoderm eggs than amphibian eggs, which may be explained by the fact that more thymidine, proportionally, is present in amphibian eggs (Sala and Conte, 1975).

Early chemical injury of oocytes can occur in the RNA. Oocytes from *Xenopus laevis* treated with the aminopiperazin radical will cease developing in a pachythene meiosis phase, ultimately resulting in the non-production of eggs (Steens, 1977).

A similarity in reaction between mammals and amphibians and reptiles was demonstrated in the lizard and the toad. Quinacrine, which interferes with sperm production in mammals, was tested for its effect on steroidogenesis in lizards and histological reactions in the toad. With the toad, the drug produced testicular lesions and changes in cell morphology. In the lizard (*Psammophilus dorsalis*), the compound caused weight loss of the testes, epididymis, vas deferens and kidneys and a total cessation of spermatogenesis. It seems to interfere with steroid biosynthesis and metabolism, indicated by the presence of accumulated amounts of the precursor of steroids, sudanophilic lipids (Shivakuma and Devaraj Sarkar, 1979).

It is well known that cadmium is extremely toxic to mammalian testes and to spermatogenesis. It has been questioned whether animals with abdominal testes react in the same way as animals with scrotal testes do. Frogs and toads were therefore exposed to cadmium by means of intraperitoneal or subcutaneous injections, followed by incubation under laboratory conditions. Sexually active frogs (*Rana tigrina*) showed a mild shrinkage of the testes after 48 hours which later regenerated, with relatively prompt production of spermatids and spermatozoa. On the other hand, with sexually inactive frogs of the same species, formation of spermatozoa was not observed until a week after injection. The effect of cadmium may bring about a release of gonadotropins which in turn initiated spermatogenesis (Matur and Ramaswami, 1976).

In toads (*Bufo melanostictus*) the injection of cadmium chloride caused a significant decrease in numbers of secondary spermatogonia and primary spermatocytes after 7 days. The suggestion of the authors is that, in the toad, cadmium suppresses spermatogenesis possibly by increasing testicular steroid hormone synthesis (Biswas *et al.*, 1976). Cadmium seems to interfere at the level of hormone regulation, although the mechanism is not well understood.

In 1926, Dilling and Healy stated that ions of lead, copper, zinc, thorium, beryllium and thallium were all suspected of disturbing the germination of the frog spawn and the growth of tadpoles. The methods were rather crude, but the conclusion was that lead was by far the most active antifertility agent.

3 EFFECTS ON EMBRYOGENESIS

The response to the herbicide preparation, Weedex, caused a total halt to reproduction in a frog pond. Weedex had been sprayed on a railway track nearby, and the spawn found in the pond were cloudy and did not hatch. Captured *Rana* frogs from the pond laid spawn in a tank, and the hatching result was poor from these also. The surviving tadpoles were three times as heavy as normal, and all died before metamorphosis. The frogs could not reproduce again until the pond was cleaned and the bottom dredged. No information was given as to spraying intensity or concentration in water. It was clear that the substance remained active in the sediment after the pond had been kept dry for a long period (Hazelwood, 1970).

Well-developed spawn of the common frog, *Rana temporaria*, was not penetrated by DDT at 0.5 p.p.m. for 24 hours. The solution was prepared by adding DDT in ethanol to Holtfreter's amphibian saline; the controls were kept in the same medium without DDT. However, when freshly laid spawn, which swells by taking in water, was treated with DDT, the hatched tadpoles showed typical hyperactive behaviour 8–13 days after hatching, and development was retarded (Cooke, 1972).

Extremes in temperature and pH will cause death of the embryos of the salamander, *Ambystoma maculatum* and *A. jeffersonianum*. Mortality occurred before gastrulation, gill formation, or hatching. The rate of development was not influenced by pH (Pough and Wilson, 1974).

Temporary ponds were the site of a field study by the same author. Embryonic mortality of spotted salamander (*Ambystoma maculatum*) was found to be correlated with a low pH caused by acid precipitation. Environmental differences, such as different soil, proximity to road, etc., were noted but not controlled (Pough, 1976).

A treatment of *Rana pipiens* eggs with copper sulphate at concentrations of 0.04–1.56 mg Cu/l did not cause death or damage; the eggs were stripped from a female and soaked in sperm suspension and then treated (Landé and Guttman, 1973).

4 EFFECTS ON LARVAL DEVELOPMENT

Copper, as noted, has little or no effect on amphibian eggs. When hatched, however, tadpoles are very sensitive to inorganic copper; growth is grossly reduced and development retarded to the point of no metamorphosis. The LD_{50} (72 hours) was estimated at 0.15 mg Cu/l (Kaplan and Yoh, 1961; Landé and Guttman, 1973).

The cytotoxic effect of copper in amphibians and reptiles does not seem to have been investigated as thoroughly as, for example, cadmium. Copper is toxic to adult frogs, but at far higher concentrations than cadmium. This may mean that copper action can be partly described as a 'metal-salt reaction', e.g. excessive mucus formation, gill coagulation, eye irritation, etc. The fact that bigger tadpoles, exposed to copper salts, have a higher survival rate than smaller individuals could be a result of a higher degree of damage to the outer gills of the small larvae and the proportionally greater surface of the small animal.

With frogs and toads, it has been demonstrated a number of times that DDT and its residues are harmful to tadpoles as well as to the adults. Treated tadpoles become hyperactive, which in turn retards development; the smaller, hyperactive tadpoles are more likely to be victims of predation than the normal tadpole. The weight loss in connection with hyperactivity is probably a result of feeding difficulties in this stage of behavioural disturbance. Also, skeletal deformities occur such as twists in the spine. With higher doses, the hyperactive stage will be followed by loss of equilibrium, lethargy and death. These experiments involved acute doses of DDT, in concentrations ranging from 0.0008 to 10 p.p.m. DDT. The solutions were made up from ethanol–DDT mixtures in amphibian saline.

There were differences in the response at different ages and at different concentrations. Tadpoles with developing hind limb-buds of both *Rana pipiens* and *Bufo bufo* were more vulnerable than others. At concentrations around 0.01–0.02 p.p.m. DDT, the typical frantic behaviour occurred as well as twisted spine. No actual LD_{50} values are calculated for the tests, but high concentrations gave rise to uncoordinated behaviour soon after the tadpoles were placed in them and mortality in the groups at 1 p.p.m. and 10 p.p.m. DDT was high.

It appears that the hyperactive stage occurs at tissue concentrations around 2–3 p.p.m. in frogs and at 3–4 p.p.m. in toads. At the tail resorption and metamorphosis stage, frog tadpoles are more susceptible to DDT residues than toads. Chronically treated tadpoles (0.0001–0.001 p.p.m. *p, p'*-DDT) showed more rapid development and growth, and no behavioural disturbances even at tissue concentrations of 2–5 p.p.m. The twisted spine was fairly common, however, among treated tadpoles. At metamorphosis these residues caused mortality among the young frog imagos, as the lipid reserves were exhausted and the DDT released. Young toads treated in the same way were not affected after metamorphosis (Cooke, 1970, 1972, 1973).

It has been suggested that insecticides lower the resistance of the tadpole to fungi, possibly implying that the agent may be only indirectly responsible for the observed deformities (Cooke, 1975a).

DDT exhibits its action through its metabolites as well, e.g. DDCN. This compound was found in the sediment of a Swedish lake and presumed to be widespread in biologically active mud and sediment. Tadpoles of the common frog were exposed to DDCN under laboratory conditions. Residues were found in the tadpoles from treated groups exposed to ≥ 0.1 p.p.m. *p, p'*-DDCN but not from lower concentrations. The residues were not detected when tadpoles were moved into uncontaminated water. At the highest concentration, 1 p.p.m., the tadpoles acted abnormally, were lethargic and very weak. Malformation of the tail occurred, a similarity with DDT-treated toad tadpoles. The deformity and the behaviour were reversible in clean water. Low levels of DDCN also seem to accelerate the development of the tadpole, as with DDT. On the whole, this compound is less toxic to frog tadpoles than DDT (Cooke, 1975b).

On exposing anuran tadpoles to DDT, a significant increase of pituitary melanocyte-stimulating hormone, MSH, was found; a direct effect of DDT upon the hypothalamus was postulated. The effect of MSH in excess is wakefulness, which can be measured from EEG data. The exposure in this case was made on *Rana clamitans* larvae in the limb-bud stage. DDT was added directly to the aquaria as a wettable powder. One group of tadpoles was exposed to 0.1–0.5 p.p.m., the other 0.5–0.8 p.p.m. DDT. Nothing is mentioned about media or temperature (Peaslee, 1970).

In a toxicity test of 19 pesticides, insecticides were, generally, 10 times more toxic than herbicides when tested on tadpoles of the frog. (*Pseudacois triseriata*). With tadpoles of the toad (*Bufo woodhousii*) the pattern was approximately the same. Some of the differences in response might be explained from differences in the ages of frogs (1 week) and toads (5 weeks) since it is known, for example, that DDT sensitivity differs with age in tadpoles. The signs of pesticide poisoning followed a predictable pattern: irritability, loss of equilibrium and death. Methodologically this experiment was thorough. It was carried out as a static bioassay, beginning with a pilot test for selecting concentration intervals. The test animals were hatched in the laboratory. The stock solutions were made in ethanol, and the tests were carried out in 5 litre aquaria (Sanders, 1970).

As with mosquitos, it appears that DDT-exposed anurans may develop resistance as, for example, in the adult cricket frogs, *Acris crepitans* and *A. gryllus*, living in the cottonfields of southern USA (Boyd *et al.*, 1963).

Resistance tests showed a possible cross-resistance between aldrin and DDT which may result from the fact that both are chlorinated hydrocarbons (Vinson *et al.*, 1963).

Tolerances to aldrin, dieldrin, endrin, toxaphene and DDT were tested on two frog species (*Acris crepitans, Acris gryllus*) and one toad (*Bufo woodhousii*). The tadpoles were collected from agricultural (pesticide-exposed) areas and from non-agricultural land in order to seek possible resistance to the agent. The relative toxicities of the five insecticides tested were consistent for all three species tested. Endrin was most toxic, followed by aldrin and dieldrin, which were about the same. DDT and toxaphene were least toxic and produced similar levels of mortality. No resistance could be detected; that is, differences in susceptibility relatable to whether the animals came from pesticide-treated as compared to untreated soils were not found. The method used was a 36-hour TL_{50}; temperature range was $80 \pm 2°F$ and the animals were of equal size (18–30 mm) (Ferguson and Gilbert, 1967).

Another pesticide Cyanatryn, chemically related to Weedex, was tested. When used at recommended levels (0.4 p.p.m.), tadpoles of *Rana temporaria* stopped feeding, acted lethargic and behaved in such a way that they were likely to become victims to the newt or other predators. The risk of magnification of concentrations or effects is obvious (Scorgie and Cooke, 1979).

5 METHODS DEVELOPMENT

With amphibians and reptiles there is an urgent need for the development of relevant tests and the identification of suitable test organisms. Many of the techniques used for fish might apply to amphibian testing; similarly, tests used with birds may, with appropriate alteration, might be useful reptiles.

It is not possible to consider reptiles and amphibians as a single group in respect to the effects of chemicals. For example, food sources differ; amphibians are often at the low end of the food chain, while many snakes can be carnivores at the upper end. Also, the yolk of the snake egg is proportionately larger than the yolk-sac of the amphibia, which means a higher proportion of the snake mother's fat will be mobilized into the egg, and with the fat may come fat-soluble substances such as pesticides. Amphibia, on the other hand, will be exposed to water during embryogenesis and the early stages after hatching. Pools and ponds are often collection and sedimentation basins for water-carried materials, such as chemicals. This may give a higher chemical exposure to animals in water than to the animals on shore.

Also, the volume/surface ratio must be considered in respect to exposure to harmful substances. A small embryo has a proportionally greater surface than a large one, and the response is likely to be more marked. In the choice between two test species, the one with the proportionally smaller embryos may have an advantage in sensitivity.

Three general approaches are available to assess effects on reproduction:

(1) acute toxicity;
(2) effects other than death, including early warning signs; and
(3) effects from chronic exposures.

With amphibians and reptiles, the tests fall mostly into group (1) or (3). The sublethal testing is by far the most interesting at the population level and, as well, for ecological understanding. The importance of early warning systems for non-target organisms is vital; animals living in water part or all of their life are not easily observed, and behavioural alteration is unlikely to be discovered. The earliest warning today is likely to come from nature enthusiasts and sportsmen which, when accurate, can only serve to confirm that harm is already done.

The selection of test animals and species include such criteria as the holding and breeding of the animals at reasonable cost, susceptibility to toxicants representative for the class or phyla, and suitability for testing, e.g. production of numerous offspring.

OECD (1979) has suggested the use of the African clawed toad for testing embryotoxicity; otherwise testing procedures for reptiles and amphibians having official or semi-official status appear to be non-existent. The hope for the future is to widen the concept of toxicity testing to keep in mind the total environment, including organisms other than the target organism. For evaluating a new product or a chemical compound, single, standardized methods for toxicity should be used, as well as tests for possible synergistic effects. After the level of toxicity is clear, the effect on the whole system would be studied to the extent practicable. The possibilities of accumulation, or long-term damage, or sublethal reproductive injury are, in the long run, far more harmful than highly toxic, acutely active substances, as the former will act in a subtle way and may cause considerable damage before it is even noticed. This is especially a danger with groups or organisms so little observed and valued as amphibians and reptiles.

6 COMMENTS. SUMMARY AND RECOMMENDATIONS

This review shows clearly that the main concern during the last 20 years has been non-target exposure of anurans to pesticides. There are very few reports on heavy metals, and poisoning of amphibians and reptiles by methylmercury is not once discussed. Compared to the mass of research on methylmercury in fish and birds in the early seventies, this can have but one explanation: amphibians and reptiles are not of sufficient interest. Economically only a few species are hunted or sought, but ecologically they have great importance as bioaccumulators in the food chain.

In the anurans it seems possible to disturb oogenesis and spermatogenesis at the DNA and RNA level. However, whether this is possible without injecting the substance into the animals is not known. Pesticides in the water can damage the eggs in at least two ways: the substance may enter the egg in the swelling phase, or it can destroy the gelatinous coating by coagulation. Copper salts seem not to damage the egg.

Tadpoles from insecticide-treated spawn show, within a week, the same signs as tadpoles treated directly with the same substance. Gill-bearing tadpoles are more sensitive than tadpoles with inner gills; tadpoles developing leg buds are even more susceptible to insecticide treatment. If residues are left in the body, the metamorphosed imago may die from the mobilization of fat containing pesticides. Frog tadpoles are generally more sensitive than toad tadpoles. Newt tadpoles are rarely tested but show the same pattern of reactions, including death. Herbicides may be less toxic than insecticides, but there are exceptions; nothing is known about possible synergism between these pesticides.

Cadmium is reported to block spermatogenesis in toads under certain conditions. Mutagenic effects from metals have been observed in other species, but extrapolation to reptiles and amphibians is uncertain. No teratogenic effects of metals in amphibians and reptiles have been described. Effects in other species have been described, but again extrapolation is uncertain.

Methods reviewed have varied widely, and it is seldom possible to compare data from one study with another. The degree of methodological refinement of toxicity studies on amphibia and reptiles is low compared to that on fish and other species.

There is an urgent need to develop more informative test procedures for examining the effects of chemicals on the reproductive function in reptiles and amphibians. Such development can receive guidance from tests developed for other organisms, especially fish and birds. Although the development of methods is still too primitive for standardization, this objective should be kept in mind.

7 REFERENCES

Biswas, N. M., Chanda, S., Ghosh, A. and Chakraborty (1976). Effect of cadmium on spermatogenesis in toad (*Bufo melanosticus*). *Endocrinologie* **68**, 349–352.

Boyd, C. E., Vinson, S. B. and Ferguson, D. E. (1963). Possible DDT-resistance in two species of frogs. *Copeia* June 14, **2**, 426–429.

Cooke, A. S. (1970). The effect of *pp'*-DDT on tadpoles of the common frog (*Rana temporaria*). *Environ. Pollut.* **1**, 57–71.

Cooke, A. S. (1972). The effects of DDT, dieldrin and 2, 4-D on amphibian spawn and tadpoles. *Environ. Pollut.* **3**, 51–68.

Cooke, A. S. (1973). Response of *Rana temporaria* tadpoles to chronic doses of *pp'*-DDT. *Copeia* **4**, 647–652.

Cooke, A. S. (1975a). Spawn clumps of the common frog, *Rana temporaria*, number of ova and hatchability. *Br. J. Herpetol.* **55**, 505–509.

Cooke, A. S. (1975b). The effects of *pp'*-DDCN on tadpoles of the frog *Rana temporaria*. *Bull. environ. Contam. Toxicol.* **13**, 233–237.

Dilling, W. J. and Healey, C. W. (1926). Influence of lead and the metallic ions of copper, zinc, thorium, beryllium and thallium on the germination of frog spawn and on the growth of tadpoles. *Ann. appl. Biol.* **13**, 177–188.

Ferguson, D. E. and Gilbert, C. C. (1967). Tolerance of three species of anuran amphibians to five chlorinated hydrocarbon insecticides. *J. Miss. Acad. Sci.* **13**, 135–138.

Fleet, R. R., Clark, D. R. and Plapp, F. W. (1972). Residues of DDT and dieldrin in snakes from two Texas agro-systems. *BioScience* **22**, 664–665.

Hazelwood, E. (1970). Frog pond contamination. *Br. J. Herpetol.* **4**, 177–185.

Kaplan, H. M. and Yoh, L. (1961). Toxicity of copper for frogs. *Herpetologica* **17**, 131–135.

Landé, S. P. and Guttman, S. I. (1973). The effects of copper sulphate on the growth and mortality rate of *Rana pipiens* tadpoles. *Herpetologica* **29**, 22–27.

Matur, U. and Ramaswami, L. S. (1976). Effect of cadmium on the testes of the Indian bullfrog, *Rana tigrina* (Daud). *Folia biol. (Cracow)* **24**, 3.

OECD (1979). *Report on the Assessment of Potential Environmental Effects of Chemicals; the Effects on Organisms other than Man and on Ecosystems.* OECD Chemicals Testing Programme, Ecotoxicology Group, December 1979.

Packard, G. C., Taigen, T. L., Packard, M. J. and Shuman, R. D. (1979). Water-vapor conductance of testudinian and crocodilian eggs (class Reptilia). *Resp. Physiol.* **38**, 1–10.

Peaslee, M. H. (1970). Influence of DDT upon pituitary melanocyte-stimulating hormone. *Gen. comp. Endocrinol.* **14**, 594–595.

Pough, F. H. (1976). Acid precipitation and embryonic mortality of spotted salamanders, *Ambystoma maculatum*. *Science (Washington, DC)* **192**, 68–70.

Pough, F. H. and Wilson, R. E. (1974). The effects of temperature and pH combination on amphibian embryonic development. *The Physiologist* **17**, 388.

Sala, M. and Conte, L. (1975). Effects of 5-bromo-deoxyuritine on the development of *Xenopus laevis* eggs. 1. Early stages of development. *Acta Embryol. exp.* **1**, 39–45.

Sanders, H. (1970). Pesticide toxicity to tadpoles of the western chorus frog, *Pseudocoris triseriata*, and Fowler's toad, *Bufo woodhousii Copeia* **2**, 246–251.

Scorgie, H. R. A. and Cooke, A. S. (1979). Effects of the triazine herbicide Cycanatryn on aquatic animals. *Bull. environ. Toxicol.* **22**, 135–142.

Shivakuma, G. R. and Devaraj Sarkar, H. B. (1979). Effect of quinacrine hydrochloride on testes and accessory reproductive organs of the lizard *Psammophilus dorsalis* (Gray). *Indian J. exp. Biol.* **17**, 1297–1300.

Steens, M. (1977). Cytotoxic effects of a reverse transcriptase inhibitor, AF/ABDPcis, on ovaries of young *Xenopus laevis*—ultrastructural and autoradiographic study. *Chem. biol. Interact.* **18**, 59–67.

Vinson, S. B., Boyd, C. E. and Ferguson, D. F. (1963). Aldrin toxicity and possible cross-resistance in cricket frogs. *Herpetologica* **19**, 77–80.

Methods for Assessing the Effects of Chemicals on Reproductive Functions
Edited by V. B. Vouk and P. J. Sheehan
© 1983 SCOPE

Methods for the Assessment of the Effects of Chemicals on the Reproductive Function of Insects

V. LANDA, B. BENNETTOVÁ, I. GELBIČ, S. MATOLÍN and T. SOLDÁN

1 INTRODUCTION

Insect reproductive function is responsive to a complex of external factors—physical, chemical, biological. The effects of external stress are variable as the fertility of insects is usually very high and the range of potential aberrations very large. The anatomy of the reproductive organs is basically simple; therefore, morphological aberrations are distinguishable in quality as well as quantity. Insect ontogeny is also known in detail, thus dynamic observation of the response of affected reproductive organs is possible. The direct effects of external factors on individual developmental stages as well as delayed effects observable in embryogenesis of the succeeding generation can be experimentally examined. Embryonic development has been well described and changes are distinct. Many species produce several generations of offspring per year, so that the effects on several successive generations can be examined. In general, all actions of the adult organism are centred on reproduction. The condition of the reproductive organs and fertility of the individual thus indicate the physiological status of the whole organism as effected by external factors.

Insect reproduction has primarily been studied along the following lines:

(1) population dynamics, especially the dynamics of pest outbreaks;
(2) effects of sublethal doses of insecticides on fertility;
(3) effects of chemosterilants and their application to insect control.

The effects of non-specific chemical pollutants in the natural environment on the reproduction of insects have not been sufficiently investigated, and reliable data are scarce. Considering that the study of insect reproduction and how it is regulated by chemicals can produce data of broad biological significance, it will be necessary to concentrate more effort on this line of research. Methods that have proved useful in the study of chemosterilants should also be employed.

415

2 CHANGES IN INSECT REPRODUCTION AND THEIR EXAMINATION

Chemicals can affect insect reproduction in any of its stages. Changes may appear in the following structures and/or functions:

(1) female reproductive organs and oogenesis;
(2) male reproductive organs and spermatogenesis;
(3) number of laid eggs and hatchability;
(4) embryogenesis;
(5) mortality during postembryonic development and variations in mortality of the following generations; changes in development and mating habits;
(6) mutagenic changes in chromosomes.

2.1 Female Reproductive Organs and Oogenesis

The condition of female reproductive organs is examined by dissecting fresh material by the usual methods. The abdomen is opened dorsally with fine scissors in physiological solutions (Pringle, Ringer or others). Fine organs are loosened by a stream of the solution from a hypodermic syringe. The usual fixatives (alcohol with acetic acid, Carnoy, Bouin, or others) may be used later, or some details can be emphasized by total staining (methylene blue, borax carmine). Whole mounts and smear preparations can be well observed using phase contrast or interference phase contrast. After fixation, histological preparations are made by the usual techniques, and sectioned materials stained with differentiating stains (recommended are Heidenhain's or Harris's haematoxylin, Pappenheim, etc.) or with specific histochemical stains (Feulgen for nucleic acids, Nile blue for lipids, mercury bromphenol blue for proteins).

Insect ovaries are paired organs situated in the abdomen consisting of ovarioles, ducts and accessory glands. Ovarioles are elongate tubes consisting distally of a germarium and proximally of a gradually formed vitellarium where oocytes grow and vitellogenesis takes place. Large numbers (up to several hundred) of ovarioles occur in Palaeoptera and Polyneoptera, several (mostly 4–7) in higher orders of insects. The germarium is the first to differentiate from primordial gonocytes (sometimes as early as during embryogenesis, e.g. in aphids). Later it contains mitotically dividing oogonia developing into oocytes or oocytes and trophocytes. The oocytes are enveloped in follicular epithelium and proceed towards the oviduct. Secretion of yolk and chorion, usually occurring prior to ovulation, is effected by follicular cells or trophocytes. According to the type of nutrition provided oocytes and corresponding structures, ovaries are categorized as atrophic (panoistic) without trophocytes in follicles, and meroistic with trophocytes either in follicles (polytrophic ovaries) or in the germarium and connected with the oocyte by fine cytoplasmic cords (telotrophic ovaries).

Oviducts consist of lateral and common oviducts into which ovarioles open through the pedicels (interfollicular tissue), and the oviductus communis is usually differentiated into organs of copulatory and sperm-storing functions, the bursa copulatrix, spermatheca, etc. Accessory glands are either of mesodermal (mesadenia) or ectodermal origin (ectadenia). Their secretions, enveloping the egg, may participate in the formation of spermatophores, or lubricate the ovipositor or eggs.

Defects caused by chemicals appear in the germarium and vitellarium of individual follicles, in uneven development of follicles, and in accessory glands and outlets. The formation of spermatophores and motility of sperm may be affected. Compounds affecting development may impair the growth of oviducts and other organs. Sterilizing effects may be manifested by conspicuous changes in the germarium which may be smaller by one-half when compared with germarium of unexposed females due to inhibition of the division of oogonia and differentiation of oocytes and trophocytes (see reviews by Campion, 1972). Sections of panoistic ovaries show that the division of oogonia has been blocked, and already developed young oocytes have died and been resorbed. In polytrophic ovaries, oocytes as well as nutritive and follicular cells are affected. The nuclei of oocytes become pyonotic, oogonia cease to divide, and the development of egg chambers is blocked. In telotrophic ovaries, the zone of dividing trophocytes is the most damaged and, consequently, follicular cells do not divide (formation of compound egg chambers). Oocytes descend either irregularly or not at all. Changes in the vitellarium show in a reduced number of egg chambers, blocked growth of follicles or production of microfollicles. Vitellogenesis is often suppressed or entirely inhibited, so that the ovaries of older females cannot be distinguished from those of teneral ones (e.g. 6-azauridine in the housefly, Rezáková and Landa, 1967; Rezábová, 1968). Egg chambers may be resorbed.

All these changes result in a reduced number of laid eggs, and, if vitellogenesis is suppressed, in complete sterility of the female. Deposition of yolk granules, indicating that vitellogenesis has begun, is easily distinguished in squash preparations of the vitellarium; phase contrast or phase interference contrast is useful, as are some stains (e.g. fast green). Changes in follicles may not be macroscopically distinct, for only in cases of serious damage are there changes in the shape and colour of unfixed follicles. However, such changes are very distinct in histological preparations. Changes in shape are characterized by alteration of the originally round or oval follicle into an irregular form; changes in colour are conspicuous as darkening of the follicle and unfixed material often grows opaque (this should be distinguished from the opaqueness of postvitellogenic follicles due to yolk deposition).

It is very important to estimate the condition of the distal follicle (i.e. the oldest one, situated distal from the germarium and proximal to the oviduct). This follicle usually is the largest, and secretion of chorion should be macroscopically distinct at the time of oviposition; occasionally this secretion is also seen in other follicles (especially in atrophic ovarioles). The absence of chorion or diminution of distal follicles indicate at least partial sterility. This does not exclude production of eggs by these follicles (e.g., microeggs in *Dixippus morosus* after treatment with juvenoids (Socha and Gelbič, 1973).

Follicular epithelium and follicular cells are very susceptible to the action of chemicals. Uncoordinated division of nuclei may take place, intercellular membranes may disappear, and tumour-like tissue with irregular clusters of chromatin may develop. Nutritive cells of polytrophic ovaries are not usually affected in this way, but pycnotic changes occur in their nuclei.

Morphological and anatomical changes are also reflected in biochemical processes. The follicular content of nucleic acids increases due to changes in follicular epithelium. The effects of chemicals on the ovaries can also be examined by monitoring changes in the activity of mitochondria. Many compounds induce a manifold increase in mitochondrial activity.

Chemical effects on accessory glands become apparent in changes in their size and the altered colour of their secretions (in fresh material). In suitably fixed material (non-alcoholic fixatives, at best formalin), the amount of secretion can be macroscopically estimated and compared with that of control specimens. In cases where much secretion is deposited on the egg surface, it is possible to estimate gland function from this point of view. A lack of secretion or minor morphological changes in accessory gland might not affect fertility, but these factors can markedly affect the activation of sperm and thus, indirectly, fertility. Profound changes in accessory glands are always accompanied by changes in germinal tissues.

In species where spermatophores are formed either outside or in the female body, it is useful to estimate the number and condition of spermatophores in the bursa copulatrix of fertilized females. The lack of spermatophores is an indication either of male sterility or of changes in mating behaviour, but even the occurrence of more spermatophores than in the unexposed control does not ensure fertilization of the eggs in oviducts. The degree of differentiation of oviducts and outer genitalia should also be examined at dissection. Some biologically active compounds may upset differentiation of these organs and thus prevent the laying of otherwise normal eggs.

2.2 Male Reproductive Organs and Spermatogenesis

The preparation and observation of whole mounts and the techniques of histological processing have been described in the previous paragraph and are applicable to examination of male reproductive organs.

Insect testes are paired organs consisting of testicle tubules (testicular follicles), ducts and accessory glands. The ducts are connected with copulatory organs. The testicle tubules are elongate, vesicular or globular organs in which germinal cells divide, grow and differentiate. The tubules number several hundred in primitive orders of insects (Palaeoptera, Polymetabola); in more advanced ones (Paraneoptera, Holometabola) there are usually only 4–7. Testicle tubules may be encased in a membranous sac (scrotum). They differentiate from primordial cells enveloped in connective and peritoneal tissues very early, often during embryogenesis or at the latest at the beginning of the pupal stage. Before the onset of spermatogenesis, the testicle tubules contain mitotically dividing spermatogonia. Some spermatogonia give rise to cyst cells with comparatively small nuclei and little cytoplasm. Spermatogonia are encased in cyst cells, divide in them and, together with the cells, produce cysts. Spermatocytes develop from spermatogonia. Spermatocytes of the first and second orders differ from spermatogonia in size, stainability of the nucleus and cytoplasm and their relative sizes. Reduction division of male gametes (meiosis) takes place in the spermatocyte stage. Spermatocytes develop into spermatids usually containing a large, easily stainable nucleus and almost no cytoplasm. These cells do not divide, but are gradually transformed into presperms and mature sperms. Cyst cells generally disintegrate only when the transformation has been completed and mature sperms descend into the seminal duct. Insect sperms, apart from a few exceptions, have one flagellum and a well-differentiated head (with a crystalline body in higher groups).

Three zones can be distinguished in the testicle tubule of a mature male: a distal zone of growth (encysted as well as free spermatogonia), a zone of reduction division (cysts with spermatocytes I and II), and, proximally, a transformation zone (cysts containing spermatids, presperms and sperms).

Ducts consist of two lateral seminal ducts and a common seminal duct passing into an ejaculatory duct of ectodermal origin and lined with a chitinous intima. Seminal vesicles serving as containers of sperm are situated at various places in the ducts. Accessory glands may be of mesodermal (mesadenia) or ectodermal origin (ectadenia). They consist of glandular and connective tissues and their secretions make up seminal fluid, sections for production of spermatophores, etc. Outer genitalia are mostly sclerotized and of very diverse shapes. Their structure, which may be relatively complex and of different nomenclature in different groups, primarily consists of an orginally paired penis and variously modified gonapophyses.

Sterilizing effects on a testis are macroscopically distinct, especially as reduction in the size of testicle tubules as well as the whole testis and derangement of differentiation of the ducts and outer genitalia. However, sterilizing effects may be manifested in a reduced number of testicle tubules or deranged differentiation of testicle tubules from primordial cells, showing either in a marked reduction of the number of testicle tubules (down to 1/3 in Polyneoptera) or occurrence of irregularly shaped testicle tubules, which in fact represent several fused together. In contrast to the ovaries, a testis in which differentiation of the follicles has been disturbed need not mean complete sterility; such a state is even physiologically common in some groups (e.g., Collembolla). Considerable differences in the size of the testis between normal and affected individuals are much more frequent; the whole testis may be reduced to one-third of its original length.

Toxic chemicals may impair differentiation of seminal ducts or development of the seminal ducts may be totally inhibited although germinal tissues have not been seriously damaged. The same consequence may occur with external genitalia. Passage of mature sperm through the ducts may be blocked, or mating prevented by defects in the copulatory organs. Macroscopic changes of accessory glands are manifested in the same fashion as in testicle tubules. Changes are primarily in size; however, the degree of filling of the ducts and seminal vesicles with mature sperm, and the amount and quality of secretion of the accessory glands must also be examined. Although the amount of sperm in the seminal ducts and seminal vesicles may not be a decisive indicator of fertility, pronounced differences in the size of seminal vesicles may be manifested in the mating ability of males, particularly in species where multiple mating is common.

Histopathological changes are often found with histological processing of the reproductive organs of males exposed to toxic chemicals. The germarium, apical part of the testicle tubule containing the zone of growth, may be shown to be damaged by the structure of the apical cell. Histopathological changes show mainly in disconnection or degeneration of cytoplasmic connections within spermatogonia which then become pycnotic, causing the whole apical cell to gradually disintegrate. The cell itself may vacuolate, or conspicuous resorptions may appear in its cytoplasm. Some compounds directly affect spermatogonia. Their effects show in inhibition of the mitotic division of spermatogonia, in disorders of the differentiation of cyst cells, or in incomplete encystation of secondary spermatogonia. Signs of necrosis, such as pycnosis of nuclei, disintegration of cytoplasm, formation of chaotic syncytia, etc., may be found in spermatogonia of the apical zone.

A marked derangement of the proportioning of spermatocytes occurs in the zone of meiotic division (layer containing spermatocytes) when reduction division has been inhibited. Meiosis is blocked by all mitotic poisons. If there is no layer containing secondary spermatocytes in a testis where the transformation zone has already been differentiated, it always means that meiosis has been blocked. Changes in the number of encysted spermatocytes are frequent. In the cyst of control individuals, there should be an accurately delimited number of cells (2, 3, 8, 16, etc.). All cysts should contain approximately the same number of cells. Greater differences in the number of encysted spermatocytes are the result of inhibited differentiation and division of germinal cells. Complete sterility is manifested by disintegration and pycnosis of the nuclei of spermatocytes, loss of their originally globular shape, or premature disintegration of cysts.

In the transformation zone where cysts disintegrate and mature sperms develop, we should especially look for disintegrating cysts and morphological changes in sperm and presperm. Disorders in transformation may become apparent in premature disintegration of cysts containing immature sperm. However, these changes need not indicate sterility, because presperm may sometimes mature only in the seminal duct. Morphological defects are rarely found in sperm and presperm; these occur only when germinal cells have been seriously damaged (pycnosis, vacuolation). Malformations can be best estimated in mature sperm, e.g., the shape of head, which is elongate in most species, may be changed, or there are changes in differentiation of the flagellum. Malformed sperms are non-functional. Their percentage can be ascertained in squash preparations, or in a Bürker chamber by the same methods used for vertebrate sperm. All sperm with the flagellum should be motile; physiological immobility of insect sperm is connected with the loss of the flagellum. Individuals whose sperm is not motile are often sterile.

Adverse effects related to histopathological changes in germinal cells can also be found in other tissues of the male reproductive system. In accessory glands, the structures of secretion epithelium are often affected (reduction of cytoplasm, pycnoses and disintegration of nuclei, vacuolation of cells) and disorders in secretion ensue. Differentiation of epithelium is inhibited, or there is a chaotic formation of syncytia in cases of serious damage. Similar changes may appear in the epithelium of the seminal duct, in peritoneal tissues and in connective tissues of the testes. Cases of proliferation resembling tumour growth, starting in the connective tissue, have been shown.

Also, the time sequence in differentiation processes in germinal cells is most important to the study of changes in the reproductive system. Transformation may be shifted without noticeable histopathological defects, but males with immature sperm will be unable to fertilize females. Therefore, it is always necessary to define accurately that stage of ontogeny in which individual zones of testicle tubules develop in order to trace a possible disharmony in the timing of individual phases of spermatogenesis.

2.3 The Number of Laid Eggs and Hatchability

Assessing the number of laid eggs and their hatchability is essentially the only quantitative method revealing changes in fecundity and fertility of insects, and this reflects the adverse effects of chemicals on various phases of development of their reproductive organs.

Insect eggs are laid either individually or in batches. Oviposition is either single (i.e. only one mating and fertilization are followed by a single oviposition at which all eggs are laid), or multiple, when a single fertilization is followed by the laying of several batches of eggs. Repeated mating is rather rare. Parthenogenesis (the laying of unfertilized diploid eggs) is relatively widespread in insects and is especially common in primitive groups and in social insects. Partial parthenogenesis also occurs quite frequently.

It is easy to investigate fecundity if the methods for the rearing of the experimental species have been well worked out. Experimental females should always be fertilized only by normal control males. If this is not possible (affected field populations), then at least by males affected to different degrees. If the purpose of the experiment is to ascertain through fertility of females to what extent the reproductive ability of males has been indirectly altered, it is necessary to mate the treated males with healthy females. The females must naturally be observed throughout their adult life because intervals between individual batches of eggs may be longer or otherwise different from those observed for control populations. It is useful always to examine a statistically significant sample of treated and control females, i.e., at least 30 individuals in each experiment. Besides the number of laid eggs, variations in their number per batch should also be noted, as should variations in the number of batches or changes in habitat preference for egg deposition and other comparable factors. The number of eggs laid under natural conditions can be evaluated only in species laying batches rather than individual eggs, and only in populations which have been demonstrably affected as a whole.

Many compounds do not alter the number of laid eggs but markedly affect their hatchability. It is possible to detect, in this way, changes in the fertility of males because unfertilized eggs do not hatch. Examination of hatchability is also the only reliable quantitative method for determining reproductive interference in parthenogenetic species in which fertilization does not affect the number of laid eggs. If incidental spontaneous or geographical parthenogenesis has been shown in a species, reproduction from such parthenogenetic individuals may distort data on the fertility of males, indirectly obtained through data on the number of eggs laid by normal females mated with the treated males. In some cases (e.g., after administration of juvenoids to *Dixippus morosus*, Socha and Gelbic, 1973), a paradoxical increase in oviposition per day may occur owing to irregularities in the maturation of individual follicles, but hatchability is minimal.

The causes of reduced hatchability vary. It is closely related to morphological defects of eggs (defective chorion enabling desiccation, defective microphyle, etc.). Hatchability may be reduced by an increase in the mortality of gametes or zygotes, by disorders in embryogenesis, and frequently by the inability of first instar larvae to leave the egg or break through the chorion.

2.4 Embryogenesis

The study of embryonic development of insects is a very subtle method of estimating the effectiveness of individual chemical agents interfering with reproduction. Changes in embryogenesis may appear even in those cases where mortality has not increased nor have adverse morphological changes in the development of reproductive organs occurred. The course of embryonic development can be observed either directly on live material or on fixed specimens. Examination of live material is facilitated by the transparence of the chorion (e.g., in water, lactic acid, oil, etc.), and by using phase contrast, infrared light, or other techniques to increase resolution.

Eggs are fixed by placing them into solutions at regular intervals in order to record all stages of embryogenesis. Carnoy can be used for whole staining and Huettner or Bouin for histological processing. The chorion must be removed either mechanically or chemically with sodium hypochlorite for whole mounts stained with borax carmine differentiated in lactic acid, toluidine blue or other stains. Before histological processing the chorion should be removed or at least punctured for better penetration of reagents and embedding medium. Sections 4–6 μm thick are stained with Heidenhain's, Harris's or Mayer's haematoxylin, Pappenheim, toluidine blue, etc. The most suitable fixation and staining should be tried beforehand for each species studied.

There are two main types of insect embryogenesis. The mosaic developmental type (Diptera) is characterized by early determination of embryonic structures. Damage to such eggs is most often revealed in malformation of or deficiency in the damaged structure. However, later determination and a considerable ability to compensate for or repair damaged structures are typical of the regulation type of development (Heteroptera). The two developmental types are not sharply delimited, the difference is rather in the time when development can still be somewhat regulated, or before which determination has already taken place. There are many intermediate examples (Lepidoptera, Coleoptera) between the two extreme types. Embryonic development is much shorter in dipteran eggs with their early determination than in eggs of those species where determination begins later.

Disorders in embryonic development may result from damage to gametes during oogenesis and spermatogenesis, or from the action of chemicals in the developing embryo. The final effect depends on the characteristics of the chemical as well as on the type of embryogenesis in the given species. The range of effects on eggs of the regulation type is much wider than in mosaic eggs because of their greater ability to repair induced abnormalities.

Damage to genetic material, i.e. embryonic lethal mutations, is most often manifested during cleavage division as a delayed effect. Karyokinesis is initiated by chromosomal aberrations during early cleavage division and, consequently, chromosomal bridges are formed. The bridges can be identified by cytogenetical methods in sections or squashes (stained with lacto-aceto-orceine). Species with diffuse centromeres are very resistant to formation of chromosomal bridges. Chromosomal fragments remain in the nuclei of daughter cells and their rearrangement gives rise to reciprocal translocations. Reciprocal translocations as well as deletions of local character (typical of Lepidoptera) often appear only in the advanced stages of embryogenesis.

Compounds producing effects of other kinds (e.g. antibiotics, analogues of insect hormones, etc.), which do not so drastically derange chromosomal material, are effective rather on the level of regulation of gene activity. Development is not inhibited during cleavage division; however, disorders in germ band formation, gastrulation, and the development of malformed miniature embryos have been caused by such compounds. Physiologically exacting processes, such as invagination of the germ band, blastokinesis and hatching, are frequently disrupted.

Other developmental stages are affected by compounds with specific toxic effects (mitotic poisons, respiratory poisons, compounds damaging the deposition of cuticle, etc.).

The results of contemporary research have shown that if hatchability is reduced by a test compound, the study of embryogenesis may yield valuable additional data of considerable practical impact, such as the effective concentrations, efficacy of various methods of chemical application, determination of the more susceptible phases of embryogenesis, and the effects on duration of the different types of embryonic development.

2.5 Mortality during Postembryonic Development and Variations in Mortality in the Following Generations; Changes in Development and Mating Habits

To quantify reproductive-related mortality, it is first necessary to distinguish the proportion of deaths due to natural causes (always higher under natural conditions than in the laboratory) and that proportion of unnatural deaths caused by factors other than those interfering with reproduction in the parental generation. This task is not always easy. Increased mortality of first instar larvae of the first filial generation is common in experiments with toxic chemicals. This effect is due to defects in embryogenesis and hatching. Evidence of abnormality may sometimes be detected in the later instars. Higher mortality in filial generations is often induced genetically through lethal mutations. There is little data supporting the idea presently, but in several cases dominant lethal mutations have been induced by chemicals (for examples see LaChance and Riemann, 1964; Valkovic and Grosch, 1968).

Sterility may be indirectly attributed to changes in the length of development, most often by slowing its rate (occurrence of supernumerary larval instars in the case of juvenoids) or to changes in mating behaviour. Mating may be shortened by various compounds thus reducing the probability that fertilization will occur. There are also a large group of compounds which impair orientation in insects seeking the opposite sex through pheromone attractants.

2.6 Mutagenic Changes in Chromosomes

Mutagenic changes induced by chemical compounds (Fahmy and Fahmy, 1954) may affect somatic cells (somatic mutations) as well as germinal cells. Only one chromatid or the whole chromosome may be damaged. Susceptibility to the mutagenic effects of chemicals depends on the number and shape of chromosomes, types of centromeres and other properties of this chromosome and specific chemical. Individual developmental stages also differ in their susceptibility to mutagenic effects. It has been found that the number of genetic defects (chromosomal aberrations) increases in proportion to increased doses of effective compounds.

3 THE TESTING OF EFFECTS OF CHEMICALS ON REPRODUCTION IN *MUSCA DOMESTICAL* L. (DIPTERA, MUSCIDAE)

Musca domestica is a suitable species for use in testing of chemical effects on the reproduction of insects. A genetically well-defined WHO strain can be used for experimentation (WHO Standard Insect Strain Reference Centre, Pavia, Italy).

Houseflies are reared in a medium consisting of groats, yeast and milk (1000 g, 3 g, 1200 ml). Pupation takes place in the upper layer of the medium; pupae are then transferred into cages where adults are fed a mixture of powdered low-fat milk and sugar (1:1) and water. Oviposition medium, the same as used in larval rearing, is placed via small cups into the cages after 6 days. The temperature of the rearing room should be $25° \pm 2°C$, RH 60–70%, photoperiod 18 L : 6 D.

Chemicals can be administered to various developmental stages. However, ovarian development in adult flies is the most suitable stage for the study of adverse effects on reproductive function. Controls reared under the same conditions are necessarily evaluated at the same time, and all parameters examined for experimental flies are compared to those of control specimens.

3.1 Tests on Larvae

3.1.1 *In the Medium*

A test chemical is mixed with the standard larval medium (mg of compound per g of dry medium) and a certain number of larvae of a defined age are placed into the mixture. Effects on newly laid eggs can also be assessed. The following characteristics are examined; survival of larvae; pupation; adult emergence; fecundity and fertility of adults; state of ovaries and testes in individual stages of the development of reproductive organs (at certain intervals); and embryogenesis.

3.1.2 *Topical Application*

A test compound dissolved in acetone (1:10; 1:100; 1:1000) is applied to the surface of the larval body (1–2 μl according to the size of the larva). Except for larvae ready to pupate, experimental animals are then placed in fresh medium. The same parameters as listed in the previous case are again examined.

3.2 Tests on Pupae

Newly formed or light brown puparia are treated with compounds dissolved in acetone at the same concentrations as in larval treatment. The following characteristics are examined: adult emergence; fecundity and fertility of adults; state of ovaries and testes in individual stages of the development of reproductive organs (at certain intervals); and embryogenesis.

For examination of adverse effects on an adult that has not yet emerged, part of the pupal case can be removed at the cephalic end and 1 μl of the compound dissolved in acetone administered.

3.3 Tests on Teneral Adults

3.3.1 *Compounds Administered in Water*

Tap water solutions at concentrations of 0.1, 0.01 and 0.001% are administered to teneral adults and replenished every 3 days. The following characteristics are examined: fecundity and fertility of adults; state of ovaries and testes in individual stages of the development of reproductive organs (at certain intervals); embryogenesis; and fecundity and fertility of F_1 generation, if necessary. If the effects of the compound are conspicuous, experiments are repeated for detailed determination of morphological and anatomical changes in the growth and development of the ovaries. A suitable method for accurately defining the time it takes a toxic chemical to act and the manner of the compound's action is by injection of 2–16 μg of the chemical in physiological solution into the upper left quadrant of the thorax followed by repeated detailed examination as described above.

3.3.2 *Compounds Insoluble in Water*

Compounds insoluble in water can be tested by topical application of acetone or other non-toxic solutions in concentrations of 1:10, 1:100 and 1:1000 once to both sexes (2 μl) 6–10 hours after emergence from the pupa. The same characteristics as in section 18.3.3.1 are then examined.

3.4 Evaluation of Changes

Changes caused by chemicals administered to any of the developmental stages are currently evaluated throughout experiments according to the parameters given above. Naturally, evaluation of developing ovaries is of prime importance,

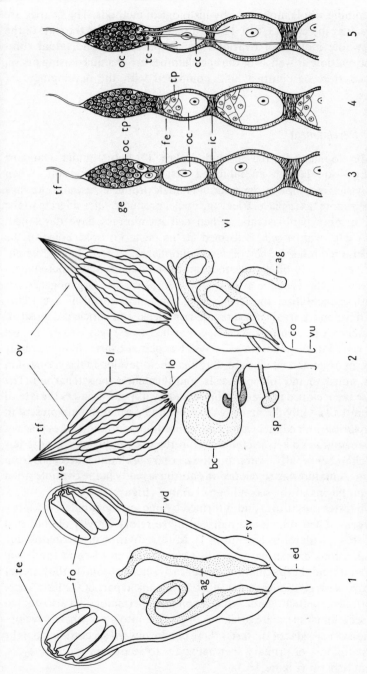

Figure 1 Sketches of internal reproductive organs of insects with details of female ovaries; male (1) and female (2) internal reproductive organs, accessory glands dotted; panoistic (3) (atrophic); meroistic–polytrophic (4) and meroistic–telotrophic (5) types of insect ovarioles. Abbreviated terminology: te, testis with peritoneal envelop; fo, testicular follicles; ve, vassa efferentia; vd, vas deferens; sv, seminal vesicle; ed, ejaculatory duct; ag, accessory glands; ov, ovaries; ol, ovarioles; tf, terminal filament; lo, lateral oviduct; co, common (median) oviduct; vu, vulva; bc, bursa copulatrix with gland; sp, spermatheca; ge, germarium; vi, vitellarium; oc, oocytes; tp, trophocytes; fe, follicular epithelium; ic, interfollicular cells; cc, cytoplasmatic cords

either by examining whole mounts or by histological methods. The ovaries are dissected at regular intervals (3, 6, 9, 12, 15, 18 and 21 days from the start of the experiment), whole mounts of ovarioles are prepared, and individual components of the ovariole as well as of the egg chamber are examined using phase, anoptral or interference contrast, and compared with the development of untreated flies.

3.4.1 *Normal Development*

Embryonic development in the housefly takes 13 hours under standard conditions. Eggs are laid in an inhibited first maturation division. When maturation division is complete, the male and female pronuclei fuse and cleavage division of the zygote takes place. Cleavage nuclei produced later migrate to the egg surface, forming periblast and, when cell membranes have developed, blastoderm. A cap of pole cells is formed at the posterior pole. Some of the cleavage nuclei remain inside the yolk as vitellophages. A germ band differentiates on the ventral side of the blastoderm. Stomodaeum and proctodaeum develop as well as the cephalic furrow and neural ridges. Organogenesis is connected with segmentation, the germ band is shortened, dorsal closure occurs and the head develops. Larval structures are completed and cuticle is deposited. The larva hatches when embryogenesis is finished (see Figure 18.4). Larval development lasts 5 days, pupal stage 7 days. The paired ovaries of a teneral fly consist of a germarium and vitellarium. Egg chambers develop in the germarium from oocytes, nutritive and follicular cells, and then enter the vitellarium. The whole ovariole is enveloped in tunica propria and by its pedicel enters the lateral oviduct (Figure 18.1). Only the first egg chamber and germarium are present in the housefly ovariole immediately after emergence (differentiation takes place in the final pupal stage). Yolk is accumulated in the oocyte during the next few days, the egg chamber rapidly grows, and the second egg chamber descends from the germarium. A mature egg enveloped in chorion is ready in the ovariole when yolk deposition begins in the second egg chamber (Figure 18.2).

Each of two testes is pyriform and is formed by one testicle tubule. Accessory glands are absent. Their function is replaced by secretory activity of epithelial cells in the ductus ejaculatorius (Figure 18.1). Mitotic division of spermatogonia and meiotic divisions of spermatocytes has already taken place in the larval stages. Spermatids and the first mature spermatozoa can be found in the testes of the pupa. The process continues in the adult. In the apical part of the testis there is a zone of primary spermatogonia while secondary spermatogonia are situated basally. The secondary spermatogonia are organized into cysts where development continues. On all sides of the testes there is a downward succession from the area of spermatogonia of primary spermatocytes to secondary spermatocytes, spermatids, and sperm (Figure 18.3).

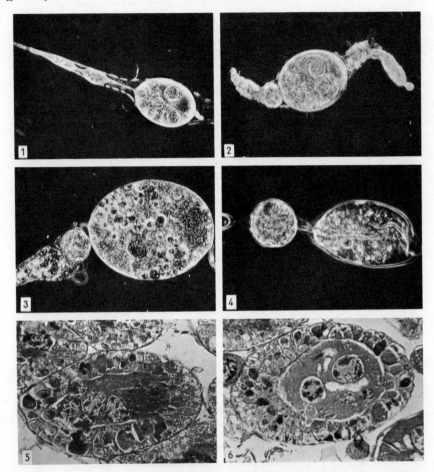

Figure 2 Normal and chemically affected development of the egg chambers. *Musca domestica*: (1) normal development of the first and second egg chambers and germarium (anoptral contrast); (2,3,4) development affected by chemicals. Resorption of the contents of egg chambers and germarium following proliferation (anoptral contrast); (5) proliferation of follicular epithelium; (6) pycnotic nuclei of nutritive cells (Heidenhain's haematoxylin)

3.4.2 Changes Induced by Chemicals

Administration of chemicals (either topical or in food) may affect the following developmental processes:

(1) survival of larvae. Larval growth in the medium larval mortality.

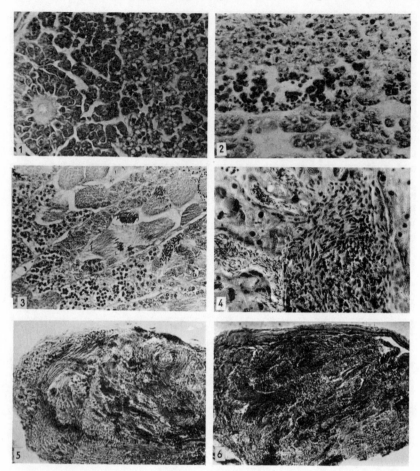

Figure 3   Normal and chemically affected development of spermatocytes. *Spodoptera littoralis*: (1) normal development; apical cell and different stages of spermatogenesis; (2) effect of chemical substances; pycnotic nuclei and necrotic spermatocytes (Harris's haematoxylin, eosin). *Leptinotarsa decemlineata*: (3) normal male; (4) section through tumour-like proliferation after treatment with chemicals (Harris's haematoxylin, eosin). *Musca domestica*: (5) normal development; (6) development affected by chemicals, absence of immature stages of spermatogenesis (Heidenhain's haematoxylin)

(2) pupation. Number of larvae which have pupated, shape of pupae (round, elongate, irregularly pigmented), their size (comparison of the weight of experimental and normal pupae is recommended in special cases).
(3) adult emergence. Number of emerging adults, conspicuous changes in their external morphology (nonstretched wings, etc.). Not yet emerging pupae are examined for the lid broken by head. The pupae that have not emerged can

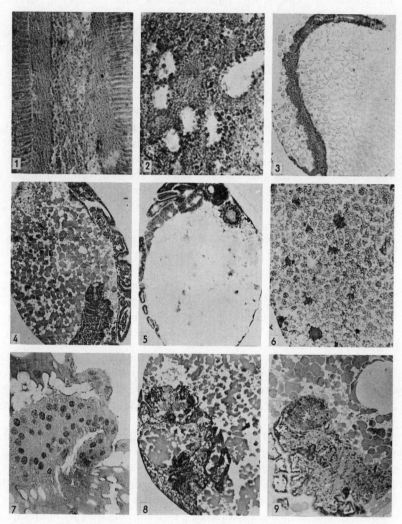

Figure 4 Normal and chemically affected development of the embryo. *Musca domestica*: (1) formation of blastoderm, normal development (after 120 minutes); (2) development inhibited in the stage of a few cleavage nuclei (after 120 minutes). *Pyrrhocoris apterus*: (3) invagination of the germ band, normal development (46 hours); (4) blastokinesis, normal development (110 hours); (5) embryo after blastokinesis, normal development (120 hours); (6) development inhibited at cleavage division; (7) development inhibited in the germ band stage; (8) embryo with a low degree of organization, cuticular structures prevail; (9) development of miniature malformed embryo

be dissected in order to find out whether the pupa is empty (death during metamorphosis).
(4) fecundity and fertility of adults. The number and hatchability of laid eggs (100 eggs are placed on filter paper in a Petri dish, larvae are counted 24 hours later; this is repeated after 48 hours and final hatchability is expressed in per cent). The number of segmented and black non-hatching eggs is recorded. The number of eggs per female can be determined in comparison with the control (individual couples are kept separately).
(5) embryogenesis. Morphological and anatomical evaluation of the state of development at various intervals, using whole mounts or histological preparations. Inhibition of development in early cleavage division, disintegration of nucleic material and later of the entire content of the egg. Death in more advanced stages of embryogenesis is exceptional (e.g. of fully developed larvae). Embryonic death is indicated by different coloration and stainability.
(6) fecundity and fertility of F_1 generation. In the case of strong mutagens, the effects of the chemicals on F_1 generation can be investigated by determining hatchability.
(7) state of ovaries and testes during development. Reproductive organs dissected in physiological solution are first examined using a binocular, then a phase microscope. Histological preparations are made by the usual methods (Figure 18.4).

Administration of low doses of chemicals results in limited hatchability of eggs (or its controlled inhibition) while the normal structure of eggs and normal course of vitellogenesis is preserved. Embryonic development may be inhibited in various phases, an extreme case being the inability of a mature larva to leave the egg.

Changes of another kind are caused by the medium range of concentrations. Typically these changes occur in individual parts of the egg chamber causing the entire structure to change during development, and no eggs are laid. The follicular epithelium, which has an important function in transport and synthesis in the growing egg chamber, is highly susceptible to chemicals. Normally the epithelium is formed by one layer of cells, which do not divide or participate in the development of chorin during the last phase of vitellogenesis. Tested compounds must be administered within 24 hours from adult emergence if effects on follicular cells are to be fully manifested. Later treatment interferes with vitellogenic processes, but the second egg chamber is entirely unaffected. The nucleus of a follicular cell begins to divide within 4–5 days after application of the compound. Mitosis does not occur. The cell grows without dividing, while the nucleic matter continues to divide. The process always begins in the oocyte region and spreads throughout the follicular epithelium. A thick belt of follicular cells with active nuclei is always formed around the egg chamber. Nutritive cells are not affected by this multiplication; however, their nuclei undergo pycnosis or chromatin forms small clusters. Cytoplasm of the nutritive cells vacuolates.

When the tumour-like proliferation of follicular epithelium and nutritive cells within the oocyte disintegrate and are resorbed, only a folded vitelline membrane with small remnants of follicular cells remain at the place of the egg chamber. Almost all egg chambers in the ovary are affected in this way, only a small percentage show signs of yolk deposition with subsequent resorption often accompanied by bizarre shaping of the growing egg chambers. Proliferation also appears in the second egg chamber, but never to such a degree as in the first because of the second chamber's low activity at the time of treatment. The highest doses of chemicals totally inhibit ovarian growth, possibly causing degeneration and resorption at the end of development. However, these effects are occurring at near lethal doses (Figure 2).

Changes in the development of male reproductive organs become apparent in an altered shape of external genitalia, deranged differentiation of reproductive ducts, inhibited development of accessory glands, and disorders in spermatogenesis. Chemicals induce pycnosis of nuclei in spermatogonia, necrosis in spermatocytes, or development of abnormal sperm. These may be malformed in various ways, or immotile (examination of whole mounts). Squash preparations display chromosomal changes, such as translocations or chromosomal bridges. Treatment of adults generally produces changes in the development of sperm or, rarely, tumours in the testes or seminal ducts.

4 THE TESTING OF EFFECTS OF CHEMICALS ON REPRODUCTION IN *PYRRHOCORIS APTERUS* (L.) (HETEROPTERA, PYRRHOCORIDAE)

Adult specimens of *Pyrrhocoris apterus* L. are reared in special cages with nylon netting on the bottom, fed on linden seed and kept at 25 °C and 18-hour photoperiod. Eggs fall from the cages into Petri dishes and are collected at 30-minute intervals. They are then placed on filter paper in a Petri dish and incubated in a thermostatically controlled atmosphere until they hatch.

4.1 Tests on Larvae

A 1 μl drop of acetone solution corresponding to 10 μg with a known concentration of an organic test substance is applied to the first abdominal segment. Development of the reproductive apparatus is examined in connection with moulting into further stages and the fecundity and fertility of adults. Compounds soluble in water are also administered as tap water solutions to experimental insects. The same criteria are examined.

4.2 Tests on Teneral Adults

Chemical compounds are administered to females in the same way as to larvae. The following parameters are then examined: oogenesis; number of eggs per female (compared with control); shape and size of eggs; hatchability; and embryogenesis.

4.3 Tests on Eggs

Either pure compounds or their solutions in acetone or oil (one drop corresponding to 10 μg of pure compound or solution diluted 1:10, 1:100, 1:1000) are applied with a fine glass stick to the anterior or posterior poles of eggs. Other eggs are dipped in the solution or put in contact with paper saturated with an acetone test chemical solution. Only the solvent is applied to control eggs.

4.4 Evaluation of Changes

4.4.1 *Normal Development*

The ovarioles of *Pyrrhocoris apterus* are of the telotrophic type. Future gametes divide and differentiate into oocytes and nutritive cells in the germarium. Yolk is deposited in the vitellarium where oocytes are surrounded with follicular cells. Oocytes in telotophic ovarioles are nurtured by nutritive as well as follicular cells. The nutritive cells remain in the anterior part of the ovariole, sending out cord-like projections through which nutrition flows to the oocytes. The oocyte grows and undergoes maturation division.

The male reproductive apparatus of *Pyrrhocoris apterus* (L.) consists of a pair of testes, each of which is formed by seven testicle tubules opening into the seminal vesicle. Each seminal duct is divided by a fine membrane into apical germarium and a part containing cysts. One, sometimes two, apical cells occur at the apex of each testicle tubule and are conspicuous by a large nucleus rich in chromatin, surrounded by a thin layer of cytoplasm. Cytoplasm is surrounded by a group of pyriform cells, rosette-forming spermatogonia, also with large nuclei and rich granulation. Cysts contain groups of germinal cells of the same developmental stage: spermatogonia, spermatocytes I and II, and spermatids. Spermatozoids are formed in the posterior part of the testicle tubule.

Cysts containing primary spermatocytes have very small, markedly stained nuclei. The lower situated secondary spermatocytes have larger nuclei in which 12 chromosomes can be distinguished. The nuclei of spermatids have large nucleoli. Spermiogenesis takes place in the posterior part of the seminal duct. The first stages of transformation occur in cysts which later burst open, releasing bundles of spermatozoids.

Male and female pronuclei fuse after oviposition and completion of meiotic division. The zygote undergoes several cleavage divisions producing cleavage nuclei. Some of these remain inside the yolk as vitellophages, while the others migrate to the egg surface forming surface periblast and, after formation of cellular membrances separating nuclei, a one-layer blastoderm. The germ band develops from the blastoderm on the ventral side of the egg, and later is invaginated. Segmentation of the embryo is connected with the development of embryonic layers. Stomodaeum and proctodaeum are formed, oral appendages and extremities begin to develop. Blastokinesis (revolution of the embryo) serves to facilitate the utilization of yolk. Dorsal closure then takes place and embryogenesis is completed. The entire embryonic development takes 168–180 hours at 25 °C.

4.4.2 *Changes Induced by Chemicals*

The effects of chemicals appear in the formation of egg chambers. Ovarian development is inhibited and the number of laid eggs is reduced, or eggs differ in size. Inhibition of mitosis in the apical trophocytes results in depletion of the nutritive tissue of older females, followed by disorders in previtellogenesis and activation of oocytes. The ooplasm of young oocytes usually vacuolates. During the division of the prefollicular syncytium, young follicular or interfollicular cells may be deranged. The follicular epithelial cells are unable to produce the nutrients essential for yolk synthesis because of their limited development. Egg chambers often contain two or more oocytes (compound egg chambers) as a result of prefollicular tissue deficiencies caused by inhibition of mitosis in the tissue. Multiplied germinal elements can also arise from the original cystoblast by its supernumerary division.

Chemicals can affect testes morphology as well as spermatogenesis and the vitality of ripe sperm (aspermia or inactivation of sperm from sterilization should be considered). All stages of spermatogenesis can be affected. Results show that spermatogonia undergoing division are the most affected, less affected are young spermatocytes, and least of all the stages of spermateliosis. Whole testes become atrophic along with destruction of germinal cells. The induction of dominant lethal mutations and the effect of compounds on spermatogenesis are often followed by a reduced vitality of sperm.

Compound and small-sized eggs do not develop. With chemicals affecting genetic material, the development of some eggs is inhibited at cleavage division. The others develop until the stage of blastoderm formation, or invagination of the germ band. Aberrations can be observed in the formation of the embryo (absence of certain structures, asymmetric arrangement, clusters of non-differentiated cells, etc.). Malformed miniature embryos frequently occur, as well as inhibition of embryo development at blastokinesis. Also, fully developed larvae die in the eggs. Embryos which ceased to develop in one of the mentioned stages sometimes survive in the egg for quite a long time. Embryonic death shows in a changed colouring of the eggs. Miniature malformed embryos often are abnormally strongly pigmented (Figure 4).

5 THE TESTING OF EFFECTS OF CHEMICALS ON REPRODUCTION IN *SPODOPTERA LITTORALIS* (BOISD.) (LEPIDOPTERA, NOCTUIDAE)

Spodoptera littoralis, the Egyptian cotton leaf worm, is a suitable, non-diapausing species for laboratory rearing. The artificial diet used for this species is composed of beans (200 g), brewer's yeast (20 g), agar (20 g), ascorbic acid (4 g), vitamin mixture (6 g), preserving solution (22 ml), sodium benzoate (1.5 g) and distilled water (1200 ml). The rearing method has been described in detail by Sehnal *et al.* (1976).

Tested compounds can be applied to larvae, pupae and adults either topically or injected in food or by fumigation (see section on *Musca domestica*).

5.1 Evaluation of Changes

5.1.1 *Normal Development*

The female reproductive system consists of two ovaries, each with four polytrophic ovarioles. Previtellarium and vitellarium consist of a chain of developing oocytes. Each oocyte contains 3–5 nutritive cells. The ovarioles develop during the pupal stage.

Testes are clear yellow, located dorsally in the fifth abdominal segment, kidney-shaped. In the last larval instar they are set closely together, surrounded with common epithelial tissue, so that prepupae, pupae and adults seem to be unitesticular. Each testis is formed by four pear-shaped testicular follicles. An apical cell can be found at the end of the testicle tubule around which spermatogonia (globular cells with large nuclei) are concentrated. The zone of encysted spermatogonia is situated dorsally. The whole development of male germinal cells through primary and secondary spermatocytes and spermatids takes place in the cysts. The process of spermatogenesis can be divided into the period of growth, two successive divisions, and a transformation period (Figure 3).

The development of male germinal cells proceeds practically throughout the larval and pupal stages. Spermatogonia multiply in early larval instars. The first primary spermatocytes are found in fourth instar larvae. The first secondary spermatocytes appear in the testes of the penultimate instar. All developmental stages of spermatozoids can be found in the testes of the last larval instar. Transformation of haploid spermatids into spermatozoa occurs in prepupal stages and the process continues in the pupa. More than 95% of mature spermatozoa can be found in adults. Accessory glands, vasa efferentia and others differentiate in the pupa.

5.1.2 Changes Induced by Chemicals

The following changes can appear in females: total degeneration of ovaries, inhibition of mitotic divisions in the germarium, disorders in vitellogenesis, degenerative changes in nutritive cells, derangement of nutritive function, proliferation of follicular epithelium and vacuolation of oocytes. In males, pycnotic nuclei occur in spermatogonia, mitotic and meiotic divisions are deranged and abnormal sperm develop. Proliferation of testicular epithelium or of epithelial cells of spermiducts can occur as well. Degeneration of accessory glands or disorders in their secretory activity take place in some cases. There are also induced changes in chromosomes (chromosomal bridges or translocations, Figure 3).

6 BIBLIOGRAPHY

Borkovec, A. B. (1966). Insect chemosterilants. *Adv. Pest Control Res.* **7**, 143 pages.

Campion, D. G. (1972). Insect chemosterilants: a review. *Bull. Entomol. Res.* **61**, 577–635.

Chang, S. C. (1965). Improved bioassay method for evaluating the potency of chemosterilants against houseflies. *J. econ. Entomol.* **58**, 796.

Crystal, M. M. and LaChance, L. E. (1963). The modification of reproduction in insects treated with alkylating agents. I. Inhibition of ovarian growth and egg production and hatchability. *Biol. Bull.* (*Woods Hole, Mass.*) **125**, 270–279.

Fahmy, O. G. and Fahmy, M. J. (1954). Cytogenetic analysis of the action of carcinogens and known inhibitors in *Drosophila melanogaster*. II. The mechanism of induction of dominant lethals by 2, 4, 6-tri (ethyleneimino)-1, 3, 5-triazine. *J. Genet.* **52**, 603–619.

Kilgore, W. W. (1967). Chemosterilants. In Kilgore, W. W. and Doutt, R. L. (Eds.) *Pest Control*, pp. 197–236. Academic Press, New York.

LaBrecque, G. C. and Smith, C. N. (1968). *Principles of Insect Chemosterilization*, 354 pages. Appleton-Century-Crofts, New York.

LaChance, L. E., Degrugillier, M. and Leverich, A. P. (1969). Comparative effects of chemosterilants on spermatogenic stages in the housefly. I. Induction of dominant lethal mutations in mature sperm and gonial cell death. *Mutat. Res.* **7**, 63–74.

LaChance, L. E. and Leverich, A. P. (1965). Cytogenetic studies on the effect of an alkylating agent on insect nurse cell polytene chromosomes as related to ovarian growth and fecundity. *Genetics* **52**, 453–454 (Abstract).

LaChance, L. E., and Riemann, J. G. (1966). Cytogenetic investigations on radiation and chemically induced dominant lethal mutations in oocytes and sperm of the screwworm fly. *Mutat. Res.* **1**, 318–333.

Landa, V. and Matolin, S. (1971). Effects of chemosterilants on reproductive organs and embryogenesis in insects. In *Proceedings of a Symposium on Sterility Principle for Insect Control or Eradication, Athens, 14–18 September 1970*, pp. 173–182. IAEA Proceedings Series STI/PUB/265.

Landa, V. and Metwally, M. M. (1974). Effects of conventional chemosterilants and juvenile hormone analogues on spermatogenesis in *Trogoderma granarium* (Coleoptera, Dermestidae). *Acta ent. bohemoslov.* **71**, 145–152.

Matolin, S. (1969). The effect of chemosterilants on the embryonic development of *Musca domestica* L. (Diptera, Muscidae). *Acta ent. bohemoslov.* **66**, 65–69.

Matolin, S., Soldán, T. and Landa, V. (1978). Effects of chemosterilants on the reproductive organs of Leptinotarsa decemlineata. *Acta ent. bohemoslov.* **75**, 102–108.

Rezábová, B. (1968). Changes in the metabolism of nucleic acids in the ovaries of the housefly, *Musca domestica*, after application of chemosterilant. *Acta ent. bohemoslov.* **65**, 331–340.

Rezábová, B. and Landa, V. (1967). Effects of 6-azauridine on the development of the ovaries in the housefly *Musca domestica* L. (Diptera). *Acta ent. bohemoslov.* **64**, 344–351.

Sehnal, F., Metwally, M. M. and Gelbič, I. (1976). Reactions of immature stages of noctuid moths to juvenoids. *Z. Angew. Entomol.* **81**, 85–102.

Socha, R. and Gelbič, I. (1973). Stages in the differentiation of ovarian development in *Dixippus morosus*. *Acta entomol. bohemoslov.* **70**, 303–312.

Sunderman, F. W. Jr. (1976). A review of the carcinogenicities of nickel, chromium and arsenic compounds in man and animals. *Prev. Med.* **5**, 279–294.

Valkovic, L. R., and Grosch, D. S. (1968). Apholate-induced sterility in *Bracon hebetor. J. Econ. Ent.* **61**, 1514–1517.

Wild, D. (1978). Cytogenetic effects in the mouse of 17 chemical mutagens and carcinogens evaluated by the micronucleus test. *Mutat. Res.* **56**, 319–327.

Wright, J. E. and Spates, G. E. (1972). Laboratory evaluation of compounds to determine juvenile hormone activity against the stable fly. *J. Econ. Entomol.* **65**, 1346–1349.

Wu, S. H., Oldfield, J. E. and Whanger, P. D. (1971). Effect of selenium, chromium and vitamin *E* on spermatogenesis. *J. Anim. Sci.* **33**, 273.

Methods for Assessing the Effects of Chemicals on Reproductive Functions
Edited by V. B. Vouk and P. J. Sheehan
© 1983 SCOPE

Methods for Assessing the Effects of Chemicals on Reproductive Function in Marine Molluscs

D.R.DIXON

1 INTRODUCTION

Marine molluscs, and in particular those from estuarine and coastal environments, are being increasingly exposed to a wide variety of chemical pollutants resulting from man's activities (i.e. oils and detergents, heavy metals, and halogenated hydrocarbons). In addition to anthropogenic pollution, these organisms also come in contact with chemical substances with biogenic (e.g. algal exudates) and terragenic/lithogenic (e.g. land run-off) origins (Roberts, 1976).

It is now recognized that a number of marine mollusc species have the ability to accumulate toxic chemical substances in their tissues, at levels often far exceeding those present in the surrounding water (Goldberg, 1978). Several of these contaminants are known to inflict damage on the tissues, with the consequence that the life processes of these organisms may become seriously impaired (e.g. Bayne et al., 1979). Such effects finally become realized at the population level as a result of reproductive dysfunction, through reduced fecundity, impaired gamete quality and reduced larval viability (e.g. Bayne, 1972, 1976; Bayne et al., 1975, 1978; Sastry, 1979).

This paper refers, for the most part, to methods relating to the reproductive stages in the life cycle of the bivalve, *Mytilus edulis* L. This has been fully intentional since the blue mussel, and other closely related species, occupies a central position in marine environmental toxicology. As a group, marine mussels are very important to many aspects of the ecology of coastal waters, notably to the productivity of the shallow-water benthos and to aquaculture. This importance is underlined by the adoption of 'marine mussels' as a theme and as subject organisms in several international, pollution-related, biological programmes (e.g. International Biological Programme, see Bayne, 1976; 'mussel watch', see Goldberg, 1978).

Figure 19.1 shows stages in the reproductive cycle of *Mytilus edulis* referred to later in the text. These reproductive stages have been identified for detailed methodological discussion:

(1) gonad (mantle tissues)—stereology;
(2) gametes, embryos and larvae (trochophore and prodissoconch I)—acute toxicity;
(3) gametes and embryos—cytogenetics.

Description is also included of a new and promising test organism for field and laboratory studies of induced embryo abnormalities, the rough periwinkle, *Littorina saxatilis*, which appears for the first time here.

No attempt has been made to give a comprehensive coverage of all methods and approaches that are recorded in the molluscan literature, and which could be applied when assessing the effects of chemicals on reproductive function in the molluscs. It will be noticed that energetic considerations have been omitted from this paper, as have the interesting concept of maternal contributed RNA and its role in early protein synthesis in the larva (e.g. Bayne, 1972; Kidder, 1976; McLean, 1976). Further details of the energetic approach can be found in Bayne (1976) and Bayne *et al.* (1975, 1978, 1979).

2 GONAD CONDITION INDEX

In *Mytilus*, gametes are produced in transitory follicles located in the mantle which lines the shell valves (Figure 1). There is a well-defined annual cycle relating to the reproductive processes in *Mytilus*, with a marked alternation between the periods of nutrient accumulation and gamete production (e.g. Lubet, 1957; Seed, 1975; Lowe *et al.*, 1982). The timing and pattern of gamete release is dependent upon climatic and geographic factors (Bayne, 1976); in Britain, populations living in the north spawn only once a year (late spring), whereas those in the south west, an area of milder winters and warmer summers, may spawn twice, once in spring and again in late summer (Seed, 1976).

This gametogenic rhythm is susceptible to disturbance from a number of physical and chemical factors in the environment. Recent studies by Lowe in this laboratory have demonstrated quantitative techniques for assessing the gametogenic cycle and its disruption by environmental disturbance. What follows is taken in large part from Lowe *et al.* (1982). Both natural (e.g. climatic) and anthropogenic (chemical pollution) stressors have been shown in the laboratory, and under field conditions, to produce quantitative changes in mantle condition in exposed populations of mussels. By measuring, with *stereological techniques*, the relative volume fractions of the vesicular cells (VC), adipogranular cells (ADG) (these two cell types comprising the nutrient store of the mantle) and the developing and ripe gametes, Lowe has been able to derive precise information relating to the reproductive status of mussels from polluted and unpolluted populations, or, by repeated sampling, obtain a quantified expression of the changes in mantle condition attributable to their exposure.

Preliminary investigations showed that the distribution of reproductive

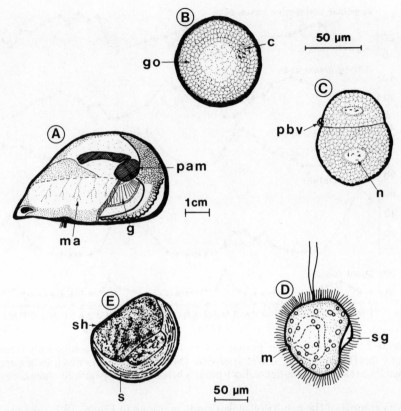

Figure 1 Life-cycle stages of *Mytilus edulis*, referred to in the text. A, adult mussel with one shell valve removed to display the internal organs; B, egg; C, 2-cell embryo showing asymmetrical first cleavage; D, trochophore larva at 24 hours (drawn from Sastry, 1979); E, prodissoconch I-stage (first shell) larva at 48 hours; c, chromosomes; g, gill; go, granular ooplasm; m, mouth; ma, mantle; n, nucleus; pam, posterior adductor muscle; pbv, polar body vesicle; s, shell; sg, shell gland; sh, straight hinge

follicles throughout the whole of the mantle is not subject to planorelated variation, i.e. are for all practical purposes distributed at random with respect to mantle orientation. Consequently, a reasonable estimation of the overall mantle condition can be derived simply from examination of a thin section taken in any one plane. In our laboratory, tissue sections at $5 \mu m$ are examined with a Zeiss (Jena) compound microscope fitted with a Weibel eyepiece graticule (Graticules Ltd) at a magnification of × 240. Point counts (Weibel and Elias, 1967) on ADG cells, VC cells, developing and morphologically ripe gametes, and areas of empty follicles resulting from spawning activity are made on five fields per animal to quantify the volume fraction of the different tissue components.

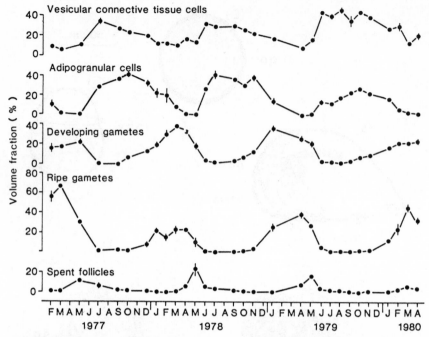

Figure 2   Volume fractions (means ± 1 s.e.) of mantle tissue components from Tal-y-foel (Menai straits, N. Wales) mussels. Only standard errors which are greater than 2% are shown in the figure. Each point is based on five separate determinations

An example of the results of such a study is shown in Figure 19.2, taken from Lowe *et al.* (1982). The factors controlling the seasonal cycle of the various cell types are complex but the cycle is susceptible to alteration by pollution and preliminary evidence suggests that quantification by stereology will provide a powerful technique for determining reproductive disturbance in this and in other species.

3 ACUTE TOXICITY TESTS WITH LARVAL BIVALVES

The larvae of a number of marine bivalve mollusca (*Crassostrea virginica* Gmelin, *Crassostrea gigas* Thunberg, *Mytilus edulis* L.) have been incorporated into standardized, short-term, acute toxicity test procedures for use in evaluating pure compounds singly or in mixtures. They can also be used to measure the acute toxicity of marine and estuarine waters, and the acceptability of salt waters for culturing and testing fish and macroinvertebrates (ASTM, 1980). The stages identified for study of toxic effects are fertilized egg, trochophore larva, and 48-hours old prodissoconch I larva ('straight-hinge' or 'D-shaped' stage) (Figure 1). The following description applies for all four species identified above.

Embryos and larvae of other planktonic-spawning bivalves (Sastry, 1979) may be used in place of these, but modifications of the adult conditioning, spawning and testing regimens frequently are required (e.g. Cain, 1973; Rhodes *et al.*, 1975).

Adult bivalves possessing developing gonads are brought to the laboratory, cleaned of all fouling organisms and detritus, and to ensure complete maturation of their gametes are held (conditioned) in circulating seawater tanks at specified temperatures several degrees above the field temperature when the adults were collected. A balanced diet is essential during this period (e.g. Bayne, 1965). Spawning is induced with one or more selected physical (e.g. temperature), chemical (e.g. KCl), or biological stimuli, as discussed later. Selected densities ($< 35,000/1$) of the embryos are exposed to the toxicant for 48 hours, during which the embryos normally will develop into fully shelled larvae (prodissoconch I stage).

Toxicity to the prodissoconch I stage is measured as the 48-hour median effective concentration (EC_{50}) based on abnormal shell development and the 48-hour median lethal concentration (LC_{50}). Other responses may include decreased fertilization, and decreases in the rates of development of specified stages (e.g. trochophore, veliger, prodissoconch I larva).

The results describe the responses of the larvae to short-term exposures to toxicant(s) under a set of environmental conditions. Temperature, pH, salinity, suspended solids, and organic metabolites from phytoplankton and bacteria are some of the water quality characteristics that may influence the effect of the toxicant by stressing the developing embryos or larvae or by altering the physicochemical form, availability, or concentration of the toxicant. Specific guidelines are laid down regarding test procedures in standard E 724–80, published by the American Society for Testing and Materials (ASTM, 1980).

4 CHROMOSOMAL ABERRATIONS AND RELATED EFFECTS

The embryos of *Mytilus edulis* are excellent material for cytogenetic analysis, and have featured in a number of studies of a cytotaxonomic nature (e.g. Menzel, 1968; Ahmed and Sparks, 1970; Ieyama and Inaba, 1974). More recently, both indirect and direct evidence has been presented for induced chromosomal aberrations in the cells of adult mussels and their embroys, exposed to chronic levels of chemical pollution (aromatic hydrocarbons) under other wise natural conditions (Lowe and Moore, 1978; Dixon, 1982). These results, coupled with information from chemical investigations conducted in the laboratory (Dixon and Clarke, 1982), indicate that the chromosomes of *Mytilus* (and other marine molluscs) are sensitive to damage inflicted by certain classes of chemical pollutants in the marine environment.

The chemical effects of pollution impinging on the genetic material of marine

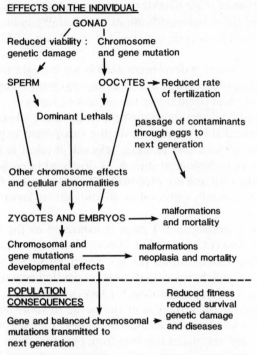

Figure 19.3   Genetic and related effects caused by toxicants impinging on the sensitive reproductive stages of a marine invertebrate. The diagram shows how the effect may be realized, as chromosome damage or otherwise, at the same stage, a closely related stage or much later on, even into the next generation

invertebrates may not always be expressed at the same stage in development as the one in which the damage was incurred. Instead, the consequences to the carrier cell, or individual may not be fully realized until some much later stage in development, even into the next generation (Figure 3).

Apart from strictly genetic effects, of a chromosomal nature or otherwise (i.e. gene mutations), there are some other types of damage resulting from pollution exposure (Table 1). When associated with the germ cells, dose–response relationships may be described in terms of fertilization rate or rates of embryogenesis. Fertilization rate measurements can be applied to both laboratory and field studies to assess either the viability of the gametes in water containing a named toxicant at a defined dose, or the condition of sperms and/or eggs originating from mussel populations exposed to pollution.

Sperm head abnormalities show a high correlation with mutagenicity for a range of chemical substances, including aromatic hydrocarbons, and could be

Table 1   The different reproductive stages of *Mytilus edulis* which can be used in testing for gentically harmful agents in seawater

Material exposed to toxicant	Maximum exposure time	Stage at which scored	Observed effects
Gonad (adult mussel)	Months	Sperms	Malformations of head
		Oocytes	Chromosome damage, e.g. translocation heterozygotes, aneuploids and polyploids
Gametes	1.5 hours (s.); 6 hour (oo.)	Fertilization	Reduced rate
Fertilized oocytes	1 hour	Same or early cleavage	Chromosomal and cellular abnormalities, e.g. abnormal polar body vesicle, septate ooplasm
Early stage embryos (< 8 cells)	7 hours	Same	Chromosomal aberrations, i.e. numerical and structural abnormalities; developmental effects, e.g. premature loss of synchrony, malformations

s., sperms; oo., oocytes

applied routinely to field monitoring of pollution-stressed mussel populations. Since this effect has its origin at some stage during spermatogenesis (as yet undefined), laboratory screening of chemicals with this technique, would require the maintenance of groups of mussels, collected from clean sites, under conditions of temperature and feeding suitable for gametogenesis to take place (Bayne, 1965; Hrs-Brenko, 1973), while in the presence of controlled levels of toxicant. Effects on synchrony of development and the different types of developmental abnormalities arising from contact with polluting substances can similarly be applied to both laboratory and field studies. Table 19.1 shows the various reproductive stages of *Mytilus* (or other similar mollusc) which have been identified for the investigation of chemical effects, the types of effects observed at any particular stage, and the range of exposure times it is possible to achieve by selecting different reproductive tissues. It is evident that the system has considerable flexibility and consequently is capable of being adapted to suit the particular requirements of the investigator; recognizing the limitations imposed only by the biological material itself.

4.1 Spawning

A large literature has grown up around this subject; for key references see reviews by Bayne (1976) and Sastry (1979). A female mussel will produce during the course of a single breeding season something in the order of 3 million eggs. These eggs are not all released at one time; spawning may be protracted, taking a period of days or even weeks, depending upon local conditions of temperature, tidal cycle, etc. In the laboratory mussels must be stimulated to spawn artificially by means of chemical or physical stimuli, or combinations of both types. The methods reported range from mechanical shaking (in a bucket), to mild electrical shocks, temperature stimuli, and various chemical techniques (for further discussion of these methods see above references).

First and foremost, it is important that the animals should be in a reproductively ripe state. Mantle squashes should reveal large numbers of mature gametes in both sexes. Ripe oocytes are large ($\simeq 70$ μm in diameter), orange in colour, and lack any sign of the stalk which attaches the immature oocyte to the follicle wall. When first released from the mantle tissues the spermatozoa are inactive, but should become motile after a few minutes contact with sea water.

Mussels containing ripe gametes can be induced to spawn artificially by first injecting 0.5 ml of 0.5 M KCl into a large central blood sinus of the posterior adductor muscle; the shell valves should be wedged apart during this procedure. After needle and wedge are removed, the mussels should be placed beneath a 60-watt lamp for about 20 minutes until the shells have warmed through. This is followed by imersion in seawater at 20 °C, taking care to release any air trapped inside the shell when doing so. Spawning should commence within the next few hours. Using this method the author has consistently obtained 50% or greater spawning success.

To avoid early fertilization of newly spawned eggs, any males which are seen to be releasing sperms should be transferred to a separate container and the water in the holding tank changed. As a further precaution, the eggs should be pipetted into small beakers and the water changed to remove any sperms which may present.   Adult mussels collected at the time of the population spawning can be kept temporarily in tanks of water at 5 °C, to prevent them from releasing gametes. Ten days before a supply of gametes is required, the mussels should be transferred, by stepwise changes (2–3 °C every 2–3 days), to water at 15 °C. It is important to feed them continuously, with a balanced algal diet (Bayne, 1976), to prevent loss of condition and concomitant resorption of gametes during this transition period.

4.2 Gamete Studies

Sperms remain viable for only 1–2 hours, depending upon the temperature, whereas eggs remain viable for up to 6 hours following their release.

Table 2   Methods for the treatment of material prior to scoring for genetic and related effects in the embryos of *Mytilus edulis*

A   Spawn adult mussels and introduce sperms to eggs (i) in sea water or (ii) sea water with toxicant added. Leave to develop for 1 hour at 10°C. Centrifuge $(1 \times 10^3$ revs/min/180 g for 2 min) and resuspend in sea water, repeat twice. Finally resuspend in original medium.
B   Allow to develop for a further hour.
C   Allow to develop for a further 2.5 hours and 6.5 hours (to allow for mitotic inhibition). Harvest embryos at the end of each period by slow centrifugation $(1 \times 10^3$ revs/180g for 2 min).
D   Replace medium with a dilute (0.01%) colchicine solution in seawater. After 2 hours dilute volume by 50% with distilled water and leave embryos in this hypotonic solution for 30 min.
E   Fix in 3 separate changes of Carnoy's fixative (ethanol, 3 parts: glacial acetic acid, 1 part: chloroform, 1%).
F   Mount in fixative and examine under medium power phase-contrast objective.
G   Mount and stain in aceto-orcein. Scan under low power and examine with high-power, oil immersion lens.

Type of effect	Field collected mussels	Embryo toxicity studies
Fertilization rate	Ai, B, E, F	Aii, B, E, F
Numerical chromosome aberrations	Ai, B, D, E, G	Aii, C, D, E, G
Structural chromosomal aberrations, metaphase analysis	Ai, B, D, E, G	Aii, C, D, E, G
Structural chromosomal aberrations, anaphase analysis	Ai, B, E, G	Aii, C, E, G
Developmental abnormalities	Ai, C, E, G	Aii, C, E, G

Sperms for sperm head abnormality investigations need to be separated from the seawater by centrifugation $(2 \times 10^3$ revs/min per 360 g for 2 min) and resuspended in 3% ammonium formate (isotonic) to remove salt contamination. Following this treatment they should be recentrifuged and fixed with Carnoy's fixative (Table 19.2E), after which they can be mounted on a slide in a drop of fixative, the edges of the coverglass need to be sealed with glycerol–gelatin (Sigma) to reduce evaporation, and examined under high power with phase-contrast microscopy. Alternatively, smears can be prepared, at the ammonium formate stage, the smears air dried, and subsequently stained with eosin as described in the method for mammalian spermatozoa by Bryan (1970). See also Bruce *et al.* (1974).

In *Mytilus* the eggs are spawned in the germinal vesicle stage, although the germinal vesicle soon disrupts and development (of the *oocyte*) proceeds to metaphase of the first meiotic division (egg maturation), where further development is delayed until after penetration by the sperm (Longo and Anderson, 1969). It follows that if sufficient time is allowed for the completion of prophase I by the newly spawned oocytes, in the absence of sperms, it is possible to score the metaphase plates for abnormal chromosome complements. Because of the reduced number of the units present at this stage, as a result of synapsis, it is not usually necessary to treat the occytes in any special manner other than fix them at fertilization + 2 hours. It is possible to see both numerical (aneuploid) and structural aberrations (translocation heterozygotes) at this stage (Figure 4A)

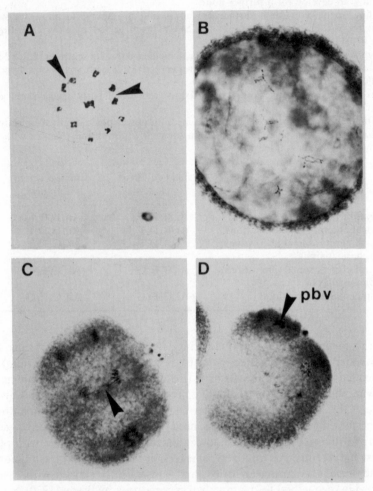

Figure 4   Normal and abnormal embryos. A, metaphase I chromosome complement with reciprocal translocation resulting in a quadrivalent configuration (arrowed); B, recently released oocyte at diplotene stage of prophase I, showing chiasmata in their primary positions; C, chromosome bridge (dicentric chromosome) linking anaphase chromatids; D, abnormal polar body vesicle (pbv), containing ooplasm, in a cell undergoing meiotic metaphase II

but the latter are better seen in freshly spawned material which is still at prophase I, (Figure 19.4B), and has yet to commence chiasma terminalization.

4.3 Fertilization Rate

Table 1 shows methods which are now being used routinely to detect chemical damage in the gametes and early-stage embryos of *Mytilus* (and other planktonic spawning marine invertebrates). Fertilization is a complex process (Monroy, 1965) involving a series of events: contact between the sperm and the egg, activation of the egg, and fusion of male and female pronuclei, which results in formation of the zygote nucleus.

Sperm penetration occurs within 5 minutes of first contact with the egg, and fusion of the male and female pronuclei after about an hour, at 20 °C. It is possible therefore to manipulate the experimental conditions to find which stage is particularly sensitive to chemical perturbation, by altering the timing and period of exposure the gametes receive. For most puposes, it is sufficient to effect fertilizations in the presence of a known concentration of toxicant and leave the eggs to develop for an hour. After this time the excess sperms are rinsed off (Table 19.2A), to prevent their remaining as contaminants on the egg surface, and the eggs left to develop for a further hour in the presence of the toxicant. By this time all fertilized eggs will have produced polar bodies, and may have commenced cleavage, and hence are distinguishable from those which are not fertilized.

With all investigations involving fertilizations, it is necessary to standardize the procedures relating to sperm and egg concentrations. It is very important not to crowd the eggs, nor to introduce too great a number of sperms (Gruffydd and Beaumont, 1970), since this can lead in decreased fertilization rate, abnormal development and polyspermy. The optimum ratio of sperms to egg is 15:1.

4.4 Chromosomal Aberrations

There are two recognized classes of chromosomal abnormalities, numerical aberrations (aneuploids, haplo/polyploids) and structural defects (achromatic gaps, chromatid deletions (open chromatid break), chromatid exchange, etc). Both classes are scorable in early stage embryos (≤ 8 cells). Later stages should be avoided due to the small size of the chromosomes and the much greater risk of overlap between adjacent cells. *Mytilus* embryos have a cell-doubling time of 90 minutes at 10 °C.

Numerical aberrations may be scored in embryos from both field- and laboratory-exposed populations (Dixon, 1982), but slightly different treatments are required in each case (Table 2). Those embryos originating from samples of mussels taken from polluted field sites need to be examined when at the first, and no later than the second mitotic metaphase (alternatively the prophase I oocytes should be examined, see above) to record aberrations in their primary state (Savage, 1975). Since the embryos have a rapid rate of cell turnover, the chromosomes do not normally achieve a state of chromatin condensation that is characteristic of more slowly growing tissues. Consequently, it is necessary to treat the cells with colchicine (Table 2D) to condense the DNA and make the individual chromosome units more easy to discern, followed by exposure to a hypotonic medium to separate them. The normal diploid number for the genus *Mytilus* is 28 chromosomes. Because planktonic spawning marine invertebrates release their young at a very early stage in their development, these organisms have not developed mechanisms for jettisoning genetically defective progeny prior to the time of their normal release (c.f. mammals). A corollary of this is that the frequency of genetically abnormal offspring amongst control groups of embryos is normally higher ($\simeq 10\%$). than is found in full-term embryos from other groups (e.g. man, Jacobs, 1972). There is good agreement however between this control value (Figure 5) and the 'primary incidence' reported for mammals (Jacobs 1972; Fraser and Maudlin, 1979).

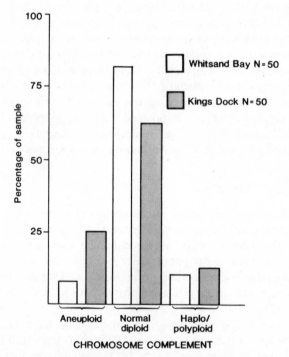

Figure 5 Percentage-frequencies of normal and abnormal chromosome complements in mussel embryos originating from polluted (King's Dock) and control (Whitsand Bay) environments

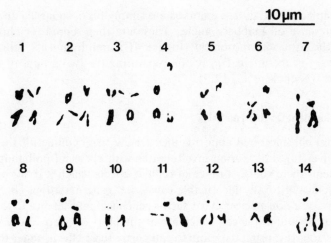

Figure 6   Karyotype for *Mytilus edulis* from King's Dock, S. Wales, based on a colchicine-treated metaphase from a 2-cell embryo. Photographed under phase contrast after staining with aceto-orcein

The normal karyotype for *Mytilus edulis* (from King's Dock, S. Wales) is shown in Figure 6, composed of colchicine-treated metaphase chromosomes from a 2-cell embryo. The chromosomes are large, homomorphic, and isopycnotic (consequently autosomal); there is evidence of balanced polymorphisms in some mussel populations (Ahmed and Sparks, 1970). The karyotype is divisible into four groups based on chromosome size (excluding centromeric distance) and position of the centromere (arm ratio): pairs 1–6 (Group A, metacentric), pairs 7 and 8 (Group B, submetacentric) pairs 9–13 (Group C, subtelocentric), and pair 14 (Group D, telocentric). With a karyotype of this type it is clearly possible to obtain detailed information relating to structural changes, and in some instances to identify the particular chromosomes affected. Methods for the treatment of laboratory and field material are given in Table 2.

It is generally recognized that metaphase analysis is particularly time consuming especially when investigating structural abnormalities, and requires a high degree of analytical skill on the part of the investigator. Detailed analysis of material collected over a few days in the laboratory may take many months of painstaking work to analyse. This has lead many cytogeneticists to opt for the simpler, anaphase method of analysis for structural chromosomal aberrations. Whilst only detailed metaphase analysis will provide comprehensive information relating to all the *visible* structural aberrations present in a cell, the reduction in sensitivity associated with anaphase analysis is outweighed by the greater numbers of cells which it is possible to analyse in a given time (Ad Hoc Committee of the EMS, 1972).

For anaphase analysis, the embryos are simply fixed, squashed and scanned for the presence of anaphase nuclei. These are then scored for chromosome bridges (dicentric chromosomes) (Figure 4C) and fragments (chromosome breaks) lying in the intercalary region separating the two groups of migrating chromatids (Nichols *et al.*, 1977).

4.5 Developmental Abnormalities

Apart from chromosomal abnormalities arising from contact of the sensitive reproductive stages of marine invertebrates with chemical pollutants in their environment, there is also a range of cellular effects which it is not possible to relate specifically to any identifiable cause, i.e. gene mutation, chromosomal aberration, or a non-nuclear event such as chemical interference to the electro-chemical gradients in the cell which are at the basis of controlled growth and differentiation. It is usual therefore to categorize these effects under the general heading of *teratogenic* effects.

As is perhaps to be expected, a wide variety of different developmental abnormalities are possible, and do occur in embryos as a result of chemical interference. These range from small effects, such as the pinching off of small amounts of ooplasm into the polar body vesicle (Figure 4D) and the premature loss of synchrony in division stages, leading to uneven cell numbers, 3, 5, 7, etc., instead of the usual 2, 4, 8 etc., to major effects such as the complete schism (separation) of sister cells, with a resultant failure to produce an integrated embryo. Other effects include the formation of false septal membranes across cells without any accompanying nuclear division—this type should be watched for when measuring embryos for fertilization rate, where it is

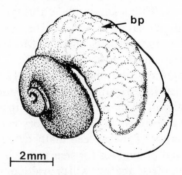

Figure 7 Female *Littorina saxatilis* removed from its shell to show the dorsally positioned brood pouch (bp) on the first body whorl

important to include only those embryos which have one or more obvious polar bodies.

I have found the gastropod *Littorina saxatilis* a convenient organism for scoring embryo abnormalities. Gastopod molluscs belonging to the *Littorina*

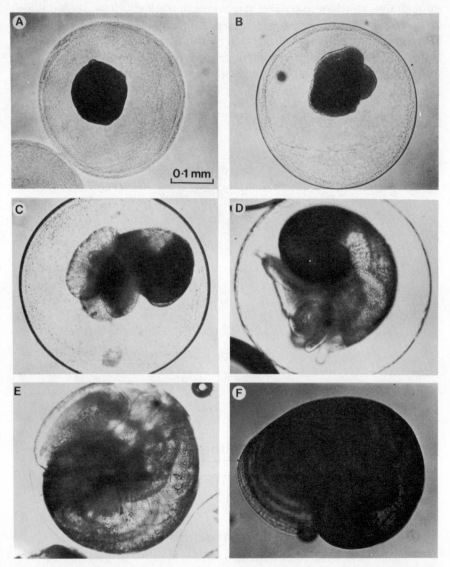

Figure 8   Normal embryonic development of *Littorina saxatilis*. A, egg (0–2 days); B, unshelled veliger (3–8 days); C, shelled veliger (9–20 days); D, late veliger (21–36 days), E, pre-emergent young (36–60 days); F, emergent stage (preserved specimen)

saxatilis 'species-complex' (Heller, 1975; Smith, 1981) retain their developing young in a specialized brood pouch, which is borne dorsally on the first body whorl of the female (Figure 7). Fertilization is internal and the fertilized eggs are passed directly from the oviduct, as batches of up to 50 in number, into the proximal region of the brood pouch, where development proceeds (Figure 8) through five, clearly recognizable stages (egg, unshelled veliger, shelled veliger (early and late), and pre-emergent young), culminating in the passive release of fully formed offspring some 60 days after fertilization (Berry, 1956; Hughes and Roberts, 1980). Adult females contain upwards of 200 embryos at any one time, with reproduction continuing throughout the year, although there is evidence of

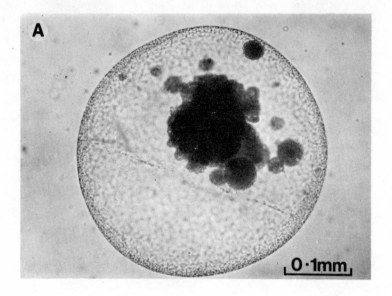

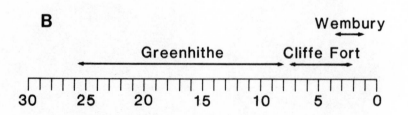

Number of abnormals per individual

Figure 9   A, Abnormal stage II *Littorina* embryo; B, frequency of abnormal embryos ($\bar{x} \pm 2$ s.e.) in three populations (N values = 20) exposed to different levels of pollution. Greenhithe is the most polluted site and Wembury is the cleanest

a summer decline in reproductive activity in some populations. Copulating pairs are to be observed at other times of the year, on the upper shore during low tide. Ovulation occurs between 17 and 48 hours following mating (Thorson, 1946; Berry, 1956).

Littorina saxatilis lives well under laboratory conditions, where it will continue to reproduce as small laboratory populations, so long as these are provided with a regular supply of algal covered rocks. Because of its brooding habit, relatively small numbers of embryos (compared to planktonic spawners such as *Mytilus*), and tolerances to salinity variation and enclosure conditions, *Littorina* is a good subject for studies of the effects of chemicals on fecundity and embryo viability (growth and development) both in the field and in the laboratory. Some preliminatry results in Figure 19.9 suggest that population differences may be considerable and can be related to environmental pollution.

ACKNOWLEDGEMENTS

I should like to express my indebtedness to the following: R. Cardwell for permission to quote from ASTM standard E 724–80, the late Clare Hawke for drawing several of the figures, D. Nicholson for photographic advice and assistance, and Roberta Grose for typing the manuscript.

This work forms part of the Experimental Ecology Programme of the Institute for Marine Environmental Research, a component of the Natural Environmental Research Council.

Appendix

Type of test	Test organism	Sensitivity	Initial cost	Running cost
Gonad condition index	*Mytilus*	Medium	Medium–high	Low
Genetic and related effects	*Mytilus*	Medium–high	High	Medium
Larval acute toxicity	*Mytilus*	High	Medium	Medium
Developmental abnormalities	*Littorina*	Not known	Low	Low

(including man-hours)

5 REFERENCES

Ad Hoc Committee of the Environmental Mutagen Society. (1972). Report of 1972. Chromosome methodologies in mutation testing. *Toxic. appl. Pharmac.* **221**, 269–275.

Ahmed, M. and Sparks, A. K. (1970). Chromosome number, structure and autosomal polymorphism in the marine mussels *Mytilus edulis* and *Mytilus californianus. Biol. Bull. (Woods Hole, Mass.)* **138**, 1–13.

ASTM (American Society for Testing and Materials) (1980). Standard practice for conducting static acute toxicity tests with larvae of four species of bivalve molluscs. In *Annual Book of ASTM Standards, E 724–80.* Philadelphia.

Bayne, B. L. (1965). Growth and the delay of metamorphosis of the larve of *Mytilus edulis* (L.) *Ophelia* 2, 1–47.

Bayne, B. L. (1972). Some effects of stress in the adult on the larval development of *Mytilus edulis. Nature (London)* **237**, 459.

Bayne, B. L. (Ed.) (1976). *Marine Mussels: Their Ecology and Physiology.* Cambridge University Press. Cambridge, London, New York, Melbourne.

Bayne, B. L., Gabbott, P. A. and Widdows, J. (1975). Some effects of stress in the adult on the eggs and larvae of *Mytilus edulis* L. *J. mar. biol. Ass. U. K.* **55**, 675–689.

Bayne, B. L., Holland, D. L., Lowe, D. M., Moore, M. D. and Widdows, J. (1978). Further studies on the effects of stress in the adult on the eggs and larvae of *Mytilus edulis* L. *J. mar. biol. Ass. U. K.* **58**, 825–841.

Bayne, B. L., Moore, M. N., Widdows, J., Livingstone, D. R. and Salkeld, P. (1979). Measurement of the responses of individuals to environmental stress and pollution: Studies with bivalve molluscs. *Phil. Trans. R. Soc. Lond. B. Biol. Sci.* **286**, 563–581.

Berry, A. J. (1956). *Some Factors Affecting the Distribution of* Littorina saxatilis *(Olivi),* 157 pages. Ph. D. Thesis, University of London.

Bruce, W. R., Furrer, R. and Wyrobek, A. J. (1974). Abnormalities in the shape of murine sperm after acute testicular irradiation. *Mutat. Res.* **23**, 381–386.

Bryan, J. H. D. (1970). An eosin-fast green-naphthol yellow mixture for differential staining of cytologic components in mammalian spermatozoa. *Stain Technol.* **45**, 231–236.

Cain, T. D. (1973). The combined effects of temperature and salinity on embryos and larvae of the clam *Rangia cunelata. Mar. Biol. (Berlin)* **21**, 1–6.

Dixon, D. R. (1982). Aneuploidy in mussel embryos (*Mytilus edulis*) originating from a polluted dock. *Mar. Biol. Lett.* **2**, 155–161.

Dixon, D. R. and Clarke, K. R. 1982. Sister chromatid exchange: a sensitive method for detecting damage caused by exposure to environmental mutagens in the chromosomes of adult *Mytilus edulis. Mar. Biol. Letters,* **3**, 163–172.

Fraser, L. R. and Maudlin, I. (1979). Analysis of aneuploidy in first-cleavage mouse embryos fertilized *in vitro* and *in vivo. Environ. Health Perspect.* **31**, 141–149.

Goldberg, E. D. (1978). The mussel watch. *Environ. Conserv.* **5**, 1–25.

Gruffydd, L. D. and Beaumont, A. R. (1970). Determination of the optimum concentration of eggs and spermatozoa for the production of normal larvae in *Pecten maximus* (Mollusca, Lamellibranchia). *Helgol. wiss. Meeresunters.* **20**, 486–497.

Heller, J. (1975). The taxonomy of some British *Littorina* spp. with notes on their reproduction (Mollusca: Prosobranchia). *J. Linn. Soc. Lond. Zool.* **56**, 131–152.

Hrs-Brenko, M. (1973). Gonad development, spawning and rearing of *Mytilus edulis* larvae. *Stud. Rev. Gen. Fish. Counc. Mediterr.* **53**, 53–65.

Hughes, R. N. and Roberts, D. J. (1980). Reproductive effort of winkles (*Littorina* spp.) with contrasted methods of reproduction. *Oecologia (Berlin)* **47**, 130–136.

Ieyama, H. and Inaba, A. (1974). Chromosome numbers of ten species in four families of Pteriomorphia (Bivalvia). *Venus Jpn. Malacol.* **33**, 129–137.

Jacobs, E. M. (1972). Human population cytogenetics. *Proceedings of the IVth International Congress on Human Genetics,* pp. 232–242. Excerpta Medica, Amsterdam.

Kidder, G. M. (1976). RNA synthesis and the ribosomal cistrons in early molluscan development. *Am. Zool.* **16**, 501–520.

Longo, F. J. and Anderson, E. (1969). Cytological aspects of fertilization in the lamellibranch *Mytilus edulis*. 1. Polar body formation and development of the female pronucleus. *J. exp. Zool.* **172**, 69–96.

Lowe, D. M. and Moore, M. N. (1978). Cytology and quantitative cytochemistry of a proliferative atypical hemocytic condition in *Mytilus edulis* (Bivalvia, Mollusca). *J. Natn. Cancer Inst.* **60**, 1455–1459.

Lowe, D. M., Moore, M. N., and Bayne, B. L. (1982). Aspects of gameto-genesis in the marine mussel *Mytilus edulis* L. *J. mar. Biol. Assoc. UK* **62**, 133–145.

Lubet, P. (1957). Cycle sexuel de *Mytilus edulis* L. et de *Mytilus galloprovincialis* Lmk. dans le Bassin d'Arcachon (Gironde). *Anée Bilogique* **33**, 19–29.

McLean, K. (1976). Some aspects of RNA synthesis in oyster development. *Am. Zool.* **16**, 521–528.

Menzel, R. W. (1968). Chromosome number in nine families of pelecypod mollusks. *Nautilus* **82**, 45–58.

Monroy, A. (1965). Biochemical aspects of fertilization. In Weber, R. (Ed.) *The Biochemistry of Animal Development.* Vol. 1. *Descriptive Biochemistry of Animal Development,* pp. 73–135. Academic Press, New York and London.

Nichols, W. W., Miller, R. C. and Bradt, C. (1977). *In vitro* anaphase and metaphase preparation in mutation testing. In Kilbey, B. J. *Handbook of Mutagenicity Test Procedures,* pp. 225–233. Elsevier Scientific Publishing Co., Amsterdam, New York, Oxford.

Rhodes, E. W., Calabrese, A., Cable, W. D. and Landers, W. S. (1975). The development of methods for rearing the coot clam, *Mulinia lateralis*, and three species of coastal bivalves in the laboratory. In Smith, W. L. and Chenley, M. H. (Eds.). *Culture of Marine Invertebrate Animals.* Plenum Press, New York.

Roberts, D. (1976). Mussels and pollution. In Bayne, B. L. (Ed.) *Marine Mussels: Their Ecology and Physiology,* pp. 67–80. Cambridge University Press, New York and Cambridge, England

Sastry, A. N. (1979). Pelecypoda (excluding Ostreidae). In Giese, A. C. and Pearse, J. S. (Eds.) *Reproduction of Marine Invertebrates,* Vol 5. *Molluscs: Pelecypods and Lesser Classes,* pp. 113–292. Academic Press, New York, San Francisco, London.

Savage, J. R. K. (1975). Classification and relationships of induced chromosomal structural changes. *J. med. Genet.* **12**, 103–122.

Seed, R. (1975). Reproduction in *Mytilus* (Mollusca: Bivalvia) in European waters. *Publ. Stn. Zool. Napoli* **39**, 317–334.

Seed, R. (1976). Ecology. In Bayne, B. L. (Ed.) *Marine Mussels: Their Ecology and Physiology,* pp. 13–65. Cambridge University Press, Cambridge, London, New York, Melbourne.

Smith, J. E. (1981). The natural history and taxonomy of shell variation in the periwinkle *Littorina rudis. J. Mar. Biol. Ass. U.K.* **61**, 215–241.

Thorson, G. (1946). Reproduction and larval development of Danish marine-bottom invertebrates. *Medd. Dan. Fisk. Havunders., Serie Plankton* **4**, 1–523.

Weibel, E. R. and Elias, H. (1967). *Quantitative Methods in Morphology* Springer Verlag, Berlin, Heidelberg, New York.

Methods for Assessing the Effects of Chemicals on Reproduction in Marine Worms

BERTIL ÅKESSON

1 INTRODUCTION

The purpose of this contribution is to describe and discuss current methods of assessing changes in the reproductive biology of marine worms caused by chemicals. Marine worms are found in several major animal taxa. As some of these taxa are dealt with in another contribution, this paper will be confined to marine annelids. Within the phylum Annelida, most of the pertinent marine research has been confined to the polychaetes.

Polychaetes are extremely varied in size and external morphology. Their structural diversity makes possible a wide range of adaptations to marine habitats. They constitute a dominant group on intertidal mud flats and in subtidal soft bottom communities. According to Knox (1977) polychaetes are a dominant or important component of soft bottom communities when measured as a number of species, number of specimens, proportion of standing crop or productivity. In a transect from a depth of 100 to 5000 m off the east coast of North America, Sanders *et al.* (1965) reported that polychaetes constituted an average of 60% of all specimens collected. The number of polychaete specimens was greatest at depths of 200–400 m. Similarly, Knox (1977) reviewed 61 community studies and reported that polychaetes averaged 44% of species number and of the number of individuals.

Benthic community analyses of polluted areas in various parts of the world have disclosed that polychaetes were the dominant group of animals and that some species, in particular *Capitella capitata*, could serve as an indicator species of heavy pollution.

Polychaetes possess a variety of feeding types with the majority being either deposit–detrital feeders or suspension feeders. They play a significant role in the food web and are important food for other invertebrates, fish and birds.

By tube building and other types of sediment reworking, polychaetes can alter the sediment characteristics in ways that may change its attraction to other organisms.

In summary, polychaetes are important members of most marine communities

459

and one of the major food resources for fish and crustaceans of economic significance. At the community level they often play critical roles in shallow water ecosystems and have been shown to respond rapidly to environmental perturbations. Methods have been developed in the last decade to utilize polychaetes in toxicity bioassay studies. In a selected number of species, the whole life cycle is available for toxicity testing.

The pollution ecology of polychaetes has recently been comprehensively reviewed by Reish (1979). Reish has devoted most of his academic carrier to pollution research, both field studies and laboratory assays. In that context he has repeatedly emphasized the role of ploychaetes in pollution monitoring.

Clark (1969, 1979) and Clark and Olive (1973) have reviewed endocrine influences and environmental determination of reproduction in polychaetes. These papers deal primarily with endocrine regulation and reproduction in healthy environments. Other aspects of polychaete reproduction have been reported by Schroeder and Hermans (1975).

2 IMPACT OF CHEMICALS ON ANNELID LIFE CYCLE STAGES

It is generally agreed that gametes, embryos and larvae represent the most critical stages in an organism's life cycle. When pollution occurs at levels which are lethal to adult animals, the larvae also have little chance of survival. Pollution at sublethal levels may leave the adults seemingly unaffected but nevertheless this stress can cause complete inhibition of reproduction. George (1971) retained for a year individuals of *Cirratulus cirratus* which had recovered from near-lethal doses of three oil dispersants (BP 1002, Essolvene, Corexit 7664). None of these worms developed gametes, whereas control worms showed normal gamete development. Ehrenström (1979) studied the effects of a 'second generation' dispersant, BP 1100 WD, alone and mixed with diesel oil on reproduction in *Ophryotrocha diadema*. The reproductive potential of these animals decreased when they had been exposed to the test solutions as larvae and subadults in contrast to that of exposed sexually mature animals. Ehrenström also demonstrated that young larvae were more susceptible than older ones. In a test series beginning with (1) newly released, (2) 1-day old, and (3) 3-day old larvae, the 96-hour LC_{50} values were 150, 270 and 370 p.p.m. respectively (dispersant only).

Bellan *et al.* (1972) and Foret (1974) studied the effects of various detergents on life cycle stages of *Capitella capitata*. In agreement with results similar to those reported above, Foret concluded that development of ovarian tissue was the stage most sensitive to pollution. In the test series, the number of spawning females was inversely related to the concentration of the pollutant, whereas the time for egg development increased with increasing concentration.

Most waste discharges contain a mixture of organic matter and chemicals.

Excess particulate organic matter may cause changes in sediment structure. Decomposition of excessive organic material leads to lowered dissolved oxygen levels in the sediment and often also in the water above the sediment. Davis (1969) and Davis and Reish (1975) studied the effect of reduced dissolved oxygen concentrations on oocyte growth and production in *Neanthes arenaceodentata*. When the dissolved oxygen level was reduced to about one-third of the control level (5.9 mg/litre), oocyte production was approximately halved. Females exposed to sublethal levels of dissolved oxygen (1.5 mg/litre) for about 2 months produced small-sized oocytes which failed to develop further even when the females were transferred to well-aerated seawater. Low levels of dissolved oxygen are a secondary consequence of organic enrichment, and is not a pollution *per se*, but when acting in concert with pollutants, even a moderate reduction may cause serious effects on reproduction.

Studies on the endocrine regulation of gametogenesis and sexual maturation in annelids have focused on the controlling influence of naturally occurring environmental agents and on brain extirpation and other laboratory manipulations of the worms.

Clark and Olive (1973) and Clark (1979) discussed the specific environmental signals which cause synchronization of sexual maturation in the population and coordination of the spawning. No research has been undertaken to relate the disappearance of polychaete species from polluted regions to failure in coordination of spawning or unsuccessful insemination. It should be kept in mind, however, that among those polychaetes which disappear early from polluted areas, many species release gametes freely into the water. On the other hand, the reproductive strategies are different in those opportunistic species which serve as pollution indicators. They usually have internal fertilization or some kind of pseudocopulation. The progeny is often protected by jelly and/or egg case membranes or kept in the female's tube during the most sensitive stages of development. Often these opportunistic species can adapt their reproductive strategy to take advantage of a new environmental situation (Grassle and Grassle, 1974, 1977).

The lethal/sublethal effects of various pollutants on larvae in the field are extremely difficult to observe. According to Thorson (1950), about 70% of marine invertebrates have planktotrophic larvae. Another fraction, less than 10%, have lecitotrophic pelagic larvae with the pelagic phase serving only for dispersal. Numerous reports have shown that pelagic larvae have a remarkably good ability to settle and metamorphose in habitats providing a suitable substratum. This literature has been reviewed by Thorson (1950), Crisp (1974) and Scheltema (1974).

Towards the end of the pelagic phase the larvae are capable of settlement and metamorphosis. In most species the planktonic stage ends with an exploratory phase during which the larvae prospect the surface of the substratum. The larvae settle and metamorphose if the environmental conditions are suitable. If not given proper environmental conditions, the exploratory phase will continue making it possible for the larvae to drift away from deteriorating habitats. In some species settlement and metamorphosis can be postponed for several weeks. It is also known, however, that developing larvae do not discriminate as much as larvae which are just ready to metamorphose. In some species, individuals may eventually accept an unsuitable substratum with increased mortality in post-metamorphosed stages as a consequence.

In the polluted habitat, the larvae of most species do not receive the correct environmental cues for induction of settlement and metamorphosis. The lack of recruitment will eventually deplete the population. In pollution literature those species which disappear at moderate levels of pollution are often stated to be more susceptible to the pollutant and therefore to die off. At least in regions of chronic pollution it is more likely, however, that larval rejection of the habitat stops recruitment and ultimately causes depletion of the population. 'The presence of a species in a polluted area may be more a question of life-history strategy than the tolerance of adverse environmental conditions' (Gray, 1979). In the estuary of the river Tees industrial pollution has accelerated during the last decades. At least four polychaete species, *Nereis virens*, *N. pelagica*, *Audouina tentaculata* and *A. johnstoni* have disappeared between 1935 and 1973 (Gray, 1979). These species all have long-lived planktonic larvae. The species which were abundant in 1973, *Polydora ciliata*, *Capitella capitata* and the oligochaete *Peloscolex benendeni*, are all brooders.

Polychaetes can respond by avoidance reactions to pollutants at levels far below those that are lethal. Vagile species may be able to avoid an area with unsuitable conditions. In choice experiments where three dorvilleid polychaetes had the choice between polluted and non-polluted substrata, they could detect and avoid the polluted substratum at levels two orders of magnitude less than 96-hour LC_{50} (Åkesson and Ehrenström, unpublished). There is no reason to assume that larvae are less sensitive; the volume ratio of nervous tissue to total body tissue is higher in larvae at the stage of metamorphosis than at any other stage of the life cycle.

3 LABORATORY STUDIES

3.1 Selection of Test Animals

The attributes of good test animals for bioassays have been discussed by several authors (Perkins, 1972; Reish, 1973b; Åkesson, 1975, 1980; Stebbing *et al.*, 1980). All writers agree that easily cultivated laboratory strains have many advantages although Perkins points to the problems of genetic drift in a laboratory strain. According to Reish (1973b, p. 46): 'The advantages of a laboratory-bred colony may be summarized as : (1) Specimens are available when needed, (2) specimens are already adapted to laboratory conditions, eliminating a conditioning phase, (3) laboratory specimens will not decimate the field populations of a desired species, a problem especially in populous areas, (4) the diet is known and controlled, which is particularly advantageous if biochemical analyses are involved, (5) many of the species of polychaetes have short life histories making it possible to study the effects of the pollutant on reproduction, and (6) specimens can be transported to other parts of the world making cooperative studies possible'. Some other properties can be added, e.g. that the test organism in question should be ecologically significant or economically important (Stebbing *et al.*, 1980), has well defined genetic composition and reproduces throughout the year (Åkesson, 1980).

Laboratory assessment of reproductive injury to marine worms has so far been confined to a limited range of test species. The most important ones are listed below together with some key references:

Capitella capitata	Reish and coworkers, several papers (lit. review in Reish, 1979), Bellan *et al.* (1972); Foret (1974); Rossi *et al.* (1976).
Cirratulus cirratus	George (1971).
Ctenodrilus serratus	Reish (1978); Reish and Carr (1978).
Dinophilus gyrociliatus	Røed (1980).
Neanthes arenaceodentata	Reish (1974); Davis and Reish (1975); Reish *et al.* (1976); Rossi and Anderson (1976, 1978); Oshida (1976, 1977).
Ophryotrocha diadema	Åkesson and Costlow (1978); Reish (1978); Klöckner (1979 and in preparation); Hooftman and Vink (1980).
Ophryotrocha labronica	Åkesson (1970, 1975); Saliba and Ahsanullah (1973); Rosenberg *et al.*, (1975); Røed (1980).
Sabellaria spinulosa	Wilson (1968a, b).

Most references given above are less than 10 years old. This reflects the new awareness that all life cycle stages should be considered in pollution monitoring. The test animals listed above (except *Cirratulus* and *Sabellaria*) have short life cycles so that research on the effects of long-term exposure to sublethal concentrations can be extended to several successive generations.

3.2 Selection of Life History Parameters to be Studied

In good test animals with sexual reproduction the following life history parameters should be available for observation:

(1) development of germ cells: appearance of ovarian tissue, percentage of fertile females, time from first appearance of oocytes to spawning;
(2) mating and spawning behaviour;

(3) spawning success, deviations from normal egg mass morphology, number of eggs per spawn;
(4) survival rate and time of development during the protected stage within the female's tube or inside egg mass membranes;
(5) survival and time of development in subsequent larval stages;
(6) growth rate and time from egg or from larval release to spawning.

The use of asexually reproducing species eliminates the 'noise' caused by genetic variation in sexually reproducting species (Åkesson, 1980). In that category, the number of new individuals and production of new setigerous segments are good parameters.

The choice of concentrations of a pollutant should be related to the 96-hour LC_{50} values of adults and larvae. If the tests are organized as two parallel series, one beginning with larvae and the other with adults, observations of sublethal effects on developing germ cells (mainly oocytes) become easier than in a single test series (Åkesson, 1975; Hooftman and Vink, 1980).

3.3 Case Studies

Rossi and Anderson (1976, 1978) studied the effects of water-soluble fractions of No. 2 fuel oil and a crude oil on life cycle stages of *Neanthes arenaceodentata*. Three successive generations were studied in a control series; larvae hatched between the ninth and tenth day of development. Hatching success and survival were inversely related to concentration and more depressed when exposure was initiated on 4-day-old larvae than when exposure began on the seventh day of development.

The growth rate of newly hatched larvae exposed during a period of 3 weeks was not reduced as much as the growth rate of juveniles. A correspondingly higher susceptibility level in juveniles was also recorded in 96-hour LC_{50} experiments. From the data provided in the two papers, it is obvious that the turning point comes at an age of about 18 days when the larvae have used up the yolk reserves and commenced feeding.

The time course of larval development from zygote to feeding stage was not affected in three successive generations, but oocyte maturation time decreased with each successive generation. In the first generation fecundity was suppressed in all concentrations. The suppression was approximately the same in successive generations.

The mortality rate from zygote to 32-setiger stage was directly related to concentration in the first generation. Brood mortality decreased with successive generations thereafter, which indicates some kind of accommodation. Mortality of the control series was as high as 36% in larvae and juveniles to the 32-setiger stage.

The body burden of both total and specific naphthalenes declined with each

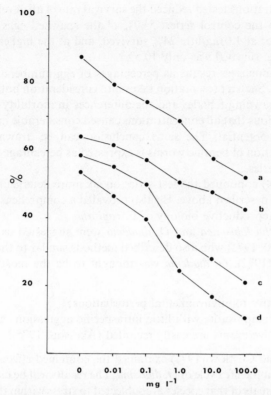

Figure 1 Effects of a polyethylene-glycol fatty acid on survival of successive larval stages in *Capitella capitata*. Results are expressed as percentages of egg numbers at different concentrations. (a) Trochophores within mother's tube. (b) Pelagic trochophores. (c) Metatrochophores. (d) Benthic worms. Data from Bellan *et al.* (1972)

successive generation which suggests some kind of adaptation not fully understood.

Bellan *et al.* (1972) studied the sublethal effects of a detergent, a polyethylene-glycol fatty acid, on life cycle stages of *Capitella capitata*. In this study data concerning most of the life history parameters listed above were recorded. The concentrations employed were 0, 0.01, 0.1, 1.0, 10.0, and 100 mg/litre.

The rate of oocyte development was inversely related to concentration as was the number of females laying eggs. The mean number of eggs per female was about the same at all concentrations except the highest. Also the rate of development of subsequent stage—trochophores, metatrochophores and young benthic worms—was inversely related to concentration.

All concentrations tested reduced the survival rate of all developmental stages (Figure 1). In the control series, 53.7% of the spawned eggs survived to the benethic stage; at 1.0 mg/litre 24% survived, and at the highest concentration, 100.0 mg/litre, survival was only 10.5%.

Table 1 summarizes results as percentages of egg numbers produced in the control series. Such a presentation takes into consideration both the decrease in number of spawning females and the differences in mortality rates. From the table it is obvious that all concentrations caused considerable impairment of the reproductive potential. The same conclusion can be drawn from Figure 2 where production of benthic worms is expressed as percentage of production in the control series.

Foret (1974) continued the test series on six more detergents employing the techniques as described above. He also provided a comprehensive review of the ecology and reproductive biology of *C. capitata*.

Ophryotrocha labronica and *O. diadema* were suggested as test animals by Åkesson (1970, 1975) who also described methods similar to those employed by Bellan *et al.* (1972). *O. diadema* was thought to be the most suitable species because:

(1) it is sensitive to environmental perturbations;
(2) it is a hermaphrodite with little intraspecific aggression; and
(3) reproductive events are easily recorded (Åkesson, 1975).

Åkesson and Costlow (1978) examined the combined effects of temperature and salinity on the life cycle of *O. diadema*. The results will be useful in bioassays where test animals of that species are subjected to stress within the ranges of their tolerance limits.

As 'part of a project on the development of methods for determining potential environmental effects of chemicals in seawater and fresh water with regard to biodegradability, toxicity, and bioaccumulation', Hooftman and Vink (1980)

Table 1   Effects of polythylene-glycol fatty acid on production of successive stages of *Capitella capitata*. Number of individuals is expressed as per cent of egg number in control series*

Detergent concentration (mg/litre)	Number of eggs	Trochophores in mother's tube	Free trochophores	Meta-trochophores	Benthic worms
0.0	100.0	87.7	64.2	58.6	53.7
0.01	89.7	71.3	55.3	49.6	41.8
0.1	74.5	55.9	43.1	37.6	29.5
1.0	75.6	57.6	42.2	28.6	18.5
10.0	51.3	29.0	23.9	14.0	16.2
100.0	26.4	11.5	9.4	4.7	2.8

* Data from Bellan *et al.*, 1972.

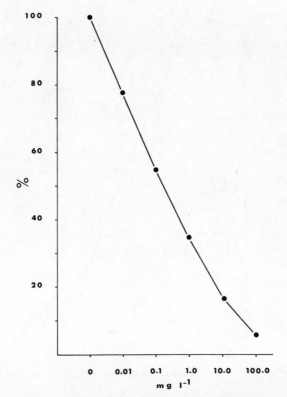

Figure 2 Effects of a polyethylene-glycole fatty
acid on production of benthic juveniles in *Capitella
capitata*. Production is expressed as percentages of
control series. Data from Bellan *et al.* (1972)

used *O. diadema* as the test animal in studies on the toxic effects of pentachlorophenol, 3, 4-dichloroaniline, and dieldrin. Methods of culturing test animals
and test procedures are extensively described in a joint report from the Central
Laboratory TNO in Delft (TNO, 1979).

Effects on reproduction were examined in two long-term tests, one starting
with newly released larvae, the other with 4-week-old adults. In both series,
concentrations of the test compounds were chosen in the range of 0.5–50% of the
96-hour LC_{50} values. Four replicate bowls with 10 animals per bowl were used
for each concentration.

In the series beginning with larvae, growth rate and time to the first appearance
of egg masses were recorded.

In both series, mortality rates, production of egg masses and number of eggs
and developing larvae per egg mass were recorded. In their tables the
summarized effect on reproduction was recorded as 'the reproductive potential',

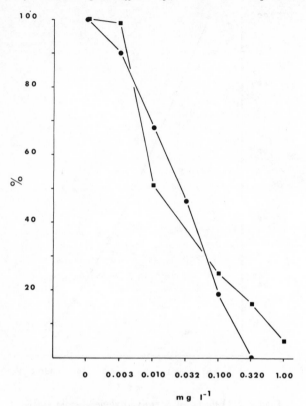

Figure 3 Effects of pentachlorophenol (●————●) and 3, 4-dichloroaniline (■————■) on the reproductive potential of *Ophryotrocha diadema*. Numbers of released larvae are expressed as percentage of control numbers. Data from Hooftman and Vink (1980)

which was defined as the number of viable larvae at each concentration expressed as the percentage of the number of larvae obtained in the control series (Figure 3).

The authors also defined the 'no toxic effect level' as the highest concentration exerting no influence on mortality, growth and reproductive potential. For larvae these 'no toxic effect levels' represent 2–3 orders of magnitude lower concentrations of the compounds than the 96-hour LC_{50} values. These concentrations are in good agreement with observations by Oshida *et al.* (1976) on *Neanthes arenaceodentata* exposed to chromium and by Reish and Carr (1978) on *O. diadema* exposed to heavy metals.

Hooftman and Vink (1980, p. 261) concluded that: '*O. diadema* can be considered as a moderately or slightly sensitive test animal if mortality is used as the toxicity criterion. If, however, in addition to mortality the influence on the reproductive potential is measured quantitatively during a test using all life-cycle stages, *O. diadema* appears to be a very sensitive test animal'.

Klöckner (1979) also used *O. diadema* when he studied the uptake and accumulation of cadmium at sublethal levels in three successive generations. Cadmium loads were extremely low in the egg masses as compared to those of the parent worms. The cadmium load of egg masses did not increase in successive generations. It is inferred that cadmium burdens in adult *O. diadema* are not transferred to the eggs. The low concentrations observed in egg masses are assumed to have resulted from absorption after egg deposition by the mucoid encapsulation layer.

In a study of the effects of cadmium on survival, growth and reproduction in *O. diadema* (Klöckner, 1977), the following life cycle events were recorded for three successive generations at cadmium concentrations of 0, 50, 100, 500 and 1000 p.p.b. employing a minimum of 50 individuals per concentration:

(1) survival rates;
(2) growth rate expressed as the increase in the number of segments;
(3) time from larval release to spawing;
(4) number of egg masses per individual produced in 100 days;
(5) cumulative number of eggs per individual in 100 days;
(6) mean number of eggs per egg mass;
(7) per cent 'successful egg masses', defined as those from which at least one viable larva was released;
(8) number of released larvae per egg mass;
(9) per cent mortality before larval release; and
(10) cumulative number of released larvae per individual in 100 days.

Observations according to (4), (7), and (10) above are summarized as 'reproductive potential' which is expressed as percentage of control series. It should be noted that Klöckner's 'reproductive potential' is defined differently from that of Hooftman and Vink (1980).

According to Klöckner, survival and somatic growth were not affected at 500 p.p.b. and lower concentrations. The reproductive potential was equal to that of the control series at 50 and 100 p.p.b. At 500 and 1000 p.p.b. the reproductive potential decreased to 34% and 4%, respectively, compared to control values.

In experiments over 21 days. Reish and Carr (1978) observed significant reproductive depression in *O. diadema* at a cadmium concentration of 1000 p.p.b., but not at 500 p.p.b.

Similarly Røed (1980) studied the effects of cadmium over three successive generations, using *Ophryotrocha labronica* as test organism. In some of the series the test animals were under additional physiological stress from lower salinity levels. Growth rate, time to sexual maturity and size at maturity were examined.

Effects on reproduction were confined to calculations of per cent egg masses from which viable larvae were released. On the other hand, Røed employed sophisticated statistics when evaluating the results.

4 FIELD STUDIES

Most field studies take into account all animal groups in the surveyed area. Benthic studies have been favoured because the fauna is largely stationary and cannot escape the pollutant. The faunal composition will therefore reflect the environmental conditions for a period of time prior to sampling. Few studies deal exclusively with marine worms, but polychaetes often constitute a dominant faunal component of the communities studied. Within the polychaetes we find a number of extremely opportunistic species which have been used as indicators of pollution.

4.1 Benthic Community Analyses

The major types of field studies can be listed as:

(1) sampling along an existing pollution gradient, i.e., harbour pollution studies or studies around discharges of domestic and industrial waste;
(2) studies on predischarge conditions before the operations of a new waste discharge system begin, followed by analyses of changes in species composition and community structure at time intervals after the discharge operations have commenced;
(3) studies on community changes after pollution abatement; and
(4) studies of effects of occasional major environmental disturbances, such as oil spill disasters or faunal depletions due to red tide.

Leppäkoski (1975) reviewed some general aspects of benthic pollution research with emphasis on brackish water studies. Reish (1979) recently published a comprehensive review on the role of polychaetes as indicators of pollution.

4.1.1 *Diversity Indices and Log-normal Distribution*

Most field studies involve the use of diversity indices to characterize the complexity of community structure. The theoretical basis for the use of diversity indices is the belief that unpolluted environments have had time to develop diverse communities of interacting species which are thought to be more stable than lower diversity perturbed communities. No one species totally dominates in these stable communities.

The diversity concept and its applicability in pollution research have been reviewed and criticized by Gray (1976, 1979, 1980) and Gray and Mirza (1979). Their major objections to the use of diversity indices concern the following facts:

(1) that the theory behind diversity indices is ignored;
(2) that the link between high diversity and high community stability is questionable;
(3) that diversity often falls during the later stages of succession;
(4) that diversity varies due to many factors other than pollution;
(5) that most diversity indices are relatively insensitive to changes in community structure; and
(6) that indices are insensitive as a measure of incipient pollution.

As a more reliable technique, the authors suggest the use of the log-normal distribution to characterize the distribution of individuals among the species. The log-normal distribution presupposes data from large samples of a heterogeneous assembly of species. The cumulative percentage of species plotted against the 'geometric class' of individuals per species gives a straight line if the distribution is log-normal.

The authors suggest that the log-normal distribution represents an equilibrium community with stabilized immigration and emigration patterns and fairly constant proportions of individuals per species. They convincingly demonstrate that even under slightly polluted conditions some species become more abundant, which causes an increase in the number of 'geometric classes' and a break in the log-normal plot around 'geometric classes' 5–9 with a shallower slope in higher classes. It is also pointed out, however, that any environmental disturbance may cause the same change of an equilibrium community structure. Even coinciding reproductive periods of several species may force the community out of equilibrium and cause a bend in the log-normal plots. Long-term monitoring on a yearly basis should therefore be reduced to sampling in midwinter when little larval recruitment occurs.

A heavy or chronic pollution may cause a return to the typical straight line log-normal distribution, but now the slope is shallower and there are more 'geometric classes' which reflects the increased dominance under polluted conditions.

A major advantage of the log-normal distribution method is that species groups can be established for future monitoring programmes. The most interesting species in this context are those in 'geometric classes' 5–9, i.e., the species around the break-point in the log-normal curve. They respond to slight pollution with increase in abundance.

To summarize, the log-normal method seems to be a suitable method for detecting slight degrees of pollution and to be more sensitive than various diversity indices. The method is not confined to soft bottom communities, it is generally applicable to any large sample of a heterogeneous community. Yet, the problem of distinguishing the effects of a pollutant (the signal) from naturally occurring variations in numbers (the noise) still remains to be dealt with experimentally.

4.1.2 Indicator Species and Life History Strategies

In many pollution studies the area under investigation can be subdivided into a number of zones, from an unaffected healthy zone to a heavily polluted and sometimes azoic zone. All zones, except the azoic one, are characterized by the community composition and often by indicator species as well.

The concept of indicator species has been disputed. Most of the discussion has been focused on the validity of the classical opportunist species, *Capitella capitata*, as an indicator species (Reish, 1960, 1972, 1973a, 1979; Eagle and Rees, 1973; Grassle and Grassle, 1974; Gray, 1979, 1980; Botton, 1979).

There is little evidence that species which decrease in number or disappear in polluted habitats really are more susceptible than species which are favoured by pollution (Gray, 1979). For instance, *C. capitata* is less tolerant of low oxygen tension than *Dorvillea articulata* and *Neanthes arenaceodentata*, both of which are considered indicators of slight pollution (Reish, 1971). *C. capitata* displays an average tolerance to heavy metals (Reish, 1978), is more sensitive to oil than *Nereis succinea* (Grassle and Grassle, 1974) and is susceptible to low levels of various detergents (Bellan *et al.*, 1972; Foret, 1974).

As discussed by Mileikovsky (1970), Grassle and Grassle (1974, 1977) and Gray (1979, 1980), life history traits, such as feeding type and, in particular, type of reproduction, determine the population success in a disturbed environment. Such opportunistic species as *C. capitala*, *Polydora ligni*, *Streblospio benedicti* and *Scolelepis fuliginosa*, all have life history strategies allowing dispersal to new disturbed areas and rapid exploitation of available resources. Comprehensive discussions of life history adaptations to an unpredictable environment are found in the papers by Grassle and Grassle (1974, 1977) and Gray (1979, 1980).

4.2 Other Field Studies

Studies on benthic communities confined to adult animals are by far the most common kind of pollution field research. Data about changes in reproductive injury are only obtained indirectly by observing changes in community structure. There are some other field approaches, however, where the research interest is more focused on reproduction, larvae and larval settlement.

Schram (1970) studied the meroplankton at five stations along a pollution gradient in the inner Oslofjord. For some polychaetes the number of larvae was inversely related to the degree of pollution. *Polydora ciliata* and *P. antennata* increased with increasing pollution. The same was true of the length of the breeding season of *P. ciliata*. Schram suggested that the presence and the number of the two spionid polychaetes are useful indicators of pollution.

Weiss (1947) exposed panels coated with antifouling paints of graded toxicity in order to study the tolerance of fouling organisms to copper and mercury. The tube worm *Hydroides parvus* appeared on the panels later than most other fouling organisms. The problem that still remains is whether settling larvae were killed or whether they rejected the painted surfaces. This problem could be solved with laboratory experiments.

Rastetter and Cooke (1979) studied the development of fouling communities in Kaneohe Bay, Oahu, Hawaii. When a new sewer outfall was constructed, they could manipulate the sewage to be discharged through the old and new outfall in alternating 2-week periods. The serpulid *Hydroides elegans* frequently settled on submerged panels when the old sewer was shut off, but was almost absent in periods when sewage was discharged.

Crippen and Reish (1969) examined polychaetes associated with fouling material along a pollution gradient in Los Angeles harbour. The results were related to chemical and physical parameters. The number of species decreased with increased pollution as did the number of individuals after numbers peaked at a site with slightly polluted conditions. The relative frequency of *Capitella capitata* was positively correlated with the levels of pollution.

Reish (1961) used sediment bottle collectors, a kind of wide-mouth glass jar, to monitor the settlement of larvae along a pollution gradient in Los Angeles and Long Beach harbours. The polychaete species composition was different at healthy, semi-healthy and polluted stations. The species diversity declined towards the inner, polluted parts of the harbour.

In another field study in the same area, Reish and Barnard (1960) used *Capitella capitata* in cage experiments. A female and a male were placed with some food in a number of plastic tubes closed at both ends with nylon netting. The cages were placed along a pollution gradient in the harbour. Survival, feeding and reproduction could be related to levels of dissolved oxygen and pollution.

Mohammad (1974) compared growth and survival of the tube worm *Pomatoleios kraussii* and other members of the fouling community at two sites in the Arabian Gulf, one of which was continously polluted with oil. The growth rate was not affected in *P. kraussii* which is the most abundant fouling organism, but in this species as in most other tube-building polychaetes settlement was slightly delayed on the oil-coated panels.

Finally, Bellan (1980) studied the relationship between the polychaete community (Serpulidae excluded) of infralittoral rocky shores and pollution in the region of Marseille. The 15 most common polychaete species were encountered at different relative frequencies at all stations facing the open sea. An 'annelid index' was proposed to characterize the degree of pollution. The index was defined as the ratio of pollution indicators (polychaetes favoured by pollution, e.g., *Platynereis dumerillii, Theostoma oerstedi, Cirratulus cirratus*) to indicators of pure water condition (e.g., syllids and *Amphiglena mediterranea*). There appeared to be a good correlation between the proposed annelid index and the Shannon–Weaver diversity index.

5 INTER-RELATING LABORATORY STUDIES AND FIELD STUDIES

'The ultimate question that must be answered concerns the ecological implications of laboratory-observed pollutant effects in the natural environment. For most laboratory studies the link between observed behavioral aberrations in the laboratory and the impact on species dynamics in an ecological system is difficult to ascertain' (Olla *et al.*, 1980, p. 175). This applies to any kind of biological assessment, studies on reproductive malfunction included. At the population and community levels, pollutants usually act in concert and also interact with naturally caused events. As reproduction is the most sensitive part of the life cycle, any pollutant at concentrations above 'safe levels' acting alone or together with other stress factors, will exert effects on the reproductive potential of the population. Therefore, bioassys examining effects of sublethal level pollutants on reproduction will be ecologically meaningful and may provide material for model studies of population dynamics.

In studies by Klöckner (1979 and unpublished) and Hooftman and Vink (1980) on reproductive impairment, *Ophryotrocha diadema* was used as the test animal. For this polychaete species, a life cycle analysis has been performed (Åkesson, unpublished). Both Klöckner and Hooftman and Vink reported:

(1) prolongation of the time to sexual maturity (an extremely important parameter in population dynamics (review by Stearns, 1976));
(2) increased mortality; and
(3) decreased reproductive rate.

Similar effects have been reported by Bellan *et al.* (1972) and Foret (1974) and seem to be general expressions of reproductive impairment caused by sublethal levels of pollutants.

In a life-table analysis of *O. diadema*, the mean life expectancy of a zygote was 29 weeks. The last individual died after 51 weeks. But calculations of the population growth parameter, the intrinsic rate of increase (*r*), from the well-known equation:

$$\sum_{x=0}^{\infty} e^{-rx} l_x m_x = 1,$$

demonstrated that individuals older than 10 weeks contributed less than 1% to the equation. In Klöckner's study (personal communication) data were provided for 14 successive weeks.

Using Åkesson's life-table data as a control, and assuming unlimited food and space, the following pollution effects were observed, all of which are quite realistic:

(1) a 10% decrease of either survival (l_x) or fecundity (m_x);
(2) a 20% decrease of l_x or m_x;
(3) the effects of (1) and (2) acting together;
(4) a 1-week delay of reproduction; and
(5) the effects of (1), (2) and (4) acting together.

The calculations are summarized in Table 2 and Figure 4. From the table it is quite obvious that a pollutant which delays the onset of reproduction affects the population growth much more than one which increases mortality or decreases fecundity. The suggested approach integrates research in applied pollution affects and population dynamic. Luoma (1977) suggested that studies of toxicant resistance in natural systems would provide a useful tool in environmental studies. 'To induce tolerance, a toxicant must be present in biologically available quantities sufficient to limit the reproductive success of a proportion of the individuals in a population (i.e. the nonresistant genotypes)' (Luoma, 1977, p. 437). Bryan and Hummerstone (1971, 1973) and Bryan (1974) reported a higher resistance to copper in the ragworm *Nereis diversicolor* from contaminated areas than in ragworms from less contaminated areas. Similar studies using polychaetes with a short life cycle over a number of successive generations would facilitate a better understanding of the development of resistance to toxic substances.

Table 2   Population effects of decreased survival (l_x) and/or fecundity (m_x) and of delayed reproduction in *Ophryotrocha diadema**

	Intrinsic rate, r	Finite rate, λ	Cohort at start	After 1 week	After 5 weeks	After 10 weeks
Control	0.880	2.412	100	241	8157	665,300
0.9 $(l_x m_x)$	0.858	2.359	100	236	7307	535,900
0.8 $(l_x m_x)$	0.834	2.302	100	230	6469	418,400
0.72 $(l_x m_x)$	0.812	2.253	100	225	5806	337,100
Reproduction delayed 1 week	0.731	2.077	100	208	3869	149,600
Reproduction delayed 1 week and 0.72 $(l_x m_x)$	0.677	1.968	100	197	2955	87,300

* Further explanations in text.

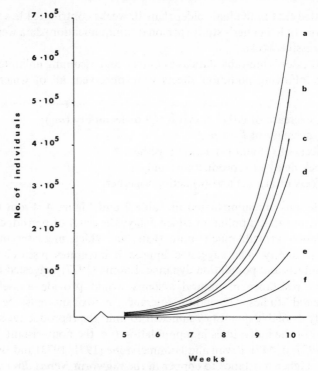

Figure 4   Effects of a pollutant on population growth in *Ophryotrocha diadema*. (a) control. (b) survival (l_x) or fecundity (m_x) reduced with 10%. (c) reduction of $l_x m_x$ with 20%. (d) reduction of $l_x m_x$ with 28%. (e) one week's delay of reproduction. (f) combined effects of (d) and (e). The cohort begins with 100 individuals

6   CONCLUSIONS AND RECOMMENDATIONS

Annelids potentially offer more test animals for long-term assessment of effects of pollutants over whole life cycles or even successive generations than most other macro-invertebrate phyla. There is no reason to rank test species now used. Any one species has its own advantages and disadvantages, and new species are continuously being suggested as sensitive test organisms for the toxicity bioassay approach. It is quite obvious, however, that the present selection of 'standard' test animals is biased towards opportunistic species, indicators of slight or heavy pollution. As these species are adapted to unpredictable environments, they can adjust themselves to polluted conditions. Originally they might have been selected because they were easily cultivated and easily transported between laboratories. Nevertheless, for long-term studies where effects on reproduction are assessed (Rossi and Anderson, 1976, 1978; Bellan *et al.*, 1972; Foret, 1974;

Klöckner, 1979 and unpublished; Hooftman and Vink, 1980) such species are well suited.

The majority of polychaetes have reproductive strategies different from the opportunists discussed above. Very commonly they have a long planktonic stage serving both feeding and dispersal. Representatives of this large group often disappear early from polluted areas.

As emphasized by Gray (1979) an early disappearance of a species from polluted regions cannot be related to an observed higher susceptibility of that species to pollutants, but rather to some factor in its life history strategy making it vulnerable. Much research is needed to evaluate the role of life history strategies in pollution studies. In this context, studies on avoidance reactions of metamorphosing larvae would be valuable. In so far as it is known, *Sabellaria spinulosa* is the only polychaete with long planktonic stage which has been experimentally used in bioassay studies. Wilson (1968 a, b) tested a detergent, BP 1002, which proved to be toxic to pelagic larvae at very low concentrations. Larvae which seemingly had recovered the initial stress died several weeks later. Sand which was soaked with the detergent and then thoroughly rinsed in seawater retained the toxic concentrations for several days.

In order to facilitate comparisons, long-term life cycle tests should be standardized. More interlaboratory calibration experiments should be performed. The first calibration test with polychate specimens (Reish *et al.*, 1978) used *Capitella capitata*, but the results were not encouraging. Specimens from an isogenetic strain were sent by air mail to the participating laboratories. Differences in test results were thought to be due to variability in shipping conditions.

When comparing results from experiments with *C. capitata* one should consider the problem of accurate identification of the test species. By employing electrophoretic techniques, Grassle and Grassle (1976) identified six sibling species from the vicinity of Woods Hole, Massachusetts. By now, the known number of sibling species has presumably doubled. For European populations, reproduction of *C. capitata* as described by Foret (1974) is quite different from

Table 3   Comparisons between reproductive data for two polychaete populations which are both identified as *Capitella capitata*

References	Foret (1974)	Warren (1976)
Collecting site	Marseille	Plymouth
Reproduction	Semelparous (one single repr.)	Iteroparous (repeated repr.)
Egg diameter	75 μm	100 μm
Number of eggs	250–300	10,000–14,500
Larvae	Pelagic	Benthic
Length of life cycle	2 months	12 months

that reported by Warren (1976) (Table 3). It is quite obvious that these two populations represent different species.

When Stebbing *et al.* (1980) listed a number of qualities required in a bioassay programme, they considered that 'the organisms cultured or collected for experiments should be as similar as possible, to minimize variability in sensitivity due to age, size, and so on'. The importance of uniform age was illustrated by Ehrenström's findings, which have been mentioned earlier and in Figure 20.5 which shows the reproductive rates of the archiannelid *Dinophilus gyrociliatus* and of *Ophryotrocha diadema*. Both species continue to grow throughout life. If test animals are picked from stock cultures, the experimenter runs the risk of picking large, seemingly fine animals which have passed the period of peak reproduction.

The log-normal method (Gray, 1976, 1979, 1980; Gray and Mirza, 1979) provides some advantages in field assessment of pollution. It is more sensitive than measurements of various diversity indices, in particular for detecting initial stages of disturbance, it can be applied to any community and seems to be labour-saving when compared to other methods.

In areas where it is feasible to use sediment bottle collectors along a pollution gradient, information can be gained about meroplankton composition and the

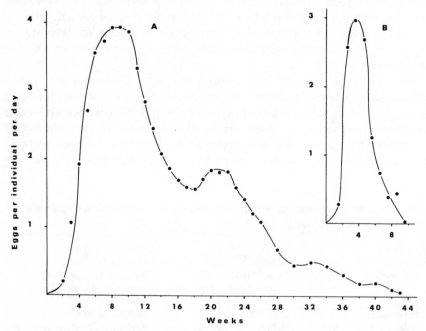

Figure 5   Relations between age and reproductive rates in *Ophryotrocha diadema* (A) and *Dinophilus gyrociliatus* (B)

attractiveness of substratum contaminated with various levels of toxicants. Furthermore, *in situ* experiments using caged animals (Reish and Barnard, 1960) and fouling panels (Mohammad, 1974; Rastetter and Cooke, 1979) are cost effective and therefore strongly recommended.

7 REFERENCES

Åkesson, B. (1970). *Ophryotrocha labronica* as test animal for the study of marine pollution. *Helgol. wiss. Meeresunters.* **20**, 293–303.

Åkesson, B. (1975). Bioassay studies with polychaetes of the genus *Ophryotrocha* as test animals. In Koeman, J. H. and Strik, J. J. (Eds.) *Sublethal Effects of Toxic Chemicals on Aquatic Animals*. Swedish-Netherlands Symposium, Wageningen, The Netherlands, Sept. 2–5, Proceedings.

Åkesson, B. (1980). The use of certain polychaetes in bioassay studies. *Rapp. P.-V. Réun. Cons. int. Explor. Mer*, **179**, 315–321.

Åkesson, B. and Costlow, J. D. (1978). Effects of temperature and salinity on the life cycle of *Ophryotrocha diadema* (Polychaeta, Dorvilleidae). *Ophelia* **17(2)**, 215–229.

Bellan, G. (1980). Relationship of pollution to rocky substratum polychaetes on the French Mediterranean coast. *Mar. Pollut. Bull.* **11(11)**, 318–321.

Bellan, G., Reish, D. J. and Foret, J. P. (1972). The sublethal effects of a detergent on the reproduction, development, and settlement in the polychaetous annelid *Capitella capitata*. *Mar. Biol.* (*Berlin*) **14**, 183–188.

Botton, M. L. (1979). Effects of sewage sludge on the benthic invertebrate community of the inshore New York Bight. *Estuarine coastal mar. Sci.* **8**, 169–180.

Bryan, G. W. (1974). Adaptation of an estuarine polychaete to sediments containing high concentrations of heavy metals. In Vernberg, F. J. and Vernberg, H. B. (Eds.) *Pollution and Physiology of Marine Organisms*, pp. 123–135. Academic Press. New York, San Francisco and London.

Bryan, G. W. and Hummerstone, L. G. (1971). Adaptation of the polychaete *Nereis diversicolor* to estuarine sediments containing high concentration of heavy metals. 1. General observations and adaptation to copper. *J. mar. biol. Ass. U. K.* **51**, 845–863.

Bryan, C. W. and Hummerstone, L. G. (1973). Adaptation of the polychaete *Nereis diversicolor* to estuarine sediments containing high concentrations of Zinc and Cadmium. *J. mar. biol. Ass. U. K.* **53**, 839–857.

Clark, R. B. (1969). Endocrine influences in annelids. *Gen. comp. Endocrinol. Suppl.* **2**, 572–581.

Clark, R. B. (1979). Environmental determination of reproduction in polychaetes. In Stancyk, S. E. (Ed.). *Reproductive Ecology of Marine Invertebrates*, pp. 107–122. *Belle W. Baruch Libr. mar. Sci. Ser. 9*. University of South Carolina Press.

Clark, R. B. and Olive, P. J. W. (1973). Recent advances in polychaete endocrinology and reproductive biology. *Oceanogr. mar. Biol. A. Rev.* **11**, 175–222.

Crippen, R. W. and Reish, D. J. (1969). An ecological study of the polychaetous annelids associated with fouling material in Los Angeles Harbor with special reference to pollution. *Bull. South. Calif. Acad. Sci.* **68(3)**, 170–187.

Crisp, D. J. (1974). Factors influencing the settlement of marine invertebrate larvae. In Grant, P. T. and Mackie, A. M. (Eds.). *Chemoreception in Marine Organisms*, pp. 177–265. Academic Press, New York, San Francisco, London.

Davis, W. R. (1969). *Oogenesis and its Relationship to Dissolved Oxygen Suppression in Neanthes arenaceodentata* (*Polychaeta: Annelida*), 62 pages. Master's thesis, California State College, Long Beach.

Davis, W. R. and Reish, D. J. (1975). The effect of reduced dissolved oxygen concentration on the growth and production of oocytes in the polychaetous annelid *Neanthes arenaceodentata*. *Rev. Int. Océanogr. Méd.* **37/38**, 3–16.

Eagle, R. A. and Rees, E. I. S. (1973). Indicator species—A case for caution. *Mar. Pollut. Bull.* **4(2)**, 25.

Ehrenström, F. (1979). De biologiska effekterna av oljedispergerings-medlet BP 1100 WD separat och i kombination med dieselolja, studerade med *Ophryotrocha diadema* (Polychaeta, Dorvilleidae) som testdjur. Mimeographed report, Department of Zoology, University of Göteborg, Sweden (in Swedish).

Foret, J.-P. (1974). Long term effects of some detergents on the development of the sedentary polychaete *Capitella capitata* (Fabricius). (Etude des effets à long terme de quelques détergents sur la séquence du dévelopment de la polychette sédentaire *Capitella capitata* (Fabricius)). *Tethys* **6(4)**, 751–778 (in French).

George, J. D. (1971). The effects of pollution by oil and oil-dispersants on the common intertidal polychaetes, *Cirriformia tentaculata* and *Cirratulus cirratus*. *J. appl. Ecol.* **8**, 411–420.

Grassle, J. F. and Grassle, J. P. (1974). Opportunistic life histories and genetic systems in marine benthic polychaetes. *J. mar. Res.* **32**, 253–284.

Grassle, J. P. and Grassle, J. F. (1976). Sibling species in the marine pollution indicator *Capitella* (Polychaeta). *Science (Washington, DC)* **192**, 567–569.

Grassle, J. F. and Grassle, J. P. (1977). Temporal adaptations in sibling species of *Capitella*. In Coull, B. C. (Ed.). *Ecology of Marine Benthos*, pp. 177–189. Belle W. Baruch Libr. Mar. Sci. Ser. 6. University of South Carolina Press.

Gray, J. S. (1976). The fauna of the polluted river Tees estuary. *Estuarine coastal mar. Sci.* **4**, 653–676.

Gray, J. S. (1979). Pollution-induced changes in populations. *Phil. Trans. R. Soc. Lond. B. Biol. Sci.* **286**, 545–561.

Gray, J. S. (1980). The measurement of effects of pollutants on benthic communities. *Rapp. P.-V. Réun. Cons. int. Explor. Mer.* **179**, 188–193.

Gray, J. S. and Mirza, F. B. (1979). A possible method for the detection of pollution-induced disurbance on marine benthic communities. *Mar. Pollut. Bull.* **10**, 142–146.

Hooftman, R. N. and Vink, G. J. (1980). The determination of toxic effect of pollutants with the marine polychaete worm *Ophryotrocha diadema*. *Ecotoxicol. environ. Saf.* **4**, 252–262.

Klöckner, K. (1977). The effect of cadmium on mortality, growth and reproduction of *Ophryotrocha diadema* (Polychaeta). In Annual Reports of the Biological Institute Helgoland, Hamburg.

Klöckner, K. (1979). Uptake and accumulation of cadmium by *Orphryotrocha diadema* (Polychaeta). *Mar. Ecol. Prog. Ser.* **1**, 71–76.

Knox, G. A. (1977). The role of polychaetes in benthic soft-bottom communities. In Reish, D. J. and Fauchald, K. (Eds.). *Essays on Polychaetous Annelids in Memory of Dr. Olga Hartman*, pp. 547–604. Allan Hancock Foundation, University of Southern California, Los Angeles.

Leppäkoski, E. (1975). Assessment of degree of pollution on the basis of macro-zoobenthos in marine and brackish-water environments. *Acta Acad. Abo. Ser. B.* **35(2)**, 1–90.

Luoma, S. N. (1977). Detection of trace contaminant effects in aquatic ecosystems. *J. Fish. Res. Board Can.* **34**, 436–439.

Mileikovsky, S. A. (1970). The influence of pollution on pelagic larvae of bottom invertebrates in marine nearshore and estuarine waters. *Mar. Biol. (Berlin)* **6(4)**, 350–356.

Mohammad, M. -B. M. (1974). Effect of chronic oil pollution on a polychaete. *Mar. Pollut. Bull.* **5(2)**, 21–24.

Olla, B. L., Atema, J., Forward, R., Kitteredge, J., Livingston, R. J., McLeese, D. W., Miller, D. C., Vernberg, W. B., Wells, P. G. and Wilson, K. (1980). The role of behavior in marine pollution monitoring. *Rapp. P. -V. Réun. Cons. int. Explor. Mer.* **179**, 174–181.

Oshida, P. S. (1976). Effects of chromium on reproduction in polychaetes. *South. Calif. Coastal Water Res. Proj. A. Rep.*, pp. 161–167.

Oshida, P. S. (1977). A safe level of hexavalent chromium for a marine polychaete. *South. Calif. Coastal Water Res. Proj. A. Rep.*, pp. 169–180.

Oshida, P. S., Mearns, A. J., Reish, D. J. and Work, C. J. (1976). The effects of hexavalent and trivalent chromium on *Neanthes arenaceodentata* (Polychaeta, Annelida). *Tech. Memo. South. Calif. Coastal Water Res. Proj.* **TM224**, pp. 1–58.

Perkins, E. J. (1972). Some problems of marine toxicity studies. *Mar. Pollut. Bull.* **3(1)**, 13–14.

Rastetter, E. B. and Cooke, W. J. (1979). Responses of marine fouling communities to sewage abatement in Kaneohe Bay, Oahu, Hawaii. *Mar. Biol. (Berlin)* **53(3)**, 271–280.

Reish, D. J. (1960). The use of marine invertebrates as indicators of water quality. In Pearson, E. A. (Ed.). *Waste Disposal in the Marine Environment*, pp. 92–103. Pergamon, Oxford.

Reish, D. J. (1961). The use of the sediment bottle collector for monitoring polluted marine waters. *Calif. Fish Game* **47(3)**, 261–272.

Reish, D. J. (1971). Effect of pollution abatement in Los Angeles Harbors. *Mar. Pollut. Bull.* **2**, 71–74.

Reish, D. J. (1972). The use of marine invertebrates as indicators of varying degrees of marine pollution. In Ruivo, M. (Ed.). *Marine Pollution and Sea Life*, pp. 203–207. Fishing News (Books) Ltd, Surrey, England.

Reish, D. J. (1973a). The use of benthic animals in monitoring the marine environment. *J. Environ. Plann. Pollut. Control* **1(3)**, 32–38.

Reish, D. J. (1973b). Laboratory populations for long-term toxicity tests. *Mar. Pollut. Bull.* **4(3)**, 46–47.

Reish, D. J. (1974). The sublethal effects of environmental variables on polychaetous annelids. *Rev. int. Océanogr. Méd.* **33**, 18.

Reish, D. J. (1978). The effects of heavy metals on polychaetous annelids. *Rev. Int. Océanogr. Méd.* **49**, 99–104.

Reish, D. J. (1979). Bristle worms (Annelida: Polychaeta). In Hart, C. W. and Fuller, S. L. H. (Eds.). *Pollution Ecology of Estuarine Invertebrates*, pp. 77–125. Academic Press, New York, San Francisco, London.

Reish, D. J. and Barnard, J. L. (1960). Field toxicity tests in marine waters utilizing the polychaetous annelid *Capitella capitata* (Fabricius). *Pac. Naturalist* **1(21–22)**, 1–8.

Reish, D. J. and Carr, K. S. (1978). The effect of heavy metals on the survival, reproduction, development, and life cycle for two species of polychaetous annelids. *Mar. Pollut. Bull.* **9(1)**, 24–27.

Reish, D. J., Martin, J. M., Piltz, F. M. and Word, J. Q. (1976). The effect of heavy metals on laboratory populations of two polychaetes with comparisons to the water quality conditions and standards in Southern California marine waters. *Water Res.* **10**, 299–302.

Reish, D. J., Pesch, C. E., Gentile, J. H., Bellan, G. and Bellan-Santini, D. (1978). Interlaboratory calibration experiments using the polychaetous annelid *Capitella capitata*. *Mar. Environ. Res.* **1**, 109–118.

Røed, K. H. (1980). Effects of salinity and cadmium interaction on reproduction and

growth during three successive generations of *Ophryotrocha labronica* (Polychaeta).
   Helgol. wiss. Meeresunters. **33**, 47–58.

Rosenberg, R., Grahn, O. and Johansson, L. (1975). Toxic effects of aliphatic chlorinated
   by-products from vinyl chloride production on marine animals. *Water Res.* **9**, 607–612.

Rossi, S. S. and Anderson, J. W. (1976). Toxicity of water-soluble fractions of No. 2 fuel
   oil and South Louisiana crude oil to selected stages in the life-history of the polychaete
   Neanthes arenaceodentata. Bull. environ. Contam. Toxicol. **16(1)**, 18–24.

Rossi, S. S. and Anderson, J. W. (1978). Effects of No. 2 fuel oil water-soluble fractions on
   growth and reproduction in *Neanthes arenaceodentata* (Polychaeta: Annelida). *Water
   Air Soil Pollut.* **9**, 155–170.

Rossi, S. S., Anderson, J. W. and Ward, G. S. (1976). Toxicity of water-soluble fractions
   of four test oils for the polychaetous annelids *Neanthes arenaceodentata* and *Capitella
   capitata. Environ. Pollut.* **10**, 9–18.

Saliba, L. J. and Ahsanullah, M. (1973). Acclimation and tolerance of *Artemia salina* and
   Ophryotrocha labronica to copper sulphate. *Mar. Biol. (Berlin)* **23**, 297–302.

Sanders, H. L., Hessler, R. R. and Hampson, G. R. (1965). An introduction to the study
   of deep-sea benthic faunal assemblages along the Gay Head-Bermuda Transect. *Deep-
   Sea Res.* **12**, 845–867.

Scheltema, R. S. (1974). Biological interactions determining larval settlement of marine
   invertebrates. *Thalassia Jugosl.* **10(1/2)**, 263–296.

Schram, T. A. (1970). Studies on the meroplankton in the inner Oslofjord II. Regional
   differences and seasonal changes in the specific distribution of larvae. *Nytt Mag. Zool.
   Oslo* **18**, 1–21.

Schroeder, P. C. and Hermans, C. O. (1975). Annelida: Polychaeta. In Giese, A. C. and
   Pearse, J. S. (Eds.). *Reproduction of Marine Invertebrates*, Vol. III, *Annelids and
   Echiurans.* Academic Press, New York, San Francisco, London.

Stebbing, A. R. D., Åkesson, B. , Calabrese, A., Gentile, J. H. Jensen, A. and Lloyd, R.
   (1980). The role of bioassays in marine pollution monitoring. *Rapp. P. -V. Reun. Cons.
   int. Explor. Mer* **179**, 322–332.

Stearns, S. C. (1976). Life-history tactics: A review of the ideas. *Quart. Rev. Biol.* **51(1)**,
   3–47.

Thorson, G. (1950). Reproductive and larval ecology of marine bottom invertebrates.
   Biol. Rev. Cambridge Phil. Soc. **25**, 1–45.

TNO (1979). *The Determination of the Possible Effects of Chemicals and Wastes on the
   Aquatic Environment: Degradability, Toxicity, Bioaccumulation.* English version of
   Report MD-N&E 77/11 of the Central Laboratory TNO, Delft, to the Ministry of
   Transport and Public Works, North Sea Directorate, Rijswijk (Z. H.), The
   Netherlands (in Dutch).

Warren, L. M. (1976). A population study of the polychaete *Capitella capitata* at
   Plymouth. *Mar. Biol. (Berlin)* **38**, 208–216.

Weiss, C. M. (1947). The comparative tolerances of some fouling organisms to copper
   and mercury. *Biol. Bull. (Woods Hole, Mass.)* **93**, 56–63.

Wilson, D. P. (1968a). Long-term effects of low concentrations of an oil-spill remover
   ('detergent'): Studies with the larvae of *Sabellaria spinulosa. J. mar. biol. Ass. U. K.* **48**,
   177–182.

Wilson, D. P. (1968b). Temporary adsorption on a substrate of an oil-spill remover
   ('detergent'): Tests with larve of *Sabellaria spinulosa. J. mar. biol. Ass. U. K.* **48**,
   183–186.

Methods for Assessing the Effects of Chemicals on Reproductive Functions
Edited by V. B. Vouk and P. J. Sheehan
© 1983 SCOPE

Methods for Assessing the Effects of Chemicals on Reproductive Function Invertebrates: Some Principles and Recommendations

K. G. Davey, A. S. M. Saleuddin, C. G. H. Steel and R. A. Webb

1 INTRODUCTION AND SCOPE

This paper deals with the following groups: Porifera, Cnidaria, Platyhelminthes, Aschelminthes (principally Nematoda), Annelida (terrestrial and freshwater only), Arthropoda (except Insecta—principally Crustacea), Echinodermata, and protochordates. Parasitic forms will not be considered in detail. This disparate assortment of taxa, including marine, freshwater and terrestrial organisms, differs widely in organizational complexity and exhibits a wide variety of reproductive patterns. Obviously it is not possible to review extensively the multitude of reproductive dysfunctions reported for each of these taxa. Rather, we have elected to adopt a generalized approach which seeks to identify similarities rather than to dwell on differences. In doing so, we first attempt to identify the various processes which contribute to reproductive function and which may be affected by environmental contaminants. We review briefly what is known about the functioning of these processes for each of the various taxa and the effect that contaminants have on them. We then attempt to identify suitable experimental systems for the study of the effects of environmental contaminants in the laboratory.

2 ORGANIZATIONAL–FUNCTIONAL LEVELS

For any metazoan, there will be a number of levels, defined in anatomical or functional terms, which function in reproduction. These various processes culminate in the fusion of the gametes and any chemical contaminant which alters any of the processes which directly or indirectly contribute to that fusion will affect reproduction. What are the various organizational–functional levels which can be discerned among invertebrates?

(1) *Gamete integrity and mobility.* Many of the organisms covered in this paper shed their gametes directly into the surrounding medium. Chemicals which

483

act on sperm mobility, or on the membrane-associated processes involved in fertilization, will affect the probability of successful fertilization.

(2) *Gamete production.* The mitotic and meiotic processes leading to gamete production may be sensitive to particular chemicals. In addition, those processes which are involved in accumulation of yolk might be affected.

(3) *Accessory secretions.* A number of accessory secretions are critical to the reproductive process. For the male, these may involve the production of seminal fluid for the maintenance of the spermatozoa or of the secretions which make up spermatophores, structures which function during the transfer of semen. For the female, the principal accessory secretion might be the yolk which may be synthesized outside the ovary in some taxa or those secretions which form egg shells or cocoons.

(4) *Control systems.* In most invertebrates that have been examined, even the most primitive, some form of hormonal control has been imposed on reproduction. While the precise details of the functioning of such systems will vary from phylum to phylum, enough is known to permit us to say that neurosecretory cells are somehow involved. Thus, any chemical which alters the functioning of neurosecretory cells may affect the reproductive process. Of course, the neurosecretory system is part of the nervous system so that neurotoxic agents may alter the activities of neuroendocrine cells in an indirect way.

(5) *Behavioural effects.* For many animals, specific behaviours are associated with reproduction, ranging from the release and detection of sex pheromones to more complex swarming and spawning behaviours. Neurotoxic agents, as well as mimics or antagonists of sex pheromones will alter reproductive activities.

This analysis of organizational–functional levels in reproduction is more than an academic exercise. It is important to note that many of the processes mentioned are quite basic and unlikely to vary in nature from taxon to taxon. Thus, it is obvious that known disrupters of the mitotic process will affect reproduction in all organisms, assuming that differences in penetration and detoxication of the chemicals can be ignored. Even at higher levels, where individual complexity might impose some degree of difference, there should nevertheless be some unity of response. For example, if a chemical has a direct effect on neurosecretory processes in one organism, then members of other taxa should also be affected in a predictable way, given that there is sufficient knowledge of the reproductive process and its control.

3 REPRODUCTION AND ITS CONTROL IN VARIOUS PHYLA

3.1 Porifera

Sponges have a well-documented ability for regeneration, and asexual reproduction plays an important role in their propagation. Most species are hermaphroditic, but the details of the sexual process are obscure. There is an apparent reponse to seasonal and daily factors in some sponges (Reiswig, 1975). The paucity of information concerning sponges is not surprising because of the difficulty of maintaining them for long periods in the laboratory (Harrison and Simpson, 1975). Any attempts to measure the effects of chemicals on the reproductive process will have to be delayed until our knowledge of that process improves.

3.2 Cnidaria

The most extensive studies have been conducted on the various species of *Hydra*, but nearly all of these have been confined to a consideration of budding and regeneration. While the basic facts of sexual reproduction are known for several species of cnidarians, we know almost nothing of the details. Sexual reproduction in *Hydra* tends to be seasonal in natural populations, while laboratory populations exhibit sporadic and unexplained periods of sexual reproduction (Reisa, 1973). Several marine hydroids have been cultured in the laboratory, the most notable of which in the present context is *Campanularia* (Stebbing, 1976). In spite of the fact that cells with some of the characteristics of neurosecretory cells exist in *Hydra*, no studies on the hormonal control of sexual reproduction exist. Strobilization in a single scyphozoan has been associated with a possible neurosecretory control (Crawford and Webb, 1972).

3.3 Platyhelminthes

The free-living turbellarians and parasitic trematodes and cestodes comprise this group. Most species are hermaphroditic and asexual reproduction is a common phenomenon. The general structure of the systems is known, but the details of mechanisms and control processes are poorly explored.

Among the triclad turbellarians, such as the familiar *Dugesia*, the oocytes develop in two ovaries situated immediately posterior to the brain. The testes in these hermaphrodites are multifollicular and numerous. Both testes and ovaries are surrounded by nerve plexi and these nerves contain neurosecretory granules which are more nymerous when the germ cells are undergoing meiosis and less so when spermatogenesis or oogenesis is complete (Grasso and Quaglia, 1971). Sexual maturation is seasonal, usually occurring in the spring, but the environmental stimuli involved are poorly known. Copulation with mutual insemination is the rule in free-living forms, but self-fertilization may occur in some parasitic forms.

Asexual reproduction by fission is common in many turbellarians, and some strains of triclad species may reproduce only by this means. Neurosecretion and complex behaviours are known to be associated with fissioning (Lender, 1974; Benazzi and Grasso, 1977), but details of the control are poorly known.

3.4 Aschelminthes

Given that nematodes are extraordinarily important in the soil fauna and that plant and animal parasitic nematodes are of considerable economic importance, it is surprising that we know so very little about the physiology of reproduction, particularly in free-living nematodes. The structure of the systems is known, and a good deal is known about the production of the gametes in some species (Bird, 1971), but we know nothing of the control of the reproductive process. Fertilization is internal, so that behavioural responses are important, and pheromones have been reported (Bone and Shorey, 1978). The spermatozoa are unusual and undergo changes in the female tract (Burghardt and Foor, 1978). The free-living *Caenorhabditis elegans* has been widely used in behavioural and developmental studies (Ward, 1976), but the fact that this species is normally parthenogenetic limits its usefulness in studies on reproductive biology. Nematodes have a neurosecretory system, (Davey, 1976), but nothing is known of the control of reproduction. We know even less about other classes of the phylum.

3.5 Annelida (other than marine forms)

Both terrestrial and aquatic oligochaetes are extremely important organisms. Terrestrial oligochaetes form a large part of the invertebrate biomass in soils where they aid in the breakdown of organic matter, assist in the mixing and aeration of soil and improve the water-holding capacity. Aquatic oligochaetes, including both enchytraeids and tubificids, are similarly important in the breakdown of organic matter in sediments and sewage. The tubificids are often used as indicators of water quality.

The biology of reproduction in earthworms has been reviewed (Edwards and Lofty, 1977). Oligochaetes are hermaphroditic, and the male and female organs are confined to a few anterior segments. Groups of spermatogonia formed in the testis pass into the seminal vesicles, where spermatogenesis is completed (Lattaud, 1980a, b).

The reproductive behaviour of earthworms, culminating in mutual copulation, is complex. While the familiar *Lumbricus terrestris* mates on the surface, other species mate below the surface (Edwards and Lofty, 1977), and pheromones may be involved in this and other processes (Rosenkoetter and Boice, 1973).

In view of their importance, it is perhaps surprising that we know relatively little about the reproductive biology of tubificids. For some species, details of the reproductive process are beginning to emerge (Poddubnaya, 1979).

Leeches are closely related to oligochaetes, and we know a good deal about their reproductive biology. Reproduction is seasonal (Sawyer, 1972; Davies and Everett, 1977). Leeches are protandrous hermaphrodites and sperm is transferred either via an eversible penis or spermatophores. Copulatory behaviour is frequently complex (Mann, 1962). Spermatogenesis, and possibly oogenesis are under the control of neurosecretory cells (Hagadorn, 1966; Webb, 1980; Webb and Omar, 1981), and the neurosecretory cells have been extensively studied (Webb and Orchard, 1979; Orchard and Webb, 1980; Webb, 1980).

3.6 Crustacea

There have been more studies of reproduction in Crustacea than in any invertebrate group other than insects. The anatomical and physiological aspects of oogenesis are reviewed by Charniaux-Cotton (1973) and its endocrine regulation by Adiyodi and Adiyodi (1970) and Kleinholz and Keller (1979). However, reproduction in Crustacea is far less well understood than the profusion of papers might suggest. The current picture indicates significant differences in control mechanisms in different groups within the Crustacea, a situation which complicates the choice of model systems for experimentation and prevents extensive generalization. The following is a highly superficial survey of some of the areas in which some generalization appears to be valid.

Most crustaceans are dioecious, though some cirripedes and isopods are hermaphrodites. Parthenogenesis is quite common in the Branchiopoda, Ostracoda and Isopoda. However, only sexual reproduction has been investigated in any detail. Although sex is determined genetically, the permanent secondary sexual characteristics are determined hormonally by the androgenic glands. Breeding is usually confined to a species-characteristic season by day length and temperature cues which regulate secretion of the hormones controlling oogenesis (discussion in Steel, 1980). These are primarily cerebral neurohormones released from the sinus gland whose action on the gonads may be inhibitory, stimulatory, or both. It is usually assumed that spermatogenesis is continuous above a threshold temperature. The sperm are often structurally complex but usually not motile. They are often transferred to the female in spermatophores where they are said to survive for several years. Fertilization is usually internal and occurs at the time of egg laying. Despite numerous reports, there is no compelling evidence for the occurrence of sex pheromones in any crustacean (Dunham, 1978).

Ovaries containing oocytes in vitellogenesis secrete a hormone which elicits the differentiation of the temporary secondary sexual characteristics seen in females during the breeding season. These consist of modified appendages which form various types of brood sacs or pouches into which the newly fertilized eggs are deposited. Thus, in most crustaceans each batch of eggs is retained attached to the mother for the duration of embryogenesis. This situation greatly facilitates assessment of the effects of chemicals on reproduction, for the viability of a complete clutch of progeny can be determined following treatments applied either to the progeny or to their mother.

3.7 Echinodermata

Most echinoderms are dioecious, but a few are hermaphrodites. Mature gametes are normally shed via gonoducts and fertilization is external except for a few species which retain eggs. No accessary glands are present. In starfish, the radial nerve contains a peptide hormone, gonad-stimulating substance, which induces in turn the production of 1-methyladenine by the follicle cells of the ovary and the interstitial cells of the testis. 1-Methyladenine in turn induces oocyte maturation and shedding of the gametes.

3.8 Protochordates and Protovertebrates

Under this heading we have grouped the phylum Hemichordata and the subphyla Acrania and Urochordata of the phylum Chordata. While this is a disparate grouping, they can be considered together in the present context largely because we know rather little about their reproductive processes.

They are all marine, and, with only a few exceptions, the sexes are separate, save in the tunicates. The gaps in our knowledge of them are large and numerous. The details of gamete formation are reasonably well known. Release of mature gametes is by rupture of the gonadal wall in Acrania, but gametes are shed via ducts in the other groups. Fertilization is external, and reproduction tends to be seasonal. Nothing is known of the control mechanisms.

4 FIELD STUDIES OF THE EFFECTS OF CHEMICALS

Our approach in this and the next section has been to conduct a computerized literature search. We have confined ourselves to those references which deal in a direct way with the effects of chemicals on those processes which lead to the production and fusion of the gametes. For most of the taxa, rather little material has been retrieved, but no attempt has been made to review all of the material involved. What follows is an attempt to provide an overview.

4.1 Porifera

No references were retrieved.

4.2 Cnidaria

Given the paucity of information concerning basic sexual reproductive processes, it is perhaps no surprise that so little literature was retrieved. One study has shown that the actinarian *Cereus pedunculata* reproduces by viviparous pathenogenesis in polluted water but is oviparous and gonochoric in a less polluted environment (Rossi and Calenda, 1974).

4.3 Platyhelminthes

No field studies on the effects of chemicals on the reproduction of free-living flatworms were retrieved.

4.4 Aschelminthes

There has been a myriad of field trials of nematicides, but all of these have dealt with population reduction, and none has considered the reproductive process in a direct way.

4.5 Annelids

Studies on the effect of environmental contaminants on aquatic oligochaetes have dealt primarily with numbers of animals in field populations. These studies are sometimes controversial. For example, while oligochaetes have long been considered intolerant to heavy metals (Aston, 1973), current studies suggest that oligochaetes are among the most tolerant benthic invertebrates (Chapman *et al.*, 1980).

There have been numerous field studies on the effect of pesticides, fungicides, heavy metals and fertilizers on various activities of earthworms, and these studies are reviewed by Edwards and Lofty (1977). Typically, these studies have involved small experimental plots with adjacent plots providing controls. Populations are assessed at the end of the experiment by soaking the plots with dilute formaldehyde, which brings the worms to the surface where they are counted. Many common pesticides are toxic to earthworms, resulting in a decreased population. Many studies (e.g. Thompson and Sans, 1974) report that after a year there is no difference between treated and control plots, suggesting, perhaps, that the reproductive capacity of survivors is unimpaired. However, such studies make no allowance for possible immigration from adjacent untreated plots (Martin, 1976).

No references to the effects of chemicals on reproduction in leeches were retrieved.

4.6 Crustacea

Although there is a large literature on the effects of various factors on reproduction on Crustacea, only four references were retrieved which dealt with effects of chemicals in the field, possibly reflecting the difficulty of obtaining useful information concerning reproduction in field studies. All four studies take the approach of counting the numbers of individuals in a polluted location and in a control location at roughly monthly intervals for periods up to 18 months. But such data do not, in themselves, say anything about reproductive processes. It is the less carefully quantified information which is potentially informative. For example, Wu and Levings (1980) report that while barnacles survive in the vicinity of a pulp mill outfall, reproducing animals are seen less often at this site. Conversely, Aston and Milner (1980) found that populations of the isopod *Asellus aquaticus* increased in organically polluted stretches of a river, a finding which they attribute to accelerated development.

4.7 Echinodermata

No references dealing with the effects of chemicals on reproduction of echinoderms in the field were retrieved.

4.8 Protochordates and Protovertebrates

No references dealing with the effects of chemicals on reproduction were retrieved.

5 LABORATORY STUDIES

5.1 Porifera

No references were retrieved.

5.2 Cnidaria

Stebbing and Pomray (1978) have described a system in which asexual reproduction (rate of budding) in *Hydra littoralis* can be used to assess the sublethal effects of environmental contaminants. In scleractinian corals, chronic exposure to crude oil led to a decrease in the number of female gonads per polyp (Rinkevich and Loya, 1979). *Campanularia flexuosa*, a marine hydroid, responds to environmental stress in a variety of ways. Of particular interest in the present context is an increase in gonozooid production which may occur at very low concentrations of contaminants (Stebbing, 1976), and this system shows considerable promise for adoption as a standard procedure.

5.3 Platyhelminthes

While chemicals are known to prevent egg-shell formation in parasitic flatworms (Bennett and Gianutsos, 1978), it is not known if these will also act on free-living forms. Chemicals, such as DDT, which affect the behaviour of platyhelminths (Kouyoumjian and Uglow, 1974) should be expected to disrupt copulatory behaviour, but no such studies have been found. In terms of asexual reproduction, it is known that chronic exposure to DDT slows the rate of fissioning and regeneration (Kouyoumjian and Villeneuve, 1979).

5.4 Aschelminthes

Rather few studies have focused directly on the reproductive system: Popham and Webster (1979) have examined the effect of cadmium on fecundity and growth of the parthenogenetic nematode *Caenorhabditis elegans*, and Weber *et al.* (1979) have shown that SO_2 applied to host plants may enhance the reproduction of plant parasitic nematodes. Samoiloff *et al.* (1980) describe a long-term toxicity assay for aquatic contaminants using the free-living *Panagrellus redivivus*, and the general field of the effect of chemicals on free-living nematodes has been recently reviewed (Samoiloff, 1980).

Among other Aschelminthes, some studies have been conducted on the effect of pH and other contaminants on egg production in a parthenogenetic gastrotrich (Faucon and Hummon, 1976; Hummon and Hummon, 1979).

5.5 Annelida

In spite of the fact that tubificids and enchytraeids are easily maintained in the laboratory, no references have been retrieved which describe the effects of chemicals on reproductive processes.

Among earthworms, only one study (van Rhee, 1975) examined the effect of chemicals directly on reproduction. This demonstrated that DDT decreased cocoon formation, that copper and mercury decreased reproductive activity and that zinc induced a loss of the clitellum.

5.6 Crustacea

In contrast with the other invertebrate groups considered in this paper, there exists a substantial literature dealing with the effects of environmental contaminants on reproduction on crustaceans. There is considerable uniformity in the methods used. Most studies have utilized *Artemnia, Daphnia* or *Gammarus* because these are small aquatic crustaceans which breed rapidly in the laboratory. Unfortunately, the details of the physiology of reproduction in these genera, particularly in terms of the role of various internal controls, are still obscure. It is thus not possible to interpret observed effects on reproduction in terms of a perturbation of any particular physiological processes.

In the great majority of cases, the chemical to be evaluated is added to the culture water (usually at several concentrations in different cultures), and some conveniently observable parameters of reproduction are measured at intervals of time ranging from 1 to 20 days. The parameters of interest consist of one or more of the following, in decreasing order of frequency of use: LC_{50} and/or longevity of parents, number of young produced, proportion of adults producing young, number of broods produced, number of eggs per brood, size of eggs. Depression in any of these parameters is interpreted as evidence of impaired reproduction. It is generally assumed that larvae liberated from the brood pouch will survive, although Cunningham (1976) also examines toxicity to *Nauplius* larvae and cysts. Linden (1976) also notes reduced incidence of precopulatory behaviour. These tests have been used to study the effects on reproduction of materials such as oil, detergents, metals (Cd, Cu, Cr, Hg), and various herbicides and pesticides.

The possibility always exists that the effects of chemicals may be expressed as an alteration in the quality or abundance of food. For example, Schwart and Ballinger (1980) have shown that changes in the species of algae supplied as food to *Daphnia* modify the various parameters listed above. Further, changes in the food supply influence the extent to which copper inhibits reproduction in *Daphina* (Winner *et al.*, 1977), indicating that indirect effects on the food supply somehow interact with direct effects on the organism itself.

5.7 Echinodermata

Since the spermatozoa of echinoderms have been used in a wide variety of basic studies on the physiology of spermatozoa, it is no surprise to find that they have been used in the assessment of the effects of pollutants on sperm mobility. Thus Nicol *et al.* (1977) have shown that aqueous extracts of No. 2 fuel oil depressed mobility of sperm and interfered with fertilization and early development in the sand-dollar and Hagstrom and Lonning (1977) have demonstrated deleterious effects on sea urchin spermatozoa of oil dispersants at concentrations as low as 0.3 p.p.b.

Echinoderm eggs have also been used in similar studies, but most of these such as the study of Kobayashi (1977) have dealt with the development of fertilized eggs, a process which lies outside the scope of this paper.

6. DISCUSSION, CONCLUSION AND RECOMMENDATION

This paper is based on a number of assumptions. The first of these is that in order to be able to assess the effects of potential chemical pollutants in the laboratory, it is important to understand at least the rudiments of the various functional levels which effect reproduction in the target organism. Given the ecological importance of some of the taxa considered in this paper, our lack of basic knowledge is a matter of urgent concern. The Cnidaria, for example, are essential for the formation and maintenance of the coral reefs of the world. Any serious alteration of the reproductive rates of the organisms which form the reefs will have profound effects. We know a good deal about the important processes of asexual reproduction (budding) in *Hydra*, a potential, though atypical, test system, but we know nothing of the factors controlling the sexual process. Nematodes are among the most common soil organisms, but we are largely ignorant of the way in which reproduction is controlled in this group. Even in those organisms which are already used in the laboratory for toxicity studies, such as the aquatic Crustacea, the test systems chosen, such as *Daphnia*, (see OECD guidelines) are frequently those which are not well characterized in terms of reproductive controls.

A second assumption is obvious: the organisms chosen as test systems must be capable of being reared in the laboratory. This sharply limits the current choice of organisms, and eliminates from consideration several whole taxa, including echinoderms, protochordates and protovertebrates.

A third assumption offers some additional room for manoeuvre. Many of the functional levels considered above are common to all organisms, and differences in absorption and metabolism aside, chemicals which affect a functional level in one organism are likely to affect the same functional level in all other organisms. For some of the functional levels, such as gamete production, sperm mobility and fertilizing capacity of the gametes, the validity of such an assumption is perhaps obvious. For higher and potentially more specialized levels, there is perhaps less merit in such an approach. Nevertheless, it is clear that for all of the taxa considered with the exception of Porifera, neuroendocrine processes play an important role in the control of reproductive processes. Since neurosecretory processes are very similar throughout the animal kingdom, chemicals which perturb the neurosecretory process are likely to affect the reproductive process. Even at the behavioural level, chemicals which affect the nervous system in one invertebrate are likely to disrupt reproductive behaviour in other invertebrates.

Given the validity of such an assumption, it should be possible to select test systems based on the functional level rather than on a particular taxon. It is true of course that there would be greater confidence in a statement that a chemical which affects neurosecretion in, for example, an annelid is also likely to affect neurosecretion in *Hydra*, than one which states the reverse: that a chemical *without* effect on one system will not affect that system in a different organism. However, that is also true for test systems based on organisms. For example, how much confidence would a responsible scientist be willing to give to a statement that because a particular compound failed to affect reproduction in, for example, *Hydra*, it would also not affect coral-forming organisms?

Against this background, then, we offer two different sets of recommendations, one set based on the concept of models of functional organisation, another based on the more conventional approach of using model organisms. These are not mutually exclusive alternatives.

The first alternative, that of using functional levels, may or may not involve taxa covered in the present paper. We recommend, however, that:

(1) Suitable systems be identified for the assay of the effects of chemicals on

the following functional levels: gamete production, sperm mobility, neurosecretion, and nervous activity.

For some of these levels, some of the taxa referred to in this paper will be most suitable. Sea urchins, for example, have been widely used in studies of sperm mobility and fertilization. For others, such as neurosecretion and nervous activity, other taxa, such as insects, will be more appropriate. An important advantage of such an approach is speed. Rather than having to rely on chronic application of chemicals, many of these phenomena can be studied on a very short time scale in a quite isolated fashion.

The second alternative, that of identifying suitable test species to represent the various taxa, involves some common principles. First, as already stated, the organisms must be capable of being reared in the laboratory. Second, it is surely obvious that the ideal model should be one which is ecologically significant, although the necessity of rearing the organism in the laboratory will require some compromises. Third, the ideal system is one in which the reproductive process is already well understood. Fourth, there will be some common methodologies to be used. These have already been addressed in the current guidelines for *Daphnia*. Against this background, we further recommend the following:

(2) That *Hydra* be developed as a test system for cnidaria. If this is to be a useful model, research on sexual reproduction in the laboratory is urgently required. Alternatively, *Campanularia* might serve as a marine organism.

(3) That *Dugesia* be developed as a model for flatworms. Once more, research on sexual reproduction is required.

(4) That *Panagrellus* be developed as a test system for nematodes and other Aschelminthes. The procedures of Samoiloff (1980) form a good basis for this work, but it should be recognized that we know very little of the processes which control reproduction in nematodes.

(5) That tubificids be developed as a model system for oligochaete annelids, although *Lumbricus* is also a candidate.

(6) That *Daphnia* continue to be developed as a model for aquatic *Crustacea* and that further research be concentrated on the physiology of reproduction in this genus.

(7) That consideration be given to the use of terrestrial isopods such as *Oniscus* as models for terrestrial crustaceans. These can be reared in the laboratory in large numbers, we know something of their reproductive processes, and crustaceans are important components of soil fauna.

(8) That, for the present, no specific test sytem for echinoderms or protochordates be contemplated. Potential effects will have to be extrapolated from other taxa.

7 REFERENCES

Adiyodi, R. and Adiyodi, K. (1970). Endocrine control of reproduction in decapod Crustacea. *Biol. Rev.* **45**, 121–165.
Aston, R. J. (1973). Tubificids and water quality: a review. *Environ. Pollut.* **5**, 1–10.

Aston, R. J. and Milner, A. G. P. (1980). A comparison of populations of the isopod *Asellus aquaticus* above and below power stations in organically polluted reaches of the River Trent in England. *Freshwater Biol.* **10**, 1–14.

Benazzi, M. and Grasso, M. (1977). Comparative research on the sexualization of fissiparous planarians treated with substances contained in sexual planarians. *Monit. Zool. Ital. (N. S.)* **11**, 9–20.

Bennett, J. L. and Gianutsos, G. (1978). Disulfuram—a compound that selectively induces abnormal egg production and lowers norepinephrine levels in *Schistosoma mansoni. Biochem. Pharmac.* **27**, 817–820.

Bird, G. W. (1971). Biology of nematodes and their phytopathogenic mechanisms. *J. Parasitol.* **57**, 87–95.

Bone, L. W. and Shorey, H. H. (1978). Nematode sex pheromones: pheromones and regulation of nematode mating behaviour. *J. chem. Ecol.* **4**, 595–612.

Burghart, R. C. and Foor, W. E. (1978). Membrane fusion during spermatogenesis in *Ascaris. J. Ultrastruct. Res.*, **62**, 190–202.

Chapman, P. M., Churchland, L. M., Thomson, P. A. and Michnowsky, E. (1980). Heavy metal studies with oilgochaetes. In Brinkhurst, R. O. and Cooke, D. G. (Eds.) *Aquatic Oligochaete Biology*, pp. 477–502. Plenum Press, New York.

Charniaux-Cotton, H. (1973). Description et controle de l'ovogenese chez les Crustaces superieurs. *Inst. Nat. Rech. Agron. Ann. Biol.* **13**, 21–30.

Crawford, M. A. and Webb, K. C. (1972). An ultrastructural study of strobilization in *Chrysaora quinquecirrha* with special reference to neurosecretion. *J. exp. Zool.* **182**, 251–270.

Cunningham, P. A. (1976). Effects of Dimilin TH-6040 on reproduction in the brine shrimp. *Artemia salina. Environ. Entomol.* **5**, 701–706.

Davey, K. G. (1976). Hormones in nematodes. In Croll, N. A. (Ed.) *The Organisation of Nematodes*, pp. 273–292. Academic Press, New York.

Davies, R. W. and Everett, R. P. (1977). The life history, growth, and age structure of *Nephelopsis obsena* Verrill, 1872 (Hirudinoidea) in Alberta. *Can. J. Zool.* **55**, 620–627.

Dunham, P. J. (1978). Sex pheromones in Crustacea. *Biol. Rev.* **53**, 555–583.

Edwards, C. A. and Lofty, J. R. (1977). *Biology of Earthworms.* Chapman and Hall, London (Wiley & Sons, New York).

Faucon, A. S. and Hummon, W. D. (1976). Effects of mine acid on the longevity and reproductive rate of the gastrotrichan *Lepidodermella squarmmota. Hydrobiologia* **50**, 265–270.

Grasso, M. and Quaglia, A. (1971). Studies on neurosecretion in planarians III. Neurosecretory fibres near the testes and ovaries of *Polycelis nigra. J. Submicrosc. Cytol.* **3**, 171–180.

Hagadorn, I. R. (1966). Neurosecretion in the Hirudinea and its possible role in reproduction. *Am. Zool.* **6**, 251–261.

Hagstrom, B. E. and Lonning, S. (1977). The effect of Esso corexit 9527 on the fertilizing capacity of spermatozoa. *Mar. Pollut. Bull.* **8**, 136–138.

Harrison, W. and Simpson, T. L. (1975). Principles and perspectives in sponge biology. In Harrison, F. W. and Cowden R. R. (Eds.) *Aspects of Sponge Biology*, pp. 3–18. Academic Press, New York.

Hummon, W. D. and Hummon, W. R. (1979). Use of life table data in tolerance experiments. *Can. Biol. Mar.* **16**, 743–749.

Kleinholz, L. H. and Keller, R. (1979). Endocrine regulation in Crustacea. In Barrington, E. J. W. (Ed.) *Hormones and Evolution*, Vol. 1, pp. 159–214. Academic Press, New York.

Kobayashi, N. (1977). Bioassay data for marine pollution using sea-urchin eggs. *Publ. Seto. Mar. Biol. Lab.* **23**, 427–434.

Kouyoumjian, H. H. and Uglow, R. F. (1974). Studies on the toxicity of DDT to planaria. *Environ. Pollut.* **7**, 103.

Kouyoumjian, H. H. and Villeneuve, J. P. (1979). Further studies on the toxicity of DDT to planaria. *Bull. environ. Contam. Toxicol.* **22**, 109–112.

Lattaud, C. (1980a). Demonstration by organ culture of a cerebral hormone stimulating the secretion of testicular androgen in the oligochete annelid *Eisenia foetida f. typica*. *Int. J. Invertebr. Reprod.* **2**, 23–27.

Lattaud, C. (1980b). Study by organ culture of a cerebral hormone stimulating spermatogenesis in the oligochete annelid *Eiseria foetida f. typica* Sav. *Bull. Soc. Zool. Fr.* **105**, 115.

Lender, T. (1974). Multiplication asexuee et sexualisation chez les planaires d'eau douce. *Ann. Biol.(Paris)* **13**, 165–172.

Linden, O. (1976). Effects of oil on the amphipod *Gammarus oceanicus*. *Environ. Pollut.* **10**, 239–250.

Mann, K. H. (1962). *Leeches (Hirudinea). Their Structure, Physiology, Ecology and Embryology*. Pergamon Press, New York.

Martin, N. A. (1976). Effect of four insecticides on the pasture ecosystem. V. Earthworms (Oligochaeta: Lumbricidae) and Arthropoda extracted by wet sieving and salt flotation. *N. Z. J. Agric. Res.* **19**, 111–115.

Nicol, J. A. C., Donahue, W. H., Wang, R. T. and Winters, K. (1977). Chemical composition and effects of water extracts of petroleum on eggs of the sand-dollar *Melitta quinqiesperforata. Mar. Biol. (Berlin)* **40**, 309–316.

Orchard, I. and Webb, R. A. (1980). The projections of neurosecretory cells in the brain of the North American medicinal leech, *Macrobdella decora*, using intracellular injection of horseradish peroxidase. *J. Neurobiob.* **11**, 229–242.

Poddubnaya, T. L. (1979). Life cycles of mass species of Tubificidae (Oligocheta). In Brinkhurst, R. O. and Cook, D. G. (Eds.) *Aquatic Oligochete Biology*, pp. 175–184. Plenum Press, New York.

Popham, J. D. and Webster, J. M. (1979). Cadmium toxicity in the free-living nematode *Caenorhabditis elegans. Environ. Res.* **20**, 183–191.

Reisa, J. J. (1973). Ecology. In Burnett, A. L. (Ed.) *Biology of the Hydra*, pp. 59–108. Academic Press, New York.

Reiswig, H. M. (1975). Natural gamete release and oviparity in Caribbean demonspongiae. In Harrison, F. W. and Cowden, R. R. (Eds.) *Aspects of Sponge Biology*, pp. 99–112. Academic Press, New York.

Rinkevich, B. and Loya, Y. (1979). Laboratory experiments on the effects of crude oil on the red sea coral *Stylophora pistillata. Mar. Pollut. Bull.* **10**, 328–330.

Rosenkoetter, J. S. and Boice, R. (1973). *Earthworm Pheromones and T-maze Learning*, 17 pages. Psychonomic Society, St. Louis, Missorri.

Rossi, L. and Calenda, G. (1974). Reproductive and sexual variability in populations of *Cereus pedunculatus activiaria Doriana* **5**, 1–6.

Samoiloff, M. R. (1980). Action of chemical and physical agents on free-living nematodes. In Zuckerman, B. M. (Ed.) *Nematodes as Biological Models*, Vol. 2, pp. 81–98. Academic Press, New York.

Samoiloff, M. R., Schulz, S., Jordan, Y., Denich, K. and Arnott, E. (1980). A rapid simple long term toxicity assay for aquatic contaminants using the nematode *Panagrellus redivivas. Can. J. Fish. Aquat. Sci.* **37**, 1167–1174.

Sawyer, R. T. (1972). *North American Freshwater Leeches, Exclusive of the Piscicolidae, with a Key to all Species*. Illinois Biological Monographs 46. U. of Illinois Press, Urbana, Chicago.

Schwart, S. S. and Ballinger, R. E. (1980). Variations in life history characteristics of *Daphnia pulex* fed different algal diets. *Oecologia* **44**, 181–184.

Stebbing, A. R. D. (1976). The effects of low metal levels on a clonal hydroid. *J. Mar. Biol. Ass. U. K.* **56**, 977–994.

Stebbing, A. R. D. and Pomray, A. J. (1978). A sublethal technique for assessing the effects of contaminants using *Hydra littoralis*. *Water Res.* **12**, 631–636.

Steel, C. G. H. (1980). Mechanisms of coordination between moulting and reproduction in terrestrial isopod Crustacea. *Biol. Bull.* (*Woods Hob. Mass.*) **159**, 206–218.

Thompson, A. R. and Sans, W. W. (1974). Effects of soil insecticides in southwestern Ontario on non-target invertebrates: Earthworms in pasture. *Environ. Entomol.* **1**, 305–308.

Van Rhee, J. A. (1975). Copper contamination effects on earthworms by disposal of pig waste in pastures. In Vanek, J. (Ed.) *Progress in Soil Zoology*, pp. 451–457. W. Junk. B. V., The Hague.

Ward, S. (1976). The use of mutants to analyse the sensory nervous system of *Caenorhebditis elegans*. In Croll, N. A. (Ed.) *The Organisation of Nematodes*, pp. 365–382. Academic Press, New York.

Webb, R. A. (1980). Spermatogenesis in Leeches I. Evidence for a gonadotropic peptide hormone produced by the supraoesophageal ganglion of *Erpobdella octoculata*. *Gen. comp. Endocrinol.* **42**, 401–412.

Webb, R. A. and Omar, F. E. (1981). Spermatogenesis in Leeches II. The effect of the supraoesophageal ganglion and ventral nerve cord ganglia on spermatogenesis in the North American medicinal leech *Macrobdella decora*. *Gen. comp. Endocrinol.* **44**, 54–63.

Webb, R. A. and Orchard, I. (1979). The distribution of putative neurosecretory cells in the central nervous system of the North American medicinal leech *Macrobdella decora*. *Can. J. Zool.* **57**, 1905–1914.

Weber, D. E., Reinert, R. A. and Barker, K. R. (1979). Ozone and sulfur dioxide effects on reproduction and host parasite relationships of selected plant parasitic nematodes. *Phytopathology* **69**, 624–628.

Winner, R. W., Keeling, T., Yeager, R. and Farrell, M. P. (1977). Effect of food type on the acute and chronic toxicity of copper to *Daphnia magna*. *Freshwater Biol.* **7**, 343–350.

Wu, R. S. S. and Levings, C. D. (1980). Mortality, growth and fecundity of transplanted mussel (*Mytilus edulis*) and branacle (*Balonus glandula*) populations near a pulp mill outfall. *Mar. Pollut. Bull.* **11**, 11–15.

Methods for Assessing the Effects of Chemicals on Reproductive Functions
Edited by V. B. Vouk and P. J. Sheehan
© 1983 SCOPE

Methods for Assessing the Effects of Chemicals on Reproduction in Higher Plants

P. L. PFAHLER AND H. F. LINSKENS

1 INTRODUCTION

The recent rapid increase in the number and diversity of chemicals released into the biosphere as a result of agricultural and industrial technology has generated much interest and concern as to the effects of these chemicals on reproduction in higher plants. Since higher plants represent a major food source and add immeasurably to our aesthetic nature, rapid, accurate tests to determine not only the immediate effect of these chemicals on reproduction but also to predict their indirect effect on evolution and ecology are vital. The development of these tests is a formidable task since reproductive ability as measured by progeny number can be altered by many physical, chemical, biological, and evironmental factors imposed for any length of time during any portion of the life cycle. Perhaps more importantly, the number and diversity of species and chemicals involved are large.

The purpose of this report is to examine the scope and complexity of the problem, to outline methods which are presently available to assess the effect of chemicals on various stages of the life cycle, and to discuss future directions which hold short-term and long-term solutions of this growing problem associated with modern technology. Since a large number of research reports are available in some areas, recent reports, books, and comprehensive review articles will be cited wherever possible for brevity.

2 SCOPE AND COMPLEXITY OF PROBLEM

Much diversity exists among the more than 150,000 species of higher plants with the following factors among the major differences contributing to their differential response to chemicals (Steward and Krikorian, 1971):

(1) method of reproduction (asexual, sexual);
(2) life cycle (type and length—annual, biennial, perennial with herbaceous or woody forms);

499

(3) flowering pattern (determinate, indeterminate);
(4) organization (monocotylodon, dicotyledon);
(5) cell characteristics (chromosome number, ploidy level, cell volume, DNA content);
(6) climatic and edaphic adaptation (tropical, subtropical, temperate in aquatic or terrestial conditions); and
(7) pollination strategy (self-, cross).

One or a combination of these factors can alter the effect of chemicals. For example, morphological variations can influence the penetration of chemicals into the plant thereby altering their effectiveness (Bukovac, 1976). Others produce biophysical, biochemical, or physiological variation which alters the effect of chemicals once inside the plant (Brain, 1964a; Crafts, 1964; Moreland and Hilton, 1976; Moreland, 1977). Still others produce developmental variation which influences the impact of chemicals (Gortner and Zweep, 1964; Kiermayer, 1964; Andel and Zweep, 1976; Linck, 1976). Factors such as pollination strategy limit the exposure of the independent but especially vulnerable mature pollen grain to chemicals present in the atmosphere. In contrast to pollen grains from cross-pollinated species, the pollen grains of self-pollinated species are completely protected from chemicals in the atmosphere by the protective floral structure. In addition, genetic differences within species which are often qualitative, simply inherited factors are known to alter sensitivity to chemicals (Nelson and Rossman, 1958; Pfahler, 1968, 1981, Hanna, 1977; Pfahler *et al.*, 1980, 1981).

An equal or even greater amount of diversity is present among potential chemical pollutants. A long list of diverse inorganic and organic chemicals in gaseous, liquid, and solid forms are known to posses phytoactivity involving numerous aspects of plant growth, development, and reproduction (Nelson and Rossman, 1958; Brain 1964a, b, 1976, Parr and Norman, 1965; Shivanna, 1972; Cartwright, 1976; Hanna, 1977; Johnson and Brown, 1978; Theurer, 1979; Pfahler *et al.*. 1980, 1981; Pfahler, 1981). Early interest in phytoactive chemicals was generated in the agricultural and forestry sectors as a means of improving yields, quality or mechanical harvest. Initially, the phytoactivity of most chemicals was determined empirically by applying highly purified compounds at various concentrations on selected species at various stages in their life cycle and observing the effects (Saggers, 1976). If some type of activity was detected by this screening procedure, an imitative approach was taken in which compounds structurally similar to the active compound were prepared in the hope of improving upon the activity of the original compound. No simple relationship between chemical structure and phytoactivity was found for most compounds (Brain, 1964b, 1976; Linser, 1964). However, a closer relationship between the chemical structure and plant auxin activity was detected (Linser, 1964; Reeve and Crozier, 1976). Apparently, chemical structure has very limited value in predicting phytoactivity in all but a restricted group of compounds. At the present time, the rational approach is increasingly used to predict phytoactivity (Saggers, 1976). This involves making detailed studies of plant biochemistry and physiology in order to more accurately predict plant systems which may be more vulnerable to certain groups of chemicals. However, this approach requires much more specific biochemical and physiological information about plant systems than is presently available or can be reasonably collected for a large number of higher plant species.

In addition to the major differences among higher plant species and phytoactive chemicals discussed above, many other factors influence the species–chemical interaction. The stage in the life cycle exposed to the chemicals greatly alters the effects. With herbicides, sensitivity decreases with plant maturity so that very little response is apparent in the reproductive stage (Aberg, 1964). Gametocides are applied at a very short period in the life cycle to induce pollen sterility. Even with this very brief period which, in some species, covers no more than a few days, remarkable differences in the effectiveness of the chemical were noted (Hanna, 1977; Johnson and Brown, 1978; Theurer, 1979). Also, more than one stage of the life cycle can be affected by the same chemical pollutant. Ozone is a gaseous chemical pollutant released directly into the biosphere as a result of industrial activity. In tobacco, ozone is known to produce weather fleck on the leaves (Dean, 1972) and also decreases *in vitro* pollen germination and tube growth (Feder, 1968, 1978).

The effect of environmental forces on both the plant species and chemical also influences the sensitivity of the species and the phytoactivity of the chemical. Plant growth, development, and reproduction are influenced by many environmental factors (temperature, wind, intensity and spectrum of light, mineral nutrition, soil moisture, plant competition, soil microbial populations) which markedly influence the plant response to chemicals (Aberg and Stecko, 1976; Muzik, 1976). The structure and phytoactivity of chemicals are known to be altered by various physical (air, soil, moisture, light, heat), chemical (reactions with other chemicals), and biological (plants, animals, microbes) forces in the environment (Crosby, 1976, 1977; Hartley, 1976; Kaufman and Kearney, 1976; Cremlyn, 1978). A further complicating aspect of this chemical–environment interaction is that some known chemical pollutants interact with the environment in such a manner that an indirect effect on plants results. This indirect effect is not associated with the structure of the chemical pollutant *per se* and cannot be detected by exposing the plant to the chemical pollutant directly. For example, chlorofluorocarbons which are used as aerosol propellants and refrigerants catalytically reduce the ozone layer high above the earth which, in turn, allows an increase in ultraviolet radiation in the B range (UVB = 280–320 nm) to reach the biosphere (Cicerone *et al.*, 1974; Cutchis, 1974; Hammond and Maugh, 1974). UVB is known to produce multiple biological effects including the reduction of photosynthetic activity and efficiency (Caldwell, 1971), induction of genetic alterations (Stadler and Uber, 1942; Swanson and Stadler, 1955), an increase in the incidence of human skin cancer (Cutchis, 1974), and a sharp decrease in *in vitro* pollen tube growth in maize (Pfahler, 1981). Another possible indirect effect of chemicals involves those species which, by necessity, must be pollinated by insects or birds (Raven, 1979). The reduction or elimination of these animal species by chemicals would alter reproduction in the vulnerable plant species.

In summary, the response of a plant species to a chemical is conditioned by at least five major components:

(1) a species component;
(2) a genetic component within the species;
(3) a stage of life component;
(4) a chemical component; and
(5) an environmental component influencing both the plant species and the chemical.

The large number of interactions possible among these components containing so many variables indicates the scope and complexity of the problem in developing adequate testing methods.

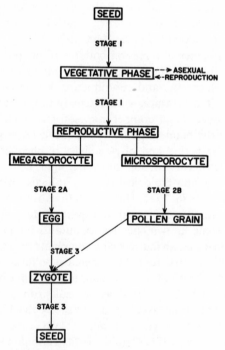

Figure 1   The stages in the life cycle of a representative higher plant

3 TESTS

An examination of the tests available indicated that three distinct stages of the life cycle were generally, involved. These three stages (Figure 1) in the life cycle of a representative higher plant are as follows:

(1) stage 1 (seed germination to the reproductive phase);
(2) stage 2 (sporogenesis); and
(3) state 3 (mature gametes to mature seeds).

The principal features, characteristics, and limitations of the tests for each of these stages will be discussed.

3.1 Stage I

Many individual reports are available regarding the effect of various chemicals on different aspects of numerous plant species (Parr and Norman, 1965; Steward and Krikorian, 1971). However, few tests specifically designed to determine the effect of a large number of chemicals on a broad spectrum of higher plant species in stage 1 have been developed. One exception is the *in vivo* standardized tests to screen chemicals for potential agricultural use and which involve a broad range of species exposed to highly purified chemicals of known structure applied at controlled concentrations (Linser, 1964; Saggers, 1976). Since these *in vivo* standardized tests represent a model approaching that required for tests at other stages, a more detailed description of these tests will be presented to indicate the factors and considerations involved in their development and application.

3.1.1 *In Vitro Tests*

In vitro tests involve the use of isolated enzyme systems or organelles, single cell cultures or selected plant tissues which can technically be derived from any stage of the life cycle but are usually isolated from stage 1 (Saggers, 1976). These tests are of particular value when a quantitative measure of a specific response is required such as inhibition of growth, photosynthesis, or respiration. They are also attractive where space and the quantity of the compound are severely limited, when speed is important, when a large number of species are to be analysed, and where strict environmental controls are necessary. The major disadvantage is that little is known about the relationship between specific *in vitro* and *in vivo* plant systems and, as a result, the projection of *in vitro* tests to *in vivo* whole plant responses is unreliable and, in some cases, very misleading.

3.1.2 *In Vivo Tests*

Controlled environment conditions A series of related standardized tests involving seedling grown in soil under rigidly controlled environmental conditions (constant 20 °C with 14 hours' day length and 8000 lux light intensity) are available which are designed primarily to recognize the many phytoactive effects of a large number of chemicals for potential agricultural use (Saggers, 1976).

The growth regulator test assesses the reaction of one species, French beans (*Phaseolus vulgaris* L. cv. Canadian Wonder), 14 days after planting. This species is particularly sensitive to chemicals which influence the growth of internodal tissue, affect dominance of the apical meristem and desiccate foliage.

The post-emergence test involves a sampling of species representing major taxonomic groups and life forms. To illustrate the range of species selected one group in use is as follows:

(1) peas (*Pisum sativum* L. cv. Onward);
(2) white mustard (*Sinapsis alba* L.);
(3) linseed (*Linum usitatissimum* L);
(4) sugarbeet (*Beta vulgaris* L. cv. Sharpe's Klein E);
(5) ryegrass (*Lolium perenne* L. cv. Westerwolthe); and
(6) oats (*Avena sativa* cv. Condor).

This group includes four dicotyledons and two monocotyledons with unprotected and protected meristems, respectively. It also includes peas with a waxy leaf surface which is difficult to wet making this species relatively resistant to many chemicals. In contrast, mustard is easy to wet, sensitive to a wide range of chemicals and is a representative of the family, Cruciferae, which contains many species. Linseed has the capacity to regrow rapidly from the leaf axils if damaged by a non-systemic chemical. Sugarbeets are a relatively sensitive species belonging to the family, Chenopodiaceae which also contains many species. None of these species must be included and could be replaced provided that the range of taxonomic and biological qualities necessary to assay some aspect of the phytoactivity of chemicals was maintained. Fourteen days after planting when the first leaf is fully expanded, the plants from each species is exposed to the candidate chemical at a known concentration. Twenty-four hours after treatment, the plants are examined for any rapid reaction to the chemicals. Seven days later, a complete assessment is made. Each species is scored on a scale of 0 to 100 with 0 = no effect and 100 = complete kill. An estimate is also made on qualitative aspects of the reaction. The nature of the qualitative response with the suspected primary site of action in parentheses is as follows:

(1) scorch or desiccant effects following loss of turgor (interference with membrane integrity);
(2) growth inhibition (upset of cell division or elongation);
(3) necrosis or a slow discoloration and death of the tissue (disruption of metabolic processes);
(4) hormone effects or growth distortion (disturbance of endogenous hormone balance);

(5) change in pigmentation such as chlorosis (blockage or chlorophyll synthesis) or anthocyanin production (sugar accumulation following a blockage of transport or respiration);
(6) leaf (abscission);
(7) growth stimulation (increase in axillary bud development or tillering);
(8) cuticular abnormalities (modification of wax formation); and
(9) root inhibition or deformities.

One or a combination of these responses show phytoactivity of the chemical, exhibited by all commercial herbicides.

The pre-emergence tests involves these species with the exception that sugarbeets are replaced by maize (*Zea mays* L.), a species which broadens the monocotyledon range and is particularly resistant to certain groups of chemicals applied in this manner. In this test, the candidate chemicals are mixed with the soil before planting. The same time schedule and types of observations are followed as in the post-emergence test.

Greenhouse conditions In these tests, the effects of chemicals over a longer period in the life cycle of the species are examined both in a qualitative and quantitative manner. Plants are grown in soil under less rigidly controlled but more normal environmental conditions than in the controlled environment tests. Usually, only a small percentage of the chemicals screened in the controlled environment tests show any phytoactivity and are examined further. Therefore, greenhouse tests involve screening fewer chemicals and more species can be included. For brevity, a listing of the species will not be presented since only the number of species within the groups given in the controlled environment tests is increased and an appropriate listing also appears in Saggers (1976).

The growth regulator test is difficult to extend to other species if activity of a chemical in this area is detected. This is because these chemicals modify the delicate balance of endogenous hormone systems and the use of species other than the French bean requires exposure of the species at the correct development stage under actual growing conditions. Empirical testing using species of special interest is necessary.

The post-emergence tests under greenhouse conditions are identical to the controlled environment test.

For the pre-emergence test, two methods of soil treatment are employed, a soil incorporation treatment similar to the controlled environment test and a soil surface treatment by overhead spray. These two methods can produce markedly different responses depending on such factors as volatility, soil mobility, absorption of the chemical, and site of uptake by the plant, i.e. root or hypocotyl. As in the controlled environment test, the species are the same and the assessment of plant response is taken during the same period. In addition, more detailed data can be collected later in the life cycle.

Field tests Chemicals identified as phytoactive in the controlled environment and greenhouse tests must be evaluated in field tests. These are essential to determine the influence of light, temperature, rainfall, soil type, and growth stage on the final expression of the phytoactivity. No standardized group of species or environments is suggested but usually the number of species, chemicals, or environments that can be included is comparatively small. Not only are field tests essential for the examination of the effects of chemicals on stage 1, but they also can be designed so that valuable information about the effects of chemicals on later stages is obtained.

3.2 Stage 2

Our present knowledge of sporogenesis was derived from a few species particularly adapted to these types of studies (Taylor, 1967). These studies suggest that no basic differences between megasporogenesis (stage 2A, Figure 1) and microsporogenesis (stage 2B, Figure 1) exist in higher plants. However, the ease of detecting any disruption in these two parallel processes differs markedly. Any disruption in megasporogenesis would be expressed as an inviable egg which is embedded in maternal tissue. This phenomena can be analysed only microscopially and with great difficulty. A similar disruption in microsporogenesis can be analysed quite readily by a simple examination of the end product of microsporogenesis, pollen grains which are easily obtained in large quantities. As a result, most of the limited information about chemical effects is associated with microsporogenesis.

No standardized tests as outlined for stage 1 have been developed for stage 2. The few tests available are quite limited as to the number of species, chemicals, and environment sampled. The *in vivo* tests for stage 2 generally are conducted under the less controlled greenhouse or field conditions since growing most species to stage 2 under controlled environment conditions is difficult.

3.2.1 *In Vivo Tests*

Tissue culture techniques involving pollen grains, microsporocytes, or anthers have been developed for a small but growing number of species (Nitsch and Nitsch, 1969). In addition to the species limitation, these techniques require a highly defined exotic medium and a rigidly controlled environment. The resulting tissues also contain extensive and unpredictable chromosome irregularities. Considering these severe limitations, tissue culture techniques do not appear adaptable to a large scale screening programme at the present time or for that matter, in the near future.

3.2.2. *In Vivo Tests*

The desire to chemically induce male sterility to produce hybrids in a limited number of agricultural species has stimulated the empirical testing of a number of chemicals for their effects on microsporogenesis (Nelson and Rossman, 1958; Kaul and Singh, 1967; Hanna, 1977; Johnson and Brown, 1978; Theurer, 1979). These tests involve highly purified chemicals of known structure and concentrations applied to plants at various stages of microsporogenesis growing under greenhouse or field conditions. The effects are assessed either by examining the number and condition of the pollen grains or counting the number of seeds produced. The results based on seed number are obviously confounded with the chemical effects on megasporogenesis producing egg abortion and on the sporophyte which may reduce the potential of the plant to produce normal seed numbers. In general, the species, stage of microsporogenesis and environment are major influencing factors. The development of standardized tests in this area would require a large number of diverse species and more basic information about the interactions involving the chemicals, sporogenesis and environment.

3.3 Stage 3

Stage 3 contains a number of sequential processes whose disruption can severely affect reproduction. The pollen grain has a much more active and demanding role in stage 3 than the egg and has a specialized structure and unique properties to fulfil this role. The pollen grain is independent of the sporophyte on which it is produced for a period of its life cycle, the length of which varies with species. The pollen grain must be transported to a receptive stigma by gravity, wind, insects or birds and must retain germinability during this transport period (Linskens, 1964, 1967; Stanley and Linskens, 1974; Raven, 1979). After attachment to a receptive stigma, the grain must compete with other grains in germination and tube growth through the style to affect fertilization (Mulcahy, *et al.*, 1975). In self-incompatible species, certain pollen grains cannot compete or participate in fertilization because of genetic factors (Townsend, 1971; Linskens, 1974; Mulcahy and Johnson, 1978). During all these processes associated with the pollen grain, the egg remains surrounded and nourished by the sporophyte, passively awaiting the arrival of the pollen tube. After fertilization, the process of seed development is also protected and nourished by the female sporophyte. Most research in stage 3 has been devoted to the pollen grain during its independent transport phase, its attachment and germination on the stigma, and its tube growth through the style in competition with other pollen grains. Very limited information is available regarding the activity of the egg during this period or seed development after fertilization. However, additional knowledge of egg maturation, embryogenesis, and seed development is critical since any disruption of these processes eliminates an individual from the next generation whereas a percentage reduction in pollen number or function does not usually reduce the number of progeny.

No standardized tests as outlined in stage 1, are available for stage 3. The limited number of procedures that have been developed involve only a few species, chemicals and environments. The *in vivo* tests for stage 3 are generally conducted in less environmentally controlled greenhouse or field conditions since growing most species to this advanced stage under rigidly controlled environments is practically difficult.

3.3.1 *In Vitro Tests*

Many *in vitro* pollen germination and tube length studies involving a limited number of species have been conducted (Stanley and Linskens, 1974). Some of these studies, especially those involving commercial species, have included chemicals and/or conditions which are not essential for pollen germination and tube growth and could be classified as potential phytoactive pollutants (Feder, 1968; Gentile *et al.*, 1971, 1973, 1978; Shivanna, 1972; Church and Williams, 1977; Pfahler *et al.*, 1980, 1981; Pfahler, 1981). Two major difficulties are encountered when *in vitro* pollen germination tests are considered to screen the effect of possible phytoactive chemicals or conditions on a wide range of species. First, the number and diversity of species that can be tested may be limited. Among almost 2000 species of angiosperms studied, about 30% shed their pollen in the trinucleate condition and 70% in the binucleate condition (Brewbaker, 1967). Trinucleate pollen grains as a group are very difficult to germinate *in vitro* and thus these species are not well adapted to these types of studies. Second, the pollen tube length obtained *in vitro* rarely equals and, in most cases, is much less than, that necessary to effect fertilization *in vivo*. From this observation, the question arises whether *in vitro* results accurately reflect the *in vivo* process (Stanley and Linskens, 1974).

In recent years, test-tube fertilization and placental pollination procedures have been refined to include more species and to improve seed set (Maheshiwari and Kanta, 1964; Zenkteler, 1967; Balatkova and Tupy, 1968, 1972; Balatkova *et al.*, 1976, 1977). Initially, the major thrust in the development of these procedures was to overcome self-incompatibility and interspecific crossing barriers by altering the critical pollen grain–stigma–style relationship in the fertilization process. However, these processes, especially test-tube fertilization, could be readily adapted to studying the effects of chemical pollutants. The major advantage of this approach is that under highly controlled environmental conditions, the whole process from pollination through seed development could be closely monitored and analysed at any stage. The major disadvantages are that, at the present time, these procedures have been developed for only a limited number and range of species and the relationship between *in vitro* results and the *in vivo* processes has not been definitely established.

3.3.2 *In Vivo Tests*

In vivo tests have been conducted in a limited number of species (Kiesselbach, 1949; Walden, 1967; Pfahler and Linskens, 1972; Pfahler, 1974; Went, 1974;

Mulcahy, *et al.*, 1975; Schwartz and Osterman, 1976; Cass and Peteya, 1979; Kroh *et al.*, 1979). The main thrusts of these studies were to examine the process in general or the effects of certain factors on pollen viability, germination or tube growth competition through the style. A large number of these studies used the number, genetic constitution, or morphology of the resulting mature seeds as a measure of the effect. Up to this time, few attempts to examine the effects of factors at any stage between pollination and mature seed production were made, although, as in test-tube fertilization and placental pollinations, these examinations are possible. The major advantage of this procedure is that the complete *in vivo* process from pollination through seed development can be closely monitored and analysed at any stage. However, the number of species adapted to this type of study is limited and the environmental conditions under which they are grown cannot be rigidly controlled.

4 ANALYSIS AND RECOMMENDATIONS

This report has clearly shown that the development of accurate, predictive tests is complicated by the extent of diversity in higher plants and the multiple effects of chemicals at all stages of plant growth, differentiation, and reproduction, in addition to the environmental influence on both the plant and the chemical. With this degree of complexity, the development of standardized multi-tiered assays which are regularly employed to predict the mutagenicity and potential carcinogenicity of chemical compounds in humans is not feasible (Epler *et al.*, 1978; Hearth, 1978). These rapid assays are based on the apparently correct assumption that any chemical which will induce mutations and/or chromosomal damage in certain microbes and mice will also induce similar effects in humans. In higher plants, the possible effects of chemical pollutants include not only mutations and chromosomal damage, but also a wide array of morphological and physiological alterations which are influenced by environmental, species, and genetic factors and can ultimately change reproductive capacity. Therefore, tests to predict the effects of chemical pollutants on the reproduction of higher plants must, by necessity, involve the actual testing of higher plant species rather than lower organisms.

Obviously, all species of higher plants cannot be tested individually so, to obtain maximum predictability, a range of species representing major taxonomic groups must be selected. The selection cannot be based solely on taxonomic group but must also consider such practical aspects as the availability of seeds or plant material for propagation, length of life cycle, reliability of seed germination, uniformity of growth patterns, and at least some insight as to the extent of genetic heterogeneity within the species (Saggers, 1976). Among all the tests outlined in this report for the three stages, the standardized tests in stage 1 included the widest range of species selected specifically for predictive purposes. However, because of practical limitations, the stage 1 tests do not include woody perennials so that any prediction in relation to this important group can only be considered speculative and would require further testing using species of interest for variation of results. Tests in stages 2 and 3 included only a limited number of species which have been selected either because of economic significance or their adaptability for a specific study.

This report indicates that the range of chemicals which are presently known to produce alterations during one or more stages of the life cycle is extremely large. In most, if not all of the studies cited here, the effects of highly purified chemicals of known structure and concentration were examined. The chemical pollutants to be tested will generally be mixtures containing numerous chemicals with unknown structures and concentrations. In preliminary screening, the testing of these complex mixtures is undersirable but probably unavoidable since rapid microbial assays cannot be used and complicated separation and identification analyses are impractical (Epler *et al.*, 1978). If phytoactivity from these mixtures is detected in the initial screening, then separation and identification of the active chemical components is essential.

Environmental effects are and will remain a major unresolved problem in interpreting and extrapolating test results over a broad spectrum of species and chemicals. The level of environmental control in plant toxicity testing varies with the type of test. Environmental conditions for *in vitro* and controlled climate tests can be manipulated artifically but projection of the results to plants in their normal habitat is complicated accordingly. The environment associated with field tests cannot be extensively manipulated; however, the results more closely reflect the conditions under which the plants grow in nature.

This report indicates that, at the present time, tests are available that could be used or at least would represent a starting point in the development of specific standardized methods to measure the effect of chemical pollutants on reproduction in higher plants. The standardized tests which were developed to screen chemicals for potential agricultural purposes in stage 1 could be adapted with little or no change. Most tests in stages 2 and 3 are severely restricted as to the number of species, chemicals and environments sampled. These techniques must be expanded in terms of the number and distribution of species that can be tested and refined to permit more rapid analysis. This expansion and refinement will require a major commitment of manpower and resources.

5 REFERENCES

Aberg, E. (1964). Susceptibility: Factors in the plant modifying the response of a given species to treatment. In Andus, L. J. (Ed.) *The Physiology and Biochemistry of Herbicides*, pp. 401–422. Academic Press, New York, San Francisco, London.

Aberg, E. and Stecko, V. (1976). Internal factors affecting toxicity. In Andus, L. J. (Ed.) *Herbicides—Physiology, Biochemistry, Ecology*, Vol. 2, pp. 175–201. Academic Press, New York, San Francisco, London.

Andel, O. M. van and Zweep, W. van der (1976). Morphogenetic responses of plants. In Andus, L. J. (Ed.) *Herbicides—Physiology, Biochemistry, Ecology*, Vol. 1, pp. 127–163. Academic Press, New York, San Francisco, London.

Balatkova, V., Hrabetova, E. and Tupy, J. (1976). The effect of sugar nutrition of *in vitro* pollinated placentae on seed set and dormancy in *Nicotiana tabacum*. L. *Experientia (Basel)* **32**, 1255.

Balatkova, V. and Tupy, J. (1968). Test-tube fertilization in *Nicotiana tabacum* by means of an artificial pollen tube culture. *Biol. Plant. (Prague)* **10**, 266–270.

Balatkova, V. and Tupy, J. (1972). Some factors affecting the seed set after *in vitro* pollination of excised placentae of *Nicotiana tabacum* L. *Biol. Plant. (Prague)* **14**, 82–88.

Balatkova, V., Tupy, J. and Hrabetova, E. (1977). Seed formation in *Narcissus pseudonarcissus* L. after placental pollination *in vitro*. *Plant Sci. Lett.* **8**, 17–21.

Brewbaker, J. L. (1967). The distribution and phylogenetic significance of binucleate and trinucleate pollen grains in the angiosperms. *Am. J. Bot.* **54**, 1069–1083.

Brian, R. C. (1964a). The effects of herbicides on biophysical processes in the plant. In Andus, L. J. (Ed.) *The Physiology and Biochemistry of Herbicides*, pp. 357–386. Academic Press, New York, San Francisco, London.

Brian, R. C. (1964b). The classification of herbicides and types of toxicity. In Andus, L. J. (Ed.) *The Physiology and Biochemistry of Herbicides*, pp. 1–37. Academic Press, New York, San Francisco, London.

Brain, R. C. (1976). The history and classification of herbicides. In Andus, L. J. (Ed.) *Herbicides—Physiology, Biochemistry, Ecology*, Vol. 1, pp. 1–54. Academic Press, New York, San Francisco, London.

Bukovac, M. J. (1976). Herbicide entry into plants. In Andus, L. J. (Ed.) *Herbicides—Physiology, Biochemistry, Ecology*, Vol. 1, pp. 335–364. Academic Press, New York, San Francisco, London.

Caldwell, M. M. (1971). Solar UV radiation and the growth and development of higher plants. In Giese, A. C. (Ed.) *Photophysiology*, Vol. 6, pp. 131–177. Academic Press, New York, San Francisco, London.

Cartwright, P. M. (1976). General growth responses of plants. In Andus, L. J. (Ed.) *Herbicides—Physiology, Biochemistry, Ecology*, Vol. 1, pp. 55–82. Academic Press, New York, San Francisco, London.

Cass, D. D. and Peteya, D. J. (1979). Growth of barley tubes *in vivo*. Ultrastructural aspects of early pollen tube growth in the stigmatic hair. *Can. J. Bot.* **57**, 386–396.

Church, R. M. and Williams, R. R.(1977). The toxicity to apple pollen of several fungicides, as demonstrated by *in vivo* and *in vitro* techniques. *J. Hortic Sci.* **52**, 429–436.

Cicerone, R. J., Stolarski, R. S. and Walters, S. (1974). Stratospheric ozone destruction by man-made chlorofluoromethanes, *Science (Washington, DC)* **185**, 1165–1167.

Crafts, A. S. (1964). Herbicide behaviour in the plant. In Andus, L. J. (Ed.) *The Physiology and Biochemistry of Herbicides*, pp. 75–110. Academic Press, New York, San Francisco, London.

Cremlyn, R. (1978). *Pesticides*. John Wiley & Sons, Chichester.

Crosby, D. G. (1976). Nonbiological degradation of herbicides in the soil. In Andus, L. J. (Ed.) *Herbicides—Physiology, Biochemistry, Ecology*, Vol. 2, pp. 65–97. Academic Press, New York, San Francisco, London.

Crosby, D. G. (1977). The environmental chemistry of herbicides. In Plimmer, J. R. (Ed.) *Pesticide Chemistry in the 20th Century*, pp. 93–108. American Chemical Society, Washington, DC.

Cutchis, P. (1974). Stratospheric ozone depletion and solar ultraviolet radiation on earth. *Science (Washington, DC)* **184**, 13–19.

Dean, C. E. (1972). *Ozone Air Pollution and Weather Fleck of Tobacco*. Florida Agr. Exp. Sta. Circ. S-218.

Epler, J. L., Larimer, F. W., Rao, T. K., Nix, C. E. and Ho, T. (1978). Energy-related pollutants in the environment: Use of short-term tests for mutagenicity in the isolation and identification of biohazards. *Environ. Health Perspect.* **27**, 11–20.

Feder, W. A. (1968). Reduction in tobacco pollen germination and tube elongation, induced by low levels of ozone. *Science (Washington, DC)* **160**, 1122.

Feder, W. A. (1978). Plants as bioassay systems for monitoring atmospheric pollutants. *Environ. Health Perspect.* **27**, 139–147.

Gentile, A. G., Gallagher, K. J. and Santner, Z. (1971). Effect of some formulated insecticides on pollen germination in tomato and petunia. *J. econ. Entomol.* **64**, 916–919.

Gentile, A. G., Vaughan, A. W. and Pfeiffer, D. G. (1978). Cucumber pollen germination and tube elongation inhibited by or reduced by pesticides and adjuvants. *Environ. Entomol.* **7**, 689–694.

Gentile, A. G., Vaughan, A. W., Richman, S. M. and Eaton, A. T. (1973). Corn pollen germination and tube elongation inhibited or reduced by commercial formulation of pesticides and adjuvants. *Environ. Entomol.* **2**, 473–476.

Gortner, C. J. and Zweep, W. van der (1964). Morphogenetic effects on herbicides. In Andus, L. J. (Ed.) *The Physiology and Biochemistry of Herbicides*, pp. 235–275. Academic Press, New York, San Francisco, London.

Hammond, A. L. and Maugh, T. H. (1974). Stratospheric pollution: Mutiple threats to earth's ozone. *Science (Washington, DC)* **186**, 335–338.

Hanna, W. W. (1977). Effect of DPX 3778 on anther dehiscence in pearl millet. *Crop Sci.* **17**, 965–967.

Hartley, G. S. (1976). Physical behaviour in the soil. In Andus, L. J. (Ed.) *Herbicides—Physiology, Biochemistry, Ecology*, Vol. 1, pp. 1–28. Academic Press, New York, San Francisco, London.

Heath, C. W. Jr. (1978). Environmental pollutants and the epidemiology of cancer. *Environ. Health Perspect.* **27**, 7–10.

Johnson, R. R. and Brown, C. M. Jr. (1978). Use of DPX 3778 to produce hybrid wheat seed. *Crop Sci.* **18**, 1026–1028.

Kaufman, D. D. and Kearney, P. O. (1976). Microbial transformation in the soil. In Andus, L. J. (Ed.) *Herbicides—Physiology, Biochemistry, Ecology*, Vol. 2, pp. 29–64. Academic Press, New York, San Francisco, London.

Kaul, C. L. and Singh, S. P. (1967). Effects of certain growth retardants on growth, flowering, and pollen viability in fenu-greek (*Trigonella foenum-graecum* L.). *Indian J. Plant Physiol.* **10**, 54–61.

Kiermayer, O. (1964). Growth responses to herbicides. In Andus, L. J. (Ed.) *The Physiology and Biochemistry of Herbicides*, pp. 207–233. Academic Press, New York, San Francisco, London.

Kiesselbach, T. A. (1949). *The Structure and Reproduction of Corn.* Univ. Nebraska Res. Bull. 161.

Kroh, M., Gorissen, M. H. and Pfahler, P. L. (1979). Ultrastructural studies on styles and pollen tubes of *Zea mays* L.: General survey on pollen tube growth in vivo. *Acta Bot. Neerl.* **28**, 513–518.

Linck, A. J. (1976). Effects on the cytology and fine structure of plant cells. In Addus, L. J. (Ed.) *Herbicides—Physiology, Biochemistry, Ecology*, Vol. 1, pp. 83–125. Academic Press, New York, San Francisco, London.

Linser, H. (1964). The design of herbicides. In Andus, L. J. (Ed.) *The Physiology and Biochemistry of Herbicides*, pp. 483–505. Academic Press, New York, San Francisco, London.

Linskens, H. F. (1964). Pollen Physiology. *A. Rev. Plant Physiol.* **15**, 255–270.

Linskens, H. F. (1967). Pollen. In Ruhland, W. (Ed.) *Encyclopedia of Plant Physiology*, Vol. 18, pp. 368–406. Springer-Verlag, Berlin.

Linskens, H. F. (1974). Translocation phenomena in the petunia flower after cross- and self-pollination. In Linskens, H. F. (Ed.) *Fertilization in Higher Plants*, pp. 285–292. North-Holland, Amsterdam.

Maheshwari, P. and Kanta, K. (1964). Control of fertilization. In Linskens, H. F. (Ed.) *Pollen Physiology and Fertilization*, pp. 187–193. North-Holland, Amsterdam.

Moreland, D. E. (1977). Mode of action of herbicides. In Plimmer, J. R. (Ed.) *Pesticide Chemistry in the 20th Century*, pp. 56–75. Amer. Chem. Soc., Washington, DC.

Moreland, D. E. and Hilton, J. L. (1976). Actions on photosynthetic systems. In Andus, L. J. (Ed.) *Herbicides—Physiology, Biochemistry, Ecology*, Vol. 1, pp. 493–523. Academic Press, New York, San Francisco, London.

Mulcahy, D. L. and Johnson, C. M. (1978). Self-incompatibility systems as bioassays for mutagens. *Environ. Health Perspect.* **27**, 85–90.

Mulcahy, D. L., Mulcahy, G. B. and Ottaviano, E. (1975). Sporophytic expression of gametophytic competition in *Petunia hybrida*. In Mulcahy, D. L. (Ed.) *Gamete Competition in Plants and Animals*, pp. 227–232. North-Holland, Amsterdam.

Muzik, T. J. (1976). Influence of environmental factors on toxicity to plants. In Andus, L. J. (Ed.) *Herbicides—Physiology, Biochemistry, Ecology*, Vol. 2, pp. 203–247. Academic Press, New York, San Francisco, London.

Nelson, P. and Rossman, E. C. (1958). Chemical induction of male sterility in inbred lines of maize by the use of gibberellins. *Science (Washington, DC)* **127**, 1500–1501.

Nitsch, J. P. and Nitsch, C. (1969). Haploid plants from pollen grains. *Science (Washington, DC)* **63**, 85–87.

Parr, J. F. and Norman, A. G. (1965). Considerations in the use of surfactants in plant systems: A review. *Bot. Gaz. (Chicago)* **126**, 86–96.

Pfahler, P. L. (1968). *In vitro* germination and pollen tube growth of maize (*Zea mays* L.) pollen. III. Pollen source, calcium, and boron interactions. *Can. J. Bot.* **46**, 235–240.

Pfahler, P. L. (1974). Fertilization ability of maize (*Zea mays* L.) pollen grains. IV. Influence of storage and the alleles at the shrunken, sugary and waxy loci. In Linskens, H. F. (Ed.) *Fertilization in Higher Plants*, pp. 15–25. North-Holland, Amsterdam.

Pfahler, P. L. (1981). *In vitro* germination characteristics of maize pollen to detect biological activity of environmental pollutants. *Environ. Health Perspect.* **37**, 125–132.

Pfahler, P. L. and Linskens, H. F. (1972). *In vitro* germination and pollen tube growth of maize (*Zea mays* L.) pollen grains. VI. Combined effects of storage and the alleles at the waxy (wx), sugary (su_1) and shrunken (sh_2) loci. *Theor. appl. Genet.* **42**, 136–140.

Pfahler, P. L., Linskens, H. F., Schoot, H. W., and Wilcox, M. (1981). Surfactant effects of petunia pollen germination *in vitro*. *Bull. environ. Contam. Toxicol.* **26**, 567–570.

Pfahler, P. L., Linskens, H. F. and Wilcox, M. (1980). *In vitro* germination and pollen tube growth of maize (*Zea mays* L.) pollen IX. Pollen source genotype and non-ionic surfactant interactions. *Can. J. Bot.* **58**, 557–561.

Raven, P. H. (1979). A survey of reproductive biology in Onagraceae. *N. Z. J. Bot.* **17**, 575–593.

Reeve, D. R. and Crozier, A. (1976). Gibberellin bioassays. In Krishnamoorthy, H. N. (Ed.) *Gibberellins and Plant Growth*, pp. 35–64. Wiley, New York, Chichester, Brisbane, Toronto.

Saggers, D. T. (1976). The search for new herbicides. In Andus, L. J. (Ed.) *Herbicides—Physiology, Biochemistry, Ecology*, Vol. 2, pp. 447–473. Academic Press, New York, San Francisco, London.

Schwartz, D. and Osterman, J. (1976). A pollen selection system for alcohol-dehydrogenase-negative mutants in plants. *Genetics* **83**, 63–65.

Shivanna, K. R. (1972). Effect of non-ionic surfactants on pollen germination and pollen tube growth. *Current Sci.* **41**, 609–610.

Stadler, L. J. and Uber, F. M. (1942). Genetic effects of ultra violet radiation in maize. IV. Comparison of monochromatic radiations. *Genetics* **27**, 84–118.

Stanley, R. G. and Linskens, H. F. (1974). *Pollen—Biology, Biochemistry, Management.* Springer-Verlag, Berlin.

Steward, F. C. and Krikorian, A. D. (1971). *Plants, Chemicals and Growth.* Academic Press, New York and London.

Swanson, C. P. and Stadler, L. J. (1955). The effect of ultraviolet radiation on the genes and chromosomes of higher plants. In Hollaender, A. (Ed.) *Radiation Biology*, Vol. 2, pp. 249–284. McGraw-Hill, New York.

Taylor, J. H. (1967). Meiosis. In Ruhland, W. (Ed.) *Encylopedia of Plant Physiology*, Vol. 18, pp. 344–367. Springer-Verlag, Berlin.

Theurer, J. C. (1979). Effect of DPX 3778 as a male gametocide in sugarbeets. *Can. J. Plant Sci.* **59**, 463–468.

Townsend, C. E. (1971). Advances in the study of incompatibility. In Heslop-Harrison, J. (Ed.) *Pollen—Development and Physiology*, pp. 281–309. Butterworth, London.

Walden, D. B. (1967). Male gametophyte of *Zea mays* L. I. Some factors influencing fertilization. *Crop Sci.* **7**, 441–444.

Went, J. L. van (1974). The ultrastructure of Impatiens pollen. In Linskens, H. F. (Ed.) *Fertilization in Higher Plants*, pp. 81–88. North-Holland, Amsterdam.

Zenkteler, M. (1967). Test-tube fertilization of ovules in *Melandrium album* Mill. with pollen grains of several species of the Caryophyllaceae family. *Experientia* (*Basel*) **23**, 775–777.

Methods for Assessing the Effects of Chemicals on Reproductive Functions
Edited by V. B. Vouk and P. J. Sheehan
© 1983 SCOPE

Methods for Assessing Effects of Chemicals on Algal Reproduction

ARNE JENSEN

1 INTRODUCTION

Reproduction in lower plants, including algae, is often quite complex, involving a series of stages of very different shape, size and function. In many cases these stages, which constitute the life cycle of the plant, have not all been identified, and their special requirements are unknown.

To illustrate the complexity of the problem, the life cycle of a macroscopic, diplobiontic, red alga is schematically depicted in Figure 1. There is ample opportunity for chemicals to interfere anywhere in this complicated cycle, and it is quite understandable that toxicologists have primarily assessed effects in terms of the simpler process of vegetative proliferation.

Relatively less complex reproductive systems are found among the microscopic algae. These species are very important since they supply the larger portion of primary production in lakes, rivers and especially in the oceans. However, the

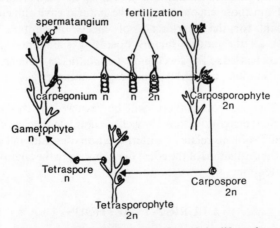

Figure 1   Schematic presentation of the life cycle
of a macroscopic, diplobiontic red algae

515

complete life cycle of many microscopic algae are still quite complex. Reproduction in these plants can remain on the simple vegetative level for very many generations before it suddenly and for no apparent reason switches a sexual stage. Since the vegetative proliferation of many microscopic algae is easily maintained in culture, toxicological and other studies, including biochemical and physiological investigations, have concentrated on this phase of algal reproduction. Current and conventional toxicological methods for the predictive assessment of reproductive injury to algae caused by chemicals are therefore normally restricted to analysis of vegetative proliferation of cells in culture.

These methods assess the influence of chemicals on the growth of algal populations, as characterized by the change in the number of cells in the populations per unit time, or by evaluating other parameters proportional to algal biomass. The results are interpreted in terms of concentrations response curve and IC 50 value, and further information on the influence of the chemical agent on the final cell density.

The major test requirements are:

(1) that desired levels of the toxicant can be prepared, maintained in the active form and measured during the test;
(2) that the cell proliferation can be followed accurately; and
(3) that the test organisms are not stressed unreasonably by the normal test conditions.

Several methods have been developed for this type of toxicological testing, and a few have been adopted nationally and even internationally as standard algal toxicity tests. These tests seem to provide satisfactory data for the ranking of chemicals according to their relative toxicity to test species; however, their virtue as a means of evaluating the real hazard of chemicals in the environment is less obvious. The rather artificial conditions prevailing in these laboratory tests are very different from those encountered in the natural environment and do not generally account for the interference of effects of multiple toxic agents interacting with all the natural factors operating simultaneously in natural habitats. This fact has led to the development of *in situ* test systems, and one such method using marine microalgae in cage cultures has been adopted internationally.

These and other current methods will be reviewed in the following presentation. The characteristic features, as well as the inadequacies of the methods, will be discussed. Problems related to interpretation of results and application of test findings to the evaluation of the effect of chemicals in the environment will be given special attention.

2 CURRENT METHODS

Bioassays based on the proliferation of microscopic algae are in routine use in a number of countries for the testing of toxic substances and for the assessment of cultural eutrophication. It is sufficient review to list chronologically the development of major algal tests: the Algal Assay Procedure Bottle Test of the National Eutrophication Research Program (US Environmental Protection Agency, 1971); the Marine Algal Assay Procedure Bottle Test of the Eutrophication and Lake Restoration Branch (US Environmental Protection Agency, 1974); the Algal Assay Procedure Batch Technique introduced in Denmark (Gargas and Søndergård Pedersen, 1974); the Dutch Water-Determination of Toxicity with Algae proposed as a standard test in 1979 (NEN 6506, 1979); and the Test with a Unicellular Alga for Determining the IC 50 Concentration suggested for inclusion in the OECD Guideline for Testing of Chemicals in 1980.

All of these tests and several other unmentioned procedure involve batch techniques and represent the conventional algal toxicity testing methods. They have been adopted as standard procedures nationally in many cases, and the EPA Bottle Tests and the OECD procedure are also in the process of being adopted on an international basis.

Continuous culture techniques, in the form of a chemostat or a turbidostat, are well established for studies of algal growth as a function of nutrients and physical factors (light, temperature, etc.), but they remain largely unevaluated as methods for toxicity testing. Cage or dialysis culture of microscopic algae seems to be the only technique which is applicable for bioassays *in situ*. The cage method is one of the few techniques available today for pollution monitoring, and its use in the marine environment has been recommended by an IOC bioassay panel (Stebbing *et al.*, 1980).

The above methods are all based on non-synchronized algal cultures, and the observed effects are related to the statistical mean of the populations. In synchronous cultures all cells divide within a very limited time range and show parallel development between the divisions. This method is in current use in biochemical and physiological studies and has been successfully applied to toxicity testing.

2.1 Batch Methods

In the batch technique several identical cultures of the test alga are exposed to systematic dilutions of the chemical to be tested. The increase in cell number is followed for each culture, and the reduction in division rate in relation to an unexposed culture (control or blank) is regarded as a measure of the toxicity. It is necessary to insure that neither nutrients nor light become limiting during the test, and that the total procedure is rigidly standardized to provide reproducible results. Accuracy corresponding to $\pm 20\%$ can then be obtained.

The test is applicable to all compounds that do not interfere directly with the counting of algal cells and do not colour the solution at test concentrations.

A fairly large number of microscopic test algae, both freshwater and marine species, are available from algal culture collections. Only a few, however, are free

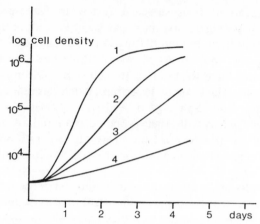

Figure 2   Expected development of a toxicity test with algae

from bacterial contamination (axenic). Axenic cultures are highly recommended for toxicological testing.

In principle the algal population is expected to grow exponentially after a short lag phase and to go gradually into a stationary state. Several techniques have been used to determine the growth rate. Counting cells under the microscope in a special chamber is the most direct method. Electronic particle counting is convenient and rapid, but it requires single cells and does not resolve algal chains or aggregates. Less direct parameters, such as turbidity, light absorption or *in vivo* fluorescence of the culture may be used to estimate growth rate in highly standardized procedures.

When cell density (number of cells per ml of culture) is plotted on a semi-logarithmic scale versus time, a graph of the type depicted in Figure 2 is expected. The curves 1, 2, 3 and 4 represent the control and test cultures receiving increasing concentrations of the toxicant.

The growth rates of the cultures are calculated from the observations, and in a new graph the reduction in growth rate relative to the control is plotted versus the logarithm of the concentration of the toxicant. The concentration estimating 50% inhibition of growth (IC 50) is read from the graph, together with the highest level demonstrating no-observed-effect.

Any one of the following detailed descriptions of this procedure is fully acceptable: the EPA Bottle Tests, the OECD Test with Unicellular Alga, or the Algal Assay Procedure used in Denmark.

2.2 Continuous Cultures

There are two types of continuous cultures, the chemostat and the turbidostat. In the former the growth rate is the independent variable, while in the latter the cell density is varied independently. Both systems are supposed to operate at steady state.

The chemostat holds the algal culture in a reactor which receives a constant flow of the nutrient solution. This flow displaces an identical volume of the culture. The growth rate of the culture is therefore identical to the flow rate when a steady state (constant cell density) is reached. In the turbidostat the cell density is predetermined and regulates the dilution rate. For both types of continuous cultures, the steady-state kinetics of growth is similar and the theory well developed. Addition of chemicals which reduce the growth rate will lead to a lowered steady-state cell density (or washout) in the chemostat, and to a reduced dilution rate in the turbidostat. Both systems are widely used in biochemical studies of nutrient requirements and in studies of the dependence of light and temperature. They have not been generally applied to studies of the influence of toxic substances on the proliferation of algal cells. They do represent, however, very promising potential toxicity testing procedures, especially since they offer constant testing conditions in regard to nutrient concentration, light level, cell density, toxicant levels and concentration of metabolic by-products. In these respects continuous culture methods are superior to the batch method.

A review of the current and future utility of continuous algal cultures in ecological research has recently been published by Rhee (1980).

2.3 Cage Cultures

In the cage culture the test alga is grown in a cage which is open to the movement of light, nutrients and most chemicals but not to the cells themselves. The cage with the culture can be placed in a tank in the laboratory through which the test medium is flowing, or it may be operated *in situ*, i.e., immersed in the lake, river or seawater. In the laboratory, control cultures are run in tanks with the control medium, and the test cultures are maintained in test tanks supplied with selected concentrations of the toxicant dissolved in the medium. *In situ* cultures are preferably operated in series of decreasing pollutant concentrations, including a control culture in a non-polluted or practically non-polluted habitat. In both systems cell proliferation is followed by cell counting or with an alternative technique as previously described.

Besides being the only known way to operate a test culture in the natural environment, cage methods ensure, through the frequent or continuous replacement of external medium, constant external conditions and a stable level of the toxicant throughout the test. The cage culture method is described in detail by Eide *et al.* (1979), and is recommended by a Bioassay Panel of IOC for *in situ* monitoring of pollution effects in the marine environment (Stebbing *et al.*, 1980).

2.4 Synchronous Cultures

Under specific conditions all cells of an algal culture may be forced to develop simultaneously, i.e., at a certain time all cells divide. The daughter cells will then grow in size for a fixed period, prepare for division and divide again in a synchronized pattern. This synchronous pattern of development offers a unique possibility for both rapid and detailed studies of the influence of chemicals on the life cycle and the proliferation of algal cells. Toxic effects of chemical agents can be detected and quantified rapidly (within hours) by means of synchronized cultures because the steps in the life cycle can be sharply defined in such cultures. It is also possible to measure the effect of the toxicant on specific processes, such as the synthesis of DNA, RNA, proteins (including specific enzymes), and carbohydrates. This method has recently been adopted by Norwegian authorities. Presently all dispersants to be used in oil spill clean-up require testing based on synchronous cultures of the green alga, *Chlamydomonas reinhardthi*, in addition to the brown shrimp and limpet tests. The test synchronous culture procedure has been described in detail by Nordland *et al.* (1978).

3 METHODOLOGICAL PROBLEMS

As long as the studies of the effect of chemicals on algal reproduction are restricted to the vegetative proliferation of cells, the risk that crucial problems in the complex reproductive cycle of algae will be overlooked always remains. It is rather likely that processes other than the vegetative division may be more sensitive to chemical interference.

In addition to this general problem, there are specific difficulties in establishing and maintaining constant biologically active doses of the toxic substance throughout the tests. For instance, heavy metals present special problems in algal test systems because the organisms frequently deactivate the toxic forms of the metal by exuding chelating substances. Light-sensitive chemicals also provide special difficulties in algal bioassays, since light cannot be excluded during the test.

A problem common to all algal tests is inherent in the need to determine increments in biomass of the growing population. Cell number is an obvious growth parameter, but average cell size frequently changes during the development of a culture. Other growth characteristics, such as increment in pigment content (chlorophyll *a*), ATP, protein, carbon, and in the levels of other chemical compounds are all dependent on the constant chemical composition of the cells during the test. However, it is well documented that the chemical composition of algal cultures vary with age, nutrient levels, light conditions and other factors that are not maintained at constant levels either within individual tests or between testing programmes.

The crucial question in all test systems of this type is the relevance of their results to chemical effects in environmental situations. This is a question of how well the test organisms represent the natural populations and how relevant the test conditions are to the situations in nature. Large differences in tolerance to heavy metals between algal species have been established, therefore, any test programme should examine a set of algal test species rather than a single population.

The relevance of these tests to effects under natural conditions is difficult to evaluate. *In situ* cage cultures are likely to be more relevant than laboratory batch cultures in this respect. There is a need for experimental tests *in situ* to establish how well estimates based on concentration–response data obtained in the laboratory predict the effects found under more natural conditions.

3.1 Batch Methods

The batch method is the simplest but probably also the least predictive technique. This is because the test conditions change significant during the test. Nutrient levels go from superabundant to below concentrations essential for normal algal growth. The light intensity is considerably reduced as the culture develops. Metabolic by-products build up, and the measurable concentration of the toxicant very often decreases during the test through various losses.

The countermeasures proposed to partially alleviate these interfering factors are use of dilute cultures, analysis of only the exponential growth phase, and completion of the test in the shortest possible time.

Extended lag periods in population response often occur in toxicological studies. Lag periods, which tend to be proportional in length to the concentration of toxic substances and which are followed by relatively unaffected exponential growth of the culture, strongly indicate that some sort of detoxification process is operating in the system. Normal dose–response effects on the growth rate and the corresponding IC 50 value cannot be determined under such response conditions. The cause of the delayed growth pattern must be identified and removed before useful bioassay data can be expected. Despite its many problems, the batch technique will presently remain the primary method for rapid screening of the relative toxicity of chemicals to algae.

3.2 Continuous Cultures

Continuous cultures of microalgae require pumps, electronic devices for control and recording, and are considerably more complicated to operate than the batch type. Both the chemostat and the turbidostat need several days of growth to establish steady state before the toxicant can be introduced, and several instruments have to be run in parallel to provide satisfactory control. It is definitely advisable to run batch experiments for localization of the effective concentrations of the toxicant prior to tests in the turbidostat or the chemostat. The provision of constant conditions, including defined concentrations of the toxic chemical throughout the test, therefore involve time-consuming operations and expensive equipment.

The use of these techniques will probably be limited to special studies of those chemicals which can be kept at constant level in batch systems only with great difficulty or for which natural detoxification processes necessitate frequent exchange of the batch medium.

3.3 Cage Cultures

Cage cultures are not commonly used for algal species, and experience with this technique is lacking in most toxicology laboratories. This method requires fairly large volumes of the test and the control media in comparison to the batch technique, and there is a need for additional space and equipment.

When the cage (bag) is composed of regenerated cellulose, toxicants with high molecular weight (> 10,000) cannot penetrate to the test organism. There is also a slight loss of light through the bag, especially toward the end of the test when the cellulose tends to become opaque.

A major problem of *in situ* tests is the growth of bacteria and foreign microalgae on the outside of the culture bag. This growth reduces the flow of nutrients and light to the test culture and may also change the concentration of the toxicant which enters the bag.

When the method is applied in the field, a power source to stir the culture is required. Problems of light and temperature shock upon transfer of the caged algae from the laboratory to the site and during sampling of the culture at the site may also arise, and it is often difficult to find suitable unpolluted sites for reference cultures. In the summer, bacteria in the water will normally break down the cellulose bags within 6–10 days; thus, at that time the test has to be interrupted. Other problems encountered are related to the high cell density developed toward the end of the growth period of many algae in cage cultures.

Several of these problems can be overcome by daily cleaning of the bags, by sampling and replacing cultures in the evening (to avoid light shock), by using other membranes instead of cellulose, and by keeping the cell density low in the test cultures.

The cage culture remains the only method applicable for *in situ* testing, and it is the simplest way to insure constant conditions during laboratory tests.

3.4 Synchronous Cultures

Synchronization of the vegetative proliferation of algal cells has been accomplished with a limited number of species. Therefore, presently only a few test organisms are available for toxicity testing utilizing this technique. The developmental synchrony may be lost quite rapidly in some cases, and when the rhythm is maintained, questions have been raised regarding the effects of stress that may result from the conditions needed to assure synchrony. The intermittent illumination/culture dilution principle used for *Chlamydomonas reinhardthi* by

Nordland *et al.* (1978) seems, however, to insure synchrony and excellent growth of healthy cells.

The technique does offer more test opportunities than can be exploited in routine toxicity testing of chemicals, for which it may appear too sophisticated. Synchrony, however, does increase the sensitivity of the test, especially when an alga which yields 12–16 new cells per cycle is used (Nordland *et al.*, 1978). The procedure developed by these authors is based on electronic counting and volume measurements of the algal cells. The cells are separated into dead and living fractions and can be used to estimate LC_{50} values when the relative lethality of the various dose levels is plotted versus the logarithm of the doses on a probit diagram. The estimated LC_{50} is not identical to the IC 50 value which is related to reduction in growth rate caused by the chemical rather than cell survival.

4 REFERENCES

Eide, I., Jensen, A. and Melsom, S. (1979). Application of *in situ* cage cultures of phytoplankton for monitoring heavy metal pollution in two Norwegian fjords. *J. exp. mar. Biol. Ecol.* **37**, 271–286.

Gargas, E. and Søndergard Pedersen, J. (1974). *Algal Assay Procedure. Batch Technique.* Water Quality Research Institute, Denmark, Søborg.

NEN 6506 (1979). *Water-Determination of Toxicity with Algae.* Ned. Normalisatie Institute Rijswijk.

Nordland, S., Heldal, M., Lien, T. and Knutsen, G. (1978). Toxicity testing with synchronized culture of the green alga, *Chlamydomonas. Chemosphere* **3**, 231–245.

Rhee, G.-Y. (1980). Continuous culture in phytoplankton ecology. In Droop, M. R. and Jannasch, H. W. (Eds.) *Advances in Aquatic Microbiology*, Vol. 2, pp. 151–203.

Stebbing, A. R. D., Åkesson, B., Calabrese, A., Gentile, J. H., Jensen, A. and Lloyd, R. (1980). The role of bioassays in marine pollution monitoring. *Rapp. P.-v. Reun. Cons. int. Mer.* **179**, 322–332.

US Environmental Protection Agency (1971). *Algal Assay Procedure: Bottle Test.* National Eutrophication Research Program, U. S. Environmental Protection Agency. US Govt. Printing Office 1972-795-146/1.

US Environmental Protection Agency (1974). *Marine Algal Assay Procedure: Bottle Test.* Eutrophication and Lake Restoration Branch, U. S. Environmental Protection Agency. US Govt. Printing Office 1975-697-829.

Methods for Assessing the Effects of Chemicals on Reproductive Functions
Edited by V. B. Vouk and P. J. Sheehan
© 1983 SCOPE

Methods for Assessing the Effects of Chemicals on the Reproductive Functions of Microorganisms

J. Howard Slater

1 DEFINITION OF REPRODUCTIVE FUNCTION IN MICROORGANISMS

In contrast to the reproductive function and systems of the animal and plant kingdoms, reproduction in the Protista must be considered in significantly different terms, basically because the reproductive unit is directly equated with the complete organism. For most prokaryotic microorganisms reproduction is viewed as growth since increase in cellular size is intimately part of the cell cycle which terminates with cell division. Thus in biosynthetic and organizational terms cell growth is directed towards replication of the genetic material, its controlled separation and its even distribution between two progeny (a process termed binary fission). Indeed for viruses and bacteriophages growth processes have been pared down to a complete minimum and the whole organism may be considered as a reproductive unit capable of its own replication (under appropriate conditions). At the opposite end of the microbial spectrum, particularly within the eukaryotic organisms, such as microalgae and fungi, morphological developments may lead to structural modifications which generate recognizable reproductive structures. Furthermore, among the more complex microorganisms differentiation into 'male' and 'female' types may be recognized: certainly reproductive events requiring the participation of + and − mating types have been described. This situation contrasts with the absence of differentiated forms in lower microorganisms.

In general, therefore, it is usual, convenient and valid to consider reproduction in terms of growth and this is the basic stance that will be adopted in this paper.

2 EFFECTS OF CHEMICALS ON MICROBIAL GROWTH

Chemicals can affect the growth of microorganisms in one of three ways.

2.1 Growth Stimulation

The compound can support or stimulate the growth of a microorganism, acting as a carbon, energy or element resource. By and large these processes are unlikely to be viewed with concern since the compounds involved usually fall within the usual category of compound exploitable for normal metabolic purposes. There may be situations, however, where gross imbalances may generate problems, such as eutrophication processes when the presence of excess inorganic nutrients may trigger the explosive growth of a limited number of species. Such events can have subsequent effects which may influence the reproductive processes of other organisms.

2.2 Growth Depression

The compound can terminate or inhibit, either generally or highly specifically, cellular function(s) which result in the cessation of cell growth and division. That is, the compound can produce a bacteriostatic effect which may be reversed subsequently, permitting normal growth to resume. In the short term these organisms are likely to be metabolically active and able to contribute to any of the processes mediated by the microbe in question: that is, they remain functionally active although unable to grow. In the longer term static organisms will lose viability and the chemical-induced response merges with the next section.

2.3 Lethal Effects

The chemical can induce rapid, lethal effects which result in cell death over a short period of time compared with the effects encountered in section 2.2. Compounds can affect many cellular functions, the precise target reflecting the nature of the compound. For example, the presence of analogues of DNA precursors rapidly affects DNA replication either inhibiting growth, producing DNA free cells or gross morphological changes (e.g. rod-shaped cells becoming filamentous); antibiotics which inhibit the synthesis of cell wall components rapidly produce cells with defective structural components leading to cell membrane rupture and lysis. In general, whatever the cellular target, the observed response normally follows the sequence of cessation of increase in cell number; gross changes in metabolic activity; cell lysis and excretion of intracellular components into the environment.

There are other processes which may be neutral in terms of the growth of microorganisms but which may influence other microbes and other life forms subsequently (for example, bioaccumulation of a compound as a result of trophic structures and food webs and chains). In other systems microbial metabolic activity may result in a transformation which may be potentially more hazardous than the primary compound, a process known as lethal synthesis. Thus, a major conclusion must be that to appreciate fully the potential effect of a compound, it is necessary to understand its complete fate in the environment irrespective of its immediate effect upon microbial growth.

The study of the effect of chemicals on microorganisms must be viewed with considerable importance because of their crucial role in establishing and maintaining the operation of the whole biosphere. Effects of chemicals, especially xenobiotic compounds, must be monitored with concern, not only at the local level but at the global level (Kornberg, 1979; Slater, 1981a).

3 METHODS OF ASSESSING THE EFFECT OF CHEMICALS ON MICROBIAL GROWTH

3.1 Standard Growth Procedures

The assessment of an effect on a microorganism is in essence simple and relies on standard microbiological procedures. As the two introductory sections have indicated, the initial measurement of an effect can be gauged in terms of the growth response of a microbial population. Growth has been recognized as the primary method in microbiology with a limited number of basic techniques involving growth in closed (batch), liquid culture; open (continuous-flow), liquid culture; and growth on solid surfaces (e.g. agar-agar added to an appropriate medium contained within a Petri dish).

In the first place the choice of growth medium (i.e. essential nutrients) is normally dictated by the type of organism to be cultured, at least for the more fastidious organisms. It is desirable, but not essential, to use defined media since this facilities reproducibility, a factor which may be particularly important in comparing data from different laboratories.

3.2 Assessment of Microbial Growth

There are many methods available to measure microbial biomass or microbial cell number concentrations. It is important to recognize that all these methods provide a mean value since microbial populations grown in traditional systems (especially closed culture and as colonies on solidified growth medium) are heterogeneous. Furthermore many environmental factors, including media composition, type of organism, physicochemical factors, substantially influence microbial biomass determinations (Herbert, 1961; Bull, 1974). Indeed it is recognized that one of the attractions of continuous-flow culture systems is that many of these variables may be controlled, leading to more accurate, reproducible estimates of microbial biomass.

3.2.1 Microbial biomass estimates by dry weight determinations

The standard method is to take a known volume of culture (sometimes treating the cells with an agent which terminates growth, such as 1% (w/v) sodium azide or formalin or gluteraldehyde), centrifuge to precipitate the organisms in a preweighed glass centrifuge tube and dry to constant weight in an oven at 105 °C. Accuracy, unless using very large culture volumes, is normally a problem and must be subjected to rigorous statistical control through appropriate replications. Variations on this procedure include filtering through preweighed membrane filters.

3.2.2 Microbial biomass estimates by turbidity determinations

The microbial biomass, under appropriate conditions particularly at lower concentrations, is some function of the amount of light scattered or absorbed by the culture. Many devices, including colorimeters, nephlometers, spectrophotometers, are commercially available to estimate either unabsorbed light or scattered light and have been described in detail elsewhere (Meynell and Meynell, 1964). An important problem with turbidity or absorbance measurements is that cell morphology, a variable parameter depending on the growth conditions, influences the values obtained. With well-characterized systems, the techniques are valuable and have the advantage over dry weight determinations in being rapid, effectively giving instantaneous results.

3.2.3 Microbial biomass estimates by specific cellular component analysis

Many cellular components including total nitrogen, protein, phosphorus, DNA, RNA and others have been assayed, usually by standard colorimetric assays and, using a known percentage composition figure, these values can be used to calculate microbial biomass in terms of dry weight per unit volume. Often the procedures are time consuming but the serious limitation is that microbial macromolecular and elemental composition is not constant and unless the precise variations as a function of, say, organism growth rate, are known, these procedures are unreliable.

3.2.4 Microbial biomass estimates by total carbon analysis

In contrast to specific components mentioned in section 3.2.3, the carbon percentage of organisms is relatively stable for most standard growth media and conditions may be used as a method of calculating biomass. Recent developments have seen the introduction of several reliable, commercially available total organic carbon analysers which are simple to use, require very small samples and provide rapid estimates of the organic carbon content of cells. This ought to be the method of choice with the major disadvantage being the cost of the equipment.

3.2.5 Total cell number estimates

The total number of microbial cells, that is, without distinguishing between viable and non-viable members of the population, can be estimated by microscopic counts using calibrated counting chambers. A variety of counting chambers are commercially available and enable the number of organisms present in a suspension (normally a growing culture considerably diluted by a known amount) to be counted in a known chamber volume. The procedure is time consuming and requires a high degree of technical accomplishment to obtain accurate and reproducible estimates. Under some circumstances, usually a highly defined organism/growth system, electronic particle counters, such as the Coulter counter, may be used to estimate total cell numbers. This procedure relies on the absence of inert or non-microbial particles in the suspension which is sometimes difficult to achieve. The procedure requires the cells to pass separately through an orifice less than 100 μm in diameter which is frequently difficult to achieve consistently.

3.2.6 *Viable cell number estimates*

For the majority of microbial experiments the significant parameter is the number of viable cells present within a population since these contribute to the overall metabolic function of the population and to the growth potential of the population. In many instances the viable count agrees closely with the total cell number estimate, especially under optimum growth conditions: that is, there are few non-viable, non-growing organisms in an actively growing population. Indeed, in many instances, the observed discrepancies are probably due to difficulties in estimating reliably the viable count. Viable counts are normally determined by preparing all appropriate dilutions of a growing culture (suitable precautions must be taken to preserve viability at this stage, for example, using buffered diluents, prewarmed diluents, rapid preparation, etc.) and evenly spreading a known volume of a known dilution over the surface of a suitable growth (recovery) medium. This distributes, ideally, single organisms over the growth medium's surface, suitably spaced. The spread plates are incubated at an appropriate temperature, leading to the development of macroscopic colonies which are assumed to have been derived from a single, viable organism orginally spread onto the surface. By calculation the number of colonies value can be used to estimate the number of viable organisms present in the original culture. The procedure is time consuming, requiring at least an overnight incubation, although variations, such as the slide culture technique, can estimate viable cell numbers more rapidly.

3.3 Growth Parameters Capable of Determination

Microorganisms generally are capable of a wide response of overall growth potential, influenced and modified by the environmental conditions. In fact in many instances microbiologists need to be aware of the variable responses made by apparently identical populations growing under apparently identical growth conditions. This is an attitude which demands appropriate replicative control and statistical analysis. Furthermore it means that searching for and quantifying the effect of a given chemical on the growth processes requires comparison with appropriate control growth systems established in the absence of the stress induced by the chemical.

In conjunction with the basic methods outlined in section 3.2, the following growth parameters can be assessed in relation to treated and untreated growth systems.

3.3.1 *The closed culture growth cycle*

In closed culture growth systems, microbial populations exhibit a characteristic sequence of growth stages or phases described in detail elsewhere (Bull, 1974; Pirt, 1975; Slater, 1979). Useful, general information may be obtained by determining the effect of a compound on the length of the various growth phases, the size of the maximum population phase culture and other parameters, such as culture viability, cell morphology and/or differentiation, and metabolic capabilities. The last factor, metabolic capabilities, is beyond the scope of this contribution since any cellular capability ranging from an overall process, e.g. the rate of oxygen uptake, to an extremely specific capability, e.g., the activity of a particular enzyme, could be assayed. It is not possible or useful to specify these processes which ought to be selected with regard to the nature of the compound under study. In some circumstances due regard may have to be taken to legislative regulation and control agency requirements. For example, the US Environmental Protection Agency requires, for pesticides, an evaluation of their effect on oxygen consumption and carbon dioxide evolution rates, nitrogen cycle reactions (where appropriate) and measurements of phosphatase or dehydrogenase activities. Variations between the control and treated growth systems as a function of the stage of the closed culture growth cycle might also provide useful information.

3.3.2 *The maximum specific growth rate, μ_{max}*

The maximum specific growth rate, μ_{max}, (units: time^{-1}), measures the optimum growth rate for a given organism under a given set of environmental conditions and is the simplest growth parameter which may be deduced from growth kinetic data. The parameter measures the rate of growth under balanced growth conditions which exist during the exponential phase of closed culture growth or during washout from a continuous-flow culture system: the methods of calculation and a detailed discussion of this parameter are given by Bull (1974) and Slater (1979). Differences in the μ_{max} values obtained between treated and untreated growth systems provide a useful and quantitative description of the overall effect of a compound on the growth of an organism.

3.3.3 *The saturation constant, k_s.*

This parameter measures the affinity an organism has for a particular, growth-limiting substrate and for most nutrients is preferably determined from continuous-flow culture (chemostat) data (Slater, 1979). The influence of a compound on the k_s value obtained may be determined but it must be stated that this requires elaborate, sophisticated chemostat equipment (especially if much credence is to be placed on the numerical values obtained); this information is technically difficult to obtain; and requires an extensive experimental programme.

3.3.4 *The inhibition constant, k_i*

From growth data, especially continuous-flow culture systems, it is possible to determine the k_i value for the chemical under test and to determine the nature of its action, i.e., competitive, non-competitive inhibition, etc. (Bull and Brown, 1979). Again these are likely to require lengthy experimental procedures.

3.3.5 *The minimum inhibitory concentration, MIC value*

An important and relatively straightforward part of a chemical's evaluation programme ought to be the determination of its minimum inhibitory concentration (MIC). Normally this may be satisfactorily evaluated in closed culture systems and ought to be tested at an early date in order to provide a set of baseline data in the light of which other experimental programmes (such as those described in sections 3.3.1–3.3.4) may be conducted; there is little point in collecting μ_{max}, k_s, k_i, etc. data using inappropriate concentrations which may be too low to have any measurable effect or too high to measure useful effects. Furthermore this baseline data is crucial in another context: it enables comparisons to be drawn between microbially harmful concentrations and concentrations known to occur, on average, in the environment. This is particularly significant since there is a tendency to over-react to datum profiles obtained at environmentally inappropriate and inconsequential compound concentrations. There is no point in curbing the use of a particular compound if the measured effect occurs at concentrations unobtainable in nature: regulatory bodies are in danger of justified ridicule through ill-considered decisions!

4 STRATEGIES FOR THE APPLICATION OF STANDARD METHODS OF CHEMICAL EFFECT EVALUATION

Section 3 outlined the basic procedures which may be employed to evaluate the effect of a chemical on the growth of a microorganism. In essence these procedures are simple and the significant features of the evaluation programme lie elsewhere. This section deals with a number of important constraints and principles which need to be taken into account if a satisfactory evaluation is to be achieved.

4.1 *Microbial Diversity*

It is perhaps an axiom but worth stating in the context of the Workshop that within the microbial world there is a wider spectrum of physiological types and metabolic capabilities than in any other group of organisms and, indeed, in the total of other organisms. This microbial heterogeneity, in terms of energy metabolism and anabolic and catabolic potential, raises a serious problem in terms of evaluating the effect of a particular chemical. Stated simply, great care must be taken in choosing a test organism since that organism must possess an appropriate cellular function as the target for the chemical. For example, evaluating the effect of a compound which specifically interferes with nitrogen-fixation processes would be pointless using a non-nitrogen-fixing organism. Furthermore the evaluation programme would similarly be invalidated if a nitrogen-fixing organism was grown under conditions where the mechanism was not elaborated (e.g. a filamentous cyanobacterium grown in the presence of ammonium ions does not differentiate to produce heterocysts and so does not fix nitrogen). Similarly, the effect of a compound which selectively impairs substrate level phosphorylation would be substantially less marked using a test organism grown aerobically compared with the same organism grown anaerobically.

Within compounds with known targets or suspected targets, the selective use of appropriate test organisms is justified. However, in the majority of instances, particularly for xenobiotic compounds, where their mode of action is not understood, then probably the only course of action would be to screen the compound against a range of metabolic types, certainly including those with major capabilities of importance to the natural environment, such as nitrogen fixation, phosphous mineralization, etc. Clearly screening programmes are labour and time intensive but, in the absence of detailed knowledge of the compounds effect, ought to be part of an evaluation programme.

4.2 Microbial Communities

Most microbiologists are imbued with an experimental approach which depends on the use of axenic cultures, i.e. the growth of a single species of microbes. This is clearly a valuable part of an evaluation programme to test effects on a selected range of known organisms with characteristic metabolisms. However, in virtually every known natural habitat, mixtures of microorganisms coexist, in some cases resulting in the formation of stable, interacting communities (Slater, 1978, 1981b). It is becoming clear that many types of interaction, ranging from the genetic to the physiological level, occur which may substantially modify the overall metabolic potential in a way which is not exemplified by any of the pure cultures alone. It is conceivable, but thus far untested experimentally, that microbial communities could transform a non-toxic compound into a toxic compound. This is an area which requires much more experimental work. On the other hand, and in fact a more likely sequence of events, is that a particular problem compound will be transformed (normally completely mineralized) more readily and more rapidly by a mixture of microorganisms acting synergistically (Bull, 1980; Slater and Godwin, 1980). That is, the long-term persistence of a compound in the environment may be considerably shorter than would be deduced from pure culture studies alone. In situations where there is a balance between the need to use a given compound and its deleterious effects, then the more rapid its degradation, the more desirable. Microbiologists in general seem reluctant to consider mixed culture studies but unless they are encouraged to do so, they will continue to furnish data which in many cases bears little relation to the processes occurring in nature.

4.3 Environmental Heterogeneity

A comparatively unexplored area, certainly in terms of chemical safety evaluation, is that of environmental variation and heterogeneity. Most simple experimental systems, such as a closed culture, depend on the homogeneous dispersion of microorganisms in a culture medium to produce a homogeneous suspension. These are conditions which rarely occur in nature: various types of surfaces and interphases occur (Marshall, 1980) and, indeed, most microbial activity occurs at these regions. Here physicochemical factors lead, for example, to major nutrient gradients which in turn affect the rate at which organisms grow. By and large heterogeneous growth systems have not been adequately explored in the present context.

4.4 Microbial Adaptation

In many instances test procedures fail to allow for adaptive processes, particularly those which may occur at the genetic level (as opposed to phenotypic adaptation or expression of a particular function). In the long term these events may be important in alleviating the effects of chemicals by the selection of mutants with desired resistance characteristics or, more importantly, by the selection of strains able to degrade the test compound. Evaluation programs ought to include some estimations of the likelihood of these events occurring but it is, of course, difficult and often a long-term programme. Nevertheless, as has been observed in other contexts, ultimately the immediate effect of the chemical may not be such a problem as was anticipated in the unadapted population (Slater, 1978).

4.5 Evaluation *in situ* and Microcosms

As indicated elsewhere in this section, one of the major experimental problems is that of relating laboratory-based experimentation—often with highly defined, simple growth systems—to the likely behaviour of the compound in natural habitats. At some stage field studies need to be undertaken to make the necessary comparisons. An intermediate stage, however, is the use of more complex growth systems, normally termed microcosms which attempt to establish a great ecosystem complexity within a laboratory-based system (Matsumura, 1979; Bull, 1980).

4.6 Microbial Systems as Models for Testing Effects of Chemicals

In much the same way as microbial systems have been analysed as convenient life forms from which the basic fundamentals of living systems may be deduced, microbial systems may, in part, serve as convenient models to test the effect of chemicals before testing on animals and plants. The relative simplicity of microorganisms, the ease of culturing and the ability to produce large quantities of material for analysis, enables them to be used in useful preliminary tests to determine likely cellular targets for the compound in question. For example, results may indicate an influence on DNA synthesis or protein synthesis inhibitor, and these results may indicate what cellular functions need to be examined in higher organisms. Clearly extrapolations of this kind need to be attempted cautiously and with due regard to the substantial differences exhibited in higher organisms. This strategy has, for example, been used as the basis of the Ames test for determining those compounds which tend to have carcinogenic effects.

5 CONCLUSIONS

The major conclusion which it is hoped is clear from the preceding test is that the basic methodologies already exist for the analysis of the effect of chemicals on microbial growth. To this author, however, there are some serious limitations to the application of these methods, especially in the range and level of complexity of the assessment tests undertaken. Much more thought needs to be given to the experimental protocols developed, taking into account the factors described in section 4.

6 REFERENCES

Bull, A. T. (1974). Microbial growth. In Bull, A. T., Laguado, J. R., Thomas, J. O. and
    Tipton, K. F. (Eds.) *Companion to Biochemistry*, pp. 415–442. Longman, London.
Bull, A. T. (1980). Biodegradation: some attitudes and strategies of microorganisms and
    microbiologists. In Ellwood, D. B., Hedger, J. N., Latham, M. J., Lynch, J. M. and

Slater, J. H. (Eds.) *Contemporary Microbial Ecology*, pp. 107–136. Academic Press, New York, San Francisco, London.

Bull, A. T. and Brown, C. M. (1979). Continuous culture applications to microbial biochemistry. In *Microbial Biochemistry, Int. Rev. Biochem.* **21**, 177–226.

Herbert, D. (1961). The chemical composition of microorganisms as a function of environment. In Meynell, G. G. and Gooder, H (Eds.) *Microbial Reaction to the Environment*, pp. 391–416. Cambridge University Press, Cambridge.

Kornberg, H. (1979). Royal Commission on Environmental Pollution. 7th Report: *Agriculture and Pollution*. Her Majesty's Stationary Office, London.

Marshall, K. C. (1980). Reactions of microorganisms, ions and macromolecules at interfaces. In Ellwood, D. C., Hedger, J. N., Latham, M. J., Lynch, J. M. and Slater, J. H. (Eds.) *Contemporary Microbial Ecology*, pp. 93–106. Academic Press, New York, San Francisco, London.

Matsumura, F. (1979). Report of task Group IV: Microcosms. In Bourquin, A. W. and Pritchard, P. H. (Eds.) *Microbial Degradation of Pollutants in Marine Environments*, pp. 520–524. US Environmental Protection Agency. Gulf Breeze, Florida.

Meynell, G. G. and Meynell, E. (1974). *Theory and Practice in Experimental Bacteriology*. Cambridge University Press, Cambridge.

Pirt, S. J. (1975). *Principles of Microbial Growth and Cultivation*. Blackwell Scientific Publications, Oxford.

Slater, J. H. (1978). The role of microbial communities in the natural environment. In Chater, K. W. A. and Sommerville, H. J. (Eds.) *The Oil Industry and Microbial Ecosystems*, pp. 137–154. Heyden and Sons, London.

Slater, J. H. (1979). Population and community dynamics. In Lynch, J. M. and Pool (Eds.) *Microbial Ecology—A Conceptual Approach*, pp. 45–63. Blackwell Scientific Publications, Oxford.

Slater, J. H. and Godwin, D. (1980). Microbial adaptation and selection. In Ellwood, D. C., Hedger, J. N., Latham, M. J., Lynch, J. M. and Slater, J. H. (Eds.) *Contemporary Microbial Ecology*, pp. 137–160. Academic Press, New York, San Francisco, London.

Slater, J. H. (1981a). *Microbes against Hazardous Compounds*. Spectrum, Vol. 175, Central Office of Information, London.

Slater, J. H. (1981b). Mixed cultures and microbial communities. In Bushell, M. E. and Slater, J. H. (Eds.) *Mixed Culture Fermentations*, pp. 1–24. Academic Press, New York.

Subject Index